Clinical Examination

John Macleod

Formerly:

Consultant Physician, Western General Hospital, Edinburgh

Consultant Physician, Royal Edinburgh Hospital

Consultant Physician, Clinic for Rheumatic Diseases, Royal Infirmary, Edinburgh

Chairman of University Department of Medicine, Western General Hospital, Edinburgh (1971-78)

Clinical Examination

A Textbook for Students and Doctors
by Teachers of The Edinburgh Medical School

Edited by
John Macleod

SIXTH EDITION

CHURCHILL LIVINGSTONE
EDINBURGH LONDON MELBOURNE AND NEW YORK 1983

CHURCHILL LIVINGSTONE
Medical Division of Longman Group Limited

Distributed in the United States of America by
Churchill Livingstone Inc., 1560 Broadway, New York,
N.Y. 10036, and by associated companies, branches
and representatives throughout the world.

First Edition 1964
Second Edition 1967
Third Edition 1973
Fourth Edition 1976
  ELBS Edition first published 1979
Fifth Edition 1979
  ELBS Edition of Fifth Edition 1979
Sixth Edition 1983

ISBN 0 443 02828 1

British Library Cataloguing in Publication Data
MacLeod, John
    Clinical examination. —— 6th ed.
    1. Physical diagnosis
    I. Title
    616.07′5   RC76

Printed and bound in Great Britain by
William Clowes (Beccles) Limited, Beccles and London

'My first point is therefore this, that in any branch of university education, including medical education, we should aim at using the methods of education rather than instruction. We must teach the student how to collect the facts, to verify them, to assign a value to them, and how to draw conclusions from them and test those conclusions; in short, how to form a judgement. As Karl Pearson said, "the true aim of the teacher should be to impart an appreciation of method rather than a knowledge of facts," for method is remembered when facts have been forgotten, and method can be used in a new situation where there are no, or too few, facts. The student learns how to learn and can go on acquiring knowledge for the rest of his life.'

SIR GEORGE PICKERING Medicine's Challenge to the Educator.
British Medical Journal, 1958 Vol. 2, p. 1117.

Preface

If medical education is to evolve it must be kept under constant scrutiny; and so it is with clinical examination. A further stimulus to critical review has been provided by the burgeoning of investigative techniques, notably imaging, with repercussions on the sharpening of clinical skills. Accordingly it became apparent that a sixth edition of *Clinical Examination* was required to ensure that the description of clinical methods and their interpretation had kept up with advances in the practice of medicine.

Since the first edition was published in 1964 it has been customary for contributors who had retired from clinical practice to give way to younger authors. This now applies to six who took part in the fifth edition; their places have been taken by Professor C. R. W. Edwards (history, general examination and external features of disease), Dr D. P. de Bono (cardiovascular system), Dr J. F. Munro and Mr D. W. Hamer-Hodges (alimentary and genito-urinary systems), and Professor Hamish Simpson (the infant and child). Dr Mawdsley has assumed responsibility for the chapter on the use of the ophthalmoscope in addition to that on the nervous system. All contributors are university teachers of undergraduate and postgraduate students and the team includes a general physician, a surgeon, a psychiatrist, a paediatrician and specialists in all the major systems. Although most chapters have been the responsibility of one person, each author has had access to the experience of his colleagues.

While many sections have been rewritten, it was not considered necessary to make fundamental changes in the successful format of the book. At the same time constructive suggestions offered by students and doctors from all over the world have been incorporated. In consequence both the text and the illustrations have been more thoroughly revised than in any previous edition.

The aim of the book is to describe diagnostic procedures which depend primarily on the clinician's trained senses and on the basic equipment generally available. The main chapters conform to a similar plan; starting with the history the reader learns how to elicit and evaluate symptoms; the methods of physical examination are then described and the significance of the findings is discussed. Indications are also given of the type of investigation which may be required as a logical extension of the clinical examination. Finally, examples are provided of the methods in practice.

The book is intended primarily for undergraduates but it has proved to be of value both to physicians in training and to general practitioners. Its international appeal has led to its selection by the English Language Book Society for publication in Africa and Asia. The sixth edition of *Clinical Examination* is closely integrated with the thirteenth edition of *Davidson's Principles and Practice of Medicine,* in which most of the contributors and the editor participate. These books in conjunction aim to provide a rational and readily comprehensible basis for the practice of medicine. An independent group of authors has also prepared 1200 MCQs[1] to help students make their own assessments of their understanding of both books.

Throughout *Clinical Examination* emphasis has been placed on obtaining accurate information by reliable methods. If we have succeeded in promoting this and the judgement to assess its value, while making the process less threatening for the patient and more enjoyable for the clinician, we shall feel amply rewarded.

Edinburgh 1983   John Macleod

---

1. Fleming P R et al 1980 1200 MCQs in medicine. Churchill Livingstone, Edinburgh

Acknowledgements

We have had generous help from many sources. We would like to express our thanks especially to Mr T. B. Hargreave (sexual disorders in the male and examples of questionnaires), Dr J. B. Scrimgeour (gynaecological examination), and Graham Birnie (preparation of the manuscript).

We are indebted to the Department of Medical Illustration, University of Edinburgh, and to Mr J. E. Pizer in particular, for assistance in the preparation of the illustrations. Original photographs were kindly supplied by Mr P. J. Abernethy (4.3A), Professor Gavin Arneil (10.3B), Dr W. A. Copland (7.1), Dr A. A. Donaldson (8.32), Elscint (GB) Ltd (7.3), Dr L. Fananapazir (5.3, 5.9 and 5.10), Dr M. C. Grayson (Plate IIIB), Professor Ian Isherwood (7.14), Dr M. V. Merrick (9.42), Dr R. E. Pfaltzgraff (4.3 C and D), Professor C. I. Phillips (Plate IIIA, C and D), Professor Eric Samuel (7.2), Professor R. E. Steiner (8.33) and Dr S. R. Wild (7.16). Other acknowledgements are made in the text.

We found some of our quotations in *Doctors by Themselves* compiled by E. F. Griffith, *The Quiet Art* compiled by Robert Coope and *The Medical Works of Hippocrates* translated by J. Chadwick and W. N. Mann. We are much obliged to these authors and their publishers for giving us permission to make use of their work.

The editor is particularly indebted to Dr E. B. French and Dr M. B. Matthews for much helpful advice in the preparation of this edition.

Contributors

Allan, N.C., M.B., CH.B., F.R.C.P.Edin., F.R.C.P.Path.
Consultant Haematologist, Western General Hospital, Edinburgh.
The Examination of the Blood

de Bono, D.P., M.D.Cantab., F.R.C.P.Edin.
Consultant Physician, Department of Cardiology, The Royal Infirmary, Edinburgh.
The Cardiovascular System

Edwards, C.R.W., M.A., M.D.Cantab., F.R.C.P.Edin., F.R.C.P.Lond.
Professor of Clinical Medicine and Chairman, University Department, Western General
Hospital, Edinburgh.
The History and the General Principles Governing the Physical Examination
The General Examination and the External Features of Disease

Grant, I.W.B., M.B., CH.B., F.R.C.P.Edin.
Consultant Physician, Respiratory Diseases Unit, Northern General Hospital,
Edinburgh. Senior Lecturer in Medicine, University of Edinburgh.
The Respiratory System

Hamer-Hodges, D.W., M.S., F.R.C.S.Lond., F.R.C.S.Edin.
Consultant Surgeon, Western General Hospital, Edinburgh.
The Alimentary and Genito-Urinary Systems
The Examination of the Breasts and Varicose Veins

Mawdsley, C., M.D.Manch., F.R.C.P.Edin., F.R.C.P.Lond.
Head of the Department of Neurology, University of Edinburgh.
The Nervous System
The Use of the Ophthalmoscope

Munro, J.F., M.B., CH.B., F.R.C.P.Edin., F.R.C.P.Path.
Consultant Physician, Eastern General Hospital, Edinburgh and Edenhall Hospital,
Musselburgh. Part-time Senior Lecturer, Department of Medicine, Western General
Hospital, Edinburgh.
The Alimentary and Genito-Urinary Systems

Robson, J.S., M.D., F.R.C.P.Edin. F.R.C.P.Lond.
Professor, Department of Medicine, University of Edinburgh.
The Examination of the Urine

Scott, J.H.S., M.B., CH.B., F.R.C.S.Edin.
Consultant Orthopaedic Surgeon, Western General Hospital and Princess Margaret Rose
Orthopaedic Hospital, Edinburgh.
The Locomotor System

Simpson, Hamish, M.B., CH.B., M.D., D.C.H., D.Obst., R.C.O.G., F.R.C.P.
Professor and Head of Department of Child Health, University of Leicester, Leicester
Royal Infirmary, Leicester.
The Infant and Child

Walton, H.J., PH.D., M.D., F.R.C.P.Edin., F.R.C.Psych., D.P.M.
Professor of Psychiatry, University of Edinburgh.
The Psychiatric Examination

Contents

1. The History and the General Principles Governing the Physical Examination   1
2. The Psychiatric Examination   16
3. The Analysis of Symptoms and Signs   30
4. The General Examination and the External Features of Disease   56
5. The Cardiovascular System   98
6. The Respiratory System   150
7. The Alimentary and Genito-Urinary Systems   189
8. The Nervous System   227
9. The Locomotor System   315
10. The Infant and Child   368
11. The Use of the Ophthalmoscope   406
12. The Examination of Urine and Blood   417
13. Appendix   445
   Stages in development of infants and children
   Desirable weights for adults
   Uses of questionnaires
   Notes on International System of Units
   A system of case recording
   Problem-orientated medical records
   Continuing medical education
Index   463

1. The History and the General Principles Governing the Physical Examination

And I place the interrogation of the patient himself first, since in this way you can learn how far his mind is healthy or otherwise; also his physical strength and weakness, and you can get some idea of the disease and the part affected.

Rufus of Ephesus (*c.* A.D. 100)

The clinical study of disease is founded on two essential processes, the history of the patient's disability, and the doctor's physical examination. 'Clinical examination' comprises both these components, each of which is based on a methodical and comprehensive routine to which the student should adhere, particularly throughout the junior apprenticeship. This chapter gives an account of the sequence which should normally be followed in the consulting room or at the bedside.

THE HISTORY

As Rufus of Ephesus pointed out almost 2000 years ago, the history is usually the most valuable part of the clinical examination in leading to a diagnosis. Every medical student is, rightly, taught this — and then spends the remainder of his or her professional life relearning the lesson. The doctor's first task is to listen and observe, not only to obtain information about the current problem but also to understand the patient as a person and that individual's life situation.

The art of obtaining an accurate history expeditiously can be acquired and developed with practice. It has three main stages, the first of which must be a satisfactory approach to the patient. Secondly, adequate opportunity must be given to the patient to tell the story. Thirdly, a competent interrogation must be made by the doctor to clarify the patient's account and, when indicated, to extract information regarding previous health, family, social and personal matters. The same sequence is followed with almost every patient, the emphasis changing in accordance with the current problem. When the basic technique has been acquired, skill will improve with experience until an efficient method is at the doctor's command, flexible enough to deal with the manifold vagaries of clinical practice.

1. The Approach to the Patient

The individual who is ill and who is possibly apprehensive when confronted by a stranger is readily disturbed if first impressions are bad, for example, if the doctor appears indifferent or unsympathetic; an emotional barrier to effective

1

communication is then erected. It is therefore essential that the patient is put at ease by being given a friendly greeting, and made to feel the centre of interest. In the consulting room it is easy to acquire the bad habit of completing notes about the previous patient at the crucial moment when the newcomer should be welcomed. Rather it should become second nature for the doctor to have all senses alert, particularly at the outset. The clinical examination begins from the moment of first contact with the doctor who must not miss the revealing, fleeting gesture, facial expression, intonation, or other body language of non-verbal communication.

Patients may be embarrassed by not knowing to whom they are speaking, and accordingly appropriate introductions should be made, for example by medical students. At the outset the clinician should do the talking while the patient adapts to the situation. Initial remarks should be about impersonal matters; a minute or so can be spent with profit in this way to help eliminate any preliminary diffidence. Any impression of hurry on the doctor's part should be avoided. Conversation can readily be built round the patient's occupation while confidence accrues. Addressing the patient by his or her name is good for the individual's self-esteem and for establishing a less impersonal relationship — a discreet glance at the notes may be necessary to prevent an embarrassing mistake. It is also wise to be sure whether it is 'Miss', 'Mrs' or 'Ms'. A satisfactory initial relationship has been achieved when the patient and the doctor have begun to get to know each other. Conditions should then be favourable for the patient to speak freely.

Students when first taking histories often feel they are imposing upon patients; however the majority of patients enjoy talking to students whose approach has been satisfactory.

2. The Patient's Account of the Current Illness

Patients should be given an opportunity to tell their story in their own way, and in order to encourage them to do so the initial question must be of a general nature, e.g. 'Now please tell me about your trouble'. If they have difficulty in starting, ask 'What was the first thing you felt wrong?', followed by 'What happened next?'. 'When were you last well?' or other prompting should encourage patients to talk. Thereafter, with attentive listening much can be learned about the symptoms and also about the patient's intellectual capacity and emotional reactions. This has, moreover, a therapeutic role, particularly when dealing with a psychiatric problem (p. 17). Wilfred Trotter has described listening in terms of 'the power of attention, of giving one's whole mind to the patient without the interposition of anything of one's self. It sounds simple but only the very greatest doctors ever fully attain it. It is an active process and not merely resigned listening or even politely waiting until you can interrupt. Disease often tells its secrets in a casual parenthesis.'

Medical students (and doctors) often make the mistake of interrupting prematurely. Intervention should be timed and planned depending on the initial assessment of the personality of the patient. While the possibilities are innumerable, certain situations commonly recur; for example, there is the intelligent person who gives a clear unemotional account, the 'good witness'. This kind of description often points straight to the diagnosis with little further aid from the doctor. The inarticulate person will require patience and help by the posing of very simple questions, whereas the verbose individual, giving irrelevant details, will need guidance to direct attention to essentials; even so, there is still a danger of interrupting too soon. The quasi-knowledgeable individual, in relation to medical matters, tends to give a diagnosis rather than an account of symptoms and speaks in terms of 'flu', 'gastritis', 'rheumatism', 'migraine', etc. Such statements must not be accepted without reviewing their basis. The emotionally disturbed patient, worried by illness or frightened in a doctor's presence, must be handled with sympathy, but the doctor must remain alert to detect sources of psychological stress which may require elucidation later. Elderly patients are liable to give the keen young doctor the answer they think will please; deafness or early dementia may add to the misunderstanding, particularly if the doctor has failed to appreciate that the patient's mental functions are impaired. Timidity, guilt or fear of disease may lead to information being suppressed. In contrast, symptoms may be exaggerated in an attempt to ensure attention. Another problem is that a patient's memory may be very fallible because of emotional stress at the time of examination. Wilful deceit is rare except by alcoholics and drug addicts; the latter are often expert at faking symptoms, as are patients with Munchausen's disease whose motive is to gain admission to one hospital after another on the basis of a convincing but mendacious tale of illness. Other examples of personality disorder are described on page 26. In Trousseau's words, *'Il n'y a pas de maladies; il n'y a que les malades.'*

3. Interrogation by the Doctor

(i) **The Current Illness.** It is first necessary to clarify the patient's account to ensure that all the symptoms have been elicited and to evaluate them. The art of interrogation, like the preceding technique, is also one which develops with practice, provided certain principles are observed. Questions should be formulated simply and clearly. When a satisfactory answer has been obtained, the same question should not be repeated later. This usually results from inattention and gives a justifiably poor impression of the carefulness of the examiner.

Many individuals are very open to suggestion and unintentionally provide erroneous information if a certain answer would appear to be expected. Biased and premature questions in conjunction with a perplexed patient open to suggestion and anxious to help the doctor, may result in a very distorted history. It is therefore important, particularly while the basic facts are being elicited, not to ask leading questions which may act as guides to the answers desired by the doctor. Later in the proceedings, however, use may be made of such questions to elucidate the patient's account provided that the potential fallacies involved are kept in mind.

The principal symptoms must be thoroughly analysed. Examples of this process are given in Chapter 3, but basically the doctor must be satisfied that accurate information has been obtained regarding the time and mode of onset of any important symptom, the circumstances in which it occurred, its duration and the existence of any ameliorating or aggravating factors. The relationship to other symptoms must be defined and a chronological account obtained of the development of the illness from the first symptom to the date of interview. If possible, exact dates should be recorded rather than vague statements such as 'last Saturday' or 'a few weeks ago'. It may be helpful to reproduce the symptoms and observe what happens; for example the patient who complains of breathlessness on exertion may be studied ascending stairs. If there is difficulty in describing a recurrent symptom of varying severity, the position may be clarified by asking for an account of the first or of the most severe attack. It is often useful to record negative findings, e.g. cough but no sputum, or breathlessness but no cough.

Elderly or ill patients easily tire during the initial history taking which should then be curtailed and completed later.

Systemic Enquiry. When a clear record has been obtained of the current complaint specific enquiries should be made about the presence or absence of cardinal symptoms suggestive of involvement of various systems, such as cough, breathlessness, indigestion (the imprecise word is deliberately used to broaden the scope), bowel, urinary or menstrual troubles, pain, insomnia or change in weight. These questions can be asked very quickly and a comprehensive view of the patient's health thus obtained. This and other information can also be elicited by questionnaires and analysed by computers but such techniques will not detect any emotional reactions which would be apparent to the alert clinician. Questionnaires, however, can usefully be exploited in selected circumstances (p. 198 and p. 451).

Drugs? Allergy? It is essential to know about any drugs taken on medical advice or otherwise. It is easy to overlook self-medication with potentially harmful preparations such as laxatives, analgesics, oral contraceptives or herbal remedies. Is there any history of drug abuse? Is the patient allergic to any substance (p. 13)?

Information from a Third Party. It is necessary to obtain information from a relative or friend when the patient is unable to supply it because of immaturity, illness, senility or mental disturbance. Corroboration is often helpful when the patient is a poor historian. Every effort should be made to procure an account from an eye-witness in the case of a person who has been unconscious or who may be suffering from a condition in which knowledge of the patient's behaviour or appearance may be useful.

Patients often give information to medical students or to nurses which has not been previously divulged, perhaps because they were unsure of its relevance or were afraid of wasting the time of a busy doctor. Social workers often obtain crucial evidence from patients or their relatives or in the course of a home visit. The hospital domestic staff can also be the source of useful knowledge not otherwise available. All these facts can readily be integrated by a well organised clinical team.

(ii) Previous Illness and State of Health. Information should be obtained about previous illness, operations and accidents and recorded in chronological order. Patients may be reminded about past illness by being asked if they have ever been in hospital or been confined to bed at home. It should be borne in mind, however, that the diagnosis supplied by the patient may not be correct, either because of misapprehension, misdiagnosis, or because, in the patient's interests, it had been judged advisable to give a less harsh explanation; a gastric carcinoma may have been described as an 'ulcer'. If medical records are not available, the examiner may have to decide about past episodes on the patient's description of symptoms and circumstances at the time, but it is salutary to realise that what may now be obvious because of the progress of the disease may have been impossible to diagnose even in the recent past. Frequently patients incriminate an accident as being responsible for subsequent troubles; any claim of this kind must be considered critically. A history of venereal disease may be suppressed, because of a feeling of guilt, and when it is suspected the individual must be asked about the possibility of infection, for example from extra-marital sexual intercourse.

Residence or travel abroad and any illness which occurred there may be relevant; a puzzling fever may prove to be due to malaria or amoebiasis contracted outside Britain. Air transport enables vast distances to be covered within the shortest of incubation periods so that infection may be transmitted to an area where it is not normally encountered. Patients will not necessarily mention their journeyings unless specifically asked if they have been abroad. The onus is on the doctor to make the relevant enquiry. It may also be necessary to know about prophylactic medication, for example for malaria, or about vaccinations or immunisations.

Previous Health. Just as knowledge of previous illness may be necessary in assessing a clinical problem, so also may information about past health. A medical examination for insurance or employment purposes would give a good basis for comparison with the present findings. In all cases it is most helpful to know the date and result of any previous radiological examination. The films should be reviewed if there is any doubt about the result.

(iii) Family History. Information regarding the age and health, or the cause of death of the patient's relatives is often valuable. The knowledge that there is a family history of diabetes, coronary artery disease, hypertension, gout or an infectious disease such as tuberculosis, should increase the doctor's awareness of the possible presence of such a condition in the patient. The symbols used in the construction of a family tree (pedigree chart) are illustrated in Figure 1.1.

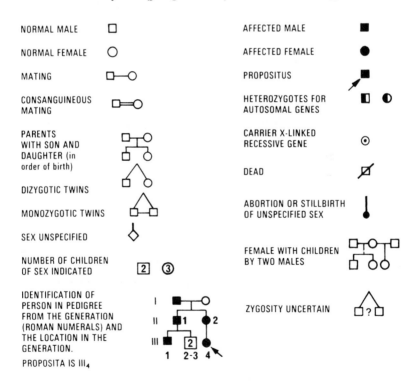

Fig. 1.1 Symbols used in pedigree charts. Drawing up a family tree begins with the affected person first found to have the trait (*propositus* if male, *proposita* if female). Thereafter relevant information regarding siblings and all maternal and paternal relatives is included.
(From Emery A E H 1982 Elements of medical genetics, 5th edn. Churchill Livingstone, Edinburgh.)

Often there is unwarranted anxiety on the patient's part lest, like a parent, some potentially crippling disease such as rheumatoid arthritis may be developing. Considerable tact may have to be deployed when asking a new patient about problems such as alcoholism or mental disorder in a close relative. Overall, however, a display of interest in the welfare of the family usually helps to secure rapport.

At this stage it is usually possible to obtain at least an impression of the individual's personal relationships but enquiry about more intimate matters, if deemed necessary, is often best postponed until after the physical examination when a good measure of confidence should have been established. However, if the patient wishes to speak about emotional disturbances at any phase of the proceedings the opportunity to do so should be taken as it may not occur again. An unhappy childhood, sexual difficulties, a broken marriage and problems with children, adolescents or elderly relatives are all very potent influences on an individual's well-being. On the other hand, the family may constitute a united group able to give substantial support to any member in difficulty.

(iv) Social History. Patients' adaptation to their occupational and social environment may, like family influences, have profound repercussions on their health. Illness may ensue directly as in the case of coalworkers' pneumoconiosis or indirectly as in malnutrition; social problems may arise as a result of illness. Much of this information may be known to the general practitioner. In contrast the doctor working in hospital sees the patient in an artificial setting and must acquire some knowledge of the individual's normal background, not only in relation to diagnosis, but also in the planning of rehabilitation. A description ('profile') of how the patient spends an average day may be helpful in determining realistic therapeutic goals. The patient's functional capacity must be assessed and related to the employment, for example in cases of heart or lung disease return to heavy work or to a polluted atmosphere may be contraindicated. Enquiry should, therefore, be made about home, occupation, personal interests and habits.

The Home. It may be necessary to know about the number of rooms and their occupants, the sanitary arrangements, the state of repair of the house and the financial obligations of the residents. The number of steps leading up to or inside the home will be relevant when planning to rehabilitate patients with angina or chronic lung disease. Neighbours may create problems or may be very helpful in times of stress. A social worker can often obtain essential information by visiting and reporting on home conditions.

Occupation. It is desirable to know not only the mere fact of the patient's employment but what it involves. It is good practice to encourage conversation about this and allied topics during the clinical examination. Useful information is obtained, the anxious patient is diverted and the doctor's interest is usually appreciated. Attention should be paid to the congeniality or tedium of the employment, to any occupational hazards, and to stresses imposed by others or by the individual's own ambitions. Frequent change of employment may indicate an inadequate personality. Unemployment or job insecurity may have an effect on the patient's health. Many married women have a part-time occupation, either because of real necessity, or because of the need to maintain hire-purchase commitments, or because of boredom at home. The type of work and the reason for undertaking it should be known. It is necessary to have at least some appreciation of the overall economic situation of the patient and the family.

Personal Interests. The doctor should also be aware of the patient's leisure pursuits, such as the amount of physical exercise undertaken, and intellectual activities.

Habits. Food, tobacco, alcohol and other drugs may have important implications in relation to nutritional problems, lung disease and psychological instability. A dietary history should be obtained if there is an obvious nutritional abnormality. In most instances an approximate assessment of the patient's food and vitamin intake will suffice but the doctor should not accept the corpulent woman's claim that she eats nothing or the statement by the girl with anorexia nervosa that she eats everything. Deficiencies of substances such as folate or vitamins C or D may occur in elderly patients whose accounts of their eating habits may not be corroborated by a neighbour or by evidence obtained from a brief inspection of the larder. Occasionally a precise evaluation by a trained dietician is required.

At this stage in the history taking, a picture should have been obtained of the individual as a whole in relation to his or her background and with discrimination the details can be elaborated as demanded by the current problem.

(v) The Psychological Assessment. In all illness it is necessary to evaluate the part played by psychological factors. The account of the history and the manner in which it is delivered usually reveal much about the patient's personality. The reaction of the individual to distressing situations in the past is also relevant, as similar patterns of behaviour tend to recur. Frequently emotional reactions during the history taking, supplemented by negative findings on physical examination, will direct attention to the need for a more detailed psychological assessment by the clinician. In the course of the clinical examination the doctor should have recognised any traumatic events, such as bereavement, separation or rejection and these should now be further explored. It is usually possible to start the patient talking about emotionally disturbing topics by such remarks as, 'You had begun to tell me about a disagreement with ——', or 'Tell me more about your mother who died last year'. If no obvious opening presents, a more direct approach is necessary; patients should be asked if anything is worrying them and thereafter any factor of possible significance must be further explored. Often specific questions must be posed about the existence of anxieties regarding financial, occupational, domestic, sexual or religious matters. Frequently fear of disease, such as cancer, is a potent source of stress, and the same fear may inhibit disclosure of what is in the individual's mind unless specific questions are asked. Many individuals have good insight into their own personalities and it may be profitable to know how they evaluate themselves, with reservations about the opinion offered.

Patients should be encouraged to talk freely about problems, and about current difficulties with people important to them, as self-disclosure to an understanding listener is of value both from the therapeutic as well as from the diagnostic aspect. When this is done, it often becomes apparent to the doctor and to the patient that the presenting symptom, apparently physical in origin, is in fact a manifestation of a psychological difficulty. Frank, unhurried discussion in privacy can be time-consuming but there is no doubt that the experienced doctor finds that it is time well spent, as many emotional problems are resolved when they are brought to the surface and ventilated in the neutral atmosphere of a consulting room. When emotional distress persists or when significant abnormalities are apparent or suspected in the patient's personality or mental processes, a formal psychiatric examination is required. The interview employed for this purpose is described in Chapter 2.

The Doctor-patient Relationship. In addition to the patient's response to the problem, the interactions between the patient and the doctor have also to be considered. This relationship is very complex as a result of the interplay between different personalities in potentially stressful situations and anything from harmony to antagonism between patient and doctor can ensue.

The patient will 'transfer' to the doctor habitual modes of behaviour, some of these deeply ingrained and learned from the parents. Thus an aggressive attitude to the doctor may represent the patient's habitual reaction to people regarded as uncompliant, in this case a doctor who does not speedily relieve painful or frustrating symptoms. An overdependent attitude is also common. The patient with hysterical symptoms characteristically masks distress by a show of 'smiling unconcern'. Other defence mechanisms include the repression of unpleasant matters, the projection of faults on to others, rationalisation and over-compensation.

Inappropriate and troublesome relationships can develop between the patient and the clinician, the best known being erotic transference. The patient comes to believe she loves the doctor and by gesture or statement conveys this to him. Occasionally, and sometimes disastrously, a clinician reacts by responding to this supposed sexual invitation. Erotic transference however is really indicative of a longing to be accepted without at the same time being exploited. The clinician is not called on to react to the overtly seductive statements but rather to the basically childlike behaviour of the patient. Thus, far from responding either on a similar level, or by rejection of the patient, the doctor can properly view the declaration of love as an aspect to be assessed as methodically and calmly as any other highly emotional communication.

The clinician should not depart from a professional position as a non-judgemental observer and should not react to troublesome patients with criticism, anger, dislike, disapproval or dismissal. In contrast, some patients strive, by flattery or other manoeuvres, to manipulate the doctor who may respond by going to excessive lengths to meet their demands. Yet other patients cause the doctor to feel helpless and inadequate; in contrast the clinician may make the mistake of treating adult patients like children. By analysis of their own feelings — i.e. the effect the patient has on them — clinicians can often gain a much clearer perception of what the patient is trying to achieve. The management of a situation can be improved when the feelings aroused by the patient are thus carefully assessed, but not acted upon. It is seldom that the doctor loses command of the position when a conscious effort is made to create an effective relationship with the patient.

The adaptation of medical students to their patients will be facilitated if they systematically give consideration to interpersonal factors of this kind and discuss problems with their teachers. Poise will come with understanding, self-awareness and self-control.

The Taking of Notes

> Hark! she speaks; I will set down what comes from here, to satisfy
> my remembrance the more strongly.
>
> Doctor of physic in Shakespeare's *Macbeth*

The human memory is far from reliable and its efficiency deteriorates with ageing and with the passage of time. It is, therefore, essential that a record be made of the findings without delay. The history should be written down as it is given; with practice this can be done quickly with little or no interruption of the patient's narrative. Some doctors develop a form of shorthand which may serve their own purposes, but notes should be legible and comprehensible if others have to use them.

It will clearly not be necessary to write down all that is said as much may be irrelevant, but the recording of the patient's own words is particularly valuable in psychiatric illness (p. 20). However, note taking may have an inhibitory effect when highly personal matters are being discussed; it may then be advisable to lay the pen aside and later record an appropriate account. An anxious patient often hurriedly jumps from one topic to another and then it is best to jot down headings and elucidate the sequence and details later. In some circumstances, for example if the history is very complicated, it may be good policy to make rough notes at the time and later elaborate these into an orderly account. This should commence by stating the presenting symptoms and their duration and be followed by a description of the development of the illness. Students will inevitably make mistakes at first, but with practice they will learn to sift the evidence, select the facts which merit prominence and record them in a coherent form.

Conclusions on Completion of History

When the history has been obtained to the doctor's satisfaction the first step has been taken towards diagnosis. The information must be appraised, taking into account the reliability of the patient as a witness. The relevant facts must be separated from the irrelevant and evaluated objectively. The logical analysis and interpretation of the evidence will usually lead to a provisional diagnosis or suggest a differential diagnosis. Only rarely can no conclusion be made. While the planning of the physical examination will be influenced accordingly, the doctor should remain unbiased and proceed to attempt to elicit further objective evidence which may confirm or refute the interpretation of the history or which may point in a wholly different direction.

THE PHYSICAL EXAMINATION

During any clinical examination attention is frequently concentrated on one or more systems. However, a review of a patient's complaints too closely restricted to a single system can lead to errors in diagnosis as important disease elsewhere may be missed. It is not always possible to make a single diagnosis to embrace all the features encountered, particularly in the elderly in whom multiple pathological lesions, not necessarily related and each requiring consideration, are commonly present.

The doctor carrying out a physical examination is entirely and solely responsible for seeking out the features of disease and must not expect them to present or depend on the patient to draw attention to them. Occasionally and for a variety of motives, patients will not reveal what they regard as stigmata of disease, but as a rule failure to recognise these signs is due to careless or inadequate examination. Shortage of time may be a contributing cause. More commonly, however, the additional factor is the natural human failing either to recognise the obvious or to remain sufficiently alert when performing repetitive tasks.

For most purposes it would not be practicable for even the most obsessional of doctors to carry out all the minutiae of examination in every patient encountered, and some degree of compromise must be accepted. The undergraduate, however, must not hurry or attempt any short-cuts, but in all cases methodically follow a careful routine until thoroughly acquainted with the procedure. It is essential for the student to become familiar with the range of normal signs before abnormalities can be confidently recognised. Discrimination comes with practice and experience allied to a logical approach to the individual problem.

Environment and Equipment

Before discussing methods, consideration has to be given to the conditions under which the physical examination is conducted and to the equipment required.

Privacy is essential and this usually constitutes no problem in the home or in the consulting-room. In some families relatives may feel it is their duty to be present in numbers which may embarrass the patient and the doctor. The tactful dismissal of all, or all but one, is desirable. In a hospital ward, screens must be drawn round the bed before the examination begins. Steps should be provided for easy access to a high couch in the consulting-room. Comfort is necessary and encourages adequate relaxation. The examination couch should have an adjustable back-rest as it is easier for the patient in the semi-reclining position to converse, and not feel at a disadvantage as when lying supine. A back support is essential for the patient with heart failure who becomes breathless when lying flat. Illumination must be good. Exposure of the area to be examined must be adequate but not to an extent that might unnecessarily embarrass or chill the patient. Both patient and the doctor should be warm; auscultation of the chest of a shivering subject and palpation of the abdomen with cold hands are common faults, for apart from the discomfort, the consequent muscle sounds and the resistance of the abdominal wall impair the efficiency of the examination. Patients have, with good reason, complained about such practices since the first century, when Martial wrote:

I'm ill. I send for Symmachus; he's here,
An hundred pupils following in the rear;
All feel my pulse, with hands as cold as snow;
I had no fever then — I have it now.

It is imperative that the handling of any painful area is gentle. Exhaustion, as a result of a prolonged examination, must be avoided; the risk of this is greatest in the frail or elderly. The needs of female patients require special consideration. While privacy is important, the presence of a relative or nurse is often desirable when dealing with a sensitive, frightened or hysterical woman and is essential when a rectal or vaginal examination is performed.

It is convenient for the doctor to carry a stethoscope, a torch, a measuring tape, and there should be access to a sphygmomanometer, an ophthalmoscope with auriscope attachment, a pin and cotton wool, a tendon hammer, a tuning fork, a clinical thermometer, disposable wooden tongue-depressors, disposable gloves, lubricant and a proctoscope. A weighing machine and a height scale should be available in the consulting-room and also facilities for procedures such as the testing of the urine described in Chapter 12.

A Method of Examination

While the doctor records the findings in terms of systems, the actual sequence of examination should be conducted primarily with the comfort of the patient in mind. After a general inspection, the hands, upper limbs, head, neck, chest, abdomen and lower limbs are usually dealt with in turn. Thus information about the heart, lungs, breasts, axillary lymph nodes and spine is generally obtained at one time while dealing with the thorax, whereas facts relating to the nervous system are usually acquired piecemeal. This compromise presents difficulties to students. At the outset of their training they should concentrate on the individual systems in turn and, later, learn to integrate their techniques. Practice may be obtained, at an early stage, by examining, and being examined by a student colleague. This will help to attain proficiency and will also give some insight into the patient's point of view. A routine is gradually acquired which should be both methodical and flexible. The experienced doctor varies the emphasis as a result of information obtained from the history. In some cases a comprehensive examination of all systems is imperative, while in other instances one system may require special attention and the remainder need only a very brief review. A word of explanation to the patient may be advisable if the examination commences at a point remote from the site of the complaint. Procedure will vary with individuals and circumstances and the method which is outlined here is intended to provide only a provisional working basis; it should be adapted as the occasion demands.

1. General inspection of the patient (demeanour, colour, physique, etc.) and surroundings, e.g. the temperature chart in hospital.
2. Feel pulse and examine hands and arms.
3. Examine head and neck.
4. Proceed now either to area mainly affected or to anterior chest (heart, lungs, breasts and axillae) and then to back (lungs and spine).
5. Examine abdomen, groins and external genitalia.
6. Examine lower limbs.
7. Record blood pressure.
8. Ophthalmoscopic examination.
9. Rectal or vaginal examination if indicated.
10. The temperature, weight and height can be recorded and a specimen of urine obtained either at the outset or at the end of the examination.

If unexpected abnormalities are elicited, a further change in emphasis in the examination may be required and it may be advisable to reassess some of the earlier findings.

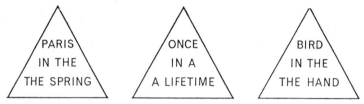

Fig. 1.2   The three triangles

Observer Error

> You see only what you look for; you recognise only what you know
>
> Merril C. Sosman, Boston

Even the most unbiased and alert doctors must be constantly critical of their clinical abilities. The scientific training of the preclinical years should have engendered an objective attitude of mind but even so the human failing of evolving preconceived ideas about one's findings is ever present. This is illustrated in Figure 1.2; when first seen most people read the legends incorrectly as 'Paris in the spring' 'Once in a lifetime', and 'Bird in the hand'. We tend to see largely what we expect to see. We also tend to pay attention to findings which we consider significant and to ignore those which we judge unimportant. We are not aware of making this judgment and if it is faulty, errors arise.

Varying interpretations of the same material are also possible as shown in Figure 1.3. Location of an apex beat or assessment of jugular venous pressure by

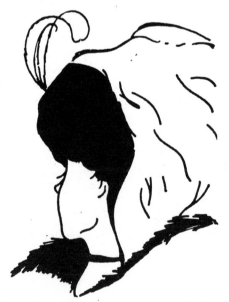

Fig. 1.3   How old is she? Some observers see a young woman, others an old one. The chin and neck of the former become the nose and mouth of the latter and vice versa. Thus different observers, confronted by the same evidence, can reach different conclusions. (E. G. Boring.)

experienced physicians often differ. Disagreements also occur in the interpretation of radiographs and electrocardiograms. Furthermore when the same evidence is reviewed at a later date by the same individuals the second reports often differ significantly from the first. The range of observer variation and error is thus wide. The junior clinician must be even more fallible, but mistakes should be fewer when there is a constant awareness of one's limitations, and a testing of conclusions against other findings. If, for example, the pulse is thought to be collapsing in nature then this should be confirmed by measuring the blood pressure. If bronchial breathing is suspected, then whispering pectoriloquy should also be present. When errors do occur they can be put to profit if the reasons for them are critically analysed.

CASE RECORDING

It is essential, whatever sequence may have been followed in the course of the physical examination, that the findings are recorded in a systematic form. When acquiring clinical experience, undergraduates should take every opportunity of examining patients in detail and of making a comprehensive written report of their findings. Later they will learn how the account may be adapted to meet the needs of the individual patient; in many circumstances quite brief notes will suffice. With most hospital patients, however, a detailed systematic report is recommended. Records of normal or negative findings often prove very helpful when comparison has to be made at a later date.

Case notes should be precise and free from any irrelevant or facetious comment which might cause embarrassment in more formal circumstances elsewhere. It is as well to remember that courts of law are empowered to demand a view of official records. The value of adequate notes, accurately and promptly recorded at the time of the illness or injury, has repeatedly been emphasised by medical defence societies.

The record must be legible and easily understood. Incomprehensible abbreviations and symbols must be avoided, but simple diagrams of the site and extent of abnormal findings are useful (p. 47). The abdomen in particular lends itself to the graphic illustration of areas of tenderness, palpable masses and enlargements of the viscera or lymph nodes (p. 203). Diagrams of neurological abnormalities (p. 330) and the effects of trauma (p. 331) are also highly informative.

Danger Signals. Drugs have dangers as well as benefits and adverse effects may arise from drug interaction. It is therefore essential to find out about recent medication and be aware that this may influence the clinical features or indeed may be the cause of disease. When a patient is found to be hypersensitive to a drug the fact should be recorded prominently on the front of the case notes. Serious repercussions and even fatalities may be prevented if, for example, *penicillin allergy* is clearly recorded. Long-term treatment is easily overlooked in an emergency and the danger of haemorrhage forgotten if a reminder is not easily available that the patient is having *anticoagulant therapy*. An even more important example is the hazard of acute adrenal failure in persons treated either currently or recently with *corticosteroids* and who are exposed to the stress of an acute infection or an operation. In circumstances such as these it is advisable for patients to carry a card giving information about their corticosteroid therapy; patients with Addison's disease or hypopituitarism should be recommended to obtain a bracelet or necklace on which the diagnosis is engraved.

Systems of Case Recording

A traditional system of case recording is given on page 454, it also outlines the main features dealt with in this and later chapters.

Problem orientated case records are discussed on page 458.

FURTHER INVESTIGATION

At the conclusion of the clinical examination it may be possible to offer either a final or a provisional diagnosis. In the latter event consideration should be given to the further investigations which may be indicated. The scope and use of these should be regarded as logical extensions of the clinical examination. The number of investigations carried out varies greatly between one doctor and another depending upon knowledge, experience or philosophy. Some are insufficiently critical of the deficiencies of clinical methods, whereas others employ a large number of routine tests and special investigations, many of which may be only remotely connected with the problem under consideration. This latter practice has become possible in Britain where the National Health Service involves no increase in expense to the individual patient. However, even the simplest test costs money; laboratories are apt to be overloaded with work and inaccuracies tend to occur; the patient may suffer unnecessary discomfort, and the doctor's clinical acumen does not develop in proportion to increasing experience. Many pitfalls are avoided if a full clinical assessment is always made before instituting any investigation, and then only those selected for a specific purpose. If in doubt it is helpful to ask oneself — 'What benefit will this be to the patient?'.

The range of investigation is ever widening. Visual examination may, by means of instruments, be extended to the optic fundus, tympanic membrane, nasal passages, larynx, trachea, bronchi, oesophagus, stomach, duodenum, pleura, peritoneum, lower gut, urinary bladder, vagina and joints. Biopsies may be obtained directly from many sites and also by aspiration methods, blindly, from the small intestine, pleura, lymph nodes, liver, spleen, kidney and other organs. Information may be obtained by recording electrical activity in the body by electrocardiography, electroencephalography and electromyography. Much help comes from the radiologist where the range of investigation is now extended by the non-invasive techniques of computed tomography and ultrasonic scanning. In the laboratory area there are contributions from the biochemist, microbiologist, pathologist, physicist and the pharmacologist with whom discussion of the problem is often most rewarding. However, all tests are prone to errors of measurement or interpretation and it should be the doctor in charge of the patient who finally weighs up all the evidence before deciding on the diagnosis and prescribing treatment.

THE METHODS IN PRACTICE

Diagnosis is an intellectual process requiring the integration of information derived from many sources. The medical student must learn first how to collect the facts and then, by analysing them, how to reach a diagnosis. With increasing experience it becomes possible at an early stage in the clinical encounter to decide on a provisional explanation. This is an hypothesis which is formulated to account for the symptoms and signs. This hypothesis is then tested systematically by further physical examination and by special investigation if necessary; these lead to the confirmation or adjustment of the hypothesis or sometimes to its total replacement. In the last event alternative hypotheses are selected and analysed in turn as further data are collected until the presenting problem is solved. The student, trained in scientific method, will recognise that this attitude conforms to the current scientific approach in studying a biological phenomenon whereby explanatory hypotheses are tested and are given up when refuted by new evidence. A series of decisions is involved, the effective taking of which characterises the thinking of the competent doctor whose knowledge is well organised.

Making and testing diagnostic judgments constitutes a strict but rewarding discipline of continuous educational value; but, in addition to the intellectual approach required to reach a diagnosis, decisions made by scientific methods must then be applied effectively to meet the needs of the individual human being.

2. The Psychiatric Examination

The most important practical skill which a student has to learn during clinical instruction in psychiatry is the use of the interview as a technique of enquiry.

Royal Commission on Medical Education 1965–1968

In the opening chapter it has been shown how clinical investigation is based on history-taking and physical examination, supplemented in many medical and surgical problems by special investigations. To detect psychiatric disorders the clinician must rely totally on the ability to take a history and examine the mental state. These skills, augmented by the clinical reasoning process, lead to diagnostic hypotheses and plans for therapy. Such medical problem-solving is the doctor's 'science', which is now recognised as definable, amendable to evaluation and which can be improved upon by appropriate teaching. Empirical investigation of doctors engaged in their clinical tasks has been promoted in part by the interest in computer approaches to medical interviewing. At the same time enormous strides have occurred in quality control of experienced doctors, audit, continuing medical education and issues of recertification. From such approaches concern has mounted that many doctors are inept in interviewing techniques and that medical students are not taught adequately how to talk to patients. When a patient sees the doctor, trust has to be gained, and once a diagnosis has been made it has to be conveyed to the patient and the treatment negotiated.

Recent studies (p. 29) have shown that medical students are seldom taught how to put patients at their ease, how to establish a proper working relationship or rapport, how to avoid medical jargon, how to extend the discussion to more personal matters and encourage the revelation of patients' difficulties and how to discern and follow up non-verbal clues to distress.

Busy junior doctors, in turn, have been found to prevent patients from giving an account of symptoms in their own way, sometimes through asking too many questions in a machine-gun style; precipitating factors of key events are rarely established. They avoid asking patients about their mood, their reactions to illness or its impact in their families.

Experienced doctors also err by failing to respond to cues given by patients about their chief concerns. They neglect to enquire systematically how patients are adapting socially and psychologically to serious physical illness; a study of patients with breast cancer showed that the surgeons detected only a fifth of those who had developed psychiatric complications in addition.

General practitioners show extreme variation in their ability to detect psychiatric illness; some identified only 20% of their patients who were thus affected, in contrast to perceptive general practitioners who detected as many as 80%. The nature of their history-taking techniques differentiated alert from imperceptive doctors; the former asked patients about the presence of psychiatric symptoms, about their families and about how they were getting on at home. Their greater detection of psychiatric disorder was not related to the amount of time spent with the patient.

Many doctors use an inflexible style of history-taking which ignores the varying levels of comprehension and responsiveness of different patients. By dominating the interview excessively they often prevent the patients from talking about the trouble that actually bothers them. A finding that is of particular concern is that these deficiences do not improve with postgraduate training or greater experience.

In addition, the rights of patients are being increasingly asserted. Many patients feel that doctors do not let them explain what is wrong and what they want. One of the most common complaints is that patients are not given enough information.

It is clear from the foregoing that competent interviewing techniques are crucial in assessing psychiatric problems. An effective method of doing so is described in this chapter.

Research into doctors' clinical abilities has clarified that the time-honoured method of clinical training, apprenticeship, does not necessarily lead to a gain in interviewing skills, in contrast to its effectiveness in teaching physical examination as, for example, the elicitations of the reflexes. Furthermore, empirical studies of the ways doctors approach patients have demonstrated repeatedly that doctors are not themselves aware consciously of the technical approaches they use in clinical work or of their efficacy. The medical student requires to be an active learner under observation when interviewing real or simulated patients. The presence of the instructor is necessary when communication skills in clinical settings are being acquired.

The psychiatric examination consists of four parts:

1. The psychiatric history
2. Examination of the mental state
3. Evaluation of the personality
4. The diagnostic formulation.

The *interview* is the method involved. While this is essentially history-taking, the process is less formal than when dealing with a purely physical problem. It also differs in that therapy is involved at an earlier stage; it is a fact that the patient is helped when encouraged to talk to an understanding listener. A series of interviews may be necessary before the clinician acquires all the information needed to comprehend both the genesis and the course of the psychiatric illness. In the first interview the goal is at least a preliminary overall history; in the course of this, prominent abnormalities of the mental state will be detected; and a working diagnosis should be possible. Moreover, a tentative assessment of the patient's personality will be obtained.

A diagnosis is a hypothesis about the nature of the illness and about its main aetiological factors. It is derived by the clinician from an informed synthesis of the facts elicited. Because diagnosis comes before therapy and because the clinician may wish to begin treatment in the course of the first interview, the aim is to reach a preliminary diagnosis as soon as possible. The initial interview takes an experienced practitioner about half an hour. Subsequent interviews may be briefer and can be arranged as required to obtain further information and to extend the psychiatric examination.

While a theoretical knowledge of interviewing procedure is essential, this process is a practical skill which can be acquired only through direct experience with patients. Furthermore, supervision is needed if technical errors are to be identified and corrected. An invaluable aid is provided by the use of videotape; the trainee interviewer has the psychiatric examination of the patient recorded, and when it is subsequently played back with the instructor both have the actual clinical data before them for review.

When conducting the psychiatric examination, clinicians inevitably make use of their own personalities; they rely on their own capacities for communication. They require to have an objective view of the extent to which they succeed in expressing themselves to the patient as intended. The instructor and such aids as tape recording and videotape help to show them whether they are accurate in their own understanding about the ways they affect patients.

The Clinician's Approach to the Interview

In the conduct of a psychiatric examination the clinician and the patient should sit in chairs placed more or less at right angles. They are then free to look at one another when they wish, without imposing any requirement for fixed stares as would be inevitable if the two participants were directly facing each other. A directorial station behind the office desk is of course altogether inappropriate. The room should be quiet and interruptions minimal.

A question and answer technique is not appropriate. The psychiatric history should flow smoothly from one topic to another in a sequence meaningful to the patient. The clinician acts as a catalyst whose primary function is to assist the patient to impart a clinically useful account of personal experience. The clinician writes steadily to obtain an accurate, factual and full record of the interaction. Any questions asked are also noted so that the verbal stimuli offered to the patient are recorded. A good history is neither nebulous nor abstract. When the patient mentions somebody, that person should be named; for example, 'I was going with a man friend at that time'. The clinician asks 'What was his first name?'. This is then recorded; if this person again enters the patient's account, in the present or a later interview, identification can be rapid.

The competent clinician does not take the patient firmly in a dull routine through each step in the historical sequence of events. The patient is left relatively free to reflect, to overcome hesitations, to go back and amplify, and to alter earlier statements as confidence is established. The clinician gently guides the patient, giving advice when inconsequential detail threatens to crowd out important events and indicating quite frankly when the patient is following a blind alley. The clinician's task is to gain possession of the necessary facts in each of the crucial areas. This apparent discursiveness is easier to permit as the clinician becomes more experienced.

It is appropriate to indicate plainly to evasive patients that the necessary information must be obtained. There is no need to encourage the patient with phrases of approval or expressions of sympathy. It goes without saying that moral censure or disapproval should never be conveyed, although unwittingly clinicians sometimes do. There is no call to become autobiographical, and tell the patient about one's own trying experiences, child rearing practices, or opinions and attitudes.

In the course of the examination the matters about which people are sensitive can be dealt with sensibly and directly as technical data. Behaviour usually regarded as wrong or unusual can be broached without equivocation, no hint of moral evaluation entering, e.g. 'Have you thought of ending your life?' Such an enquiry may be welcomed by a depressed patient as a much needed opportunity to disclose distressing impulses towards suicide; the very process of speaking about these intentions may effectively serve to deter the patient from making a suicide attempt. Sexual experience is discussed in terms which the patient is sure to understand, checking where necessary the patient's term for a part of the body or a sexual activity. Nowadays the patient will almost certainly know what 'masturbation' means, but not always; the clinician will often perceive that more explicit explanations or simpler words are needed to obtain the information sought.

While the patient is not constrained to give a formal, chronological and precisely sequential account, the clinician examining the psychiatric patient has a technical task to complete, a schedule of operations to be performed. The aim is to do this as methodically as in any other clinical sector, the neurological system for example. Thus if the ocular fundus has not been examined or if the plantar reflexes have not been tested, the trained clinician knows that the examination is incomplete. Similarly with the psychiatric assessment if, for example, the clinician has not found out about the patient's family relationships, understanding of the patient's personality is deficient; if the patient's job record has been neglected, the history is also incomplete. The psychiatric examination is a technical skill, within the competence of all clinicians. One can know about a person's mind with more or less certainty according to one's ability to carry out the relevant clinical procedures.

1. THE PSYCHIATRIC HISTORY

Description of the Patient. The patient's name, age, occupation, marital status, sometimes the religious affiliation and finally the method of the referral are facts the clinician will want to record. Eliciting such relatively neutral information may be a useful way of starting the history-taking; while replying, the patient is able to settle in the chair as comfortably as possible, and to assess the situation and size up the clinician as the examination begins.

Reason for the Consultation. The clinician then ascertains why the patient has come, and what the patient requires of the doctor. The reason for the interview may on occasion be straightforward, for example on account of a phobia, or at times bizarre. The police may send a patient, as occurs when a psychiatrist is asked to examine a woman who has harmed her children physically and has then attempted to kill herself. It may be a relative who brings the patient, as occurs when a mother tells the clinician she has been worried recently about her small son, and describes mannerisms which alarm her. The presenting reason for the referral of course may be merely the introductory gambit, to be extended when the clinician has gained the patient's confidence: a man complaining initially of indigestion may later disclose that he has actually come on account of impotence.

Present Illness. Having established why the patient has requested to be seen, the clinician then obtains a detailed account of the patient's symptoms. Each complaint should be recorded scrupulously, in terms close to the patient's own. If the patient mentions a pain in the heart, that is to be noted as the symptom; it should not be translated into clinical jargon, such as 'precordial pain'. Rephrasing the patient's description into medical terminology impairs the clinician's grasp of the patient's experience. An adequate description of the illness has been reached when the clinician has traced chronologically each manifestation of the disorder.

Many patients prefer to start the consultation by describing the present illness. However, there are certain patients who deny their main difficulties (as occurs commonly in patients with alcoholism or anorexia nervosa), and complain initially of secondary problems. Other patients do so with the cautious aim of ascertaining whether the doctor will not be offended if they divulge their real worries. Once the patient is relaxed and more confident, a useful account of the illness can be elicited, not necessarily in chronological sequence. Any circumstances which may have precipitated the illness are explored, the time and mode of onset are established, and the progress of the disorder is established. The severity of the illness and its likely prognosis can often be tentatively decided when the present illness has been described.

Family History. This consists of a verbal sketch by the patient of both parents and of all the brothers and sisters. 'You mentioned your *father* — what sort of person is he?'. The question causes some patients to pause in perplexity, until after hesitation they describe the father as one of the best, or portray him as strict but perfectly fair, or as a mean man who terrorised the family when drunk at weekends, as the case may be. The clinician can usually determine whether the father was perceived positively, in a neutral light, or negatively. The importance of this information is that it conveys the role which a parent took in the formation of a patient's personality; a concept of each parent is incorporated during growing-up, forming an aspect of the patient's self.

The *mother* has also to be characterised and this can usually be done with less trouble. A patient may say of her that she was kind and gentle, or two-faced, or a virago who started her persecution before the patient's birth by striving to obtain an abortion. Again, in describing the mother the patient is disclosing a significant relationship which contributed to personality structure. The description of the parents usually discloses whether either of them was violent, or unduly punishing, or inconsistent or inappropriately lenient.

It is useful to ask the patient to list the *brothers and sisters*, in order of seniority, with an indication of the patient's relations with each of these siblings. The position in the sibship may by important. If he was an only child, alone with his mother until 5 years of age when his father was demobilised from the army, then to have a baby sister arrive on the scene, the patient may proceed to describe a rivalry which agitated his childhood and coloured his subsequent social relationships in adult life with envy and competitiveness. The clinician's perception of the parental family is filled out when the patient is asked to comment on the general atmosphere which existed in the home. Finally, the patient is asked to give details of any psychiatric illness suffered by the parents and other near relatives.

Personal History. This can follow naturally from the account of the parental family. The clinician finds out if the patient was a wanted child, whether control of the bladder and bowels was acquired at the usual age, whether in infancy admission to hospital occurred or if a parent was away from home — but these crucial facts are seldom elicited by blunt questions. To grasp in addition whether the patient separated from the mother without difficulty and managed to start school attendance without anxiety, whether there was an early conduct disorder like stealing, or a neurotic illness such as a childhood obsessional state, calls for an ability on the part of the clinician to empathise with patients, so that they realise how accurately they are being understood.

One then discovers from the patient about the onset of puberty, the development of sexual awareness and information, and the form of erotic imagery. The patient tells whether there was a chum, a first close friendship. Progress at school is studied to obtain information about intellectual ability, and about relationships with teachers and other children and involvement in recreational activities. The course of adolescence discloses whether gradual separation from the parents to become an independent individual was achieved, and whether this social growth — if it occurred — was relatively untroubled, or took the form of rebellion against a parent. Identity-formation proceeds rapidly from the middle teens, and if arrested the youngster does not arrive at an understanding of personal potentiality nor about appropriate future work, nor a definition of values to be adopted. A boy may be greatly troubled about sexual aspects of this stage of maturation, with prolonged or recurrent fears about homosexuality or masculine inferiority. A girl may reject aspects of femininity. In the later teens the capacity for close relation with another person begins to develop if personal maturation is proceeding smoothly, the individual finding greater purpose when deeply fond of somebody else. Discussion about adolescence should disclose any experimentation with drugs, and involvement with the police or undetected delinquent behaviour.

Details of any higher education or special qualifications are sought.

The clinician then inquires about courtship, marriage and each of the patient's own children. The patient may tend at first to deny any sexual or personal difficulties in the marriage, revealing these only later, when confidence in the doctor has been gained. It may be important to know about extramarital sexual relationships. The account of the personal history is completed by following the jobs the patient has had during the course of a working life and noting the quality of the patient's relationships with employers, workmates and acquaintances beyond the family circle. Retired or unemployed people, who make up an increasing section of the community, should be asked how they occupy themselves and how contented they are. The inquiry about personal adjustment will convey the patient's present occupation, living arrangements, interests and leisure activities. Such facts may be crucially important about bereaved or elderly people.

Previous Illnesses. These are then studied; physical disorders are described more readily by the patient and can be rapidly surveyed. They can of course have emotional consequences, especially if they occurred early in life or left a disability which interfered with the patient's social participation.

Previous psychological disorders are sometimes more difficult to track down. They are often revealed if careful questioning is directed to the major stressful epochs in the biography, namely the start of schooling, puberty, later adolescence, courtship, marriage and the onset of middle life with the realisation of advancing years. Any previous psychiatric disorders and the way they were managed are recorded in order of occurrence.

Previous Personality. This is especially relevant in undertanding the patient's illness. Thus obsessional traits or hysterical mechanisms may have been prominent throughout the patient's life. In contrast, the onset of serious disease or psychosis may constitute a break with the patient's former self. Suddenly, unheralded, the delusion took form; the cheerful, busy man altered to become anxiously preoccupied and troubled by groundless convictions that he suffered from cancer.

The previous personality is important not only to define the time of onset of illness. It is also important, because from understanding it, the clinician can identify special strengths — perhaps obscured by the symptoms of illness — which the patient will be able to call on when recuperating; values and habits of mind, initiative, friendships and other social relationships, membership of groups, clubs and organisations, and special interests may be useful assets at this time.

Recording the History. As the patient speaks, the clinician writes. The transcript of the interview may not be orderly, but when the material is recast in systematic form, data will have been obtained in each of the important sectors of the patient's biography.

2. EXAMINATION OF THE MENTAL STATE

Many of the clinical signs characterising the mental state of the patient will have become apparent during history taking. The clinician now sets out to study systematically the different aspects of the mental state which can now be given special further attention.

General Appearance and Behaviour. The patient is described tersely but exactly, to provide a record which will suffice to call the individual to mind in terms of posture, expression, clothes, mannerisms, reactions to the clinician, and mode of presentation. In the case of a mute or stuporose patient this aspect of the mental state may be among the most revealing. The patient's non-verbal behaviour is then all there is to go by, and such features as mode of dress, gait, motor activity including mannerisms, and social manner are of diagnostic relevance.

Thought Processes. Talk is externalised thought; thus the clinician notes how ideas are handled and the manner in which the patient arranges and expresses concepts. The major abnormality may be in this psychological sector. It may be disclosed in disordered syntax, as when a schizophrenic patient juxtaposes apparently unrelated references to a portion of the body and the river lived close to as a child: 'This is my arm and the Thames is in England'.

A sample of talk is written down, in the patient's own words, to convey major preoccupations and ways of expression.

Mood. The clinician has probably already obtained much evidence about the prevailing affect from the facial expression, the posture and gestures, and the emphases during history-taking. The patient can then be asked, 'How do you feel in yourself?' or 'What is your mood like?'. The patient may reply in dispirited tones that nothing that takes place means anything any more — 'It's all flat'. Depressed mood is often accompanied by early wakening, loss of interest, poor concentration, hopelessness, guilt, low self-esteem and suicidal impulses. In some instances sadness is not mentioned directly; instead the patient talks of a dead sensation in the chest or an emptiness in the head, or the deeply pessimistic patient describes the surrounding world as grim and hopeless. In contrast, the hypomanic patient feels elated, full of energy, 'on top of the world'. An anxious mood consists of pervasive fear without any obvious reason, and is often accompanied by breathlessness, palpitations, sweating, faintness and tremor.

Delusions. Patients may disclose that they have developed false beliefs which they adhere to firmly despite proof to the contrary, misinterpreting everyday events as specially significant or attributing unwarranted intentions to people with whom they come into contact. Such persons are wrongly seen as intensely concerned with pestering or maligning or scorning the patient. Others may consider themselves under the control of outside influences: 'I know from the way I've been feeling that there is some evil force that is directed onto me by supernatural powers'. A delusion cannot be corrected by argument on the part of the clinician, nor will the patient give up the false belief if offered proof to the contrary.

Hallucinations. When a patient perceives visual, auditory or tactile sensations in the absence of any actual external stimulus, the mental experiences which may have been extremely startling are firmly but wrongly believed to be originating outside the patient:

> During the morning of the 10th of March I was de-frosting my refrigerator when I distinctly heard my husband in his office, which is completely away from our house in an entirely different street. I heard him having consultations with three different people and then dictating letters to his secretary. During the early afternoon I was most disturbed to hear a strange male voice which was loud and clear. I got absolutely no peace from this voice which was accompanied by music and a mixed choir.

This patient had alcoholic hallucinosis. In schizophrenia hallucinations also occur in a setting of clear consciousness, whereas in delirium they are accompanied by altered awareness. The hallucination has all the properties of a real perception. This total lack of insight is in contrast to a *pseudo-hallucination,* as can occur in bereavement, when the person recognizes the perception, e.g. the dead person's utterance, as unrealistic. Hallucinations have also to be differentiated from *illusions,* which are misinterpretations of an external stimulus, as when an apprehensive person out at night mistakes a shadow for a person.

Obsessions. These are thoughts — ideas or images — which the patient regards as foreign or silly and tries to dispel, but which nevertheless persist:

> The idea keeps coming back that I may be pregnant. I've never had sexual intercourse and my periods never stopped, so with my logical mind I know it's impossible. I think over and over again that I may be having a child. I've sent away to an agency for a pregnancy test, and saved up for an abortion.

Obsessional thoughts are distressing, often to do with sex or violence, and are repellent to the patient, e.g. fears of harming someone the patient loves, blasphemous thoughts in religious patients are experienced as horrifying.

Compulsions are repetitive acts, the motor counterpart of obsessions in overt behaviour. An example is the repetitive hand washing accompanying morbid cleanliness. The patient is impelled to perform the action frequently, however pointless and silly it is recognized to be. The ritual may take the form of avoiding contact with people or certain things such as doorhandles or knives.

Evidence of Intellectual Defect. When there is either acute or chronic brain impairment, leading respectively to temporary (delirium) or permanent intellectual defect (dementia), disorders of the following functions may be detected:

ORIENTATION. An estimation of the patient's capacity to orient in time and space emerges as the history is taken and more accurate assessment is gained by testing the patient. The following five questions can be used, a score of one point being awarded for each correct answer: What year is this? What month is this? What day of the month is this? What is the place you are in now? In what town is it?

MEMORY. This is tested by assessing the patient's ability to recall remote and recent events. The clinician may already have noted gaps or inconsistencies in the patient's account. An unimaginative but effective question is to ask what was had for breakfast.

ATTENTION AND CONCENTRATION. These are attributes of a normal person whose sensorium is intact. In delirium, in contrast, alertness and attentiveness are clearly deficient. Less obvious impairment may be revealed by the patient's inability to calculate an arithmetical sum correctly. The 'serial sevens' is a classical test. The patient is asked to subtract seven from 100 and to continue to take seven from what remains as rapidly and as accurately as possible. Most people will complete this task within one minute and will make no more than two mistakes.

GENERAL INFORMATION. This is tested by asking questions about current affairs, e.g. national politics and international problems.

INTELLIGENCE. This is assessed from the detail and subtlety of the patients' accounts of themselves, their capacity to reason, the extent of their knowledge, and the level of their occupational attainment. Accurate measurement is made by use of standardised intelligence tests. These can be carried out by the clinician, or by a clinical psychologist and are expressed as the patient's Intelligence Quotient (I.Q.), the normal range of of which is 80–120.

Insight and Judgment. This is the final sector in the examination, and deals with the extent of the patients' recognition that they are ill, their grasp of the nature of the disorder, and the realism of their judgment about their future.

---

3. EVALUATION OF THE PERSONALITY

The personality may be defined as the totality of a person's actions and reactions; it is the individual as he or she appears to others, by reason of those persistent behaviour patterns which distinguish them from their fellows, and which form the basis of predictions about how they can be expected to act. Abnormalities of personality are expressed particularly in the individual's relationships with other people and these are unusual, in specific ways, when the personality is disordered.

The clinician diagnoses the personality by two clinical techniques. The first is applied during the history-taking. At the same time as facts are gathered about the illness, note is taken of the characteristic behaviour which the patient describes — e.g. a man may give repeated instances of gross and passive dependence, first on his mother and later on a teacher, an employer, his wife, etc. Patients may ask for special tonics, may indulge in special pleading for another appointment in the very near future, may comment on the extent of their reliance on the doctor to take good care of them, etc. The clinician registers mentally, as these specimens of the patient's social responses are recorded, that a morbid pattern of clinging passivity appears to be emerging.

The second procedure depends on the use of the clinician's own personality as an instrument in the clinical interaction. Clinicians know — or should know if adequately trained in interviewing — what effect they have on people — i.e. what behaviour is customarily evoked. They know from experience what reactions are exceptional, as when a patient becomes unduly aggressive or when excessive demands are being made. A man with abnormal passivity may convey by his behaviour in the interview that he will become a burden to the doctor, a 'dead weight'. The tentative personality diagnosis which may have been suggested by the patient's own account will then have been supported by his dependent mode of relating to the doctor, a characteristic which impairs the patient's social adaption. The doctor has observed his or her own personal responses to the patient, and made use of these as clinical information.

A third possible step to confirm these two sources of clinical information about the personality structure is to request formal personality testing, to be carried out by a clinical psychologist. Tests commonly used evaluate neuroticism (anxiety proneness), extraversion-introversion (sociability), hysterical and obsessional traits, and the level of aggression.

---

4. THE DIAGNOSTIC FORMULATION

The fourth part of the psychiatric examination is a technical decision-making procedure. The doctor coordinates all the data derived from the patient, decides on the relative weighting to be given to the different elements in the case and arrives at a diagnosis. In psychiatry this consists of two parts:

The Naming of the Disorder (or nosological diagnosis). The term to be applied to the illness depends on the most prominent symptoms and signs in the case, together constituting one of the psychiatric syndromes or patterns of disorder laid down in the International Classification of Diseases and described in standard psychiatric texts, e.g. manic-depressive psychosis (p. 28) or schizophrenia (p. 28).

The Psychodynamic Formulation. The second part of a psychiatric diagnosis lists, in a coherent sequence, the pattern of factors which the clinician considers to have contributed to bring about the illness, e.g. 'The patient, the submissive member of an identical twin pair, is less attractive than her sister; during childhood her mother discriminated against her, and the patient is now resentful and hostile.

She tried to suppress these impulses in order to win affection from those to whom she forms overdependent attachments (e.g. twin sister, husband) Her illness began when she found evidence in her husband's wallet that he was associating with another woman.'

Because in successive examinations the patient may communicate fresh biographical material, the psychodynamic formulation becomes gradually fuller as confirmation is obtained about less immediately evident aspects of the patient's adaptive pattern. The nosological diagnosis may also in some cases have to be revised. The formulation of the illness can well be tested — in many cases — by communicating it to other members of the medical team who have also had contact with the patient. The value of concensus is also evident, for example, when the formulation is discussed with a general practitioner who has close knowledge about the patient and that person's environment.

THE METHODS IN PRACTICE

1. THE RECOGNITION OF ABNORMAL PERSONALITY

This example has been chosen because it is important that the clinician should be aware of the clinical presentation of the main types of abnormal personality. Such deviations can be identified from the information obtained by the method described on page 24. Two degrees of severity can be recognised, the lesser being the personality disorders and the more severe being known as sociopathy.

Personality Disorders

There are four types of personality disorder:

Obsessional personality. Obsessional persons are rigid, over-attentive to details, and prefer to have everything predictable and orderly. They are over-careful, methodical, concerned with neatness and orderliness. They are meticulous, punctual, and over-organised, and become upset if their fixed routines are disturbed. They may work compulsively, check things more than once or twice and be unable to use opportunities for relaxation.

Schizoid personality. Schizoid persons are solitary, aloof and detached from other people. They may be preoccupied with some impersonal activity in such realms as electronics, physics, mathematics or engineering. The personality deviation is recognised from the person's quietness and shyness, a disinclination to mix socially and a preference for solitary pursuits.

Hysterical personality. Such people crave attention and appear insincere. They are characterised by excessive displays of emotion. They like to be the centre of attention and find it easy to act a part. The clinician diagnoses the disorder from the patient's showiness, histrionic manner and dress, and need to be appreciated. Speech is superficial, with ample exaggeration. The hysterical man cannot form any enduring attachment to one woman. The hysterical woman is often frigid sexually.

Paranoid personality. Persons of this type are enduringly suspicious and mistrustful. They do not get on with other people, perceive offence where none is intended, and feel constantly picked upon. They are often self-conscious and view themselves as underestimated and misused. They are envious, blaming others for their shortcomings, and are argumentative. Such people need particularly precise and careful explanations from doctors whom they consult when physically ill.

Sociopathy

This is the most severe degree of abnormality of personality. Sociopaths have serious defects in their capacity for feeling. They have a severely defective conscience, and are often described as affectionless. They cannot form satisfactory relationships and major failures repeatedly occur in marriage, work and social life. They are seen as indifferent, loveless and destructive. They come into conflict with the customs and laws of the community. They do not learn from failures, nor are their social transgressions corrected by punishment. Social ineptitude causes them to be persistently in trouble. Many sociopaths are superficially likeable and charming, and initially mislead well-meaning people, whom they subsequently disappoint and distress. A characteristic of sociopathic behaviour is impulsiveness. Uncontrolled emotional outbursts occur in the absence of sufficient provocation.

Sociopaths may be punished repeatedly for the same unacceptable behaviour, continuing an antisocial behaviour pattern despite the harm it does them. They disregard possible consequences of their actions, and give scant consideration to the welfare of those on whom they depend. There are two types of sociopathy:

Aggressive Sociopathy. Persons of this type make hostile attacks on other people, cause damage to property and often come to legal attention because of thefts or fraud.

Passive Sociopathy. A person of this type is seriously inadequate and chronically dependent and passive. Some are placid and responsive while others are cold, withdrawn and apathetic. They may adapt at so poor a level as to exist as aimless drifters to be found in places where hoboes congregate. However, if the family is accepting and supportive, the inadequate sociopath may manage a sheltered existence under the protection of relatives.

2. THE RECOGNITION OF PSYCHIATRIC ILLNESS

Analysis of the various forms of abnormal personality just described does not call for the detection of any signs or symptoms, but for the recognition of certain traits, qualities present also in normal people. These traits are found in excess in abnormal individuals, e.g. too much aggressiveness, or too high a degree of dependency.

To diagnose psychiatric illness, in contrast, the clinician requires the presence of symptoms or signs, i.e. new manifestations which are not present in normal people, such as those set out in the examination of the mental state (p. 22). For example, patients are psychiatrically ill when they have compulsions, suffer from delusions or are hallucinated.

Psychosis. The first step in the diagnostic process is to identify or exclude psychosis. By this is meant what the layman calls madness, and what used to be termed insanity. The patient's whole personality is affected by the illness. It has often come out of the blue, not being precipitated by some personal setback. Contact with reality is grossly impaired. Patients consider they are drastically changed (unless they have no insight); a break has happened in their life, so that they no longer regard themselves as the person they used to be.

Psychoses are either organic or functional.

ORGANIC PSYCHOSIS. This condition, when acute, is termed *delirium,* or a toxic confusional state. In the United States it is known as the *acute brain syndrome.* The person is hallucinated, deluded, seriously restless and the sensorium is impaired by some blunting of consciousness. The last feature is often diagnostic but may be so subtle as to be evident only to trained observers. Delirium runs a short course lasting only a few days.

Dementia is the chronic organic psychosis. It is characterised by impairment of memory, chiefly recent memory. The patient has no difficulty recalling remote events, and may answer readily a question about childhood but not one about news in the morning paper or the name of the head of State. In addition to amnesia, the patient with intellectual deterioration will have some disorientation for person and place, will show blunting of finer sensibilities so that the personality in time becomes a caricature of its former self, and the person so deteriorated as to be unable to give any accurate account of his or her present condition or of the surrounding realities. Dementia is progressive and irreversible.

FUNCTIONAL PSYCHOSIS. The psychotic illnesses not associated with organic cerebral changes are sub-divided according to the prominent symptoms and signs. *Manic-depressive psychosis* is characterised, in the depressive phase, by a lowering of mood, so that the person is morbidly sorrowful, to the extent of depressing the clinician also. Such persons believe all is hopeless, the future black; they are self-reproachful and often suicidal. In the manic phase such patients are unduly elated, with hyperactivity, unwarranted optimism, high physical drive and conspicuous lack of insight.

The second great category of functional psychosis is the *schizophrenias.* In these disorders the chief symptoms and signs are in the sector of thought. The patient's disordered thought may show as a lack of expected connections between spoken phrases, so that a sense of incomprehension is generated in the clinician. The bizarre behaviour may be accompanied by blunting of feeling. In addition to thought disorder and emotional blunting, the patient is detached from reality. These symptoms are not confused with acute organic psychosis, because the state of consciousness in schizophrenia is absolutely clear.

Psychoneuroses. These are the minor psychiatric illnesses. Here only part of the personality is involved, so that only rarely is admission to hospital necessary. The housewife can manage many of her duties and the man his job. Insight is not impaired, as is the case with the psychoses. The illness follows a special psychological stress; this setback is not always stated plainly but becomes evident to the clinician, and often to the patient also, only after detailed exploration. The essential clinical feature is the presence of a psychoneurotic syndrome, i.e. a characteristic constellation of symptoms and signs typical of each type of psychoneurosis. Depending on the symptoms and signs which are most prominent the neurotic illness diagnostically may be one of the following: (i) anxiety neurosis; (ii) hysterical neurosis either of conversion or dissociative type, depending on whether the symptoms are somatic or, in the latter type, consist of altered awareness such as occurs in psychogenic amnesia; (iii) phobic neurosis; (iv) reactive depressive illness; (v) obsessional psychoneurosis.

As indicated at the outset the clinician may find the psychoneurotic patient is helped considerably by the mere communication of distressing experiences during the course of the interview.

REFERENCE

Editorial 1982 History-taking. Medical Education 16:245

3. The Analysis of Symptoms and Signs

If there is a fault in us bred of familiarity it is, I believe, the old fault of omitting to probe sufficiently deeply into causes; the fault of accepting the fact of common symptoms without trying to explain them.

John A. Ryle (1948).
The Natural History of Disease. Oxford University Press, London.

A comprehensive account leading to a complete understanding of all symptoms is not only outside the scope of this textbook, but is beyond the limits of the present state of knowledge. The object of this chapter is to demonstrate by a few examples how to obtain in full and to analyse in detail the information which may be derived from a symptom or sign. Three symptoms have been selected because they are common and important, because they illustrate different but fundamental points, and because they are not solely within the province of any single system subsequently described. *Pain* is a purely subjective complaint. *'Black-outs'* show among other things the importance of the interrogation of eyewitnesses. *Breathlessness* is often associated with objective findings and can, if necessary, be reproduced.

Two signs have been chosen; *swellings* because they require systematic examination and because they may be encountered in almost any part of the body; *oedema* because it provides a simple example of the clinical application of physiological and pathological knowledge.

The junior student may find that the understanding of this chapter will be facilitated after reading about the examination of the major systems.

PAIN

General Considerations. The importance of pain in diagnosis cannot be overestimated. Its subjective nature is such that it is only through personal experience of pain that a doctor can have insight into the meaning of the descriptions given by patients. Further understanding may be acquired by careful enquiry and by observation. Sudden or severe pain may be accompanied by objective signs such as the withdrawal of a limb when the skin is pricked or the muscle spasm which accompanies deep pain. Examples of the latter are the sudden fixation of the lumbar spine in flexion at the onset of lumbago, the catching of the breath due to pleurisy or the rigidity of the abdominal wall in the presence of peritoneal inflammation. Other signs may include pallor, sweating, vomiting or fainting, an involuntary shout evoked by pain of abrupt onset, screaming attacks due to intestinal colic in children, and groaning due to protracted pain. Relief may be sought by characteristic actions such as the adoption of specific postures, the application of heat to the affected area or the use of appropriate medicines such as aspirin or alkalies. Pain as a symptom is poorly suited to investigation by animal experiments. Much of our knowledge has been gained by clinical observation and extended by experiment in human beings.

The distribution of pain resulting from the injection of hypertonic solutions at various sites has been studied. In addition many observations, particularly those made upon the raw bases of artificial blisters, have led to the identification of certain pain-producing substances. Among these, in concentrations which may be achieved in pathological circumstances, are hydrogen ions, potassium ions, acetyl-choline, histamine, 5-hydroxytryptamine and various polypeptides such as bradykinin. It is of interest that many of these substances are present in combination in the stings of nettles, wasps, hornets and other insects.

It is assumed here that the student is conversant with the anatomical and physiological facts about sensation. The nervous pathways for the conduction of pain are described on page 278. Briefly it may be recalled that while several sensations arise from the skin, pain is the main conscious feeling originating in the deep structures. In the skin, pricking, cutting, pinching and extremes of heat and cold cause pain, whereas considerable stretching fails to do so. In the viscera spasm of smooth muscle or distension may cause pain, but the other stimuli mentioned above do not produce any sensation. Ischaemia induces pain in all types of muscle, while the parenchyma of several structures including liver, spleen, kidneys and brain is completely insensitive. Rapid stretching of the capsules of the liver or kidney may cause pain such as that which arises from the liver in acute cardiac failure or the kidney due to sudden ureteric obstruction.

The solution of a clinical problem may demand that every aspect of a pain is elicited from the history. There will be many occasions when the cause of a pain is obvious without entering into details, but even then it is good practice, when time permits, to make a full enquiry. The experience gained through the variations which are encountered will improve diagnostic accuracy in difficult cases.

The Analysis of a Pain

The patient should be encouraged to describe the features of the pain in detail without interruption. Thereafter further information should be obtained by a system of analysis of pain based upon questions about the undernoted 10 features:

1. Main site	6. Frequency and periodicity
2. Radiation	7. Special times of occurrence
3. Character	8. Aggravating factors
4. Severity	9. Relieving factors
5. Duration	10. Associated phenomena.

1. Main Site of Pain. With the eyes shut, it is possible to point precisely to the site of a pinprick on a finger-tip, yet on the skin of the back a spot several centimetres away from the point pricked may be indicated. Similarly two pinpoints can be distinguished from one when they are separated by about 3 mm over the finger-tip, yet the distance required between them may be as much as 50 mm on the leg or back. Localisation is proportionately less accurate in structures from which sensory stimuli rarely reach consciousness. For example, pain arising in the lower thoracic spine may be felt in the hypogastrium, whereas a kick on the shin bone is correctly localised. Misinterpretation of the source of pain in the muscles of the trunk can be demonstrated by injecting hypertonic saline into the erector spinae on one side. This will cause an immediate pain in the back, poorly localised by pointing. The pain soon radiates through anteriorly on the same side. Muscle spasm and localised tenderness may then appear in front, signs which in other circumstances might lead to the erroneous supposition that an inflammatory lesion lies somewhere immediately beneath the examining finger.

By contrast with skin, normal viscera rarely give rise to conscious sensation, and localisation is poor. The oesophagus is, however, sensitive to extremes of temperature, and the bladder and rectum arouse charactersitic sensations when they are full. To some extent therefore we are trained in the knowledge of the position of these organs, and for this reason pain arising in them tends to be correctly orientated. Localisation of pain originating in other viscera is far less accurate or specific. Pain arising in unpaired organs is not always referred to the midline. However, a useful rule is that midline pain always arises from single structures while paired organs never cause symmetrical midline pain. Unpaired structures such as the heart, pericardium, alimentary tract, liver, biliary system, pancreas, bladder and uterus tend to give pain deep in the midline anteriorly. Such mal-localisation could well be called referred pain, but the term is more conveniently reserved for spread beyond the main site. Paired structures such as muscles, bones and joints, eye, pleura and renal tract cause unilateral pain on the affected side. The localisation of pain in limb joints is usually accurate, presumably owing to training through sense of position, but a notable exception is the frequency with which pain from a disorder of the hip is referred to the knee, through mutual innervation by the obturator nerve.

While studying the main site of any pain it is often helpful to find out whether it is localised or diffuse, and at the same time to note any gesture made by the patient. For example, the epigastric pain of peptic ulcer is often indicated by three fingers or just one finger localising the affected area. The palm of the hand rubbed diffusely over the epigastrium may be used to indicate the pain of biliary colic or acute hepatitis. Characteristic gestures are also used to describe angina pectoris (p. 100).

The common sites of pain arising from the various organs and structures of the body are mentioned in the appropriate chapters.

2. Radiation of Pain. Two main aspects of the radiation of pain from the site of the initial lesion must be considered, namely referred pain and spread of pain due to extension of disease.

REFERRED PAIN. In contrast to pain arising in the skin, deep pain may sometimes be felt in or may spread to areas remote from the main site or point of origin, and the distribution of such a referred pain may be highly characteristic. Diaphragmatic pleurisy, for example, or involvement of the undersurface of the diaphragm by acute peritonitis may be referred, through the phrenic nerve, to an area of skin over the shoulder-tip. Local lesions of the skin or of the fourth cervical root may give pain in a similar distribution, while in a few patients with biliary colic or acute cholecystitis pain may similarly be referred to the tip of the right shoulder through involvement of some twigs of the phrenic nerve supplying the gall bladder.

The distribution of referred pain may be more complicated and less readily explained than in this example. Thus the pain of myocardial ischaemia may spread beyond the main retrosternal site to any or all of the following areas: the left pectoral region; down the left arm to the finger-tips (often mostly felt in the elbow and the wrist); the throat; up the left side of the neck to the lower jaw and the tongue; through to the back; sometimes down the right arm and up the neck to the right side of the jaw. The pain may radiate symmetrically to both arms, or to the right arm only. Rarely it may be felt in the epigastrium. Sometimes referred pain may be felt without the main pain, and diagnosis then depends on other features. Thus pain in the left forearm could be due to cervical spondylosis, the carpal tunnel syndrome or perhaps even a hiatus hernia, but regular induction by exercise and relief by rest would point to myocardial ischaemia as the cause.

Pain due to pressure upon a nerve root or to sensory nerve involvement by a disease (e.g. herpes zoster) is referred to the corresponding dermatome. For example, compression of the fifth lumbar nerve root by a prolapsed intervertebral disc may cause pain in the buttock, the posterolateral aspect of the thigh, the anterolateral aspect of the leg and the dorsum of the foot. However, the pain may be felt only in the buttock, leg or ankle, of there may be a pain-free gap. In fact, nerve root pains may be indistinguishable from pains originating in the viscera or other deep structures.

SPREAD OF PAIN DUE TO EXTENSION OF DISEASE. Appendicitis is most readily diagnosed when pain, first felt in the umbilical area, moves after some hours to the right iliac fossa, where it is accompanied by tenderness and muscle guarding. Extension of the inflammation to the serous surface of the appendix with involvement of the overlying parietal peritoneum accounts for this change in site. Less frequently pain and tenderness due to extension of the inflammation may occur elsewhere, according to the position of the appendix.

Pain due to extension may be the first indication of a latent disease. For instance, peptic ulceration may occur without causing pain. Hence the condition may remain symptomless until pain from penetration into surrounding structures develops. Diagnostic difficulties and errors will result unless such a possibility is borne in mind.

3. Character of Pain. As the result of carefully controlled studies in man it has been shown that all pain arising in the skin has a pricking quality if brief or has a burning quality if protracted. However, it is common experience that pains due to a pinprick, burn, cut, pinch or wasp sting can be distinguished, mostly by the context in which they occur, but also by the intensity, duration and distribution of the pain, and by various associated sensations such as heat or traction.

Deep pain is a diffuse aching sensations such as that reproduced by squeezing the tendo achillis; yet its site and duration lead to variations which are described in comparable terms by different patients. Sometimes these descriptions are highly imaginative, and such expressions as 'like being in a vice', or 'like an iron band round the chest' frequently replace the common terms 'tight', 'heavy', 'crushing', 'pressing', or 'like a weight' which are used for the retrosternal pain of myocardial ischaemia. It is remarkable how seldom such a pain is described in any other terms. Yet when myocardial pain is felt in areas of reference elsewhere it does not have this special quality. It appears to be the retrosternal site which determines the character of this pain. A similar crushing pain may be due to pericarditis, dissecting aneurysm of the aorta, pulmonary embolism, collapsed thoracic vertebra, fractured sternum, peptic ulcer or hiatus hernia.

The epigastric pain of peptic ulcer on the other hand is never described in these terms, but is usually said to have a gnawing, aching or dull quality. Pain across the epigastrium which is described as burning should lead to suspicion of a psychogenic disorder.

Likewise, headaches of organic origin are described in terms of pain which is intermittent, felt mostly over the frontal, occipital or occasionally temporal regions and usually relieved by suitable analgesics. By contrast, psychogenic headaches are often indicated by the flat of the hand pressed down on top of the head; they are described in terms of a pressure or perhaps a tightness or lightness, they are continuous and the patient may frequently resort to an analgesic in spite of the experience that it has no effect upon the headache.

4. Severity of Pain. In some diseases pain is characteristically severe, while in others it is mild or may vary in severity. Thus in most cases of perforated peptic ulcer, acute pancreatitis, biliary and renal colic, and dissecting aneurysm of the aorta, the pain is normally so bad that is unusual to obtain a description of quality. Pain due to trigeminal neuralgia, glaucoma, toothache, earache, pleurisy and myocardial infarction is often severe. However, individuals vary so much in their tolerance to pain that a mere statement of severity is unsufficient; it is the doctor's responsibility to form a reasoned judgement on the evidence available. In doing so it must be remembered that the intensity of a pain depends greatly upon the patient's state of mind. Thus a remarkable indifference to pain my be observed in states of mania, religious fervour and hypnosis or after prefrontal leucotomy. Endorphins, opiate-like substances which are present in the brain, play a part in the neural transmission of pain. Fluctuations in the concentration of these may be one explanation of variations in the appreciation of pain. Pain suffered on the football field is apt to be borne much more easily than that due to an injury of similar severity inflicted in the home. On the other hand, mental depression, anxiety and introspection tend to aggravate the severity of pain. Such observations must be familiar to the reader; similar influences affect the appreciation of all subjective symptoms. For example, the tick of an alarm clock may irritate some people to the extent of interfering with sleep, yet others may not hear either the tick or the alarm bell at the bedside. Similarly the incessant sounds (tinnitus) which may accompany disorders of the cochlea and its connections may make life miserable for some patients, yet others can ignore these noises so successfully that they are no longer aware of them without consciously trying to hear them.

The behaviour of the patient while pain is present may be of great help. In biliary and renal colic, patients are usually restless and, having unsuccessfully sought relief by lying down in all sorts of positions, they try sitting, standing or walking. By contrast, the perforation of a peptic ulcer tends to make the patient lie still. Severe pain is commonly associated with pallor, sweating, vomiting, an increase in the pulse rate and blood pressure and a leucocytosis. Hysteria or acute anxiety may lead to restlessness and groaning, but the other features are absent and diversion by conversation may immediately calm the patient. With very little experience a reasonably accurate judgement of the true intensity of a pain may be made if the patient is seen during its occurrence. An account of the pain and details of the patient's behaviour, supplemented if possible by evidence from witnesses, may enable a retrospective assessment of severity to be made. When all these factors are taken into account, an assessment of the severity of a pain, though sometimes misleading, is usually of considerable diagnostic value.

5. Duration of Pain. Estimations of time without actual measurement are often very inaccurate. Yet the duration of pains of various origins may range from less than a second to several days, so that even approximations may be helpful. Thus the lightning pain of the now rare tabes dorsalis, or the excruciating jabs of trigeminal neuralgia, last for less than a second at a time. Each of the griping pains of intestinal colic is felt for less than a minute. The pain of angina of effort ceases two or three minutes after resting, whereas that of a myocardial infarct may continue for hours. The head pain of migraine may be relieved in an hour or so, or it may persist for days.

6. Frequency and Periodicity of Pain. In some instances pains may occur at regular intervals every few minutes as in labour or intestinal colic. At the other extreme the recurrence of pain may be unpredictable as in biliary colic, which may return more than once in a day, though an interval of days, weeks, months or even years may elapse between two attacks. On the other hand, the symptoms of peptic ulcer recur in attacks lasting for one to several weeks, interspersed with pain-free intervals of weeks or months. During an attack the pain usually appears at predictable times on more than one occasion during the 24 hours. Trigeminal neuralgia is another example of a disease with spontaneous remissions. These may last for months and naturally the last remedy given often gets the credit.

The information about the severity, duration and frequency of a pain may be usefully summarised in the form of a time-intensity diagram (Fig. 3.1).

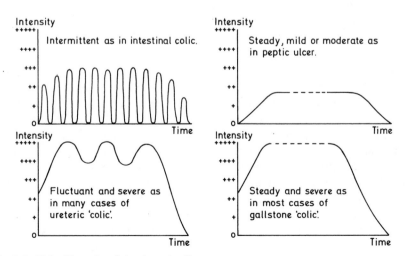

Fig. 3.1 Pain. Examples of time-intensity diagrams.

7. Special Times of Occurrence. It is important to ask if the pain recurs at any special times. Are symptoms present on wakening? Do they occur in the forenoon, afternoon, evening or night? The results of such interrogation may lead to the recognition of a rhythm which can then be related by the doctor to activity, meals, posture, etc.

Migraine, for example, may occur especially in the morning, or every weekend, or at the menses. Most other headaches are intermittent but some occur at special times. That associated with arterial hypertension is often present on wakening, whereas the headache of frontal sinusitis is usually at its peak a few hours after rising. The pain of duodenal ulcer may waken the patient in the early hours of the morning, yet is very rarely present at the ordinary hour of wakening, although it may reappear at predictable times in the forenoon, afternoon and evening. Pain due to bone disease is commonly worse when the patient is warm in bed.

8. Aggravating Factors. The patient should first be asked if any aggravating factors are known. Positive replies must then be assessed for reliability. For example, if bending is alleged to bring on a pain, some specific examples should be sought. It may have happened once only and position may have been incorrectly blamed. On the other hand, if bending to tie shoe-laces brings on a pain regularly, then posture is an acceptable cause. Indeed, the patient may take to putting the foot up on a chair to tie the laces. If no aggravating factors have been noticed, a few suitable questions should be asked. These should be framed in such a manner that 'yes' or 'no' cannot supply a complete answer. For instance, 'Does posture make any difference?' is preferable to 'Does bending make the pain worse?' Sometimes, however, it may be necessary to resort to leading questions to clarify a vague history. Particularly in these circumstances, it is essential to obtain further information as an extra check when a positive association has been elicited. For example, a housewife might spend a vigorous week cleaning her home and then incidentally develop acute appendicitis. With a natural tendency to rationalise symptoms, a clear statement might be made that unusual exercise involving repeated bending has been the cause of the pain. Such false deductions can be eliminated only by enquiry into the precise time relationships.

9. Relieving Factors. Similar caution must be exercised before accepting patients' statements about relieving factors. Many pains subside spontaneously, and the evidence upon which the patient's belief is based must be obtained in detail and carefully considered. For example, epigastric pain due to peptic ulcer is relieved by alkali in 5 to 15 minutes, but never immediately nor in an hour or more, and even half an hour is a suspiciously long time. Yet the patient may deduce that alkali has helped a pain if there is slight relief after a week's treatment or complete relief after two hours, but in either case the doctor can assume that the deduction is incorrect. A combination of faith and gratitude may convince a patient that the condition has improved as a result of treatment which has in fact had no real effect.

10. Associated Phenomena. Some pains may be accompanied by other manifestations which are of diagnostic value. Migraine, for example, is often preceded by visual disturbances and accompanied by vomiting, thus giving rise to the lay terms 'blinding headache' or 'bilious attack'. Rarely, premonitory symptoms such as hunger, an unusual sense of well-being or depression, may precede the attack by a day or so. Added to these characteristics there are usually other members of the family who suffer from recurrent headaches. Further examples are the rigors and pyuria of acute pyelonephritis, the haematuria which may accompany renal colic, or the brown urine, pale stools and yellow sclerae which may follow a bout of pain due to gallstones.

Conclusion

Almost any pain can be analysed in relation to these 10 features. An example is given of the application of the method in the assessment of chest pain (p. 100). When these principles are employed not only will progress be made towards a solution of the problem but the diagnostician's own store of knowledge will often be increased.

BLACKOUTS

The complaint of blackouts is common, and presents a challenging diagnostic exercise since the causes range from the trivial to the serious. In the clinical approach it is first essential to understand what the patient means. Although the term 'blackout' is most frequently used to describe some form of lapse of consciousness, it is also sometimes employed to denote attacks of vertigo, of weakness and of psychiatric disturbances such as fugue-like states.

The nature of episodes wherein consciousness is lost is best diagnosed by a trained observer who has witnessed such an attack. However this is not often possible and the interpretation has to be inferred from the patient's accounts of the events which precede and succeed the attack, supplemented whenever possible by interrogation of a witness of the incident.

Most blackouts are due either to a reduction of blood flow to the brain or to epilepsy. There are a number of miscellaneous causes, but these are quantitatively far less important.

1. Reduction of Blood Flow to the Brain

Disturbance of consciousness may be due to a temporary decrease in the flow of blood to the brain as a result of a number of mechanisms.

Simple Faints (vasovagal attacks). In spite of the name, these are caused by a complex series of reflexes which induce cardiac slowing and at the same time vasodilatation, particularly in skeletal muscle. The result is a sudden fall in blood pressure. The stimuli which trigger the fainting reflex are complex and not fully understood, but receptors in the left ventricle which are activated when the systolic volume of the ventricle falls below a critical value are probably involved. Circumstances in which there is increased sympathetic tone (which enhances ventricular contractility) combined with reduced cardiac filling pressure (as a result of haemorrhage or dehydration) are particularly likely to lead to fainting. Pain, fright, anxiety, intense emotional stimulation or a hot crowded environment are common precipitating factors. Fainting most often occurs when the patient is standing; it is uncommon in the sitting position and very rare when lying. Faints almost never occur during excercise, but may happen when vigorous exercise is suddenly stopped. There is usually a prodromal period which often lasts for several minutes before loss of consciousness, and during which the patient may complain of weakness, nausea, sensations of heat or coldness, sweating, buzzing in the ears or blurring of vision.

The sufferer rarely falls precipitately, but rather sinks to the ground. During the attack the patient is limp and pale, and pallor persists after recovery. The period of unconsciousness rarely lasts longer than a minute, unless the patient is prevented from lying down — in which case prolonged unconsciousness and even grand mal fits may supervene.

Fainting on standing up (postural syncope) is a feature of impairment of the vasomotor reflexes (p. 117) and can occur when arterial hypertension is over-treated. Postural hypotension occurs in the elderly, and in autonomic neuropathy (e.g. diabetic), but it is readily overlooked unless the blood pressure is measured with the patient standing as well as lying flat. Those who are liable to this symptom suffer more severely after being confined to bed; indeed it is a fairly common complaint at any age, on rising from bed after prolonged illness.

Syncope associated with movements of the head suggests either a hypersensitive carotid sinus reflex or insufficiency of the vertebro-basilar arterial flow. In the former, confirmation should be obtained by observing whether a brief pressure on one or other carotid sinus (p. 109) causes extreme bradycardia. Lapses of consciousness due to insufficient blood flow in the vertebro-basilar arteries are often attended by other features of brain stem ischaemia such as double vision or vertigo. Syncope is apt to occur on turning the head or on looking upwards.

Cough syncope refers to a transient loss of consciousness at the end of a purple-faced paroxysm of coughing in some patients with chronic bronchitis and is particularly liable to occur in obese, thick-set men, overindulgent in tobacco and alcohol.

Micturition syncope is rare and occurs in the male who leaves a warm bed at night; the upright position and straining are contributory factors.

The *fainting lark* is a trick learnt by some schoolboys whereby they contrive to reduce the blood flow to the brain to the point of syncope. It consists of a series of manoeuvres, the first of which is to squat, which traps blood in the legs. Simultaneously the subject over-breathes; hyperventilation is known to produce peripheral systemic vasodilatation and cerebral vasoconstriction. Standing erect and performing a Valsalva manoeuvre, i.e. forceful expiration against resistance (p. 117), reduces the cardiac output to such an extent that syncope follows. Those who wish to try it for themselves should take precautions against injury!

Syncope on exertion is found in some patients with extreme limitation of cardiac output due to severe obstruction at the aortic or pulmonary valve, the signs of which would usually be evident; it may also occur in patients under treatment with drugs which block the sympathetic nervous system.

Syncope resulting from Cardiac Arrhythmias. Syncope may result from either excessively fast or excessively slow cardiac rates. Patients suffering from syncope caused by tachycardia may notice palpitation before losing consciousness, but this is not constant. If the tachycardia is very rapid, a pulse may not be palpable during the attack. Frequent extrasystoles or short bursts of tachycardia may be noted on examination of the patient between attacks, but these findings are increasingly common with advancing age even in a 'normal' population. Tachycardia-associated syncope is sometimes precipitated by exercise, and recording an electrocardiogram (ECG) during exertion may be helpful.

Syncope resulting from excessive bradycardia or asystole characteristically occurs without premonitory symptoms. The patient collapses suddenly, is pale and pulseless, and may seem dead. There may be grand mal fits. Recovery is often rapid, and may be accompanied by a pink flushing of the skin. Examination of patients between attacks may reveal underlying complete heart block, or the features of the sick sinus syndrome. In many patients no abnormalities can be detected.

The diagnosis of syncope resulting from cardiac arrhythmias has been greatly helped by the availability of equipment which can continuously record the ECG on magnetic tape over a 24 hour period or longer, and is small enough to be carried by the ambulant patient. The technique is sometimes called Holter monitoring after one of its originators.

2. Epileptic Attacks

An epileptic fit is a transient disturbance (not necessarily a loss) of consciousness due to a brief, excessive electrical discharge of cerebral neurones. The abnormal electrical discharge may remain localised to a small area of the brain, or it may become generalised.

Fits may occur at any time and in any situation. Sometimes, however, in an individual they run to a pattern; some epileptics have fits only during sleep, or when they are pyrexial or during menstruation. A minority of patients develop seizures in response to specific stimuli such as flashing lights or noise. It is important to explore these relationships and precipitants during the taking of the history.

Characteristically an epileptic fit is of abrupt onset. The features of a *grand mal* fit with its tonic phase ushered in by a cry or groan followed by the jerking movements of the clonic phase, are so distinctive that most lay observers can diagnose such an attack. During the tonic phase the eyes remain open and deviated to one side. The arms are flaccid, the legs extended and the face becomes congested and cyanosed. In the absence of an observer the patient's history will often be indicative as the fall may cause an injury and there is frequently incontinence of urine, or tongue biting during the attack.

The very short lived 'absences' of *petit mal* when clearly described by an observer present an easily recognisable pattern. The sufferer, almost always a child, is described as looking vacant or blank for a few seconds. Petit mal seizures are usually very frequent; scores of attacks may occur daily.

In some varieties of *focal epilepsy* consciousness is not entirely lost and the clinical features may be unusual or bizarre. Seizures which originate in the temporal lobe (the commonest type of focal epilepsy) may give rise to diverse manifestations, depending on the site of the initial electrical abnormality and the extent to which it spreads. In the most characteristic variety the onset is associated with a hallucination of smell which is almost always unpleasant. On occasion the prodromal features of a temporal lobe fit are manifest by the patient developing an intense feeling of familiarity with the surroundings—the '*déjà vu*' phenomenon. Visual hallucinations of a specific organised nature occur; miniscule men or animals may be seen in one part of the patient's visual field. Less commonly the patient may describe auditory hallucinations; voices or music may be heard.

These and allied phenomena will be accompanied by variable loss of consciousness and commonly attacks will go on to complete loss of consciousness. When consciousness is retained to some extent patients may carry out motor acts of a bizarre or even antisocial nature. They may appear to the outside observer to be in control of their actions, but the patients afterwards have no memory of their behaviour. Sometimes too this form of *automatism* occurs after the major events of a fit are over.

In *Jacksonian attacks* also patients can retain contact with their environment. They may be able to describe involuntary movements beginning in one area and spreading. The fit may then cease or consciousness may be lost and the features of a grand mal seizure supervene. Occasionally after a Jacksonian fit the affected parts of the body exhibit a temporary paresis, rarely lasting for more than one or two hours.

The Cause of Epilepsy. The recognition that a patient's blackouts are epileptic is the first stage in the diagnostic process. The underlying cause of the fits must then be determined. Epilepsy may be due to genetically determined factors of unknown nature, to any intracranial injury or disease, or to a variety of systemic illnesses or metabolic disturbances. Close attention should, therefore, be paid to the age of onset of the fits, the family history, the previous medical history, associated symptoms and the results of neurological as well as the general systematic examination. In practice one is particularly concerned to define the group of epileptics whose fits arise from a potentially curable cause.

A history of generalised fits which began in childhood and which have been present for many years in a patient who knows of relatives similarly affected, strongly suggests that there is no underlying structural lesion. Fits of recent onset and focal nature, developing for the first time in an adult raise the possibility of a primary cause such as an intracranial tumour. Associated features such as headache or focal neurological signs would reinforce this suspicion. Fits which occur only in the early morning before breakfast or after prolonged fasting should evoke consideration of an insulin-secreting tumour resulting in periodic hypoglycaemic fits. Clinical features of renal or hepatic failure may point to the underlying cause of epilepsy.

It is becoming increasingly important always to explore the possibility that fits may be drug induced. Some drugs, such as L.S.D., are epileptogenic. The sudden withdrawal of many hypnotic drugs, including alcohol, after their long continued and regular ingestion may result in epileptic fits.

3. Miscellaneous Causes of Blackouts

Narcolepsy and cataplexy may sometimes mimic epileptic attacks. *Narcolepsy* is characterised by attacks wherein the patient has an irresistable desire to sleep. These episodes often occur in situations which normally produce drowsiness such as sitting in front of a fire, watching television, or sitting for long periods in a lecture theatre. But they occur too in most inappropriate circumstances as when eating a meal, or driving a motor car. Sometimes narcolepsy may be accompanied by *cataplexy* wherein the patient suddenly becomes intensely weak and may fall to the ground but throughout remains fully conscious.

Hysterical attacks are often bizarre in their manifestations and are rarely accompanied by the stigmata of tongue biting and incontinence of urine. Interviewing an eye witness would reveal none of the features of deviation of the eyes, or cyanosis which are observed in epileptic attacks. Hysterical seizures usually take place in the presence of others, and create maximal disturbance. Movements of the limbs often occur in hysterical episodes but these are coordinated and may be aggressively directed towards other people.

Conclusion

The approach to blackouts exemplifies how a clinical problem may be clarified by the analysis of a single symptom in meticulous detail, seeking evidence from diverse sources, notably in this instance from the interrogation of eye witnesses.

BREATHLESSNESS

A complaint of shortness of breath (dyspnoea) implies that the act of breathing has become a conscious effort. Although many dyspnoeic patients breathe rapidly, there is no direct correlation between the observed rate of breathing and the subjective sensation of dyspnoea. Patients with acute pneumonia, especially children, may take as many as 60 breaths per minute without experiencing respiratory discomfort, while in other conditions, such as respiratory paralysis, a feeling of shortness of breath may not be accompanied by any increase in the rate of breathing. There is also considerable variation in what might be called the 'dyspnoea threshold'. Some patients with objective evidence of gravely impaired respiratory function may complain of relatively mild dyspnoea, while others with only slight disturbance of function may experience quite severe respiratory distress.

Factors contributing to the Production of Dyspnoea

While *hypoxia* and dyspnoea frequently co-exist, hypoxia *per se,* unless it is severe, plays a relatively minor part in the production of dyspnoea. Many patients with severe dyspnoea are not hypoxic, while in hypoxic patients dyspnoea is not always a conspicuous symptom. There is a similar lack of direct correlation between dyspnoea and *hypercapnia.* Although a rise in the carbon dioxide tension of arterial blood immediately causes hyperventilation and dyspnoea in normal subjects, it may not do so in patients with chronic ventilatory inadequacy in whom the respiratory centre may have become unresponsive to carbon dioxide or to an increase in hydrogen ion concentration.

The disturbances of respiratory function which may contribute to the production of dyspnoea are now well recognised. The most important of these are an increase in the work of breathing, increased pulmonary ventilation, and weakness of the respiratory muscles. Each of these disturbances has a variety of causes, and there are thus many factors which may operate, singly or in combination, to produce dyspnoea in an individual case.

1. Dyspnoea associated with an Increase in the Work of Breathing. Airflow limitation, decreased pulmonary compliance ('stiff lungs') and restricted chest expansion all increase the work of breathing.

Airflow limitation is the main cause of dyspnoea in patients with obstructive lesions of the larynx, trachea and main bronchi, bronchial asthma, chronic bronchitis and emphysema. Those conditions in which *decreased pulmonary compliance* may contribute to the production of dyspnoea include all forms of diffuse interstitial lung disease, including interstitial pulmonary oedema, which is the main cause of cardiac dyspnoea. Pneumothorax, pleural effusion and pleural thickening may also restrict pulmonary expansion and produce disturbances in respiratory function similar to those caused by decreased pulmonary compliance. Dyspnoea due to *restricted chest expansion* may occur in patients with severe pleural pain, kyphoscoliosis, ankylosing spondylitis and gross obesity.

2. Dyspnoea associated with Increased Pulmonary Ventilation. An increase in the respiratory dead space, severe hypoxia and metabolic acidosis, may all be responsible for an increase in pulmonary ventilation. Hyperventilation may also be a manifestation of hysteria.

An *increase in the volume of the physiological dead space* occurs in massive pulmonary embolism as a result of a drastic reduction in blood flow through capillaries perfusing well ventilated alveoli. Patients who survive a massive embolism for a few hours may exhibit a striking degree of hyperventilation ('air hunger'), but this is usually overshadowed by the effects of a sudden severe reduction of cardiac output, such as hypotension and syncope.

Severe hypoxia, in conditions such as pneumonia, pulmonary oedema and interstitial lung disease, increases pulmonary ventilation by reflex stimulation of the respiratory centre via the aortic and carotid chemoreceptors.

In *metabolic acidosis,* caused for example by diabetic ketoacidosis or renal failure, the respiratory centre is stimulated by the increased hydrogen ion concentration in the blood, and the resultant hyperventilation may produce the sensation of dyspnoea.

Hysterical hyperventilation is also accompanied by a sensation of breathlessness. Breathing is often irregular, and may be sighing. If the hyperventilation is sufficiently severe and prolonged, it may lead to tetany, or even to an epileptic fit.

3. Dyspnoea associated with Weakness of the Muscles of Respiration. Neuromuscular lesions, such as high spinal cord injuries, poliomyelitis, polyneuropathy and myasthenia gravis, may cause partial or complete paralysis of the muscles of respiration, with the result that the patient is no longer able to meet the ventilatory requirements.

4. Dyspnoea associated with Multiple Factors. In some cases a single factor may be chiefly or even entirely responsible for the dyspnoea, as for example in patients with airflow limitation or with respiratory paralysis. In most conditions, however, the mechanisms responsible for the production of dyspnoea are more complex. Two examples are given:

(i) In *pneumonia* the restriction of chest expansion by pleural pain is probably the chief cause of dyspnoea in the early stages of the illness; later, if the lungs become extensively consolidated, dyspnoea is mainly due to a combination of decreased pulmonary compliance and increased pulmonary ventilation caused by hypoxia.

(ii) *Pulmonary oedema* of cardiac origin begins in the alveolar walls and causes dyspnoea by reducing pulmonary compliance and increasing the work of breathing. Later, intra-alveolar transudate aggravates the dyspnoea, at first by increasing pulmonary ventilation in response to hypoxia, and then by producing airflow limitation.

Clinical Forms of Dyspnoea

The sensation of dyspnoea is apparently the same, whatever its cause, but its mode of presentation varies considerably. There are, however, two main patterns, which may occur either independently or together, namely *paroxysmal dyspnoea* and *exertional dyspnoea*.

1. Paroxysmal Dyspnoea. This usually develops when the patient is at rest, but in some conditions is provoked by exertion. It is by definition acute in onset and may be intense and alarming. An acute attack of dyspnoea is usually due to the rapid development either of airflow limitation or of a restrictive lesion of lungs or pleura. Rarely, as in massive pulmonary embolism, it may be associated with a sudden increase in the volume of the physiological dead space. The differential diagnosis therefore includes the following conditions:

    (i) Obstruction of the larynx, trachea or main bronchi by exudate or vomitus, or by an inhaled foreign body

   (ii) Retention of secretions in the air passages of a patient with respiratory paralysis

  (iii) Inhalation of gastric acid during coma or anaesthesia

  (iv) Bronchial asthma

   (v) Left heart failure

  (vi) Massive pulmonary embolism

 (vii) Spontaneous pneumothorax

(viii) Pleural effusion accumulating rapidly.

HISTORY. A carefully taken history is often of great help in identifying the cause of an acute attack of dyspnoea. In children the possibility of a *foreign body* in the larynx or of membranous exudate obstructing the air passages should not be forgotten. In adults unable to cough effectively because of weakness of the respiratory muscles, the *retention of secretions* may produce acute dyspnoea, as may the *inhalation*, during coma or anaesthesia, of acid gastric secretions, with the production of a chemical pneumonia.

An attack of *bronchial asthma* is in most cases readily recognised. As airflow limitation in this condition is maximal during expiration, the latter is slow and laboured while inspiration is relatively rapid but at the same time restricted because the lungs may already be almost fully inflated. Wheeze and rhonchi are almost invariably present and are predominantly expiratory. If, as is often the case, there have been previous episodes, these will probably have responded promptly to a bronchodilator drug. It is more difficult to recognise from the history alone a patient's first attack of asthma. This is particularly a problem in the child, as anxious parents are often unable to give an accurate account of the episode. The diagnosis usually becomes obvious, however, when a subsequent attack is witnessed by a trained observer.

Attacks of dyspnoea occurring during the night (paroxysmal nocturnal dyspnoea) may be due to bronchial asthma, but in middle-aged and elderly patients pulmonary oedema secondary to *left heart failure* is the most likely cause. Although the term 'cardiac asthma', used to describe paroxysmal dyspnoea of cardiac origin accompanied by wheeze, has now fallen into disrepute, it serves to emphasise the difficulty which may occasionally arise in distinguishing this condition from bronchial asthma. In most cases, however, a previous history of exertional dyspnoea can be elicited and patients will often state that they sleep more comfortably in the upright position, supported by several pillows. The attack usually develops in the early hours of the morning as a result of sliding into the recumbent position during deep sleep. They then waken with intense breathlessness, which often produces feelings of suffocation and panic. The usual reaction is to sit upright with the legs over the side of the bed, and the hands clutching the back of a chair if one can be found. Patients may even struggle to an open window in the hope that cool fresh air will ease their breathing. In most cases the attack subsides spontaneously in about half an hour, but it is an acute medical emergency which may occasionally be fatal.

Paroxysmal nocturnal dyspnoea is seen most frequently in left ventricular failure secondary to hypertension, coronary heart disease or aortic valvular lesions. It is uncommon in mitral stenosis except during pregnancy or as a result of a change in cardiac rhythm. In the later stages of left heart failure paroxysms of dyspnoea may develop whenever the patient lies down. Such intolerance of the recumbent position is known as *orthopnoea*. Some patients with severe emphysema are also orthopnoeic, but for a different reason. In left heart failure the recumbent position is avoided, possibly because it is liable to induce pulmonary oedema by increasing cardiac output. In emphysema, on the other hand, the upright position is more comfortable because it improves pulmonary ventilation by facilitating the range of movement of the thoracic cage.

Paroxysmal dyspnoea may also be experienced during the phase of hyperpnoea in Cheyne-Stokes breathing (p. 168).

The dyspnoea which follows *massive pulmonary embolism* produces a sensation of suffocation in which the patient feels desperately short of air, although, in fact, breathing may be deep ('air hunger'). It is invariably accompanied by profound circulatory collapse caused by a fall in left ventricular output, and by pulmonary hypertension and right ventricular failure. The differential diagnosis from myocardial infarction may be very difficult or even impossible by clinical methods, particularly in the elderly who may experience similar pain in the two conditions; if the dyspnoea is of the character described above and no crepitations are heard on auscultation of the lungs, pulmonary embolism is the probable diagnosis.

Dyspnoea caused by *spontaneous pneumothorax* usually develops suddenly, not infrequently in the morning when the patient wakens or shortly after getting out of bed. In other cases the dyspnoea is slight at first but becomes more severe following exertion or a bout of coughing. Unilateral chest pain or 'tightness' typically precedes or accompanies the onset of dyspnoea.

Fluid in the pleural space produces acute dyspnoea only if it accumulates very rapidly. Massive intrapleural haemorrhage is probably the only condition in which this occurs and can usually be recognised without difficulty, as the dyspnoea is accompanied by features of acute blood loss.

PHYSICAL EXAMINATION. The following findings are of particular value in the differential diagnosis of acute dyspnoea. These are described in detail in Chapters 5 and 6 but are summarised here for convenience.

1. Clinical features indicating a possible cause for left heart failure, e.g. diastolic hypertension, myocardial infarction, aortic or mitral valve disease.

2. An increase in jugular venous pressure (p. 113) which is usually raised in acute dyspnoea of cardiac origin and in massive pulmonary embolism.

3. Central cyanosis (p. 105) which is a relatively late feature in acute dyspnoea of cardiac origin but develops at an early stage in severe airflow limitations of all types. In massive pulmonary embolism cyanosis is chiefly of the peripheral type (p. 105) which, in combination with intense cutaneous vasoconstriction, imparts a slate-grey colour to the lips and cheeks.

4. Hypotension, which occurs in massive pulmonary embolism and also in extensive myocardial infarction, and may be associated with acute dyspnoea in both conditions.

5. Physical signs indicating either a primary abnormality in bronchi, lungs or pleura, or a pulmonary abnormality secondary to a cardiac lesion:

(i) Expiratory rhonchi which, if the sole clinical abnormality, strongly suggest a diagnosis of bronchial asthma.

(ii) Markedly diminished or absent breath sounds on one side of the chest, accompanied by hyperresonance on percussion in spontaneous pneumothorax and by stony dullness in massive pleural effusion or haemorrhage. When sufficiently gross to cause severe dyspnoea, both these conditions are easily recognised from the physical signs. Failure to discover a spontaneous pneumothorax in such circumstances is usually the result of inadequate examination of the chest in the stress of the emergency.

(iii) Basal crepitations which, produced by pulmonary oedema, are almost invariably present in acute dyspnoea of cardiac origin.

When the cause of acute dyspnoea cannot be clearly identified from the history and clinical examination, a portable chest radiograph and an electrocardiograph may provide information which will enable a precise diagnosis to be made.

2. Exertional Dyspnoea. When dyspnoea on exertion is the dominant complaint it is usually due to heart failure or chronic lung disease, although it may be aggravated, or even caused, by obesity, anaemia or hyperthyroidism. Its severity can be assessed only by reference to the level of physical activity at which it is induced. A series of standard questions to grade the severity of dyspnoea can be used as follows:

Grade 1. The patient can walk at a normal pace on level ground and can walk up mild inclines and stairs without feeling short of breath.

Grade 2. The patient can walk at a normal pace on level ground but becomes short of breath on walking up mild inclines or stairs.

Grade 3. The patient cannot walk at a normal pace because of shortness of breath but can walk on level ground for a distance of a mile or more at a slow pace.

Grade 4. The patient cannot walk for a distance of more than 100 yards without having to stop to regain breath.

Grade 5. The patient becomes short of breath on taking a few steps and while washing or dressing.

HISTORY. Patients with sustained exertional dyspnoea should be asked whether it is increasing in severity, stationary or improving. If it varies spontaneously in degree, this may provide a lead to its cause, as in the case of chronic asthma, while an improvement following treatment with a diuretic will suggest that the dyspnoea is of cardiac origin. The nature of the patient's other symptoms may also be of value in identifying the cause of exertional dyspnoea.

PHYSICAL EXAMINATION. The clinical investigation of exertional dyspnoea calls, in particular, for a detailed examination of the cardiovascular and respiratory systems. Amongst the abnormalities which should be looked for with special care are, in the cardiovascular system, increased jugular venous pressure, peripheral oedema, cardiac enlargement, left ventricular hypertrophy, hypertension, valve lesions, arrhythmias, added heart sounds and pericardial effusion, and in the respiratory system, severe chest deformities, airflow limitation and emphysema, interstitial lung disease, pulmonary oedema, pleural effusion and pneumothorax. In some cases, however, clinical examination fails to elucidate the cause of exertional dyspnoea and further investigation, such as radiological examination of the heart and lungs, electrocardiography and respiratory function tests (including arterial blood gas studies), is then necessary to reach an exact diagnosis.

Conclusion

Breathlessness may be the presenting complaint in a large number of important cardiovascular and respiratory diseases. A correct assessment of its significance requires a clear understanding of the disturbances in physiology with which it is associated, and of the pathological processes by which these disturbances are created. By means of a carefully taken history the possible causes of dyspnoea in an individual patient can usually be narrowed down to two or three conditions, and a final diagnosis can often be made from the physical signs. In some cases, however, special investigation, such as radiological examination of the chest, ECGs or tests of respiratory function, may be required.

Breathlessness illustrates how an important symptom is analysed. Other complaints may be interpreted in a similar way by correlating their physiological and pathological basis with the clinical findings.

THE EXAMINATION OF SWELLINGS

A swelling is a common presenting feature. In reporting the discovery of a lump, a patient often makes an erroneous deduction that it has appeared recently because nothing had been noticed previously. Similarly physical examination may reveal a lump whose presence is unknown to the patient. An open mind must always be kept about the apparent duration of a lump or gross errors about its nature will be made.

By systematic attention to detail it should be possible to determine the origin of a swelling if the examiner is aquainted with the anatomy of the region. The local findings should also give at least some indication of the pathological nature of the swelling — whether this is due to trauma, inflammation or neoplasm.

In the first place, inspection may show the position, the approximate size and shape, and any unusual colour of the mass. By palpation, further information should be obtained about its position, size, and shape; tenderness may be elicited, the mobility, consistency, surface texture, and type of edge of the mass may be determined, and any enlargement of the regional lymph nodes can be detected. Other methods of examination, such as auscultation, are usually much less informative. The examination of a goitre (p. 81) provides a good example of the methods in practice.

Inspection and Palpation

Position. The anatomical situation of a mass must be defined as accurately as possible. Frequently this will present little or no difficulty, as in the case of a swelling in the breast, in the thyroid, or in the parotid gland. Elsewhere, however, the precision with which a lump can be located will vary in spite of the most careful palpation, especially with some masses in the abdomen. In these circumstances, other features, such as its shape or mobility, will help to identify its anatomical origin.

Size. The size of a swelling should always be measured. A diagram, indicating the dimenions, position and shape of the swelling should be recorded and dated (Fig. 3.2). In this way, significant changes, which may occur later, can be recognised. In contrast, vague statements about size, such as large, medium or small, or comparisons with fruit, eggs or vegetables, are inaccurate and misleading.

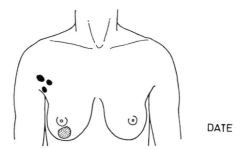

Fig. 3.2 The use of diagrams in case recording. Lump in right breast and axillary lymphadenopathy in patient with carcinoma of the breast.

Shape. Many swellings have characteristic shapes, as, for example, diffuse enlargement of the thyroid gland with its two lobes linked by the isthmus. The swollen parotid gland of mumps fills in the hollow between the posterior border of the mandible and the mastoid process, and often lifts up the ear and extends forward on to the cheek below the zygoma as the accessory parotid gland. The characteristic outline of a mass in the appropriate position should simplify the recognition of an enlarged spleen or liver, a distended bladder, or the fundus of the uterus in the later months of pregnancy. Even with these familiar examples, however, errors can arise, and some additional evidence may be required, such as the disappearance after catheterisation of a swelling when this was due to a full bladder.

Colour and Temperature. The skin over acute inflammatory lesions near the surface is usually red and this may be accompanied by a rise in temperature due to an increase in blood flow. A vascular skin tumour may range in colour from red to blue or purple according to the proportions of reduced haemoglobin present and the depth of the layer of skin through which it is seen. Other colour changes over swellings may occur, for example in haematomas the pigment from extravasated blood may produce the range of colours caused by various breakdown products of haemoglobin so familiar in a bruise. Melanin deposition may be responsible for brown pigmentation in the skin over swellings when there is any undue pressure from clothing and other causes. A brown or black colour is common in melanomas, though some are not pigmented. A xanthoma is a small skin nodule which may be identified by its yellow colour due to the lipids it contains.

Tenderness. Inflammatory swellings are characterised by tenderness. While this sign must be deliberately sought, palpation should be particularly gentle whenever the patient complains of pain. Many large tumours, in contrast, are entirely free from pain or tenderness, partly because they carry no nerve supply and also because they may have developed in an area where tissue tension is low and where a mass can be accommodated without subjecting any structure to undue stretching. Tumours eroding bone or growing into nerve roots and plexuses are capable of causing severe persistent pain of a most intractable type, and this is often worse at night.

Movement. The mobility of a mass must be tested in order to determine whether it is part of, attached to, or free from adjacent structures, such as skin or bone. So far as the skin is concerned, this may be tested by attempting to pick up a fold of skin over the swelling and comparing this with the mobility of the skin over other structures in the vicinity. Fixation of the skin may be associated with a fine dimpling at the opening of the hair follicles resembling 'pigskin' or 'orange skin' when there is lymphatic obstruction. Such a change is most commonly due to malignant disease.

Fixation to deeper structures such as bone or muscle will be recognised by attempting to move the swelling in different planes relative to the surrounding tissues. For example, with a tumour in the breast, the patient is asked to press the hand firmly on the hip of the affected side. The mobility of the mass may then be tested in relation to the contracted and immobilised pectoral muscle. Again it may be difficult to decide whether a mass is situated in the abdominal wall or within the abdominal cavity. This distinction is made by noting the effect of contraction of the rectus and other muscles on the accessibility of the swelling, as described on page 82. In the case of the thyroid, most goitres will move up and down on swallowing.

Adherence to adjacent structures such as a blood vessel, a nerve or a viscus, may cause pulsation, paralysis, pain or obstructive symptoms. Pulsation of a lump will readily be appreciated if the palpating hand is kept still for a few moments. It is then necessary to determine whether this is the expansile pulsation of an aneurysm or a vascular tumour, or whether the movement is transmitted from an artery nearby.

An impulse on coughing is characteristically felt in certain swellings within which a rise in pressure may occur because their contents communicate with the thoracic or abdominal cavity. The commonest example is an inguinal hernia.

Consistency. The consistency of a swelling may vary from soft and fluctuant through increasing degrees of firmness until this may be so striking as to merit the term 'stony hard'. Very hard swellings are usually malignant or calcified, or consist largely of dense fibrous tissue.

Fluctuation indicates a fluid-containing swelling, such as an abscess or a cyst. Soft tumours such as lipomas may also show some degree of fluctuation. The sign is elicited by detecting with one finger the bulge created by compressing the swelling suddenly with another finger placed at a distance. Fluctuation should be detectable in two planes before the sign is regarded as positive.

Surface Texture. The surface of a swelling may vary widely from the uniform smooth to the grossly irregular, as is commonly illustrated in enlargements of the thyroid gland and the liver. The surface of a simple goitre and of some primary toxic goitres is usually uniformly smooth, whereas other goitres, especially those of long standing, may be so irregular in outline that they are described as nodular. A similar variety of texture may be noted on palpation of the liver, ranging from the smooth surface usually found in congestive cardiac failure, through the fine irregularity of portal cirrhosis, to the gross degreee of nodular change in some cases of metastatic tumour. However, a thick abdominal wall may make it impossible to appreciate these variations with confidence.

Ulceration. Lesions which arise within the skin, such as squamous or basal cell carcinomas, or lesions which lie close to the skin, such as breast cancer or malignancy in axillary lymph nodes, may ulcerate. The character of the edge, the size and shape of the ulcer and the nature of its base should all be noted. Similar observations should be made of visible or palpable ulcers in the mouth or rectum.

Margin. The edge or margin may be well or ill-defined, regular or irregular, sharp or rounded. The margins of enlarged organs such as the thyroid gland, liver, spleen or kidney can usually be defined more clearly than those of inflammatory or malignant masses. The indefinite margin of a mass is sometimes a valuable indication of an infiltrating malignant growth as opposed to the clearly defined edge of a localised benign tumour.

Associated Swellings. The nature of a lump can sometimes be inferred by identifying others with similar characteristics. Conditions in which multiple swellings occur include neurofibromatosis (Plate I), lipomatosis, metastases in the skin, lymph nodes in reticuloses, and nodules in the breast in chronic mastitis. The suspicion that a tumour is malignant should invariably lead to a thorough examination for evidence of involvement of the lympth nodes draining the area concerned.

Additional Methods of Examination

Percussion. This technique is of very limited value in the examination of a swelling, although occasionally it may be helpful in defining an abdominal mass (p. 208).

Auscultation. *Vascular Sounds.* If the blood supply through a tumour is very large, a systolic murmur (bruit) may be audible over the swelling. A murmur is commonly present over vascular goitres and, if it is sufficiently marked, a thrill may also be palpable. Systolic murmurs may also be heard over arterial aneurysms, while over the very rare swellings due to arteriovenous aneurysms there is a continuous murmur, often accompanied by a thrill, similar to the bruit of a persistent ductus arteriosus (p. 134).

Fetal Heart Sounds. These may be audible over the pregnant uterus after the 30th week.

Bowel Sounds (p. 209). These may be heard over a hernia which contains intestine.

Friction. This may sometimes be heard over an enlarged spleen or liver when fibrinous perisplenitis or perihepatitis is present.

Transillumination. This is occasionally a useful test in distinguishing between a swelling composed of solid tissue and one consisting of transparent or semi-transparent liquid which may be under such tension that fluctuation cannot be elicited. The sign is sought in darkened surroundings by pressing the lighted end of an electric torch into one side of the tumour. A cystic swelling will light up like a lantern if the fluid within it is translucent provided that the covering tissures are not too thick. The sign is useful in helping to distinguish a hydrocele from a solid tumour of the testis, though it must be borne in mind that a testicular tumour may lie within the hydrocele.

Further Investigation. *Radiographs* may define a mass either directly or by the use of various contrast media and *ultrasonography* distinguishes between a solid and a cystic swelling (Fig. 7.16 p. 220).

Biopsy is often required and must be carried out if there is any suspicion of malignancy.

Conclusion

The examination of a swelling illustrates the value of a strictly methodical approach, making particular use of two of the basic procedures in physical examination, namely, inspection and palpation. The same principles are applied in defining the physical characteristics and in deducing the nature of any mass wherever it may be situated.

OEDEMA

Oedema means swelling of the tissues due to an increase in interstitial fluid. It may be generalised due to a disorder of the heart, kidneys, liver, gut, or diet, or it may be local from venous or lymphatic obstruction, allergy or inflammation. Sometimes, as is explained later, oedema may be postural and relatively unimportant. An appreciation of the physiological and pathological background is required in order to understand the significance of oedema.

Clinical Manifestations of Oedema

The doctor may be consulted because of swelling of the ankles, face or abdomen, breathlessness or a rapid gain of weight. When oedema is due to generalised fluid retention, for whatever reason, its distribution is determined by gravity. Thus it is usually observed in the legs, back of the thighs and the lumbosacral area as in cardiac failure in the semi-recumbent patient If a patient can lie flat quite comfortably, it may readily be seen in the face and hands as in many children with acute glomerulonephritis. Regional rises in venous pressure also determine the distribution of oedema fluid as exemplified by pulmonary oedema in left heart failure or by ascites when there is portal hypertension.

The cardinal sign of subcutaneous oedema is the indentation or *pitting* made in the skin by firm pressure maintained for a few seconds by the examiner's fingers or thumb. The pitting may persist for several minutes until it is obliterated by the slow reaccumulation of the fluid which had been displaced. However, pitting on pressure may not be demonstrable until an increase in body weight of as much as 10 or 15 per cent has occurred; day to day alterations in weight usually provide much the most reliable index of progress or response to treatment.

Myxoedema, in contrast to oedema, is characterised by swelling which does not pit on pressure and which is due to infiltration of the tissues by a firm mucinous material. Chronic lymphoedema may also fail to pit on pressure for reasons that will be described later.

The Genesis of Oedema

Generalised oedema is bound to occur if, after allowing for water loss through the skin, the breath, the stools or discharges, the fluid intake exceeds the renal excretory capacity. The latter may be reduced by disease of the kidneys or renal function may be altered by extrarenal factors. For example, a fall in renal blood flow leads to a reduction in glomerular filtration rate and an increase in obligatory water absorption by the proximal tubule as in the early stages of cardiac failure. Renal tubular reabsorption of water may be greater when a rise in circulating aldosterone enhances the reabsorption of sodium as occurs in some patients with hepatic cirrhosis, the nephrotic syndrome or cardiac failure. The retained fluid dilutes the plasma and so causes a drop in the osmotic pressure of the proteins and consequent oedema (Fig. 3.3). However, many instances of generalised oedema and all forms of local oedema are due to alterations in the factors which control the formation and disposal of interstitial fluid at capillary level. In some types of oedema, such as that due to advanced cardiac failure, the genesis is multifactorial.

The Formation and Disposal of Interstitial Fluid. Interstitial fluid is formed as the result of filtration through the capillary walls, and it is removed partly by reabsorption into the capillaries and partly by drainage along the lymphatic channels. It is convenient to regard the capillary wall as a semi-permeable membrane although the full explanation of the transport of water and solutes across it is much more complicated. The main force causing filtration is the hydrostatic pressure within the vessels; in addition, there is the osmotic pressure of the proteins in the interstitial fluid. The latter is normally very low as albumin in a concentration of not more than 20 mg per cent escapes through the intact capillary.

In inflammatory, allergic and lymphatic oedema, on the other hand, there is a high concentration of protein which retains tissue fluid by its osmotic effect. Reabsorption of the fluid is determined by the osmotic pressure of the plasma proteins (oncotic pressure) with an additional effect from tissue pressure depending upon site and position. These factors are shown diagrammatically in Figure 3.3.

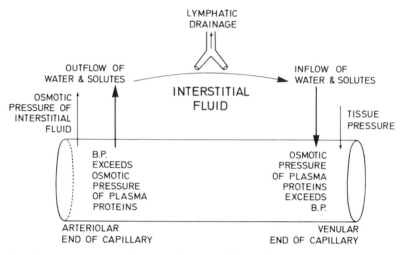

Fig. 3.3   The formation and disposal of the interstitial fluid.

The hydrostatic pressure within the capillaries varies widely at different sites. The mean pressure in the pulmonary capillaries, for example, during recumbency is less than 10 mmHg, while that in the glomerular capillaries is about 75 mmHg. Thus the lungs are well protected from oedema in spite of the low tissue pressures, while the kidneys are adapted to a high filtration pressure. Another example, is the effect of the erect posture in which, owing to the effect of gravity, the pressure in the capillaries of the scalp falls, while that in the feet rises. It can readily be calculated that the mean capillary pressure in the feet of a person of average height during quiet standing is at least 110 mmHg. It is not surprising that some swelling of the feet at the end of a day's work may be normal. Indeed, the swelling of the feet would be much greater were it not for the fact that contractions of the muscles pump the venous blood and lymph towards the heart and because of the valves in the veins this reduces the capillary venous pressure to some 20 mmHg. Similarly, some puffiness under the eyes for a short time after rising in the morning is an unflattering sight familiar to many. This is due to the rise in capillary pressure during recumbency in areas where the tissue is lax.

The Types and Causes of Oedema

Oedema may be generalised or localised and it results from factors disturbing the physiological control of body fluid.

Generalised Oedema. The causes of generalised oedema (anasarca) may conveniently be considered under three headings, namely, hypoproteinaemia, cardiac failure and renal causes. As will be seen, several factors may contribute in some instances.

1. HYPOPROTEINAEMIA. The oncotic pressure is mostly due to the serum albumin so that a fall in the concentration of this protein in particular predisposes to oedema. One or more of five mechanisms may lead to hypoproteinaemia:

(i) *Inadequate intake* of protein may be responsible as in kwashiorkor, the most important and widespread nutritional disorder in the world. Famine conditions, the diet of food faddists, or pyloric obstruction with vomiting, may also impair the protein intake.

(ii) *Failure of digestion* of dietary protein results from impairment of the exocrine secretion of the pancreas, as in chronic pancreatitis.

(iii) *Failure of absorption* of the products of digestion may occur after resection of considerable lengths of small intestine or in diseases such as gluten induced enteropathy.

(iv) *Reduced synthesis* of albumin is found in diseases of the liver, such as cirrhosis. When the portal venous pressure is high, ascites is a more prominent feature than dependent oedema.

(v) *Excessive loss* of protein may occur, especially in the urine in the nephrotic syndrome. Protein may also be lost into the gut in a variety of disorders from the stomach to the colon. Although in gastric lesions the protein lost is digested and reabsorbed, the rate of loss exceeds hepatic synthesis. The syndromes are grouped as protein losing enteropathy. The repeated removal of ascitic fluid by paracentesis or drainage of an empyema or other discharge will also cause depletion of protein.

The low intravascular volume induced by any of these five mechanisms may cause secondary hyperaldosteronism via the renin-angiotensin system, promoting sodium retention and an increase in the oedema.

2. CARDIAC FAILURE. The causes of oedema in cardiac failure are multiple and are not fully understood. Significant factors are:

(i) *Impairment of Renal Blood Flow.* In cardiac failure a 'rationing system' gives priority to the maintenance of the coronary and cerebral circulations at the expense of other organs. Reduction in renal blood flow, alteration in the pulsatile pattern of renal perfusion, and possibly alteration in the distribution of blood flow within the kidney promote excessive reabsorption of salt and water — these are the main causes of 'cardiac' oedema. Rest, which diverts blood away from the muscles, and diuretics, which counter the excessive salt and water reabsorption, are the most effective treatments.

(ii) *Increased Venous Pressure.* In cardiac failure there is a rise in venous pressure proximal to the failing chamber. Thus in right-sided failure the increase in venous pressure can be measured by inspection of the neck (p. 113). In left-sided failure, pulmonary venous congestion is inferred from the symptoms of dyspnoea and cough and from the auscultatory findings of crepitations in the lungs. It is possible to measure the rise in pressure by a catheter wedged in a branch of the pulmonary artery. However, the heights of these rises in venous pressure do not correlate with the degrees of oedema and it is clear that the hydrostatic effect does not account for the major part of the fluid retention.

(iii) *The Effect of Aldosterone.* In some cases of cardiac failure secondary hyperaldosteronism occurs and contributes to the oedema.

(iv) Antidiuretic Hormone. There is evidence of an increase in antidiuretic substances in the urine of some patients with cardiac failure.

(v) Lymphatic Factors. Lymphangiectasis, incompetent valves, and poor lymph drainage have been demonstrated in cardiac failure.

(vi) Oncotic Pressures. A combination of chronic passive congestion of the liver reducing albumin synthesis, a poor appetite, and loss of protein into the oedema fluid and the urine may account for a significant drop in the concentration of the serum albumin in some cases.

Acting in the opposite direction is an increase in the protein content of the interstitial fluid. In cardiac failure, this may rise to as much as 1 g % compared with only 0.02 g % in normal interstitial fluid. This change has sometimes been interpreted as evidence for an increase in capillary permeability supposedly due to ischaemia, but it is likely to be mainly due to lymphatic failure.

(vii) Vasodilatation. In wet beriberi (vitamin B_1 deficiency) the extremities are characteristically hot and oedematous. An abnormal accumulation of carbohydrate metabolites causes peripheral vasodilation, and high output cardiac failure often ensues. The vasodilatation leads to a rise in capillary pressure which contributes to oedema formation just as very hot weather induces swelling of the feet and hands in unacclimatised persons.

3. RENAL CAUSES. The oedema of the nephrotic syndrome has been discussed under hypoproteinaemia. In acute glomerulonephritis inflammatory swelling of the glomeruli leads to a fall in the glomerular filtration rate, a relative increase in tubular reabsorption and consequent reduction in urinary volume. Should normal fluid intake be maintained, oedema results. This also applies to any condition in which urine production is diminished (oliguria) or negligible (anuria).

Localised Oedema. This may be due to venous, lymphatic, inflammatory, or allergic causes.

1. VENOUS CAUSES. External pressure upon a vein, venous thombosis or incompetence of the venous valves due to varicose veins may each contribute to a rise in capillary pressure in the areas of drainage. A common example is thrombosis in a leg vein complicating an operation, pregnancy, or an illness which confines a patient to bed. Venous return will also be impaired if the normal pumping action of the muscles is diminished or absent, and accordingly oedema may occur in an immobile bedridden patient, in a paralysed limb, or even in a normal person sitting still for long periods as, for example, during air travel.

2. LYMPHATIC CAUSES. The small quantity of albumin filtered at the capillary is normally removed through the lymphatics. In the presence of lymphatic obstruction, the water and solutes are reabsorbed into the capillaries as the tissue pressure rises, but the protein remains until its concentration approaches that in the blood. Ultimately, fibrous tissues proliferates in the interstitial spaces and the whole part becomes hard and no longer pits on pressure.

Lymphatic oedema is common in some tropical countries due to obstruction by filarial worms. One or both legs, the female breast, or the external gentalia in either sex, are the parts most frequently involved. The skin of the affected area may eventually become very thick and rough — elephantiasis. Lymphatic oedema is comparatively rare in Britain. It is the cause of the peau d'orange appearance (p. 48) in some instances of mammary carcinoma. It may be due to congenital lymphangiectasis or hypoplasia of the lymph vessels of the legs (Milroy's disease) and may affect an arm after radical mastectomy and irradiation for carcinoma of the breast.

3. INFLAMMATORY CAUSES. As a result of damage to tissues by injury, infection, ischaemia, or chemicals such as uric acid, there is liberation of histamine, bradykinin, and other factors which cause vasodilatation and an increase of capillary permeability; the inflammatory exudate, therefore, has a high protein content which upsets the normal balance of forces. The resulting oedema is accompanied by the classical signs of inflammation, namely, redness, heat and pain. Testing for pitting on pressure in inflammatory oedema causes pain and should be avoided.

4. ALLERGIC CAUSES. Increased capillary permeability also occurs in allergic conditions but, in contrast to inflammation, there is no pain, there is less redness, and eosinophil cells rather than polymorphs and red cells make their way into the exudate, which has a high protein content. Angio-oedema is a specific example of allergic oedema; it is particularly prone to affect the face and lips. The swelling develops rapidly, and it is pale or faintly pink in colour. The condition may constitute a serious threat to life by suffocation if the tongue and glottis are affected.

Conclusion

In analysing the pathogenesis of oedema, it is desirable to think particularly in terms of disturbance at the capillary level, where the fluid exchanges are taking place. Thereafter, further evidence should be sought from the associated clinical features in order to determine the primary cause. Physiological principles can be applied along similar lines to the interpretation of many other clinical signs.

4. The General Examination and the External Features of Disease

> The trouble with doctors is not that they don't know enough, but that they don't see enough.
>
> Corrigan (1853)

The object of this chapter is to describe those aspects of clinical examination which it would be inappropriate to assign to any single system. These include the observations made on first meeting the patient, while the history is being taken. Several other important elements of a general examination are also described, for example, study of the hands, the head and neck, the lymphatic system, the breasts and the skin. It is during this phase of the examination that much useful information can be gathered about the endocrine system and notably about the functioning of the pituitary, thyroid and adrenal glands.

The general examination begins as soon as the patient enters the consulting room or the doctor approaches the bedside. Early impressions will certainly be formed while taking the patient's history and all the doctor's faculties should be on the alert from the outset. The aphorism which heads this chapter serves to emphasise the importance of inspection and this will be evident, not only throughout this chapter, but also particularly in the chapter devoted to the examination of the infant and child. At the start of the formal examination an analysis is made of the patient's demeanour, complexion, physique and the other features which together constitute the individual's appearance. Thereafter the hands, head and neck are examined in turn. With constant practice this part of the examination can be dealt with expeditiously. At first students must be prepared to take their time and develop a methodical routine. With increasing experience, facility and speed will gradually be acquired as well as the ability to discriminate between the details of examination that are vital in one case and superfluous in another. To compromise too early in this respect is to invite disaster.

GENERAL OBSERVATIONS

Demeanour

Early impressions of the patient's condition are compounded from many factors including the greeting, handshake and dress. The handshake of a patient with acromegaly, for example, may arouse suspicion because of the size of the hand and the excessive palmar sweating. The gait may indicate neurological or locomotor disturbances (p. 235). The posture of the patient in bed can be informative. Can the position be adjusted spontaneously or is help required? Does the patient sit up or lift the head spontaneously when addressed or have to be supported or propped up on several pillows? Does the patient tend to slip helplessly into some awkward position and seem to disregard the attendant discomfort?

Facial expression may serve as an initial guide to physical or mental disorder. A look of pain, fear, excitement, anxiety or grief does not require a medical training for its recognition. More subtle, however, is the appreciation of such features as the agitation of hyperthyroidism or hypomania, the apathy of hypothyroidism and of some types of depression and the poverty of facial movement in parkinsonism. However, without in any way intending to deceive, the more intelligent patients will often manage to conceal their apprehension, or may cloak their feelings in an air of feigned cheerfulness. They may occasionally make light of their symptoms or signs, or deal facetiously with features about which they feel the most anxiety; the doctor should avoid adopting the patient's light-hearted attitude, but on the other hand should not be too ponderous. The inexperienced doctor will do well to behave naturally and so eliminate risks of misunderstanding.

Complexion

Everyday experience leads to familiarity with the wide variety of the physical characteristics of the face. Among these, abnormalities of complexion may be the first to be noticed by patients or by their friends or relations. When these simple observations are reinforced by medical training, complexion may become a remarkably sensitive index of disease. It must be remembered, however, that lighting conditions affect the appreciation of colour. This is well enough known to shoppers when choosing clothes and cosmetics, but the effect of light on the complexion is not so widely appreciated. For instance, jaundice deep enough to be obvious to anyone in daylight, may be undetectable in artificial light.

The colour of the face depends upon variations in oxyhaemoglobin, reduced haemoglobin, melanin and, to a lesser extent, carotene. Unusual colours, excluding those which have been applied externally, are due also to abnormal pigments such as sulphaemoglobin and methaemoglobin (bluish tinge), carboxyhaemoglobin in carbon monoxide poisoning (pink), jaundice (yellow or greenish), and uraemia (sallow with a brownish tinge).

Haemoglobin. The contribution of haemoglobin to the normal complexion is largely determined by the amount which is present in the subpapillary venous plexuses and the proportion which is oxygenated or reduced. Abnormal pallor may be due to vasoconstriction as in fright, or to draining of blood from the face as when the upright subject faints, or it may be due to anaemia. It is common knowledge that a sallow face is not necessarily an indication of anaemia, but it is not so widely recognised that vasodilatation may produce a deceptively pink complexion in spite of a severe degree of anaemia. An unduly plethoric complexion may be seen in some chronic alcoholics (alcohol may produce a pseudo-Cushing's syndrome), in

Cushing's syndrome itself or in polycythaemia. Cyanosis is discussed on page 105.

Melanin. This pigment is normally formed in the deepest layer of the epidermis and colours the skin brown or even black according to the amount present. The colour is largely determined by hereditary influences but may be modified by a number of factors. The pigment diminishes or increases in amount with withdrawal from or exposure to ultra-violet light. Absence of melanin from the skin may occur in patches, described as vitiligo (Plate II); these depigmented areas are often associated with autoimmune disease. Total absence of pigmentation occurs in albinism as a result of a genetically determined failure to form tyrosinase in the melanocytes, and this may occur in any race. An acquired form of failure to synthesise pigment is largely responsible for the pallor which is so characteristic a feature of hypopituitarism in the white races.

In Addison's disease reduction in the output of adrenocortical hormones is associated with excessive production of adrenocorticotrophin (ACTH), β-lipotrophin (β-LPH) and N-terminal pro-opiocortin (N-POC) by the pituitary gland. These peptides all contain a melanotropin core sequence and their overproduction is accompanied by the development of brown pigmentation of the skin, particularly in creases, in recent scars, overlying prominent bones and on areas exposed to pressure from belts, braces and tight clothing. Melanin may also be deposited in the mucous membranes of the lips and of the mouth where it results in a slaty grey pigmentation. In both Addison's disease and hypopituitarism vasoconstriction occurs in the skin, so that pigmentation and pallor respectively are accentuated by the absence of the normal red background. Pregnancy is also commonly associated with a blotchy pigmentation of the face, the so-called pregnancy mask — chloasma gravidarum — and melanin is also formed in the areolae, the linea alba and around the genitalia. Increased melanin formation can be induced by heavy metals deposited in the skin, as for example, iron in haemochromatosis. Local over-production of melanin is responsible for freckles and for the pigmentation of moles.

Carotene. This yellow pigment is unevenly distributed and is seen particularly in the face, palms and soles but not in the sclerae. A distinct yellow colour of the face may appear in hypothyroidism because of impaired metabolism of carotene in the liver. Carotenaemia occasionally occurs in vegetarians or in food faddists, particularly in those who elect to eat excessive quantities of raw carrot.

Bilirubin. In haemolytic (acholuric) jaundice, the sclerae and skin are a lemon-yellow colour. The stools are dark and the urine looks normal, but contains an excess of urobilinogen (p. 424). This form of jaundice is due to an increase in circulating unconjugated bilirubin which is not excreted in the urine.

In hepatocellular or obstructive jaundice bilirubin has been dissociated from plasma albumin and is conjugated with glucuronic acid by the liver. It is water soluble and readily passes through the renal glomerular filter (p. 424). The urine is brown like beer and the stools tend to be pale in colour like putty, because of the reduction in the amount of bile in the faeces. If the jaundice is deep and of long standing a distinct greenish colour becomes evident in the sclerae and in the skin due to the development of appreciable quantities of biliverdin. Scratch marks may be prominent on the skin in obstructive jaundice as a result of the pruritus which is believed to be due to the retention of bile acids.

Abnormal Movements

Involuntary movements may be due to organic disease of the central nervous system, particularly when the extrapyramidal system is involved (p. 269). Disorders of movement may also result from primary disease elsewhere. The 'flapping tremor' of encephalopathy due to hepatic failure is such an example but may not be apparent unless deliberately sought by inspecting the outstretched arm with the hands dorsiflexed. The sign consists of jerky movements of the hands due to flexion and extension of the wrists and fingers in a manner somewhat resembling the action of a bird's wing, though less regular and rhythmical. Similar twitching movements not unlike those seen in liver failure may occur in renal failure ('uraemic twitchings') and in respiratory failure with carbon dioxide retention. In thyrotoxicosis there is exaggeration of the normal physiological tremor and the patient is also often very restless or fidgety, a state of affairs sometimes described as hyperkinetic. Other causes of tremor are described on page 269.

Abnormal Sounds

Sounds which are heard either by the doctor or the patient or another witness, may be of considerable value in diagnosis. Foremost amongst such is the information to be gained by attention to peculiarities of voice and speech.

The factors which contribute to the production of the voice include the ability to expel sufficient air from the lungs as well as the integrity of the mucosa, muscles and nerve supply of the larynx. Normal speech depends also upon the tongue, lips, palate and nose. The neurological abnormalities which cause disturbances of voice and speech are described on page 234. Many of the other causes can be recognised by inspection, for example a cleft palate, nasal obstruction, loose dentures, or a dry mouth (xerostomia). Hoarseness of the voice, again excluding neurological causes, may be due to laryngitis of infective origin, or it may result from excessive smoking. The chronic alcoholic is frequently hoarse, but in such cases there are probably several factors concerned, including that of cigarette smoking.

The voice in myxoedema may be so characteristic that the diagnosis can be made without seeing the patient, perhaps even over the telephone. The normal inflections of tone disappear, speech is low-pitched, slow and deliberate, and seems to require more effort than normal; it sounds 'thick', in that it flows less freely than normal, and the patient may stumble over individual syllables. Many of these changes in myxoedema are due to infiltration of the tissues concerned in voice production.

Several other types of sound may be heard, especially in connection with the respiratory system. Wheezing, rattling or stridor may help in the differentiation of dyspnoea. The character of a cough may be revealing (p. 152). Witnesses may give an account of a whoop suggestive of pertussis or the cry of an epileptic fit. Loud noises of cardiovascular origin and various sounds arising from the alimentary tract are described in the appropriate chapters.

Abnormal Odours

Though the olfactory sense is poorly developed in man, there are occasions when the smell is so offensive that it is tempting to give the patient a wide berth. Some odours are sufficiently characteristic as to be diagnostic, like the sickly 'fetor hepaticus' of liver failure, or the sweetness of acetone in the breath in diabetic coma, which is so obvious to some observers but is not appreciated at all by others. Apart from their value in diagnosis, bad smells may be a source of great embarrassment to patients. One of the major sources of malodour in any patient, apart from dirty clothing and general soiling, is the skin, particularly of the axillae, under the breasts, of the external genitalia and the feet. In most highly organised communities with access to the usual amenities, odour due to dirt should not occur, except in the very young, the elderly infirm who are incapable of looking after themselves and their toilet, and some of the mentally defective, for whom adequate provision outside an institution may not have been made. Nevertheless, from time to time one comes across patients who have access to the necessary facilities but who are too lazy or incompetent to take the trouble to keep themselves clean, and who show little if any embarrassment at what is sometimes the filthy state of their skin, and particularly of their feet.

Halitosis is an affliction which is less readily avoided. Malodorous breath often passes unrecognised by the patient but may be particularly offensive to others. This condition may be associated with decomposing food wedged between the teeth, carious teeth, gingivitis, stomatitis, atrophic rhinitis, and tumours of the nasal passages, as well as pulmonary suppuration. Less acute disease such as bronchiectasis may be associated with offensive breath, and in some cases the patient may notice that expectorated sputum tastes foul. In patients with gastric outlet obstruction from scarring or carcinoma of the stomach, foul-smelling eructations may occur, but probably the most offensive odour of this type is associated with a gastro-colic fistula, due to the faecal contents of the stomach. It should be noted that some individuals are afflicted with halitosis for which no adequate explanation can be found.

The *smell of alcohol* may prompt the doctor to ask appropriate questions about the patient's habits, but it should also be remembered that a comatose patient may have been given whisky or brandy as a remedy by a well-intentioned layman, and that alcohol may not be responsible for the patient's condition.

The source of other smells is usually only too easy to identify if the cause is excessive sweating of the feet, gangrene, chronic suppuration, necrotic tumours or some skin disorders.

Anthropometry

A routine examination should include the measurement of *weight* and *height,* both for their immediate value and for future reference. Other measurements such as *span, sitting height* and *pubis to ground height* are made occasionally when a more precise evaluation of growth and development is required. The special measurements applicable to infants and young children are given on page 379.

The *weight* of an adult patient taken in the outpatient department or consulting-room should include normal indoor clothing without shoes. Patients in hospital should be weighed in pyjamas and dressing-gown, again without shoes. The *height* should be recorded with a suitable rigid arm sliding on a vertical scale, and with the patient standing on an even floor surface, so that the heels, calves, buttocks, shoulders and occiput can be aligned against the vertical plane. Under certain circumstances, such as when children with short stature are being measured, a more accurate device is required; one such is called a stadiometer.

Increase in Height. Gigantism as a feature of hyperpituitarism is very uncommon, but the appearance of some patients with hypogonadism and of patients with Marfan's syndrome may give the impression that they are disproportionately tall. In hypogonadism the limbs continue to grow for longer than is appropriate because of the absence of sex hormones which normally serve to close the epiphyses after puberty. Thus the sitting height of the patient (head, neck and trunk) will be considerably less than half the height of the patient measured standing. Alternatively, the height from the top of the symphysis pubis to the ground can be recorded and this measure of the length of the lower limbs will be found to exceed the sitting height. The span of the arms measured fully extended will be found to exceed the height standing or, more significantly, twice the sitting height, thus once more emphasising the disproportionate length of the limbs in contrast to the trunk.

In Marfan's syndrome the appearance of the patient is rather similar, that is to say, the limbs are longer than is appropriate to the length of the trunk. As a rule there are additional features to distinguish the patient with Marfan's syndrome from the hypogonadal patient, in particular long slender hands (arachnodactyly Fig. 4.1) and narrow feet, a high arched palate, dislocation of the lens or dilatation of the aorta causing aortic regurgitation.

Short stature may be due to many causes; from among these the most striking contrast to the conditions just described is provided by achondroplasia. Gross shortening of all four limbs with a normal trunk length is a constant and characteristic finding. The stunted growth of rickets is usually associated with some limb deformity, particularly genu valgum (knock knee) or varum (bow leg). If cretinism has remained untreated or has been inadequately treated for sufficiently long for growth to be restricted, there will usually be some other signs of persistent hypothyroidism, particularly impairment of mental development.

Nutritional Status

Life is shortened by being overweight or severely underweight. Obesity leads to many complications besides the disability from breathlessness on exertion. Tables of ideal weight in relation to height and frame (body build) will be found in the appendix (p. 450). Many of the standard tables in common use are less suitable as they were prepared from life insurance figures obtained from individuals belonging to social and occupational classes in which the average weights were usually in excess of the ideal.

The amount of fat can be estimated by measuring the skin fold thickness over the triceps or below the scapula by means of a special pair of calipers. Such a measurement, of course, includes two thicknesses of skin and subcutaneous fat. A simple clinical estimate can be made by picking up the skin fold between the finger and thumb.

Although the majority of adults in Britain requiring dietetic advice are suffering from the effects of overeating, some are too thin due to undereating or starvation. Undereating results from the anorexia accompanying many organic diseases and some psychological disorders such as anorexia nervosa. In Britain starvation due to poverty is rare, but it is all too common in many parts of the world; iron deficiency is more frequent in women than men. Specific deficiencies of protein and vitamins are rare in Britain and when they occur are usually caused by a visceral disorder. For example vitamin B_{12} is not absorbed in pernicious anaemia due to failure of the production of intrinsic factor by the atrophic stomach; fat soluble vitamin K is not absorbed in obstructive jaundice and multiple deficiencies occur in generalised diseases of the small intestine. Scurvy affecting elderly people living alone is almost the only vitamin deficiency disease of dietetic origin seen in British adults. In Asian immigrants vitamin D deficiency is not uncommon and probably results from differences in dietary intake and absorption of the vitamin and decreased formation in the skin. Deficiencies conditioned by visceral disorders may cause anaemia, cheilitis, smooth tongue, bruising and skin abnormalities as their external manifestations.

Abnormalities of Fat

In the normal individual fat is stored mainly in the mesentery and in the subcutaneous tissues. In the *common type of obesity*, excess fat is widely but not always uniformly distributed. In more gross cases, the abdomen is predominantly affected and fat deposits may be so great as to make palpation of the abdomen uninformative. The hernial orifices may remain relatively accessible, since the tightness of the skin about the flexural folds, including the inguinal region, restricts the accumulation of fat in these areas. Next in order, the breasts, the buttocks, and the thighs will usually show signs of undue accumulation of fat. As a rule, the amount of fat deposited on limbs is greatest nearer the trunk and tapers towards the wrists and ankles, very little excess being deposited on the hands or feet. In some the excess of fat may extend uniformly to just above the wrist or ankle, where it ceases abruptly, producing on the legs an appearance like Turkish trousers. The neck and face usually share in the accumulation of fat.

The distribution of fat in the body, particularly excess fat, may be abnormal in *Cushing's syndrome*. This syndrome results from prolonged elevation of free (i.e. non protein bound) corticosteroid levels. It can result from the administration of supraphysiological amounts of glucocorticoids such as cortisone or prednisolone, injections of adrenocorticotrophic hormone, or from excessive endogenous secretion of cortisol. These hormones increase the appetite and may lead to a mixture of a simple form of obesity, together with the more striking changes due to excessive corticosteroid production or administration. Under the influence of these hormones fat deposition tends to be restricted to the trunk, neck and face, together with an increase of the normal pad of fat over the lower cervical and upper thoracic vertebrae. The limbs remain relatively thin or are actually wasted, the whole impression giving rise to the descriptive term of 'buffalo obesity'. The complexion often becomes florid, the face round and the neck thick. The so-called 'mooning of the face' is the earliest and sometimes the only change to appear (Fig. 10.3).

Osteoporosis causing collapse and wedging of the thoracic and lumbar vertebrae leads to shortening of the spine, increased protuberance of the abdomen, and further exaggeration of the abnormalities described. The thickness of the skin is decreased due to atrophy of collagen in the dermiṣ. Bruising is more common and stretching of the skin, especially over the abdomen, thighs and upper arms, may result in purple striae.

Localised deposits of fat which are sometimes tender, may form on the limbs particularly in middle-aged females. Lipomas are commonly found around the trunk and are rather soft, circumscribed, lobulated swellings.

The term *progressive lipodystrophy* is used to describe a rare condition in which subcutaneous fat disappears sequentially from the face, neck, arms, chest and trunk. Fat remains or may even be deposited in excess on the lower trunk and thighs, the line of demarcation varying from case to case. Diabetes mellitus is a common accompaniment.

Localised atrophy of subcutaneous fat may occur occasionally in diabetics in areas where insulin is habitually injected. This does not seem to occur when highly purified monocomponent insulin preparations are used.

The Significance of a Change in Weight. A history of a recent change in weight must be regarded critically until it has been explained.

Loss of weight may be due to inadequate intake, malabsorption or a metabolic disturbance. A coincident loss of appetite in a middle-aged person who has previously enjoyed eating should bring the possibility of an underlying malignancy to the doctor's mind. Emaciation may occur in young women suffering from anorexia nervosa; these patients frequently take a great deal of trouble to conceal the fact that their diet is grossly inadequate. Anxiety at any age and depression in later years are common causes of loss of appetite and weight.

Alimentary disease, with malabsorption as a feature, may be expected to cause some loss of weight. Rarely protein loss from the bowel may result in hypoalbuminaemia and oedema and the latter may conceal the change in weight. This may also occur in patients with cardiac cachexia and oedema.

Weight loss accompanied by a history of increased or unchanged appetite suggests the possibility of diabetes mellitus or hyperthyroidism. The former would usually be readily confirmed by examination of the urine for glucose. This diagnosis may, however, be missed if the renal threshold for glucose is elevated. In patients with hyperthyroidism there are usually other symptoms apart from weight loss, e.g. heat intolerance, emotional lability, excessive sweating and palpitations. Informed examination and appropriate biochemical investigations will confirm the diagnosis once the possibility has been suspected.

Radiological examination of the chest should invariably be carried out if weight loss is unexplained, since pulmonary tuberculosis and primary or metastatic malignancy do not always produce symptoms indicating chest disease.

A *gain in weight* is frequently encountered in hypothyroidism, in patients treated with corticosteroids or during adolescence, following pregnancy or at the menopause. Endocrine causes of obesity are, however, extremely rare. A change of food intake, giving up cigarette smoking or moving from an active to a sedentary job are much more common explanations. A very rapid increase over a period of days is often due to fluid retention, for example in patients with cardiac failure.

The State of Hydration

The state of hydration should be assessed in all cases of fluid loss, notably from vomiting, diarrhoea, sweating and polyuria. Unless the possibility of dehydration is given special thought, its existence may be overlooked or its severity underestimated. A detailed history of the nature and quantity of fluid loss is of first importance. If the patient's usual weight is known, much the most satisfactory assessment is obtained by weighing. A dry tongue is apt to be deceptive as it may be due to mouth breathing alone. In an adult, after 4 to 6 litres have been lost, the blood pressure may be low and the skin dry, loose and wrinkled. Loss of elasticity of the skin can be demonstrated by pinching up a fold which then remains as a ridge and subsides abnormally slowly. The eyeballs are soft, due to lowering of the intraocular tension (p. 74).

All these methods, except weighing, are crude and inaccurate. If it is known that the patient was not anaemic previously and has not lost blood, finding a high haemoglobin concentration or an elevated packed cell volume (p. 439) will be helpful, and serial readings will indicate when treatment of the dehydration has been adequate. Plasma osmolality measurements are even more informative.

Temperature, Pulse and Respiration

Examination of the pulse and respiration is discussed on pages 106 and 168 respectively. Body temperature is estimated for clinical purposes by taking readings beneath the tongue or in the rectum. For convenience some use the less accurate sites of axilla, groin or natal cleft. Rectal temperature is usually about 0.5°C higher than the mouth which in turn is 0.5°C higher than the axilla. Rectal readings are more reliable and should be recorded when there is any doubt about the authenticity of recordings from the mouth or axilla.

The normal oral temperature is 37°C. Circadian variations of about 0.5°C occur, the lowest in the early morning. Fever is usually due to organic disease, though occasionally this is not the case. An otherwise inexplicable transient rise may be due to a recent hot drink or a hot bath. Malingerers sometimes falsify their temperatures by a variety of tricks, including the use of hot-water bottles, in order to feign illness.

The warmth of the skin to the touch usually provides a remarkably good indication of fever, but gives a totally unreliable estimate of normal or low body temperature. The skin of a patient with a normal temperature may feel remarkably cold, and an apparently normal skin temperature does not exclude hypothermia. When hypothermia is present, it is commonly overlooked because the ordinary clinical thermometer reads only as low as 35°C and it is not always shaken below this level before a patient's temperature is measured. Clinical thermometers which record down to 30°C are readily available and should be used routinely. Rectal temperatures as low as 27°C are not uncommon in patients left exposed to cold such as after the onset of a cerebrovascular accident of sufficient severity to immobilise the patient and in patients with hypopituitarism or hypothyroidism. The deliberate reduction of body temperature to points approaching these figures is used in cardiac surgery.

THE HANDS

After the history has been obtained and advantage has been taken of the opportunity that this provides for making an early general appraisal of the patient, the more formal physical assessment usually begins with examination of the hands and pulse. This first physical contact with the doctor is the one expected by the patient.

The hand, directed by the mind, is largely responsible for the dominant position of man in the animal kingdom. It is such a highly developed structure that its area of

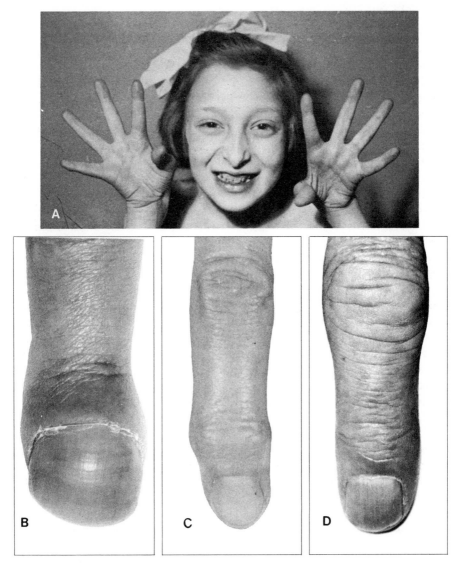

Fig. 4.1 The fingers as a diagnostic aid. (A) Arachnodactyly in Marfan's syndrome. (B) Advanced finger clubbing. (C) Heberden's nodes of osteoarthrosis. (D) Fusiform swelling of proximal interphalangeal joint in rheumatoid arthritis.

representation on the cerebral cortex is appropriately extensive. While the palmist reads more from the hand than is justified, critical inspection supplemented by palpation can in fact provide much reliable general information. In inspecting the hands, attention should be paid first to general features and then to detailed consideration of individual structures on an anatomical basis. The examination of the function of the hand is described on page 330, and the significance of right or left handedness on page 231.

General Features

Grip. The firm determined grip or the soft flabby handshake may reflect the personality of the patient.

Movements. *Gestures* can be most informative while the history is being given (p. 2). There is, for example, the hand pressed flat on top of the head accompanying a complaint of headache and suggesting that this is a psychogenic symptom, 'something weighing on the mind'.

Tremors are studied with the hands at rest and then outstretched; causes include anxiety, hyperthyroidism, alcoholism, parkinsonism and liver, respiratory or renal failure. Characteristic tremors are described on page 269.

Tetany may be recognised by the presence of carpal spasm (p. 296).

Posture. This may be almost diagnostic as exemplified by the flexed hand and arm of hemiplegia or the wrist drop of radial nerve palsy. In long standing rheumatoid arthritis there is often ulnar deviation of the fingers.

Shape. Trauma is the commonest cause of deformity of the hand. Other examples of unusual shapes include the long thin fingers of arachnodactyly (Fig. 4.1) while a short fourth metacarpal, best seen when making a fist, would strongly support a diagnosis of Turner's syndrome in a woman complaining of amenorrhoea. Short metacarpals, especially the fourth and fifth, are found in patients with pseudohypoparathyroidism in which the tissues are resistant to the effects of parathyroid hormone.

Size. Large, broad hands may provide useful clinical corroboration of a diagnosis of acromegaly which has been suspected from the facies. Rings which were previously loose may not now be removed or there may be a history of rings having to be cut off or enlarged. The increase in bulk consists largely of soft tissues; these are also thickened in myxoedema. Oedema may be part of a generalised process or be local from venous or lymphatic obstruction or, more commonly, disuse as with a hemiplegia. The increased blood flow through the paralysed limb is probably also a factor.

Colour. Pallor of the nails and palmar creases supports pallor of the mucosae in the clinical assessment of anaemia. White hands with a smooth soft wrinkled skin are seen in conjunction with similar changes in the face in hypopituitarism. Conclusions regarding pigmentation are similar to those applying to the skin in general (p. 58). The brown staining of the fingers from smoking should be reconciled with the history of cigarette consumption. Coal miners may have small blue tattoo marks in the skin of their hands and in other sites where particles of coal dust have been embedded in the scars of minor injuries. It is worth bearing in mind that professional tatooing within the previous few months may have been the source of an acute type B viral hepatitis. The nature of the tatoo may be informative about the personality of the patient (Fig. 4.3). In both miners and professional tatooing the blue colour is due to black particles (carbon or Indian ink) changed in appearance by the scatter of light as it passed through and is reflected back from the skin. The same effect explains why normal veins look blue, while in the elderly, with very thin skin from atrophy of collagen, the true red colour of the blood may be seen. The significance of cyanosis is considered along with temperature.

Temperature. In a cold or cool climate the temperature of the patient's hand is a good guide to the mean blood flow through it. If the hand is warm and cyanosed it can be deduced that arterial oxygen saturation is reduced. In most patients with heart failure the hands tend to be cold and cyanosed due to vasoconstriction in response to a low cardiac output. If they are warm the cause of the heart failure may well be hyperthyroidism or cor pulmonale.

Sweating. The warm moist palms of hyperthyroidism may be contrasted usefully with the cold, clammy hands of the anxious patient. Palmar sweating is also increased in acromegaly.

Detailed Features

Skin. The smooth, hairless hands of a boy should change to the lined and hairy hands of the adult male unless hypogonadism is present. Manual work may produce specific callosities due to pressure at characteristic sites. In contrast, disuse results in a soft, smooth palmar skin like that of an infant, just as occurs in the soles following prolonged recumbency.

The skin may feature a wide variety of specific skin disorders or dermatological manifestations of systemic diseases (p. 94). An example of the former is dermatitis due to an external irritant. Scleroderma is an example of the latter as it may be a sign of progressive systemic sclerosis. The skin has a shiny, glazed appearance and is tightly stretched over the underlying tissues, limiting the movement of the fingers which are held in a semi-flexed position.

Nails. The fact that well manicured nails are things of beauty and a social asset may account for disproportionate distress when an abnormality is present. Injury is by far the most common cause of changes in the nails and may permanently impair their growth. A transverse groove at a similar level on each of the nails dates a systemic disturbance and occasionally indicates a previous illness which has not been mentioned.

In long standing iron deficiency the nails become brittle and then flat and, ultimately, spoon-shaped (koilonychia, Fig. 4.2). Splinter haemorrhages (Fig. 4.2) are a feature of infective endocarditis (p. 106). The fact that one or two may occur in healthy subjects has wrongly discredited this sign. The nails may be pitted by psoriasis (Fig. 4.2) which may also discolour and deform them so as to cause confusion with fungal infection. Small isolated white patches (leuconychia) are often seen in the nail plates of normal persons. Whitening of the nail beds is much less common but may occur in hypoalbuminaemia (Fig. 4.2). Bitten nails suggest that anxiety neurosis may have to be considered in the final assessment.

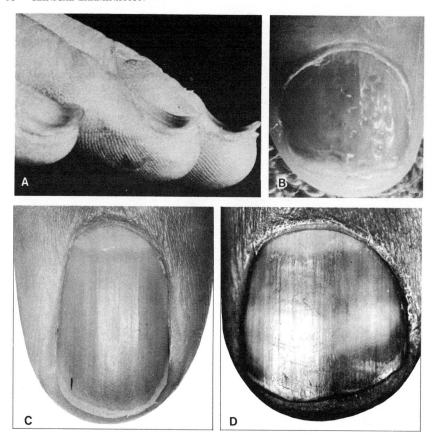

Fig. 4.2   The nails as a diagnostic aid. (A) Advanced koilonychia. (B) Pitting of nail in psoriasis. (C) Splinter haemorrhage. (D) Whitening of nail bed in hypoalbuminaemia.

Subcutaneous Tissues. In Dupuytren's contracture there is thickening and shortening of the palmar fascia resulting in flexion deformities of the fifth, ring and middle fingers. It may be found more commonly in chronic alcoholics than in teetotallers. Firm, painless subcutaneous nodules occur in rheumatoid disease but they are much more frequently found over the upper end of the ulna than on the hands. Finger clubbing (Fig. 4.1) is discussed on page 161.

Joints. The two commonest types of arthritis frequently involve the hands so that when a patient complains of arthritis, a glance at the hands may provide the diagnosis. Rheumatoid arthritis (Figs. 4.1 and 4.3) affects the proximal interphalangeal, metacarpophalangeal and carpal joints and causes pain, stiffness, swelling, restriction of movement and ultimately, often gross deformity. Osteoarthrosis affects mainly the terminal interphalangeal joints and causes little or no disability. At this site the characteristic changes are Heberden's nodes (Fig. 4.1) which are visible and palpable osteophytes projecting from the dorsal surface of the base of the terminal phalanx. If the terminal joints are affected by a diffuse swelling along with apparent rheumatoid changes in other joints, then psoriatic arthropathy should be suspected and skin and nail lesions should be sought.

Muscles. Wasting is common in rheumatoid arthritis. It also occurs in lesions of the lower motor neurone; causes in this category include syringomyelia, poliomyelitis, lesions of the first thoracic nerve root and motor neurone disease in which fasciculation (p. 268) is also most often seen. Specific muscle groups are involved in lesions of the ulnar or median nerves, e.g. in leprosy (Fig. 4.3). In the

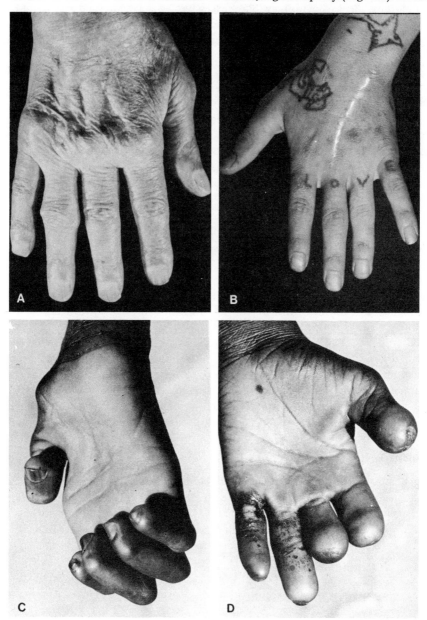

Fig. 4.3   The hands as a diagnostic aid. (A) Rheumatoid arthritis; swelling of one proximal interphalangeal and of all metacarpophalangeal joints; wasting of small muscles of hand.
(B) Aggressive sociopath; scars and pornographic tatoos were also present elsewhere. (C) Leprosy; late median and ulnar nerve lesions causing thenar and hypothenar wasting and claw hand.
(D) Leprosy; extensive sensory damage has permitted trauma and sepsis to destroy tissue.

carpal tunnel syndrome there may be selective wasting of the thenar muscles when the median nerve is compressed and this in turn may be a consequence of a generalised disorder such as myxoedema, acromegaly, premenstrual fluid retention or rheumatoid arthritis.

Tendons. Tenosynovitis may follow excessive use of a tendon and may result in a 'trigger finger' (p. 332). A tendon may be ruptured from its involvement in hypertrophied synovial membrane on the dorsum of the hand in rheumatoid arthritis.

Bones. Fractures are usually obvious, a notable exception being the scaphoid when the only finding may be tenderness localised in the anatomical snuff-box. Occasionally the bones of the hand, particularly the phalanges, may be involved in granulomatous or other generalised disorders such as sarcoidosis or hyperparathyroidism. Acute dactylitis is characteristic of sickle cell disease in children.

Nerves. Motor changes have already been described. In polyneuropathy there is a characteristic sensory impairment of a glove distribution affecting both hands; the feet are usually also involved. An example, common in the tropics, is the late result of dimorphous or lepromatous leprosy. Secondary infection through abrasions leads to gross deformities from absorption of the phalanges or from loss of fingers by ulceration (Fig. 4.3). In tuberculoid leprosy the lesions are likely to be asymmetrical or unilateral.

Blood Vessels. Palmar erythema is a mottled, bright red cutaneous vasodilatation often seen mainly over the hypothenar and thenar eminences. Though it is found in normal persons, it is useful confirmatory evidence of liver failure in the appropriate context. Osler's nodes (p. 106) occur in infective endocarditis and are probably due to arteritis which is also found in connective tissue disorders; it causes small necrotic lesions around the base of the nail most commonly in systemic lupus erythematosus. Raynaud's disease is due to arterial spasm and is described on page 136. Occlusive arterial disease due to atheroma is rare in the hands especially when compared to its frequency in the legs.

Conclusion

Much information can be gained from thorough inspection of the hands. The principle of considering every detail should also be applied elsewhere, particularly to the mouth, eye and skin where inspection is paramount. Looking does not always lead to perception but a methodical approach helps. In contrast, important clues will be overlooked in a cursory examination.

THE HEAD

For purposes of convenience, the examination of the various components of the head is described in topographical sequence from above downwards — the cranium, hair, face, eyes, ears, nose and mouth. In practice the examination will probably commence with the structure mainly involved.

The Cranium

The examination of the cranium in infancy and childhood can be most informative (p. 380). This is in striking contrast to the paucity of positive findings in the adult. In the latter, inspection may reveal generalised enlargement in Paget's disease or localised bony bossing overlying a meningioma. In cranial arteritis the temporal arteries are often visibly and palpably enlarged and tender. On auscultation a bruit may occasionally be detected in the presence of an arteriovenous malformation (p. 297). Breath sounds can be easily heard when a stethoscope is placed on the cranium of a patient with Paget's disease.

The Hair

While the examination of the hair of the scalp and face is being described it is convenient to refer to abnormalities of the growth of hair in other sites.

The Scalp. In the normal adult male after puberty, the hair margin of the forehead tends to recede, or at least to become thin, particularly at either side; this is described as temporal recession. When present in females, particularly if they show other evidence of virilisation, it may be of some significance. Loss of hair over the frontal region is an almost constant finding in the rare condition myotonic dystrophy. Alopecia totalis is a striking and distressing condition in which all hair may disappear permanently.

The most common local disease of the hair of the scalp is alopecia areata in which the hair falls out in patches; hairs shaped like exclamation marks are found at the periphery of the bald area which is clean and smooth in contrast to fungus infection in which the area is covered with hairs which are broken off close to the skin. Lice and nits of *Pediculus capitis* may also be found (p. 93).

Facial and Body Hair. *Hirsutism* is an excessive growth of hair on the face, trunk and limbs. It is a common complaint among young women and although it may be possible to demonstrate an excess of circulating androgens or a deficiency of sex hormone binding globulin in some, in many others no explanation can be found. Racial and other genetic factors may play a role in these patients.

In any form of adrenocortical or gonadal dysfunction in the female associated with virilisation, the distribution of the hair usually changes in the direction of a masculine appearance. Hair appears on the beard or moustache areas, and when this is dark in colour, it may cause serious embarrassment. In addition, the pubic hair may spread from its normal flat topped distribution up towards the umbilicus, this being described as a male escutcheon. Hair may also appear on the limbs. At first this is most marked on the forearms and on the thighs, but later the normal hair on the legs may also become more conspicuous.

Secondary sexual hair on the face in the male, and in the axillae and on the pubis of both sexes, may fail to develop normally in hypogonadism; it may diminish in quantity in old age or be lost in hypopituitarism or as a result of hepatic cirrhosis. In severe hypopituitarism the loss is ultimately complete, including the hair follicles, so that the axillae and pubis return to the smooth appearance seen in childhood (Fig. 4.11). The early development of pubic hair is related to adrenal androgen production and is called the adrenarche. This occurs in the absence of gonadotrophin secretion. Thus patients with isolated gonadotrophin releasing hormone and hence gonadotrophin deficiency may have early pubic hair but no other signs of pubertal development.

Eyebrows. The amount of hair here varies very widely. Although the statement is frequently made that thinning of the outer third of the eyebrows is a feature of myxoedema, this is so common in normal people as to be of little value in diagnosis.

The Face

Some facial appearances are pathognomonic of disease, for example the immobile stare of parkinsonism, the startled appearance of hyperthyroidism, the pale, puffy face of nephritis, the coarse features of myxoedema or the eyes of the mongol. To the experienced observer the briefest glimpse of one of these patients will suffice. In addition, a patient's face, rather like the clothing, may serve to indicate some features of the personality. This perhaps applies with greater force to women, and the evidence of time, expense and care devoted to a person's appearance may be informative. In children, study of the facial appearance is particularly rewarding (Figs. 10.2 and 10.3).

In most cases the characteristics which blend to form the facies must each be considered separately. While no attempt will be made to offer a complete compendium of facial characteristics, some examples of the more common and more significant findings will serve to illustrate the importance of this aspect of the examination of a patient.

The Eyes and their Surroundings

In addition to numerous purely ocular disorders, there are many other diseases which may have manifestations in and around the eyes. These include conditions involving the respiratory system (p. 161), the nervous system (p. 245) and those found in children (p. 382). The present section deals with features which are not considered in these more specialised fields.

While the history is being taken, the patient's eyes will be under observation. Any asymmetry should be noted. These differences may affect the whole or part of the globe and the eyelids, and include squint, abnormalities of the conjunctiva, iris or pupil, exophthalmos or enophthalmos, lid retraction or ptosis and oedema or other affections of the lids.

The Eyelids. When the patient is alert, the eyelids are normally held in such a position that, with the individual looking directly ahead, the upper and lower margins of the iris are partly covered. In bright light the orbital fissure narrows, while pain, particularly when this involves the eye, may cause spasm of the eyelids, *blepharospasm,* which can be so intense that retractors or the use of a local anaesthetic may occasionally be required before the eye can be properly examined. Conditions in which there is a reluctance to face the light (*photophobia*) include meningitis, painful conditions of the eye and migraine.

Retraction of the eyelids, especially the upper, is a common feature of hyperthyroidism. The upper lid retraction means that the sclera is visible above the iris while the patient is gazing straight ahead. In hyperthyroidism, when gaze is directed from above downwards, there may be delay in the downward movement of the upper lid; this is a useful confirmatory sign known as *lid lag.*

Swelling of the eyelids occurs readily owing to looseness of the peri-orbital tissues. Swellings due to trauma and inflammatory lesions are sufficiently common to be familiar to the layman. Periorbital oedema is often due to drugs or to contact dermatitis from cosmetics or hair dyes. Possible systemic causes of swelling of the eyelids include glomerulonephritis (Fig. 10.3), hypothyroidism, angio-oedema, infection with *Trichinella spiralis* (trichinosis) and in South Americans or travellers from that continent, infection with *Trypanosoma cruzi* (Chagas' disease). Swelling of the eyelids may be quite conspicuous in patients with right ventricular failure who are sufficiently free from dyspnoea as to be able to lie flat. The swelling will be greater on the side on which the patient has been lying.

Swelling of the eyelids may occur in thyrotoxicosis but is almost always present in myxoedema due to the accumulation of mucinous material together with water and electrolytes. This material infiltrates between the cellular elements of the dermis and accumulates in the subcutaneous tissue. It does not pit on pressure.

A *meibomian cyst* is a painless swelling due to blockage of a tarsal gland on the internal surface of the lid. A persistently *watering eye* suggests that a nasolacrimal duct is blocked; the opening of the upper ends of these ducts can be seen at the medial end of each lid. The lacrimal glands lying in the upper and outer quadrant of the orbits are not normally visible.

Xanthelasmas consist of yellowish plaques of lipid. They are fequently present in the skin at the medial ends of the lids and may be associated with hypercholesterolaemia. Xanthomatosis is described on page 95. The most common site of *rodent ulcers* (p. 95) is on or near the eyelids, though they are frequent elsewhere on the face.

The Eyelashes. Many common abnormalities of the eyelids result from disorders affecting the eyelashes. Thus a *stye* is due to staphylococcal infection of a hair follicle and *blepharitis* is the term applied to chronic infection of the edges of the lids; *ectropion* refers to eversion of the lids and *entropion* to inversion; both conditions predispose to conjunctivitis and in the latter the eyelashes tend to damage the cornea.

The Conjunctiva. The palpebral conjunctiva of the lower lid may readily be inspected if the lid is gently everted while the patient looks up. The colour gives an approximate assessment of the patient's haemoglobin level. If there is any doubt, the haemoglobin must be estimated (p. 430) as significant anaemia is easily overlooked, particularly in the elderly.

The upper lid may be everted by using the upper margin of the tarsal plate as a hinge. The patient looks down and the lashes and free margin are grasped between the index finger above and the thumb below. By a twisting movement the tarsal plate can be made suddenly to turn back to front (Fig. 4.4). The bulbar conjunctiva can be readily inspected at the same time. The two most common abnormalities are conjunctivitis and foreign bodies. *Conjunctivitis* is commonly accompanied by photophobia, excessive lacrimation and adhesion of the lids by purulent exudate on

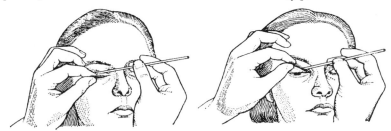

Fig. 4.4 Eversion of the upper lid.

wakening. Exudate does not accompany the painful, red, subconjunctival injection of scleritis which otherwise closely resembles conjunctivitis. It should be borne in mind that conjunctival injection at the limbus (corneoscleral junction) is also a feature of iritis and glaucoma.

Pingueculae are triangular yellow deposits with their base at the limbus and may develop with advancing years beneath the conjunctiva between the canthus and the edge of the cornea. In the same area a progressive fibrosis may develop and encroach upon the cornea (*pterygium*), particularly in tropical countries.

Chemosis is oedema of the conjunctiva and its causes include malignant exophthalmos, alcoholism, chronic respiratory failure and obstruction of the superior vena cava; these will be differentiated by other features of the primary condition.

Subconjunctival haemorrhage may obscure the greater part of the sclera and alarm the patient. A bright red colour persists for several days until the blood is absorbed. In the adult it commonly has no obvious cause and may be recurrent. Sometimes it results from coughing, especially whooping cough in a child. Occasionally it may be due to a fractured skull or a bleeding disorder.

Calcium deposition may sometimes be found in the conjunctiva in hypercalcaemic states.

The Sclera. Normal sclera is uniformly white in colour and is the most suitable site for the early detection of jaundice as bilirubin is strongly bound by the plentiful elastic tissue there. It appears blue in fragilitas ossium, a rare hereditary disorder of connective tissue in which the sclerae are thin; the blue colour is caused by the choroidal pigment beneath. In elderly patients scleromalacia often allows the choroidal pigment to be seen as small brown patches on either side of the iris. This condition may also be found in rheumatoid arthritis and may lead to perforation — scleromalacia perforans.

The Cornea. Normal cornea is perfectly transparent, and even considerable damage to its surface or small embedded foreign bodies may be difficult to recognise without the assistance of fluorescein; with this any breach of the surface will be stained yellow. Opacities of the cornea due to scarring may follow trauma or infection. A white ring at the outer margin of the cornea (*arcus lipidus or corneal arcus*) is commonly present in elderly patients. If it is observed in young subjects it may indicate hypercholesterolaemia and early coronary atheroma. A yellow or brown deposit of copper (*Kayser-Fleischer ring*) at the periphery of the cornea is pathognomonic of hepatolenticular degeneration (Wilson's disease). Corneal calcification found at the corneo-scleral junction is a useful sign suggesting hypercalcaemia, especially in younger patients. It is not uncommonly found in normocalcaemic elderly individuals.

The Iris. This is inspected while the pupillary reactions are tested. Iritis is often a manifestation of systemic disease. Symptoms of iritis include pain in the orbit or over the nose or forehead, photophobia and excessive watering of the eye. The vessels of the bulbar conjunctiva at the limbus are dilated and the detailed pattern of the iris is blurred. The pupil may be irregular, especially when dilated by a mydriatic (p. 407), due to adhesions of the iris to the lens (posterior synechiae) which are likely to be permanent.

Examination of the *lens, vitreous body* and *retina* is described on pages 407–412.

Intraocular Tension. This can be tested digitally but at best only a very

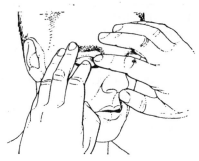

Fig. 4.5 Testing intra-ocular tension.

approximate assessment can be made without using a tonometer. The importance of detecting the rise in pressure in acute glaucoma is emphasised by the fact that vision is likely to be lost permanently unless treatment is instituted rapidly. The discovery of a low intraocular pressure, though of no importance as regards the eye itself, is useful confirmatory evidence of dehydration. The middle, ring and little fingers of both hands of the examiner should be placed on the patient's brow in order to steady the hand and the two index fingers are used to test the tension of the globe by eliciting fluctuation (Fig. 4.5). Unless this is done gently, there is some danger of causing retinal detachment, especially if the intraocular tension is high.

The Ears

The size, shape and form of the auricle normally vary widely between individuals. Some congenital deformities involving the ears are of genetic origin. In Down's syndrome the auricles are usually small and the lobule may be rudimentary or absent. The helix of the ear is a recognised site of gouty tophi, white chalky nodules consisting of sodium biurate crystals deposited in the cartilage.

Auriscopic Examination. The external auditory meatus and the tympanum may be inspected through an electrically lit auriscope (p. 407). An improved view of the drum and the meatus will usually be obtained if during inspection the auricle is drawn upwards, backwards and slightly laterally in order to straighten the external meatus as much as possible (Fig. 4.6). Wax commonly obscures the view and may be removed by syringing with warm water. A history of middle ear disease or perforation of the drum precludes syringing by the inexperienced. Hard wax may require to be softened by applying a few drops of warm olive oil for two or three nights before removal.

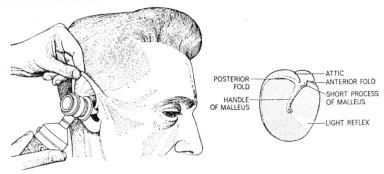

Fig. 4.6 Auriscopic examination and the tympanic membrane.

The normal drum appears pearly-grey in colour, with the handle of the malleus visible and lying almost vertically near the centre of the tympanic membrane. A cone of light is reflected from its lower end downwards and forwards to the periphery of the drum (Fig. 4.6).

Acute otitis media usually causes earache which may be severe, but in infants it may present as an acute febrile illness without local pain. The common abnormalities on inspection of the drum are acute inflammation and perforation (p. 382). Foreign bodies lodged in the external meatus are not uncommon in children.

The Nose and Sinuses

In spite of its conspicuous position and excepting the overlying skin, the information to be gathered from inspection of the nose as part of a general examination is limited. It may be deformed as a result of an old fracture, or enlarged, red and bulbous (rhinophyma) in the late stages of rosacea. The severe rhinitis of congenital syphilis may produce a characteristic flattening of the bridge of the nose known as saddle-nose. The nose may be narrowed when there is chronic obstruction of the airway in childhood and this associated with mouth breathing produces the 'adenoid facies'. Widening of the nose is one of the early features of acromegaly.

As a test of patency each nostril should be closed in turn by finger pressure and the patient asked to breathe through the other with the mouth closed. The airways should then be examined by direct inspection, preferably with the aid of a nasal speculum. The state of the mucosa and the anterior ends of the inferior turbinates can be visualised; the pearly-grey smooth surface of a polyp or a bleeding point on the nasal septum are two common abnormalities which may be seen. Sniffing of cocaine by addicts may cause ulceration of the nasal mucosa and perforation of the septum.

Infection of the frontal air sinuses may cause a headache which characteristically reaches a peak within two or three hours of rising and then spontaneously subsides as the day proceeds. Involvement of the maxillary sinuses may simulate toothache. A purulent nasal or post-nasal discharge is often present and there may be tenderness on pressure over the affected sinus.

The Mouth

Routine examination of the mouth must include inspection of the lips, teeth, gums, tongue, palate, tonsils, mucosa of the cheeks, floor of the mouth and the oropharynx. Any of these structures may be involved by local disease or may show lesions which are part of a systemic disorder. If a mirror is required to examine the nasopharynx and the larynx, then this procedure should be postponed until near the end of the physical examination. The technique of indirect laryngoscopy is described on page 164.

The Lips. Exposure to cold commonly causes dryness followed by desquamation and cracking of the lips. Somewhat resembling this is the much rarer cheilosis of riboflavine deficiency causing red, denuded epithelium at the line of closure of the lips, peeling towards the mucocutaneous junction. A similar appearance may follow the use of lipstick to which the patient is hypersensitive.

Angular stomatitis, consisting of painful inflamed cracks at the corners of the mouth, is often caused by ill-fitting dentures allowing saliva to dribble out of the mouth, followed by infection with *Candida albicans;* this condition may also be due to deficiency of iron or riboflavine.

A fissure of the lip in an elderly patient, which fails to heal within two weeks in response to treatment, should be regarded as a possible epithelioma. Intractable lesions of this type may require biopsy.

The Teeth. The deciduous teeth are discussed on page 386. Only too often the 32 so-called 'permanent teeth' also have a relatively short life. Inspection of the teeth will give some indication of the patient's attitude to hygiene in general, as well as to that of the teeth. The three principal findings are discoloration, caries and missing teeth. Discoloration is usually due to staining from tobacco or from poor hygiene, but devitalised teeth also gradually become grey. Caries may be kept in check for many years by regular dental treatment with fillings. Missing teeth are most commonly the molars, and as these are used for grinding rather biting, their absence is important in connection with dyspepsia. If dentures are worn, enquiry should be made as to whether they are used for eating or only on social occasions. Elderly patients often discard their dentures because they have become ill fitting as a result of atrophy of the gums. They often think it is not worth while obtaining a new set and the repercussions on digestion or nutrition may be considerable.

The teeth may be pitted and mottled yellow in fluorosis, notched, separated and peg-shaped upper incisons occur in congenital syphilis (Hutchinson's teeth), and poorly developed (hypoplastic) in juvenile hypoparathyroidism. Eruption of the teeth may be retarded as part of any disorder responsible for delayed development, especially rickets.

The Gums. Gingivitis is very common. At first bleeding is apt to occur, and a narrow line of inflammation can be seen at the free border of the gum, and the interdental papillae are swollen. If the condition progresses, food debris, bacteria and pus tend to accumulate between the teeth and the gum margin (pyorrhoea alveolaris). Halitosis may be apparent and the teeth may become loose. A further hazard is that pus may be aspirated into the bronchial tree and initiate pneumonia. Badly affected gums are associated with frequent transient bacteraemia due to *Streptococcus viridans* which is a particular danger in patients with valvular heart disease. Painful ulceromembranous gingivitis may be due to Vincent's infection (p. 80).

Phenytoin used for the treatment of epilepsy gives rise in some cases to a firm hypertrophy of the gums which may make it desirable to change to some other anticonvulsant. Other abnormalities, due to systemic disease are rare, but examples include the soft, spongy, haemorrhagic gums of scurvy, the hypertrophied bleeding gums of acute leukaemia and the blue line of chronic lead poisoning.

The Tongue. Inspection of the tongue has probably always been a rite with doctors and their patients. The layman frequently attaches great weight to the appearance of the tongue and may readily develop obsessions about its cleanliness and the significance of any real or imagined changes. These convictions in turn can lead to forms of self-medication which may be harmful, for example, persistent purging can produce potassium deficiency.

MOVEMENT AND SIZE OF THE TONGUE. The response to the command 'put out your tongue' may provide information about much else besides the movement of the tongue and mandible; for example, a stuporous patient who responds obviously hears and understands. Even the extent to which a tongue can be protruded may be important; neurological disease, tight frenulum, modesty or a painful condition of the mouth may restrict the movement of the tongue. The symmetry, the size and the shape of the tongue should be noted. Fasciculation (p. 268) may be seen in motor neurone disease and should be observed as the tongue lies at rest within the mouth. Wasting of half of the tongue occurs with lesions of the hypoglossal nerve (p. 265) and it is protruded towards the affected side. The tongue is enlarged in some cases of primary amyloidosis, in acromegaly and in myxoedema. If the organ is asymmetrical, then the possibility of a unilateral lesion must be considered.

THE SURFACE OF THE TONGUE. This normally varies greatly both in regard to colour and to the appearance of the surface. Shades of pink and red, with a range of grey or even yellow or brown towards the centre, may be acceptable as normal. Variations in colour may be due to foods, particularly coloured sweets, or they may be due to quantitative or qualitative changes in the haemoglobin. Central cyanosis can best be assessed clinically by inspection of the tongue (p. 105).

Small, red, flat elevations can be seen on the surface, especially at the tip and edges; these are the fungiform papillae. The filiform papillae are more numerous at the centre and give rise to the fur. Transient denuded islands give rise to the term geographical tongue, usually a symptomless change of no known significance. Iron or vitamin B deficiency cause a smooth clean looking tongue from diffuse atrophy of the papillae.

Excessive furring, by contrast, is of little diagnostic significance. It occurs when a soft or milky diet is eaten, and in fever or dehydration. Leukoplakia is characterised by grey opaque areas interspersed with a few red inflamed patches. Occasionally this precancerous condition may be due to syphilis.

Separating the anterior two-thirds from the posterior third of the tongue are the circumvallate papillae (p. 255) set in a wide V with its apex pointing backwards to the foramen caecum. Patients who discover these relatively prominent papillae for themselves are often alarmed by the thought that they might be cancerous. Congenital fissuring of the tongue occurs in varying degrees but has no pathological significance.

The Palate. The hard palate comprises the anterior two-thirds, and the soft palate with the uvula lies posteriorly. Deformity such as cleft palate may be noted, and a narrow high arched palate may be found. The latter is of little importance by itself, but may be associated with other varieties of congenital abnormality. The uvula varies much in size and shape; it seldon presents clinical problems except as a source of anxiety to the patient with obsessional disorders focused in the mouth. The examination of movement of the soft palate is described on page 263.

The Tonsils. The tonsils are masses of lymphoid tissue which lie beneath the mucous membrane between the pillars of the fauces. In common with lymphoid tissue elsewhere, the tonsils enlarge to reach a maximum between the ages of 8 and 12 years, after which involution takes place. There can be little doubt that failure to recognise this normal phase of lymphoid hyperplasia has led to many erroneous recommendations for tonsillectomy. Streptococcal tonsillitis must be distinguished from less common causes of sore throats such as infectious mononucleosis, Vincent's infection (p. 80) and diphtheria (p. 80).

Tumours of the tonsils may also occur either in isolation or as part of lymphatic leukaemia or lymphoma.

The Pharynx and Buccal Mucosa. To see the oropharynx adequately it may be necessary to depress the tongue with a spatula and ask the patient to say 'ah' in order to elevate the soft palate. The gag reflex (p. 262) may simultaneously be noted. Small lymphatic nodules can normally be observed on the posterior wall. Mucus or pus consequent on infection in the nose may sometimes be visible trickling down the back of the throat. The nasopharynx can be inspected only with the aid of a suitable mirror and good illumination. After these areas of the mouth and pharynx have been examined, the remainder of the buccal cavity should be checked. Any dentures should, of course, be first removed. A good light or a torch is essential and a spatula is required to separate cheeks and tongue from the teeth and gums. Characteristic abnormalities to be seen here include Koplik's spots (p. 80), secondary syphilitic ulcers (p. 80) and pigmentation.

Pigmentation in the Mouth. Melanin deposition in the buccal mucosa is normal in negroes and is proportionally less common as the skin becomes lighter, so that usually it is not seen at all in fair-skinned, fair-haired subjects. Pathological pigmentation in the mouth occurs in Addison's disease. If there are no other suggestive features of this rare conditions, the pigmentation is most likely to be congenital in patients with black hair and brown eyes. Other causes which would have to be considered, particularly in fair persons, are chronic cachexia, the malabsorption syndrome, haemochromatosis or the rare Peutz-Jegher syndrome of polyposis of the small intestine with pigmentation around and in the mouth and particularly on the lips and fingers.

The Salivary Glands. In the course of the examination of the mouth the opening of the parotid duct may be seen on the buccal mucosa as a small papilla opposite the second upper molar tooth. The openings of the ducts of the submandibular salivary glands seldon require identification, but may be found near the midline in the sublingual papilla, adjoining the root of the frenulum of the tongue. Each of these openings is more readily seen if a free flow of saliva is provoked by something tasty. Purulent infections of the salivary glands may be investigated by culturing pus expressed through these orifices.

Salivary calculi form very much more often in the submandibular glands. Obstruction of the duct may cause intermittent swelling with pain while eating or lead to infection of the gland. Other causes of enlargement of the parotid gland include mumps, sarcoidosis and tumour.

The Recognition of Some Diseases of the Mouth

Carcinoma may be found on the lips, the tongue, the fauces, or the floor of the mouth, usually in the form of an ulcer. The only compelling evidence in favour of the diagnosis of neoplasm may be the chronicity of the lesion. In the later stages of disease, enlargement of the regional lymph nodes, fixation of the mass, and other signs of malignant disease may appear, but in the earlier stages any indolent ulcer for which an adequate explanation is not forthcoming provides a clear indication for biopsy.

Stomatitis may be a local disorder or an oral manifestation of disease elsewhere. Thus an ulcerative stomatitis may complicate acute leukaemia or agranulocytosis, since these deprive the patient of the normal cellular defence mechanisms against infection. In acute leukaemia the gums often bleed and may be so swollen that the teeth may be largely obscured. Agranulocytosis may present as a sore throat which may progress to an ulcerative form of stomatitis. Unless vigorously treated with antibiotics, a fatal pneumonia is likely to supervene.

Aphthous stomatitis is characterised by ulcers on the inner sides of the lips, the edges of the tongue, the insides of the cheeks or on the palate. In the earliest stages a small vesicle forms which is quickly destroyed, leaving a shallow ulcer usually surrounded by a red margin. Such ulcers can cause intense discomfort and while they may heal quickly in the course of a day or two, they may progress to form multiple deep indurated ulcers which heal slowly, and may then leave a small scar. The lesions tend to occur in crops; a patient may be free from ulcers for months at a time, only to suffer a relapse. The cause is obscure. They are often seen in patients with ulcerative colitis.

Ulcerative stomatitis (Vincent's infection) is due to the combination of a spirochaete and a fusiform bacillus which can be seen in a smear taken from one of the ulcers. The condition is painful and foul smelling.

Thrush may occur in the infants of mothers who carry infection with *Candida albicans* in the vagina; it also occurs, particularly in the elderly, in association with febrile or debilitating diseases. It is common in patients being treated with antibiotics, corticosteroids or immunosuppressive drugs. The fungus may be seen as individual or coalescent white deposits adhering to the mucous membrane of any part of the mouth. There is very little evidence of inflammation unless bacterial infection has been superimposed.

Syphilis, in the secondary stage, causes highly infective mucous patches consisting of shallow ulcers with a narrow edge and a surface covered by a thin white membrane described as resembling snail tracks. The primary ulcer or chancre of syphilis may also occur on the lips, and sometimes in other parts of the mouth.

Specific fevers with associated rashes often also show lesions of the oral mucosa. In measles small white spots on an erythematous background are distributed over the mucosa of the cheeks opposite the molar teeth and sometimes throughout the mouth. These *Koplik's spots* are of particular diagnostic value as they appear before the rash.

The membrane of diphtheria is liable to form on any part of the mucous membrane of the mouth, nose, pharynx, larynx or trachea and particularly in the region of the tonsils. The affected area bleeds if attempts are made to remove it. The causative organism can be identified on a direct smear and its pathogenicity determined by bacteriological examination.

THE NECK

Physical abnormalities in the neck are so common that careful inspection and palpation should be undertaken in any systematic physical examination.

Inspection of the neck will show deformities, abnormal movements, or restriction of movement. Any changes in the skin will be noted, such as scars, unusual pigmentation, rashes, spider telangiectases, abnormal growth of hair, arterial and venous pulsations, or tumours.

Systematic palpation should then be carried out, bearing in mind the salivary glands, the lymph nodes and the thyroid gland. From the front the examiner can palpate the back and sides of the neck. The patient should then sit up and the examination continues from behind. Palpation is carried out successively beneath the mandible, over the tonsillar lymph nodes, over the anterior triangles, above the clavicles and especially deep to the sternoclavicular attachments of the sternomastoid muscle where lymph node enlargement may be associated with disease particularly in the chest, and occasionally in the abdomen or pelvis.

Auscultation over the blood vessels may reveal a murmur due to stenosis in a carotid or subclavian artery (p. 138).

The Thyroid Gland

Enlargement of the thyroid gland (goitre) is a common occurrence. It is best observed with the neck slightly extended and identified by its movement when the patient swallows. Palpation is, however, easier from behind with the patient sitting or standing (Fig. 4.7). As a rule it is possible to define the two lobes of any goitre.

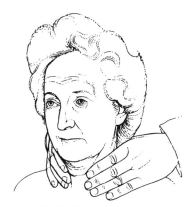

Fig. 4.7 Palpation of the thyroid gland.

A goitre should be examined like any other swelling as described on page 46 and attention paid to the undernoted features.

The *position* of a goitre is usually characteristic, but it should be recalled that it may extend into the superior mediastinum, or indeed may be entirely retrosternal, and so not be detected on clinical examination. Rarely, the gland may be located along the line occupied by the thyroglossal duct. When it is situated near the origin on the dorsum of the tongue, the structure is referred to as a lingual goitre. In this situation its nature may be confirmed by histological examination, or by the ability of the swelling to concentrate radioiodine.

The *size* of a goitre can only be roughly estimated by palpation, but change in the circumference of the neck measured over the point of maximum swelling may be used as an indication of alteration in size. Another method of following changes in thyroid size is to make a frontal plane scan. A ball-point pen is used to outline the goitre and an impression of this is then made on paper moistened with methanol. The paper is then dried and kept as a permanent record in the notes.

The *shape* of the gland is usually symmetrical in primary hyperthyroidism (Graves' disease) whereas it is irregular in a secondary or nodular toxic goitre. Simple goitres may be relatively symmetrical in their earlier stages, but usually become irregular with time.

Colour changes over a goitre are most unusual, unless it is very big, when distended veins may be responsible for a dusky blue appearance. After exceptionally large doses of radioiodine, thyroiditis occurs and may be associated with slight reddening of the skin, tenderness and perhaps transient dysphagia.

Pain and *tenderness* may occur in other forms of thyroiditis, particularly the subacute or giant cell variety and may be associated with transient episodes of fever. Dysphagia may also be present.

The *mobility* of the gland is a characteristic feature. The fact that the thyroid gland is ensheathed by the pretracheal fascia determines its movement on swallowing and distinguishes a goitre from other tumours. However an invasive thyroid carcinoma may lead to fixation of the gland to other surrounding structures and very large goitres may be immobilised because they expand to occupy all the space available in the root of the neck.

The *consistency* of a goitre may vary from soft to 'stony hard', the latter usually attributable to carcinoma. Furthermore the texture of the gland may vary from one part to another, just as does the smoothness of its surface. Nodules in the substance of the gland may be large or small, single or multiple.

Enlarged lymph nodes near a goitre will suggest the possibility of carcinoma of the gland particularly if they are firm or hard.

On *auscultation* a bruit indicates an abnormally large blood flow. In the untreated state this usually implies hyperthyroidism, but the use of antithyroid drugs may promote an increase in the blood supply sufficient to produce a murmur. Precautions should be taken to ensure that a murmur arising in the carotid artery or transmitted from the aorta, or a venous hum (p. 134) originating in the internal jugular vein is not mistaken for a bruit in the thyroid gland.

Radiological examination of the neck may reveal calcification in the thyroid, narrowing or displacement of the trachea, or a retrosternal goitre.

Scanning. A mediastinal swelling is proven to be thyroid if it takes up radioiodine. Radionuclide scanning is also useful in estimating the amount of tissue present, and in detecting 'hot' or 'cold' nodules in the gland which concentrate radioactive iodine more or less than the surrounding glandular tissue.

Ultrasonography can usually distinguish between a cystic and a solid tumour (p. 220).

THE LYMPHATIC SYSTEM

The lymph nodes should be palpated as a routine in the course of each regional examination. The sites which should be examined include the following: pre- and post-auricular, submental, tonsillar, occipital, and posterior and anterior triangles of

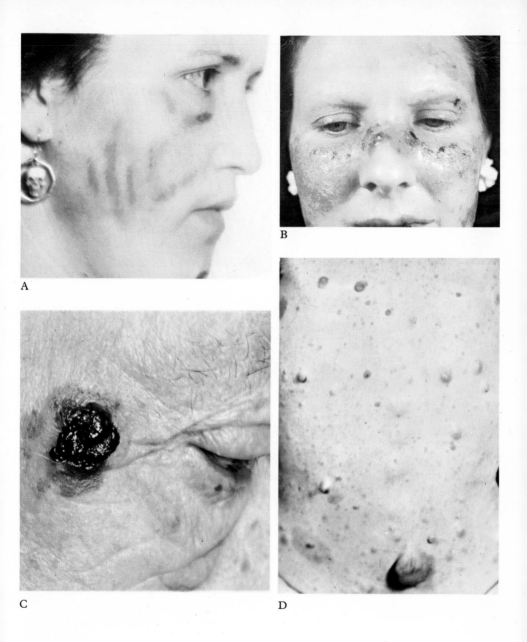

Plate I The skin as a diagnostic aid. (A) Dermatitis artefacta; unusual symmetrical lesions with clear-cut margins in an accessible site. The earring is also significant. (B) Lupus erythematosus showing characteristic butterfly distribution of facial rash. (C) Malignant melanoma. (D) Neurofibromatosis; café au lait pigmentation in lower left corner and many nodules.

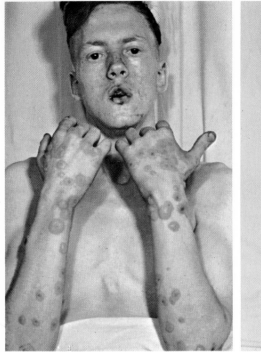
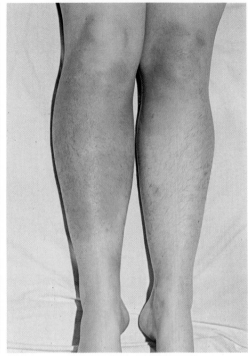

A

B

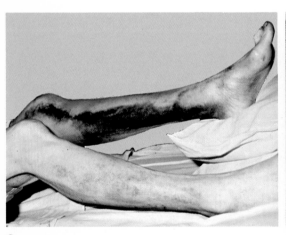
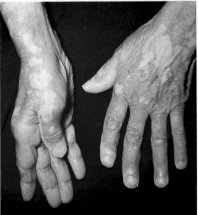

C

D

Plate II The skin as a diagnostic aid. (A) Erythema multiforme caused by sulphonamide.
(B) Erythema nodosum due to sarcoidosis in a women aged 30 years; the lesions on the right leg
have become confluent. (C) Scurvy in an old man living alone; vitamin deficiency is often overlooked
in the elderly. (D) Vitiligo in a patient with autoimmune disease.

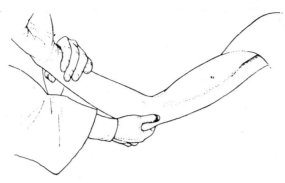

Fig. 4.8 Palpation of the epitrochlear lymph node.

the neck as described on page 162. The epitrochlear lymph nodes are conveniently felt under the thumb if the patient's right elbow is grasped by the examiner's right hand and vice versa for the left (Fig. 4.8). The procedure is facilitated if, with the other hand, the examiner suspends the patient's arm by the wrist and flexes it at the elbow. The examining hand should then be slid up the inner side of the arm to the axilla, for some lymph nodes lie along the brachial vessels. The right hand should then be used to palpate the vault and medial wall of the left axilla and the left hand for the right axilla (Fig. 4.9). Lymph nodes in the groin and those extending a short distance along with the femoral vessels must also be palpated, though interpretation of the findings in this region is difficult unless enlargement is considerable or change in consistency is unequivocal. While palpating the abdomen it may sometimes be possible to feel gross enlargement of para-aortic or iliac lymph nodes.

Apart from enlargement, there is much diagnostic information to be gained by noting the consistency of the nodes and the presence or absence of tenderness or fixation in accordance with the scheme for the examination of any mass (p. 46).

When there is no obvious local cause for enlarged lymph nodes, it may be helpful to review the reticulo-endothelial system as a whole, including palpation of the liver and spleen. If the outcome points to diffuse involvement, examination of the blood and bone marrow and biopsy of a lymph node may also be required. Biopsy of an enlarged node also is used in the diagnosis of bubonic plague, trypanosomiasis and sometimes in kala azar.

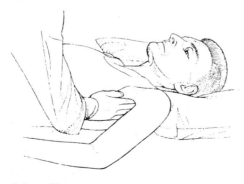

Fig. 4.9 Palpation of the axilla.

THE BREASTS

General Considerations. The female breast is liable to be affected especially by acute pyogenic abscess, fibrocystic disease and simple and malignant tumours. Since the breast is the most frequent single site of carcinoma in women of all age-groups, a general examination is incomplete unless both breasts have been included. Any mass detected must be regarded as a potentially malignant tumour until this has been excluded.

Breast abscesses are usually preceded by damage to the nipple during the early phase of lactation and seldom cause diagnostic difficulty. In fibrocystic disease, irregular areas of nodularity, usually bilateral, are often combined with tenderness either locally or over a wider area. Fibro-adenomas will also have to be considered. If these changes are localised it may be impossible to exclude carcinoma on clinical examination alone.

Carcinoma characteristically consists of a solitary and often irregular nodule that is firm or hard and usually painless, contrasting sharply in consistency with the surrounding breast tissue. In more advanced disease there may be evidence of infiltration into the adjacent tissues, fixation to the overlying skin and underlying muscles and enlargement of the regional lymph nodes. Patients with carcinoma of the breast, afraid of cancer, may use denial as a defence mechanism, and occasionally conceal the tumour for many months (Fig. 4.11).

A blood-stained discharge from the nipple may be the only indication of an intraductal tumour which may be so small as to be impalpable. Inversion of the nipples is a common abnormality. Unilateral inversion should be an indication to examine the breasts with special care. Retraction or deformity, especially when associated with an eczematous change, developing in a previously normal nipple, is a diagnostic feature of carcinoma.

Gynaecomastia (enlargement of the male breast, Fig. 4.11) occurs when oestrogens are used in the treatment of prostatic carcinoma and may also be caused by other drugs, e.g. spironolactone. It is a feature of Klinefelter's syndrome. Carcinoma of the male breast occurs at a rate of about 1% of that in women.

Galactorrhoea may be an important physical sign in that it suggests that prolactin levels may be elevated. There is usually associated Montgomery tubercle hyperplasia. Spontaneous milk production is uncommon and often galactorrhoea is found only by trying to express milk.

Anatomical and Physiological Considerations. For the purposes of examination and description, the breast may be divided into the nipple, the areola and four quadrants, upper and lower, inner and outer, with the axillary tail projecting from the upper and outer quadrant. The adult nipple consists of erectile tissue covered with pigmented skin which is shared with the areola. The openings of the lactiferous ducts may be seen near the apex of the nipple. The breasts are normally symmetrical. The size and shape of the breast in healthy women vary widely in accordance with hereditary factors, sexual maturity, the phase of the menstrual cycle, parity, pregnancy and lactation, and the general state of nutrition. The amount of fat and stroma surrounding the glandular tissue largely determines the size of the breast except during lactation, when the temporary enlargement is almost entirely glandular.

Swelling and some tenderness of the breasts commonly occur in the week before and at the time of menstruation. This engorgement is sometimes attributed to fluid retention associated with fluctuations in the secretion of ovarian oestrogens and progesterone. Palpation may show that the glandular elements of the breasts are more readily detected then than at other times, and they give an impression of radiating strands of firm tissue with a variable degree of granularity. The ease with which the glandular elements of the breast can be felt also varies with the age of the patient, the prominence of the glandular tissue and the quantity of the surrounding fat. There is also a tendency for the strands to be less obvious towards the periphery.

Procedure for Examination. Whenever the presence of a carcinoma is suspected, the full procedure detailed below should be carried out. If the breast is being examined as part of a general systematic examination, it may be acceptable to use a less complete procedure, bearing in mind that many an early carcinoma has first been recognised in the course of a thorough routine examination and before the patient has been aware of any abnormality.

An adequate examination of the breasts requires that the patient should be completely undressed to the waist and initially should be seated on a chair. The doctor should sit opposite the patient in a good light. Occasionally special care may be required to avoid offending the unduly modest patient, but this should never prevent a complete examination.

Before proceeding to palpation, a systematic inspection of both breasts should be undertaken. Any asymmetry should be sought, together with changes in the skin, the nipple and the presence of any local swelling. In order to emphasise any local change, and in particular the presence of a mass or an area of fixation, the patient should be asked to take up each of several positions in turn.

1. The patient's hands are resting on the thighs so that the pectoral muscles are relaxed as shown in Figure 4.10a.
2. The hands are firmly pressed on to the hips ensuring contraction of the pectoral muscles (Fig. 4.10b).
3. The arms are raised above the head, stretching the pectoral muscles as well as the skin overlying and surrounding the breast (Fig. 4.10c).
4. The patient leans well forward so that the breasts are pendulous (Fig. 4.10d).
5. Finally, the breasts are examined while the patient is lying flat on a couch or bed, with the side under review raised by a pillow (Fig. 4.10e).

In each of these positions the breast is inspected, followed by palpation of the four quadrants and the axillary tail in turn. The breasts should be examined with the palm of the hand and the tissue rolled gently against the chest wall. This will have the effect of accentuating a tumour, while the diffuse nodularity of fibrocystic disease becomes barely palpable. If a mass is noted or suspected it should also be felt with the finger-tips so as to elicit the other characteristics of any lump, as described on page 46. One of the most characteristic features of carcinoma of the breast is

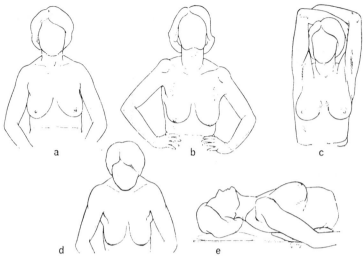

Fig. 4.10 Positions for the examination of the breasts. Note in (b) that the patient is not symmetrically positioned and that this is reflected in an apparent difference in the breasts.

'tethering' of the skin. This may not be obvious at first, but if the breast is elevated gently by the hand, the area of dimpling overlying the tumour becomes visible immediately.

A complete examination of the breasts must include palpation of the regional lymph nodes. The examination of the axillae should be undertaken first with the arms relaxed in order to explore the apex of the axilla and then with the hands on the hips in order to tense the axillary fascia and to contract the pectoral muscles. Finally, evidence of any involvement of the supraclavicular lymph nodes should be sought.

The nature of a lump in the breast can often be determined with reasonable certainty by the application of these methods, but in spite of this, it is unusual for a final decision to be reached on clinical grounds alone. On most occasions a biopsy will be required.

THE SKIN

Structure and Functions

The skin consists of a thin, superficial, avascular, cellular layer (the epidermis) and a deeper, tough fibro-elastic layer (the dermis) which also contains nerves, blood vessels, sweat glands, sabaceous glands and hair follicles. Beneath the skin there is a layer of areolar tissue containing fat. The amount of fat varies widely in different parts of the body and from one individual to another.

The skin protects the deeper parts from trauma, from infection and from extremes of heat and cold. Vitamin D_3 is formed in the skin from 7-dehydro-cholesterol in response to ultra-violet light, and harmful effects of this form of radiation are reduced by the melanin pigment also formed in the skin. Mammals are insulated against cold and wet by hair and by the secretions of the sebaceous glands,

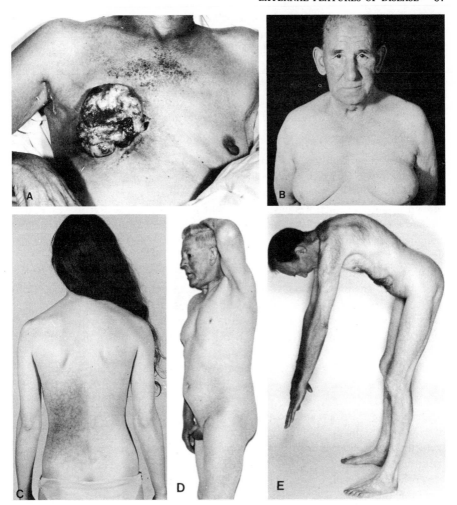

Fig. 4.11 The trunk as a diagnostic aid. (A) Carcinoma of breast, concealed by patient for many months, denial being used as a defence mechanism. (B) Gynaecomastia due to oestrogen therapy for prostatic carcinoma. (C) Erythema ab igne in an unusual site where heat has been applied for chronic pain. (D) Loss of body hair and pallor of the skin in hypopituitarism. (E) Advanced ankylosing spondylitis with marked loss of flexion of spine.

and heat loss can be minimised by erection of the hairs consequent on contraction of involuntary muscle fibres — the arrectores pilorum. A vestige of this reaction is seen in man in the form of 'goose-flesh'. The skin is also of vital importance in dissipating heat by vasodilatation and sweating, and it conserves heat by vasoconstriction aided by the insulating effect of the subcutaneous fat. It serves also as a channel for the excretion not only of water and electrolytes, but also of normal and abnormal metabolites and drugs.

Disease ensues if any of the main structures of the skin are missing or cease to function. Thus breaches of the surface are liable to infection; ultra-violet light causes sunburn in unpigmented skins; failure of sweating results in death from hyperpyrexia in hot climates; vasodilatation in a cold atmosphere may result in death from hypothermia, a combination which is apt to occur in coma from excess of alcohol; loss of nerve function may result in trophic ulcers; cuts and burns of the skin of the hands accompany the absence of pain and temperature sense in syringomyelia. In addition there is a wide variety of primary disorders of the skin and there are many dermal manifestations of systemic disease.

Examination

When examining the skin, attention must be paid to abnormalities of its structure and function and to any pathological lesions present. The discovery and differentiation of disorders affecting the skin depend largely upon inspection, though palpation sometimes has a useful part to play. Normal practice, especially when the main complaint appears to be a dermatological disorder, should include examination of the whole body surface. This is usually carried out in stages as the various systems are examined.

Colour. Localised or generalised variations in colour are similar to those described for the complexion (p. 57). *Pigmentation* has already been discussed in this context (p. 58). The body may also be somewhat pigmented in the unclean, especially in those instances in which there is infestation with body lice (*Pediculus corporis*). Chronic inflammation, as is often seen in varicose eczema, may give rise to pigmentation. Some localised colour changes are produced by fungal infections and numerous other skin diseases. In a patient who has been resident abroad the possibility of tuberculoid leprosy should be entertained if depigmented anaesthetic patches are found.

The climate in Britain leads to another striking form of pigmentation, *erythema ab igne*, or, more colloquially, 'Granny's tartan'. This is commonly seen on the legs of women who sit close to a fire for long periods, and is therefore more commonly found in the elderly and in the inactive. The pigmentation is at first red and later brown in colour, and follows the distribution of cutaneous venous plexuses, thus providing the appearance of a coarse net. Even patients with hypopituitarism whose facial pallor is so characteristic, are liable to this form of pigmentation, and indeed these and hypothyroid patients may be specially susceptible because of their sensitivity to cold. The discovery of a similar pattern on the skin of the abdomen or elsewhere, due to the local application of heat, should lead to enquiry about the possibility of chronic pain (Fig. 4.11).

Texture and Sebaceous Secretion. Normal skin has a fine texture and a slightly moist surface. A relatively common disorder is the dry, scaly skin of congenital ichthyosis (fish-skin). In myxoedema the skin also becomes dry and coarse. In contrast is the greasy skin often noted after puberty with its liability to acne vulgaris. Over-active and hypertrophied sebaceous glands become blocked by comedones (blackheads) which consist of plugs of semi-solid secretion capped by horny debris darkening on oxidation. This may be succeeded by an inflamed papule and then by a pustule which ultimately bursts. Larger lesions result in permanent scarring. Acne is characteristically distributed over the face, back of the neck, and the front and back of the chest.

Sweating. Diffuse sweating counters the rise of body temperature liable to occur in hot atmospheres, during exercise, in fevers or in hyperthyroidism and failure to sweat in a hot climate may cause death from hyperpyrexia (heat stroke). Episodes of sweating occur in fainting, in shock, with severe pain, during menopausal flushes, in acute hypoglycaemia or during acute hypertensive episodes caused by a phaeochromocytoma. Sweating on the face, palms, soles and in the axillae is often due to anxiety. Interruption of the sympathetic nerve supply, as in Horner's syndrome (p. 248) or following sympathectomy, causes a local loss of sweating. Rarely there may be a congenital absence of sweat glands.

Sweat contains most of the solutes of blood, but their concentration is much less than in a filtrate of plasma. In cystic fibrosis a characteristic increase can be demonstrated in the concentration of sodium chloride in the sweat (p. 402). In diabetes mellitus the glucose content of sweat is high, and this predisposes to skin infections, particularly with fungi and pyogenic organisms.

A febrile patient, though not sweating visibly, may lose a considerable amount of water. Even more serious account must be taken of visible sweating, which may be responsible for the daily loss of several litres of water containing electrolytes in a concentration of about one-third of that in the plasma.

Hyperhidrosis, or excessive and inappropriate sweating, is usually confined to the axillae, the palms, and the soles and its odour may cause considerable embarrassment. Hyperhidrosis predisposes to fungal infection between the toes characterised by painful cracks in thick, white, sodden skin.

Skin Temperature. Differences in temperature between symmetrical regions can be detected with remarkable accuracy by the back of the examiner's fingers, provided that the hand is not cold. Excluding the recent application of heat to the part, a local rise in temperature is due to an increased blood flow. This may be due to inflammation, to Paget's disease of underlying bone, or to tumours with a large blood supply. It may also be due to a recent deep venous thrombosis with a shift of circulation into the skin vessels, or to chronic arterial block which has resulted in the opening up of collateral circulation through the skin.

In contrast to local increases of temperature, local cooling, particularly of a limb or part of a limb, raises the possibility of arterial occlusion (p. 136). In some circumstances, for example with a 'saddle embolus' lodged on the bifurcation of the aorta, both lower limbs might be equally cool.

Nails and Hair. Abnormalities of these structures are discussed on pages 67 and 71 respectively.

Lesions of the Skin. The skin is no exception to the rule that method is necessary for the study and description of its pathological lesions. The history is obtained in the usual way, but specific points may require special attention, for example, the possibility of contact with infectious disease like childhood fevers, scabies, syphilis or leprosy. Contact with animals or occupations involving the handling of animal products introduces the possibility of unusual infections of the skin such as animal ringworm, orf, erysipeloid and anthrax. The distribution of the lesions may suggest contact dermatitis, when special enquiry must be made about work, the purchase of new clothing, jewellery, or the application of new cosmetics or hair dyes. Another important factor may be the potential adverse effects of medicaments which may have been applied with or without medical advice. To add to the diagnostic difficulty, many variants of the typical appearance and distribution of the lesions may be seen and further differences may arise from the effects of scratching, secondary infection or inappropriate treatment.

When examining the skin and assessing the significance of the abnormalities noted, not only must account be taken of their type and distribution but also whether associated lesions are to be found, for example in the mucous membrane of the mouth or nose, the conjunctiva, or the genital area. Enlarged lymph nodes in the appropriate drainage area may result from inflammatory or neoplastic conditions of the skin.

DESCRIPTIVE TERMS. Most abnormalities can be defined by one or more of the following terms:

Erythema means reddening of the skin, and the term is usually qualified by an adjective such as diffuse, punctate, macular or papular. A *macule* indicates a small circumscribed spot such as a freckle. *Papular* lesions are by definition raised above the surrounding surface of the skin and this can easily be confirmed by running the finger-tips over the affected area. *Vesicular* lesions (blisters) may be superimposed on the changes already mentioned, and consist of collections of fluid in the epidermis or the dermis. Vesicles vary in size, the larger being described as *bullae*. If the fluid within vesicles becomes purulent the lesions are known as *pustules*. *Urticaria* is a raised pale area of skin, varying in width from a few millimetres to several centimetres. It is caused by an increase in interstitial fluid with a high protein content due in turn to increased capillary permeability. The lesions are surrounded by a flare resulting from arteriolar dilatation through an axon reflex. A similar mechanism affecting the subcutaneous tissues gives rise to the less well-defined swelling of *angio-oedema*.

Visible *scaling* or *desquamation* due to abnormal growth of the skin is a feature of many chronic skin lesions. The superficial keratin layer remains nucleated and no longer rubs off imperceptibly. Removal of the epidermis when the lesion is scaly may help to distinguish between psoriasis which leaves a dry surface with bleeding points, and eczema in which a moist, weeping area is exposed.

Linear markings known as *cutaneous striae* may sometimes be seen around the abdomen, shoulders, buttocks and thighs. Those of recent origin are pink, while older striae are white or opalescent. They are found in healthy adolescents after sudden increments in weight, in pregnancy and in obesity. In Cushing's syndrome the striae tend to be darker red in colour and more conspicuous than in other conditions.

The observation of *scars* may remind patients of operations which have been forgotten. Puncture marks of hypodermic injections may be noted in diabetics, but, if not adequately accounted for, should raise suspicions of addiction to drugs such as heroin or cocaine.

Some Common Dermatological Abnormalities and their Significance

Examination of the skin seldom fails to reveal some abnormality. Many are of limited significance, for example callosities, moles, freckles, erythema ab igne, warts and acne. The importance of some of these is in the eye of the beholder. A few acne pustules on the face of a teenage girl is of no relevance from the point of view of physical health, and the doctor is aware that the condition will clear up spontaneously in a few years. From the girl's view-point, however, this disfigurement is a social embarrassment which may well influence her behaviour and colour her whole outlook on life. Medically trivial skin lesions should be treated with a respect and sympathy which may seem disproportionate to their gravity. The student can soon become familiar with common abnormalities by paying attention to the skin in every patient. By so doing, the less usual and sometimes far more important conditions will also be noticed. Some of the more common lesions encountered are discussed separately but briefly under the headings of vascular abnormalities, infections, hypersensitivity reactions, cutaneous manifestations of generalised disease, and primary skin disorders, including tumours. Such an outline provides a general perspective of the range to be covered and gives some indication of what can be learned from a careful study of the skin. The importance of this examination in childhood is discussed on page 378. For a detailed description of individual lesions, the student should consult a textbook of dermatology (p. 97).

Vascular Abnormalities of the Skin

Purpura and Ecchymosis. Spontaneous bleeding into the skin may be manifest as purpura of various sizes and shapes, or in the subcutaneous tissues it may be visible as ecchymoses (bruises).

Petechiae are the most common manifestations of purpura. They are red or blue lesions of about 1 to 3 mm in diameter visible in the skin deep to the epidermis. Since they consist of extravasated blood they fail to disappear on pressure or on stretching the skin in the affected areas. By contrast, lesions with an intact vasculature can be made to fade and on release of the pressure the colour returns as in spider telangiectasia. Petechiae tend to occur in crops, and unless replaced by fresh lesions, disappear in three or four days or less. They should be regarded as evidence of abnormal capillary fragility. This can be demonstrated by *Hess's test* in which a sphygmomanometer cuff is applied to the upper arm and maintained at a pressure midway between the systolic and diastolic levels for five minutes. Many purpuric spots appear on the forearm when capillary fragility is increased.

Senile purpura is common in elderly patients and is usually confined to the dorsal surfaces of the forearms and hands. The lesions are dark red in colour and remain so until they disappear; they may be as much as 2 cm or more in diameter, and persist for many days or even weeks before they are absorbed. Thereafter a small white scar usually persists permanently, and sometimes many of these are to be seen on the forearms. The lesions are produced by shearing strains on the skin, associated with loss of collagen from the affected skin. Similar changes occur in younger patients on long-term treatment with supraphysiological doses of corticosteroids.

Ecchymoses or bruises usually result from trauma, but their significance increases in proportion to the triviality of the injury which has produced them. Spontaneous bruising for no demonstrable reason occurs more often in women than in men. An acquired liability to bruising from minor injury, as in the case of petechiae, indicates the necessity for a full investigation of the blood clotting mechanism. Ecchymoses persist longer than petechiae and usually undergo a series of colour changes in the skin from blue to green, yellow and brown as the extravasated blood is broken down.

Significance of Purpura and Ecchymosis. A liability to bleed into the skin or subcutaneous tissues may be due to one of many defects in the process of blood clotting, to a vasculitis as in Henoch's purpura, to inadequacy of the capillary intercellular cement substance as in scurvy or to toxic damage to the small blood vessels. The last may occur in uraemia, from drugs such as co-trimoxazole, or in infections such as meningococcal meningitis. The size and the distribution of the lesions may be very useful guides to the cause of the bleeding. Thus generalised bruises and petechiae, combined perhaps with evidence of bleeding elsewhere in an otherwise healthy patient, are suggestive of thrombocytopenic purpura. Petechiae in a patient who is obviously unwell might suggest leukaemia, infective endocarditis or uraemia. A raised purpuric eruption, usually distributed symmetrically and mainly over the extremities, suggests the Henoch-Schönlein syndrome if associated with abdominal pain or arthralgia. Massive painful bruising of the legs with induration of the muscles, and perifollicular haemorrhage, in an elderly person living alone, are almost pathognomonic of scurvy (Plate II).

Dilatation of Blood Vessels. Obstruction of the blood flow through main vessels may lead to the development of a *collateral circulation*. Venous collaterals are observed much more frequently than arterial because superficial veins are normally visible and are more obvious when distended. Arterial collaterals are seldom detected in conditions other than coarctation of the aorta (p. 137). Dilatation of the small veins (*telangiectasia*) of the face is not necessarily pathological; such an appearance is, however, liable to develop in chronic alcoholics and in those exposed constantly to the rigours of the weather. Small irregular telangiectases also accompany the pigmentation and scarring which follow radiation damage to the skin, and they may be a feature of a number of skin disorders.

Spider telangiectases are characterised by a central arterial dot from which radiate several dilated vessels, all of which are readily obliterated by central pressure. Refilling commences from the central arteriole feeding the vessels. These lesions occur on the face, arms and upper part of the body and are particularly common in patients with hepatic cirrhosis, though they may also be seen frequently in relatively small numbers in pregnancy and hyperthyroidism and occasionally in normal people.

Hereditary haemorrhagic telangiectasia is an uncommon disease in which dilated blood vessels present as dark red spots or larger swellings up to 1 or 2 mm in diameter. They refill readily after being emptied by finger pressure. The lesions occur especially about the face and on the mucous membranes of the mouth and nose, and also at the finger-tips. Epistaxis is common and severe iron deficiency anaemia may develop.

Haemangiomas (Campbell de Morgan spots) commonly develop on the chest and abdomen with advancing years. They consist of firm, bright red to purple swellings, about 1 to 2 mm in diameter, usually raised slightly above the surface of the skin. Only with difficulty can they be obliterated or made to fade on pressure. They have no recognised significance as indicators of other disease, nor ar they in any way harmful themselves.

A congenital diffuse angioma on the face, colloquially known as a port wine stain, is not uncommon. The disfigurement alone is serious enough for the patient but the lesion may also be associated with a calcifying intracranial angioma causing epilepsy, as well as glaucoma and cataract.

Infections and Infestations of the Skin

The *exanthemata* such as scarlet fever, measles, rubella and chickenpox have characteristic skin eruptions. This is also true of *syphilis* in its secondary stage.

Herpes simplex consists of a vesicle or a group of several vesicles on an erythematous base. A dark scab may form as the vesicles dry. The lesions are usually found on the mucocutaneous junction round the mouth but they may occur occasionally anywhere on the skin or mucosae. The condition is due to a viral infection and in susceptible subjects may recur during trivial fevers such as common colds or even as a result of excessive exposure to sunlight. Herpes simplex is also a frequent accompaniment of pneumococcal, meningococcal and malarial infections.

Herpes zoster, ('shingles'), is caused by infection of the posterior root ganglion with the varicella/zoster virus. The thoracic nerves or the ophthalmic division of the trigeminal nerve are commonly affected and the latter may lead to corneal ulceration. There may be a prodromal period of several days characterised by pain in the distribution of the appropriate nerve mimicking conditions such as pleurisy, cholecystitis, sciatica, or sinusitis. Thereafter the skin in the same area develops an irregular erythema upon which groups of vesicles appear. These in turn ulcerate, and in the course of two weeks or more dry up and are replaced by crusted lesions which finally separate. Permanent scarring of the skin is common and may be the only sign in patients with post-herpetic pain, which is sometimes severe and persistent, particularly in the elderly. The incidence of herpes zoster is high in patients whose immune mechanisms are impaired by leukaemia or lymphoma or by immunosuppresive drugs. Occasionally it may cause a lower motor neurone lesion such as a facial palsy.

Bacterial infections of the skin are commonly due to *Staphylococcus aureus* or to *Streptococcus haemolyticus.* The former causes focal lesions such as boils; the latter produces spreading lesions like erysipelas or cellulitis. Both are potent sources of cross infection which may readily become disseminated in surgical wards, children's hospitals, schools and among debilitated persons. Much less common bacterial infections of the skin include diphtheria, tuberculosis, anthrax and erysipeloid.

Infestation of the skin and hair by lice and other insects is not uncommon, and is easily overlooked. Ticks and mites may be acquired from contact with crops or with domestic animals, and their presence should be suspected if bites or itching follow such exposure. Ticks are readily seen. The head is buried in the skin and the body swells as it distends with blood. In *scabies,* a mite (*Sarcoptes scabiei*) burrows beneath the epidermis, particularly into the fine skin of the web of the fingers, the wrists, feet and penis, and often leaves a shallow linear track. Itching, especially at night, is a cardinal feature, and scratch marks are common, sometimes in turn becoming secondarily infected. The parasite can be identified under the low power or a microscope if it is picked out of the burrow in the skin with a needle and placed in a drop of 5% potassium hydroxide on a microscope slide.

One species of flea, *Pulex irritans,* is fully adapted to man. Infected fleas from rodents are responsible for transmitting plague and endemic typhus fever.

Infestation with *Pediculus capitis* (the head louse) is most readily recognised by the presence of the eggs (nits) on the hair of the host. These superficially resemble flakes of dandruff, but are found to be firmly fixed to the hair. Once eggs are seen the lice can usually be found by using a fine toothed comb.

Pediculus corporis (the body louse) is found upon the trunk and in the axillae and the ova are laid on the underclothes. *Phthirius pubis* (the crab louse) may be found on the pubis, in the axillae, on the chest wall or on the eyebrows. It is very much smaller than the head or body louse. It may burrow into the epidermis and may easily be overlooked because it remains virtually immobile. Undisturbed, it presents after feeding on blood as a blue spot, and when fasting as a light brown spot about 1 mm in diameter. Infestation with crab lice is transferred only by close contact, and its acquisition can be classed as a venereal infection.

Cutaneous Hypersensitivity Reactions

The antigen may reach the skin by the blood stream or may react with the skin through external contact. Both immediate and delayed types of hypersensitivity occur, as exemplified by urticaria and dermatitis. A specific food such as shellfish may occasionally be incriminated, but nowadays drugs are more usually responsible for immediate hypersensitivity reactions. Enquiry should therefore be made not only about drugs and injections but also about any self-medication. Drugs such as aspirin can easily be overlooked.

An external agent should be suspected from the distribution of a rash; it may be detected by considering the patient's occupation or by obtaining a history of contact with a new garment, cosmetic, soap, watch strap, etc., in accordance with the possibilities raised by the areas involved.

Cutaneous Manifestations of Generalised Disease

It will be clear from the foregoing that some vascular, infective and allergic lesions will be part of a general rather than a local disturbance. A few examples will be given of other disease processes in which the importance of the dermatological changes lies in the information they give about disease elsewhere. Skin manifestations often supply part of the evidence of *vitamin deficiency*, as for example follicular hyperkeratosis (vitamin A), cheilosis, angular stomatitis (riboflavin), pellagra (nicotinic acid) and bleeding into the legs in scurvy (vitamin C).

The skin is frequently involved in the *connective tissue disorders*, especially in scleroderma (p. 67), dermatomyositis and systemic lupus erythematosus. In the last named condition an erythematous eruption may be present over the bridge of the nose and adjacent part of the cheeks (butterfly rash, Plate I). *Sarcoidosis* may involve the skin producing papules, nodules or plaques, and is also one of the causes of *erythema nodosum* — a series of red, painful, tender, indurated swellings, varying in size from a few millimetres to several centimetres in diameter (Plate II). They are to be found most constantly over the front of the legs, though they may also extend over the knees and on to the thighs, and may even be found on the extensor surface of the arms or forearms. The tenderness may sometimes be sufficiently marked to make even the weight of bedclothes intolerable. In children and young adults primary tuberculosis or streptococcal infection is more often responsible. Erythema nodosum, like *erythema multiforme* (Plate II), may also be precipitated by drugs such as sulphonamides.

Xanthomatosis is characterised by yellow lesions of varying size, distributed widely on the trunk and limbs. The extensor surfaces of the elbows and knees are often involved as are tendons. Identical lesions can occur in biliary cirrhosis but jaundice precedes the xanthomatosis. Hypercholesterolaemia and hyper-triglyceridaemia are usual and the condition may be associated with diabetes mellitus.

Dermatitis artefacta (Plate I) is found in patients with personality disorders. It is usually characterised by linear and sharply defined lesions with an artificial appearance at sites readily accessible to the patient. In *self poisoning* from barbiturates and other drugs, tense bullae may appear on the hands and feet within 24 hours of ingestion of the drug.

These few examples serve to demonstrate that cutaneous lesions are often present in a wide range of systemic disorders. The skin manifestation may provide the main diagnostic clue in common conditions such as the exanthemata or in rare disorders like xanthomatosis. The important lesson is to learn to look at the skin and to question the significance of every abnormality that can be observed.

Primary Disorders of the Skin

Psoriasis is one of the commonest primary skin disorders. The characteristic lesions are usually clearly defined, scaly, erythematous patches with a predilection for the extensor surfaces of the elbows or knees. When the patches are scratched numerous distinctive silvery scales are produced. Involvement of the finger-nails (Fig. 4.2) and joints occurs in some cases (p. 67).

Both benign and malignant skin *tumours* may occur. In a *papilloma* all elements of the skin are involved, while other benign tumours may be derived from the individual tissues comprising skin, for example sebaceous cysts, lipomas, neurofibromas and vascular naevi. *Sebaceous cysts* can be distinguished by the fact that they arise in the dermis and therefore move freely with the skin and are attached to it near the central point where a comedo (blackhead) may be present. The swelling, if not too tense, may be indented by pressure. *Neurofibromas* are relatively rare but most frequently arise from small branches of cutaneous nerves causing dermal nodules of varying sizes, some of which may become pedunculated. They are usually associated with scattered patches of brown (café au lait) pigmentation (Plate I). They are important not only because of the disfigurement they cause, but also because they are occasionally associated with tumours of nervous tissue elsewhere, for example, on spinal nerve roots, accoustic neuromas, meningiomas or the tumours of chromaffin tissue forming phaeochromocytomas. *Naevi* are congenital lesions which include *angiomas* (port wine stain) and *melanomas* (moles). The latter may become malignant (Plate I). Any change in a melanoma or any irregularity in its colour, outline or surface may signify malignancy.

Basal cell carcinoma or *rodent ulcer* is a locally malignant tumour which is very frequently seen about the face in elderly persons. These growths start as pearly-white nodules which slowly enlarge until the centre becomes crusted or ulcerated.

The *squamous cell carcinoma* or *epithelioma,* in contrast, is a rapidly growing tumour which may spread to adjacent tissues and to the lymph nodes at an early stage. *Metastases* to the skin from distant sites such as the lung, the breast, or the kidney may be of only passing interest when the primary diagnosis has already been made. Sometimes, however, a carcinoma will first present as a cutaneous metastasis, and if this is suspected biopsy should always be undertaken.

THE METHODS IN PRACTICE

THE RECOGNITION OF DRUG ADDICTION

This example is chosen because of the prevalence of drug addiction and because it illustrates the need for alertness on the part of the clinician if the condition is to be recognised.

The increasing variety of preparations on which patients become dependent, coupled with the implications that this carries for the doctor who may encounter such patients unexpectedly, makes it important that the few signs which may be present are recognised without delay. Drug addicts commonly are sociopathic (p. 27) and disturbance of behaviour may be apparent particularly when supplies are short or withdrawal is in progress. This is most familiar to doctors in the patient dependent upon alcohol, but corresponding features characteristic of the individual drug may be seen on withdrawal in many other forms of dependence, for example when narcotics, cannabis, barbiturates or amphetamines are involved. These may be used in isolation or in various combinations.

The withdrawal syndrome is usually characterised by irritability, restlessness, tremor, sweating, lacrimation, nausea and abdominal pain. An overdose of a powerful narcotic such as heroin may lead to coma with constricted pupils, depressed or periodic respiration, hypotension, and with recovery, vomiting. Evidence may be found of needle punctures, thrombosed veins, ulcers at injection sites, skin sepsis or hepatitis transmitted by infected needles.

The addict will use any subterfuge to obtain drugs such as, for example, feigning illness at a doctor's surgery or at the hospital casualty department. Individuals dependent on drugs are often very knowledgeable about medical and hospital procedures and pass from one doctor or hospital and one town or city to another taking advantage of every opportunity to obtain the drugs they require. Nowadays clinicians should be on the watch for such patients, and be prepared to undertake a careful search for evidence of addiction.

Conclusion

The general examination provides a wealth of opportunity for diagnosis largely by the simple techniques of inspection and palpation. These basic procedures are also fundamental components of the examination of the individual systems. Where supplemented by auscultation and, to a lesser extent, by percussion, they meet the needs of many clinical problems. With easy access to ancillary methods of diagnosis, doctors may tend to limit the use of their special senses and fail to base their diagnostic decisions on information gained by taking a patient's history with care and thereafter performing a thorough physical examination. It is only on such a background that logical and economical use can be made of the investigative methods now widely available.

REFERENCE

Mackie R M 1981 Clinical dermatology: An illustrated textbook. Oxford University Press, Oxford — A concise text supplemented by many good colour photographs.

5. The Cardiovascular System

No man's opinions are better than his information.

Paul Getty (1960)

Clinical examination of the cardiovascular system is particularly rewarding in that the symptoms and signs elicited can often be explained in terms of basic physics, anatomy and physiology, and will frequently allow an accurate diagnosis to be made at the bedside. Increasingly sophisticated techniques of cardiac investigation, including echocardiography, phonocardiography, nuclear cardiography and cardiac catheterization have in no way supplanted clinical examination, but have frequently given fresh insights into the mechanism and significance of physical signs. As understanding has increased, the student's work at the bedside has become more rational and hence more enjoyable. At the same time, the increasing scope of cardiac surgery has set new standards for accuracy and completeness of diagnosis.

Information is of limited usefulness unless it can be communicated. During the long history of clinical examination there has evolved a certain verbal shorthand, of phrases which epitomise in a few words a clinical picture which would otherwise take many paragraphs to describe. Like any living language, it is liable to abuse and corruption. The student needs not only to understand it but to use it critically and carefully. For example, 'the left side of the heart' is a term used to describe the left atrium, left ventricle and the mitral and aortic valves. 'Left heart failure' is a useful if not very elegant extension of this to describe a clinical picture which includes a reduced cardiac output and pulmonary oedema. If we know that impaired left ventricular function is responsible we can use the more precise term left ventricular failure, but it would be wrong to do so if the pulmonary oedema might in fact be a consequence of mitral stenosis.

THE HISTORY

THE PRINCIPAL SYMPTOMS OF HEART DISEASE

Dyspnoea, pain, oedema and palpitations are the principal manifestations of heart disease, and are discussed in detail as their analysis depends on an understanding of their origin and significance. It is the symptoms which provide a measure of functional capacity. However, it is important to appreciate that severe heart disease may be asymptomatic, and come to light only when a complication arises, as, for example, when an arterial embolism occurs.

The general principles which are involved in the assessment of the severity of a symptom have been described in Chapter 1. It is a common practice in the field of cardiology to use the term 'functional grade' to denote the degree of incapacity caused by pain or dyspnoea (p. 45). Though such a classification may be a useful abbreviation it is no substitute for a succinct record of the patient's description of the symptoms. Questions which often prove helpful include the following: 'What do you now find difficult which you used to be able to do easily?'; the housewife generally gives up scrubbing and polishing first — but in an age of mechanisation there may be other reaons for this! 'When you are walking, can you talk at the same time?'; or 'Do you now keep others back?'; or, when there is difficulty in establishing when a symptom occurs (e.g. cardiac pain), it is often useful to say — 'If I wanted to see you with the pain, what could you do to bring it on?'.

Dyspnoea

The analysis of breathlessness is discussed on page 41, but some elaboration is necessary here from the cardiac aspect.

Dyspnoea on effort is usually the first symptom of left heart failure. Exercise leads to increased venous return, and the relatively normal 'right side of the heart' (right atrium and ventricle and the tricuspid and pulmonary valves) transmits this increase through the pulmonary circulation. In the presence of left heart failure the result is pulmonary venous congestion. This stimulates fine nerve endings around the terminal alveoli, and causes a sensation of breathlessness. At the same time, pulmonary interstitial oedema begins to develop. When exercise is stopped, venous return diminishes, congestion subsides and dyspnoea is relieved. Very occasionally severe unaccustomed exercise in the presence of incipient left heart failure leads to progressive pulmonary oedema.

Paroxysmal nocturnal dyspnoea (p. 44) is a characteristic symptom of left heart failure. It is traditionally attributed to a rise in venous pressure as the patient slips down the pillows to a more recumbent position during the night's sleep. This may be an oversimplification. Paroxysmal nocturnal dyspnoea requires a special search for a cause of increased left ventricular work, such as hypertension or aortic stenosis. In the absence of such a cause it is usually an indicator of disease of the left ventricle. Paroxysmal nocturnal dyspnoea is a rare symptom in mitral stenosis, except during pregnancy or at the onset of atrial fibrillation. The drop in pulse rate during sleep may help left heart function in mitral stenosis, and, in patients with chronic mitral valve disease, thickening of the alveolar walls and dilatation of the pulmonary lymphatics may protect against pulmonary oedema. Abrupt blockage of the mitral valve by left atrial thrombus or a left atrial myxoma may also cause paroxysmal nocturnal dyspnoea, but this is very rare.

Breathlessness demanding the upright position, *orthopnoea*, when due to heart disease, is a symptom of persistent pulmonary oedema and indicates that the heart disease is advanced. With improvements in therapy it is now much less commonly seen. In attacks of *acute pulmonary oedema* there is persistent severe breathlessness of sudden onset, accompanied usually by coughing and, generally, considerable alarm. Unless treatment is prompt and effective, the cough, initially repetitive and unproductive, may produce copious watery, frothy and often blood-tinged sputum.

Breathlessness is not a common feature of pure 'right heart failure' (p. 145). However pulmonary hypertension, whether 'primary' or caused by chronic thromboembolic pulmonary disease, is often accompanied by severe dyspnoea, possibly as a consequence of the altered pattern of blood flow within the lungs.

Pain

The most common cardiac pain is that due to myocardial ischaemia. Less frequently pain may arise from the pericardium or as a result of aortic disease.

Angina Pectoris. This term was originally used by Heberden in 1772 to describe a characteristic chest pain occurring on exertion which we now know to be the principal symptom of myocardial ischaemia. By extension, the term angina is also used for pain caused by myocardial ischaemia under other circumstances, for example during coronary artery spasm, but 'angina' without further qualification generally means angina of effort. Since it is frequently the sole symptom, and often unaccompanied by abnormal physical signs, it must be evaluated precisely by analysing the pain along the lines described on page 30.

SITE. In describing the symptom the patient often places both hands on the chest with fingers meeting on the lower sternum, or presses the palm or a clenched fist there.

RADIATION. A feeling of heaviness or uselessness in one arm, usually the left, or both arms often accompanies the sensation in the chest. Aching in the wrists, or in the jaw or neck, and less often in the back of the chest may be volunteered or elicited. Any of these places of reference may be involved without discomfort in the chest, and the relationship to exertion is then the indication that the pain is probably of cardiac origin.

CHARACTER. The pain is characteristically like a tight band round the chest, or a feeling of constriction or heaviness. The description depends so much on the personality of the patient that other features are more reliable, such as the circumstances under which the symptom occurs and the gestures which the patient uses. The pain is often attributed wrongly to indigestion. The patient may describe the sensation as a discomfort rather than a pain or may regard it as a form of breathlessness.

SEVERITY AND DURATION. Cardiac pain produced by exertion usually begins at about the same place in the course of a regular walk. It generally demands a rest, or the adoption of a slower pace, so that the patient does not allow it to become severe. With rest the pain usually disappears in two or three minutes. Sometimes a 'second wind' effect occurs — for example a patient who develops mild angina during the first hole of a game of golf may not have it subsequently despite encountering steeper hills.

AGGRAVATING FACTORS. Walking uphill, particularly in a cold wind, or exercise after meals is often noted as likely to result in angina pectoris, or to bring it on more easily. Angina pectoris is often produced by excitement, stress of fear. Boxing matches on television, sexual intercourse, or outbursts of rage may provoke it. In some patients angina occurs mainly at night, sometimes in association with vivid dreams (including those induced by beta-blocker therapy). Patients with coronary artery disease and incipient left ventricular failure may get angina on lying flat — *decubitus angina*. Pain which is typical of angina in site and character, but not related to effort nor a symptom of acute myocardial infarction is often attributed to coronary artery spasm. Such pain is sometimes called *variant* or *Printzmetal angina*. Coronary artery spasm is very difficult to confirm by any technique short of coronary angiography, but it may be associated with Raynaud's phenomenon (p. 136) and is much more common in cigarette smokers.

Typical attacks of angina provoked by less and less exertion, and/or attacks of chest pain like angina occurring at rest with increasing frequency, constitute the syndrome of *crescendo angina*, which may precede myocardial infarction.

RELIEVING FACTORS. Pain persisting significantly longer than about five minutes after the end of exercise is very unlikely to be angina pectoris. A sense of time, however, is not always reliable, especially in the presence of pain, and severe pain may seem to last for several minutes wheres its true duration is much shorter. Glyceryl trinitrate hastens the relief of anginal pain, but is also effective in relieving the pain of oesophageal spasm, and its action cannot be regarded as specific.

ASSOCIATED PHENOMENA. Dyspnoea is a usual accompaniment, as can be readily appreciated by walking with a patient who has angina pectoris, but is usually not mentioned by the patient. Belching is common, and often appears to relieve the pain; it may misdirect medical interest towards the stomach.

Angina pectoris can be provoked by anaemia, obesity or hyperthyroidism; in some cases it may be a symptom of aortic stenosis, hypertrophic cardiomyopathy or syphilitic aortitis.

Other Chest Pains of Cardiovascular Origin. The pain of *myocardial infarction* generally differs from that of angina pectoris in that it is more severe and oppressive and occurs or persists at rest; its type and radiation are similar. The pain or discomfort is often accompanied by a sense of apprehension or of impeding death. The patient tends to lie still and is generally quiet and pale, and often sweats. The pain usually reaches a maximum in minutes, or over an hour or so, and then may be persistent for hours until relieved by analgesics. Occasionally the pain is intermittent or remittent even without treatment. Myocardial infarction is not always painful, and electrocardiographic (ECG) or post-mortem evidence of 'silent infarction' may be found in patients who have never had typical symptoms.

Prolonged cardiac pain at rest mimicking that of myocardial infarction may result from attacks of paroxysmal tachycardia, especially in patients with diseased coronary arteries; the patient may be aware of palpitation, or the doctor may find tachycardia during an attack.

The pain of *pericarditis* is often mistaken for that of myocardial ischaemia. The features in common are that it is retrosternal and may radiate to shoulders, neck or upper arms. However, it is usually accentuated by or may be present only during inspiration; this is not a feature of pain arising from the myocardium, but pericarditis frequently follows a few days after a myocardial infarction and at this stage there may be pain associated with breathing. The pain of pericarditis may also be provoked by swallowing or by change of position.

Rapid accumulation of fluid in the pericardial space gives rise to a sense of retrosternal oppression, usually indistinguishable from that of myocardial ischaemia. The development of a haemopericardium in a patient with myocardial infarction, and under treatment with anticoagulants, may also be mistaken for a further episode of infarction. Other signs of acute cardiac tamponade (p. 110) may allow a diagnosis to be made on clinical grounds and echocardiography (p. 142) or chest radiography may help to confirm it.

Pain from *dissecting aneurysm of the aorta* is usually of dramatically sudden onset and in the upper chest posteriorly more often than anteriorly. Spread of the dissection to the abdominal aorta may account for abdominal pain. There is often a sensation of loss of power in the legs. *Syphilitic aneurysm of the aorta*, which is now uncommon in Britain, may produce pain when there is erosion of bone, usually a persistent interscapular or upper retrosternal ache, often worse at night.

A momentary jab of pain at about the site of the cardiac apex is a common experience in normal subjects and is sometimes called *precordial catch*; it never indicates organic heart disease.

Various bizarre discomforts are described by those subject to *anxiety* and can usually be readily distinguished. However, patients who have organic pain and are prone to use colourful descriptions may require considerable patience from the clinician if the symptom is to be interpreted correctly.

Oedema

Oedema is the most characteristic feature of fluid retention in cardiac failure; together with ascites and pleural transudates, it is dealt with fully on pages 50 to 55.

Other Symptoms

Palpitation, or awareness of the heart beat, is a common feature of anxiety and can be produced by sympathomimetic drugs such as adrenaline, or isoprenaline; panic attacks are commonly confused with paroxysmal tachycardia. Patients can often say whether the heart beat seems to be regular or irregular, and by tapping with the finger can sometimes indicate the approximate heart rate. Such evidence is of help in diagnosing paroxysmal tachycardias when normal rhythm has returned before the patient is seen. Continuous ambulatory ECG monitoring (p. 39) is of great value in detecting paroxysmal arrhythmias.

Cough, which is repetitive, dry, unproductive and accompanied by tachypnoea, is the herald of pulmonary oedema in some cases. Cough may also be a symptom of aneurysm of the aorta. Compression of the trachea or a main bronchus sometimes gives this a trumpeting quality.

Haemoptysis is a feature of pulmonary infarction which is a frequent sequel to pulmonary thromboembolism in bedridden patients, and can also result from pulmonary artery thrombosis in patients with pulmonary hypertension.

Syncope, which is defined as loss of consciousness accompanied by a fall in blood pressure, has numerous possible cardiac causes, and is discussed in detail on page 37.

Tiredness is a common symptom in severe heart disease, particularly in the presence of cardiac failure. Its unexpected appearance in a patient with congenital or rheumatic heart disease should arouse a suspicion of infective endocarditis. However it is a common symptom of other disorders; for example the patient with mitral valve disease who complains of tiredness is more likely to be depressed than to have infective endocarditis.

The *eyes* may be affected in various forms of cardiovascular disease. Sudden unilateral impairment of vision may result from retinal haemorrhage in severe hypertension, or from emboli to the retina in cases of valvular heart disease. Often, retinal haemorrhages do not cause noticeable impairment of vision, but are revealed on routine examination with an ophthalmoscope. Unilateral visual distrubances may also result from retinal artery or retinal vein thrombosis (Plate III), or from cranial arteritis. Disturbances of vision affecting both eyes, usually in the form of a homonymous field defect (p. 240), may follow occlusion of a cerebral artery. Patients starting on therapy with a potent diuretic sometimes notice transient visual blurring, possibly related to changes in the hydration of the lens.

Gastrointestinal Symptoms. Nausea and vomiting are often features of acute myocardial infarction. They are also the most common presenting symptoms of digitalis intoxication. Sometimes nausea and vomiting accompany worsening cardiac failure, perhaps as a consequence of hepatic or gastric congestion. Diarrhoea may be a result of digitalis toxicity; conversely constipation may result from the dehydration caused by excessive diuretic therapy. Electrolyte disturbances produced in this way can also present as drowsiness, muscle cramps, or muscular weakness.

Renal function is dependent on cardiac ouput, and severe cardiac failure, for instance that resulting from pericardial tamponade, leads to oliguria or anuria. In less severe cardiac failure the usual diurnal rhythm of urine output may be reversed, with more urine being produced at night than during the day. Acute polyuria sometimes accompanies paroxysmal supraventricular tachycardia.

Other Aspects of the History

The progress of heart disease should also be analysed as accurately as possible, i.e. 'When was heart disease first suspected?'; 'When was the rhythm first noted to be irregular?' and 'When did symptoms first develop, and what were they?' With experience it will be learned that symptoms are relatively early in some diseases, e.g. mitral stenosis, and almost terminal in others, e.g. aortic stenosis.

Certain medical contexts have also to be recognised, such as the liability of patients with Marfan's syndrome (p. 61) or coarctation of the aorta to acute dissection of the aorta, or of patients with Friedreich's ataxia to cardiomyopathy. Arterial occlusion, whether peripheral or coronary, is abnormally frequent in diabetics, in cigarette smokers and in patients with hypercholesterolaemia (e.g. with xanthomatosis). Recurrent urinary infections may lead to chronic pyelonephritis and explain the development of hypertension. The rare carcinoid tumour with hepatic metastases can produce unusual flushing of the skin and signs of tricuspid and pulmonary valvular disease.

It is traditional, and important, to enquire of patients with valvular heart disease whether they have had rheumatic fever or chorea, but the patient's diagnosis should not be accepted uncritically. Echocardiography suggests that many patients given the 'label' of chronic rheumatic heart disease actually have congenital or degenerative lesions.

Obstetric History. The development or exacerbation of symptoms during past pregnancies must be carefully noted, and may be of great relevance with respect to a subsequent pregnancy.

Family History. In rheumatic heart disease, hypertension and premature ischaemic heart disease, a family history of the same complaint is very common.

Social History. A precise enquiry into the patient's home circumstances, and the requirements of his or her work, is as important for cardiac as for other categories of patient. A diagnosis of cardiac abnormality may have important implications for patients in certain occupations, such as airline pilots or drivers of heavy goods vehicles.

Smoking habits, and particularly cigarette smoking, must be recorded because of their relevance to coronary artery disease and cor pulmonale. It is often valuable to make a rough estimate of the total number of cigarettes smoked during life (number per week × 50 × number of years). Many patients claiming to be non-smokers have stopped only at the onset of symptoms. Alcohol consumption should also be assessed, and perhaps corroborated with relatives.

Drugs. A complete list of all medications is essential, and it must include drugs used for 'noncardiac' conditions. Apart from the association between high-oestrogen contraceptives and thromboembolism, other associations include tricyclic antidepressants with cardiac arrhythmias, appetite suppressants with pulmonary hypertension and liquorice derivatives or anti-inflammatory drugs with fluid retention.

THE PHYSICAL EXAMINATION

The emphasis placed on different aspects of the physical examination will depend on the history and on the mental list of differential diagnoses which the examiner draws up as the history is being elicited. The student will however need to develop, and then adhere to, a routine of examination which ensures that nothing important is overlooked. This routine will include, as a minimum, attention to the following points:

1. General inspection;
2. Hands and face;
3. Arterial and venous pulses;
4. Measurement of the blood pressure (p. 112).
5. Examination of heart and lungs by inspection, palpation, percussion and auscultation;
6. A search for oedema, ascites and hepatomegaly;
7. Examination of the optic fundi (p. 411).

1. General Inspection

This should begin even before the examiner starts to take the history, as the patient's appearance, gait, attitude and clothing may all be relevant. A short walk with the patient to the examination room may give valuable information about exercise tolerance. Features such as severe anaemia, Paget's disease, hyper- or hypothyroidism may be apparent at once, or detected only after careful examination.

Cyanosis. This is a bluish or purplish tinge of the skin or mucous membranes which results from the presence of an excessive amount of reduced haemoglobin in the underlying blood vessels. It may be due either to poor perfusion of these vessels (peripheral cyanosis) or to a reduction in the oxygen saturation of arterial blood (central cyanosis). For cyanosis to be observed, there must be a minimum quanity of reduced haemoglobin (about 5 g/dl) in the blood perfusing the skin; cyanosis may thus not be detectable in patients with severe anaemia even if they are gravely hypoxaemic.

Peripheral cyanosis is a familiar sight in the hands, cheeks, lips and ears in cold weather, as a consequence of cold-induced vasoconstriction. It is seen also in patients with a greatly reduced cardiac output, when differential vasoconstriction diverts blood flow from the skin to other organs such as the brain. Peripheral cyanosis is seldom seen in the tongue or buccal mucosa because they are well perfused except in advanced circulatory failure. It can usually be assumed that when cyanosis is present in these sites it is of central (cardiopulmonary) origin. The same assumption can be made when the hands are cyanosed and warm.

Central cyanosis can usually be detected when the oxygen saturation of arterial blood falls below 80–85%. It may be due to respiratory (p. 161) or to cardiac causes. The most common 'cardiac' cause is pulmonary oedema, with its associated symptoms of dyspnoea and cough, and the physical sign of crepitations at the lung bases. A less common cardiac cause is an intracardiac or intrapulmonary 'right to left shunt', where venous blood bypasses the lungs and is shunted into the systemic circulation. This is seen in pulmonary arteriovenous fistulae, in Fallot's tetralogy and other rarer forms of congenital heart disease. Patients with a right to left shunt show little or no increase in arterial oxygen saturation when given oxygen to breathe, whereas patients with hypoxaemia from pulmonary oedema or respiratory causes usually show an improvement. Sometimes, hypoxaemia results from pulmonary thromboembolism.

Very occasionally, cyanosis is due to the presence of the *abnormal pigments* sulphaemoglobin or methaemoglobin in the bloodsteam. In these cases, arterial oxygen tension is normal, and the diagnosis can be confirmed by spectroscopic examination of the blood.

2. Hands and Face

These areas particularly repay attention in cardiac patients. In practice, their detailed inspection is usually integrated with the examination of the peripheral pulses and the search for oedema, but for convenience the points of special interest are collected here.

The *hands* provide valuable information about the patient's occupation and smoking habits. It is useful, as well as polite, to begin the physical examination by shaking hands with the patient. Warm hands indicate peripheral vasodilatation, cold ones vasoconstriction, and sweaty palms reflect increased sympathetic nervous activity either from anxiety or cardiac failure. A blue tinge to the hands may be due to arterial desaturation, but it can also be due to a reduced cardiac output or to stasis of blood in dilated superficial vessels. It should not be regarded as pathological without corroborating evidence. Chronic arterial desaturation, particularly that due to cyanotic congenital heart disease, causes finger clubbing which is also a classic, if rather late, sign in infective endocarditis. This last condition may also be associated with splinter haemorrhages (Fig. 4.2, p. 68) under the finger (or toe) nails, or with small, tender Osler's nodes in the finger pulp. In patients with ischaemic heart disease and hypercholesterolaemia, xanthomas may be palpable as small lumps in the tendons of the extensor digitorum muscle, or in the tendons around the elbow.

Face. Many varieties of congenital heart disease are associated with abnormalities of the facial skeleton — for example, the high-arched palate of Marfan's syndrome, the hypertelorism (wide-set eyes) sometimes seen in pulmonary stenosis, and the elfin facies (receding jaw, flared ·nostrils and pointed ears) of supravalvar aortic stenosis. Usually, however, the heart disease draws attention to the facial abnormality rather than vice versa. Some patients with mitral stenosis and a reduced cardiac output have pallid faces with patches of rather dusky erythema over the cheek bones. Although sometimes called the mitral facies, this appearance is not specific as it may be seen in other forms of heart disease and not infrequently in normal subjects.

The *teeth and eyes* should be inspected. Dental disease or its treatment may be responsible for infective endocarditis. Edentulous patients, however, may sometimes develop endocarditis if ill-fitting dentures cause a portal of entry for bacteraemia. Xanthelasma (p. 73) and, in young adults, an arcus lipidus (p. 74) may be indicators of hypercholesterolaemia. Ophthalmoscopic examination is particularly informative in hypertensive patients (pp. 413—415).

3. Arterial and Venous Pulses

The arterial pulse wave which is felt by the examining fingers is imparted to the column of arterial blood by the contraction of the left ventricle and takes between 0.2 and 0.5 seconds to reach the feet; the blood takes ten times as long to make the same journey. The form of the pulse wave is largely determined by the quantity of blood ejected into the aorta, the speed of ejection, and the rigidity of the arterial system. The arterial pulse is routinely examined for rate, rhythm, volume and form of the pulse wave. Several peripheral pulses are available for examination, and while virtually any pulse gives information about rate and rhythm, volume and waveform are more reliably assessed from the more 'central' pulses such as the carotid, brachial or femoral.

The Radial Pulse. This is the most accessible of the peripheral pulses. A technique for palpating the radial pulse is shown in Figure 5.1. Occasionally the radial artery follows an aberrant course, traversing the 'anatomical snuff box' and passing over the dorsum of the first metacarpal bone. It is good practice to palpate both radial pulses simultaneously, as weakness or delay in one may give a clue to more proximal arterial disease. The radial and femoral pulses should also be checked for synchrony if coarctation of the aorta is suspected (p. 111).

The Pulse Rate. This is measured by counting the pulse for a measured period:

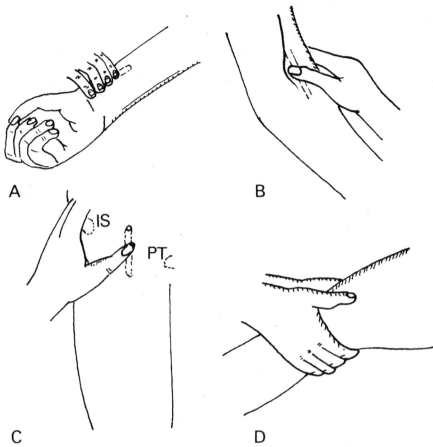

Fig. 5.1 Methods for palpating peripheral pulses. (A) radial; (B) right brachial; (C) femoral; (D) popliteal. Note that the thumb is shown being used to feel the brachial and femoral pulses. When searching for a very weak pulse, as in the presence of peripheral vascular disease, it is better to use the fingers rather than the thumb, as very faint pulsation in the examiner's thumb may be mistaken for the pulse being sought. Note that the femoral artery lies midway between the anterior superior iliac spine (IS) and the pubic tubercle (PT) and that the popliteal pulse is felt with the fingertips of both hands.

fifteen seconds is usually adequate. Experienced doctors often estimate the pulse rate rather than time it, but this is not recommended to students. Counting the heart rate by auscultation is an acceptable alternative, and more accurate at fast rates; the ECG is better still.

Tachycardia is sometimes defined as a pulse rate faster than 100 per minute, and *bradycardia* as a rate slower than 50 per minute, but the appropriateness of the tachycardia or bradycardia is more significant than its absolute value. Sinus tachycardia is appropriate during exercise or in a febrile patient. It accompanies anxiety, shock and most forms of cardiac failure, and it is a normal finding in infants or young chidren. Sinus bradycardia is common during sleep, and often occurs at rest in healthy and athletic young people. On the other hand it may be a feature of the 'sick sinus syndrome', of hypothyroidism or hypothermia, or of raised intracranial pressure. Ectopic beats (extrasystoles), when they alternate with normal beats and produce no palpable pulse, may cause an illusion of bradycardia, but auscultation will reveal them.

In *complete heart block* the pulse rate is usually less than 40 per minute, and may fall as low as 20. In *paroxysmal supraventricular tachycardia* the pulse rate is usually between 140 and 180 per minute, and may be more rapid in children. Carotid sinus massage (p. 109) may terminate the attack, or cause a transient but abrupt fall in pulse rate. *Atrial flutter* is a variant of atrial tachycardia with a rapid atrial rate of about 300 per minute. The ventricles usually respond to alternate atrial beats (2:1 atrioventricular block) giving a regular pulse of 150 per minute, but carotid sinus pressure may cause a sudden reduction to 100 per minute (3:1 block) or slower. Atrial fibrillation is considered under pulse rhythm.

Ventricular tachycardia may produce a rate so rapid that the pulse is impalpable and the patient becomes syncopal. At slower rates it may be difficult to distinguish from atrial tachycardia without the help of the ECG. Carotid sinus pressure does not affect the rate in ventricular tachycardia, but this is not a reliable point of distinction as some cases of atrial tachycardia also fail to respond.

Pulse Rhythm. The commonest irregularity is *sinus arrhythmia* — this is an acceleration of the pulse during inspiration and a slowing at the beginning of expiration. It is particularly prominent in adolescents or athletic young adults, or in circumstances of increased vagal tone. It is not found in patients with cardiac failure, with autonomic neuropathy (e.g. in diabetes) or with a large atrial septal defect.

Ectopic beats are recognised by their prematurity; they occur earlier than the next expected regular beat. The more premature the ectopic beat, the smaller the pulse volume, and very premature beats may not be detected at the wrist. Ectopic beats are followed by a compensatory pause, and because of this the succeeding pulse may be of greater than normal volume; it is this beat, rather than the extrasystole, which is often noticed by the patient. In theory, atrial and ventricular extrasystoles can be distinguished by the length of the compensatory pause, but the ECG is easier and more reliable. In some patients extrasystoles disappear on exercise as the heart rate increases, but in others, and especially in patients with ischaemic heart disease, they may be induced by exercise.

Intermittent heart block causing 'dropped beats' may also cause an irregular pulse, although much less often than extrasystoles. Atrio-ventricular conduction may fail sporadically and unpredictably, or there may be a regular numerical relationship between atrial and ventricular beats (Wenckebach block). In the latter, it is as though succeeding atrial beats found it increasingly difficult to 'get through' to the ventricle, until one beat fails to do so and a pause results which allows the conducting system to recover (Fig. 5.2). The resulting pulse cadence is accurately described, in Wenckebach's own expression, as a 'regular intermission of the pulse'.

Atrial fibrillation is classically described as causing an 'irregularly irregular' pulse. At the onset of fibrillation the ventricular rate is characteristically rapid, averaging 150 to 180 per minute. At these rates some of the pulse beats may be too weak to feel at the wrist, and the true ventricular rate must be determined by auscultation or the ECG. The difference between this rate and that counted at the wrist is called the *pulse deficit*. As the ventricular rate slows, either spontaneously or under the influence of digoxin, the pulse deficit tends to become less. Note that it is

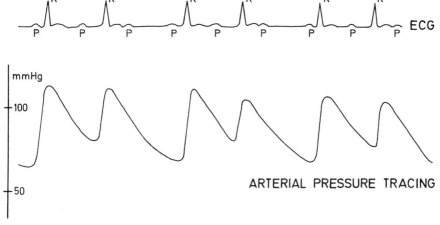

Fig. 5.2 The Wenckebach Phenomenon. ECG and pulse trace showing 3:2 atrioventricular block; every third P wave on the ECG is not followed by a QRS complex, and a pulse beat is 'dropped'.

the ventricular rate which slows as a result of an increased degree of atrioventricular block; the atrial rate remains rapid. Sometimes the pulse rhythm is so close to being regular that its true nature is appreciated only if the pulse is examined for a prolonged period.

Pulse Volume and Character. Invaluable information about left ventricular function and left-sided valvular lesions can be gained from a careful assessment of the volume and character of the pulse. The 'closer' to the heart the pulse is palpated the less it is likely to be modified by the properties of the peripheral vessels. The carotid, brachial or femoral pulses are thus more useful for assessing pulse volume and character than the radial pulse.

The *brachial pulse* is most conveniently felt using the examiner's thumb (Fig. 5.1). There is a prejudice against using this digit for feeling pulses which may be justified when searching for a faint peripheral pulse but is inappropriate here, where the excellent proprioceptive and kinaesthetic sense of the thumb make it ideal for the purpose. *The carotid pulse* is also best felt with the thumb, which is placed adjacent to the trachea in the lower part of the neck, and pressed gently backward until carotid pulsation is felt between it and the cervical vertebrae (Fig. 5.6). *Carotid sinus massage* is a useful manoeuvre for transiently increasing vagus nerve activity. It is helpful in the diagnosis and treatment of tachycardias and sometimes in the assessment of blackouts and 'funny turns' (p. 37). It depends on stimulating the blood pressure receptors in the carotid sinus, which lies at the bifurcation of the common carotid into internal and external carotid arteries. Sometimes this bifurcation lies quite low in the neck; more commonly it lies just beneath the angle of the jaw (Fig. 5.6). Carotid sinus massage should be gentle, and only one side massaged at a time. It should always be done with the patient lying on a couch because there is some risk of syncope in patients with a sensitive reflex and it is wise to take this precaution even when this pulse is simply being felt to assess its character.

The *femoral* pulse may be felt with either the thumb or the forefinger. It lies halfway between the pubic tubercle and the anterior superior iliac spine at the level of the inguinal ligament (Fig. 5.1). It cannot be felt satisfactorily through layers of clothing.

Pulse volume reflects left ventricular stroke volume: it is increased during or after exercise, in the presence of a fever, or when there is increased 'run off' from the arterial tree through a persistent ductus arteriosus or other arteriovenous fistula. In aortic regurgitation the 'run off' is back into the left ventricle itself during diastole. Conversely, the pulse volume is small in the presence of poor left ventricular function or during tachycardia.

The commonest cause of a change in pulse volume from beat to beat is arrhythmia, for after a longer diastole there is an increase in stroke volume and vice versa. A regular succession of large and small pulses is called *pulsus alternans*, and occurs in severe left ventricular failure. It needs to be distinguished from the alternation of pulse volume caused by coupled ventricular ectopic beats, which is much more common.

Pulsus paradoxus is a real or apparent decrease in pulse volume during inspiration and increase in expiration. One variety of 'pulsus paradoxus' occurs in severe asthma, where excessive swings in intrathoracic pressure are superimposed on the arterial pressure. In this case systolic and diastolic pressures rise and fall in parallel so there is no consistent change in pulse pressure — but this can be appreciated only with the aid of a continuous intra-arterial recording. In the other variety, or 'true' pulsus paradoxus, there is not only a fall in systolic pressure but a true diminution of pulse volume during inspiration (Fig. 5.3). Although a minor variation in pulse volume in this way occurs in normal subjects (so the term 'paradoxus' is a misnomer) its occurence in such an exaggerated fashion that the changes can be detected by palpation is virtually diagnostic of *cardiac tamponade* — cardiac compression by a tense pericardial effusion. Normally, the physiological changes in intrathoracic pressure during the respiratory cycle are transmitted equally to the four chambers of the heart, so that the swings in left atrial pressure are accompanied by almost identical changes in left ventricular diastolic pressure. In the presence of a tense pericardial effusion, the left ventricle is prevented from responding to the lower intrathoracic pressure during inspiration, its filling is impeded, and stroke volume falls. The right ventricle on the other hand is connected via the right atrium and vena cava to the extra-thoracic systemic veins, and its filling can increase at the

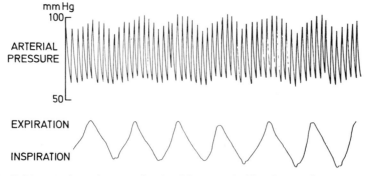

Fig. 5.3 Pulsus paradoxus in a case of pericardial tamponade. Note that systolic pressure and pulse volume are both reduced during inspiration (*courtesy of Dr L. Fananapazir*).

expense of the left ventricle. The resulting shift in the interventricular septum can sometimes be detected by echocardiography (p. 142). When the increased right ventricular stroke volume is eventually transmitted via the pulmonary veins it tends to accentuate the cyclical variation in left ventricular output.

In patients with a very low cardiac output as a result of cardiac tamponade the radial and brachial arteries may be barely palpable, and pulsus paradoxus is better detected in the carotid or femoral pulses. Sometimes the abnormality is found while the blood pressure is being measured, and this is a good way of confirming an impression of paradoxical pulse gained by palpation.

Delayed Pulse. If there is obstruction to blood flow between the heart and the site at which the pulse is felt, pulse volume will be diminished, and the pulse wave itself will be delayed. Delay can be appreciated clinically only if there is another pulse at a similar distance from the heart which can be used for comparison: for example, the femoral pulses are delayed relative to the radial pulse in coarctation of the aorta, and the left brachial pulse might be delayed relative to the right in the presence of left subclavian stenosis.

The Form of the Pulse Wave. When there is increased 'run off' from the arterial tree (p. 132) the pulse wave may rise normally but then declines abruptly. This is termed a *collapsing pulse,* and the most common association in a resting adult patient is with aortic regurgitation. In children, a collapsing pulse may be more readily felt in the femoral arteries, and may be an indication of a persistent ductus arteriosus.

A slow rising pulse, best detected in the carotids, is characteristic of aortic stenosis. Turbulence as blood is forced through the narrowed valve is felt as a carotid thrill or shudder. Sometimes the rate of left ventricular ejection is so slowed as a consequence of beta-blocker therapy that a slow-rising pulse is produced, but without a thrill or murmur.

Increasing rigidity of the arteries gives a more rapid upstroke to the pulse; in the elderly, this can help to obscure the diagnosis of aortic stenosis.

In hypertrophic obstructive cardiomyopathy, left ventricular ejection is initially unimpeded, but is then suddenly 'throttled' by contraction of a muscular ridge in the left ventricular outflow tract. This results in a distinctive 'jerky' quality of the carotid pulses.

Pulsus bisferiens, that is, a pulse with two humps (Fig. 5.4) is sometimes felt in

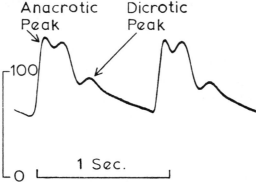

Fig. 5.4 Bisferiens pulse. Intra-arterial tracing from a patient with aortic stenosis and regurgitation. The two palpable elements in this ulse are the anacrotic peak and the second peak.

patients with aortic stenosis and regurgitation. The earlier explanation was that the first, or 'anacrotic' peak represented the force of left ventricular contraction transmitted through the aortic valve, and the second peak was due to the actual ejection of blood into the aorta. A more recent suggestion is that the 'dip' in the pulse is the result of energy dissipation in the production of a loud systolic murmur.

Blood Pressure

Ideally, blood pressure should be measured with the patient as relaxed as possible, that is, at the end of the physical examination. However it is often helpful to be aware of an abnormal pressure at an earlier stage, and there is also some risk that if left to the end this very important measurement may occasionally be forgotten. It is the author's practice to measure the blood pressure immediately after palpating the brachial pulse, and then to repeat the measurement at the end of the examination if there is any suspicion of hypertension.

Blood pressure is usually measured by the cuff method; this is generally taught in the physiology course, so only a few points of technique will be considered here. The normal cuff width for adult use is 12 centimetres — a wider cuff is used for the leg, or for exceptionally fat arms, and a narrower one for children. Too narrow a cuff causes a spuriously high estimate of blood pressure, and this also results if the patients makes a muscular effort in holding up the arm. On the other hand failure to remove tight clothing from the upper arm gives a falsely low estimate. The cuff should be smoothly applied with the centre of the rubber bag over the inner side of the arm. The stethoscope should then be applied over the brachial artery previously palpated and the cuff pressure allowed to fall slowly until the first Korotkov sounds are heard. This corresponds to the systolic pressure, and the radial pulse becomes palpable shortly afterwards. In this way it is possible to avoid an underestimate of the true systolic pressure resulting from the 'auscultatory gap' phenomenon, where the Korotkov sounds transiently disappear between systole and diastole. As pressure in the cuff continues to fall, the sounds become louder and 'ringing' in nature, then suddenly muffled. This point of muffling is called 'phase IV', and in Britain has traditionally been used to indicate the diastolic pressure. It does indeed correlate well with diastolic pressure as measured by intra-arterial recordings, but epidemiological studies have shown that there is less variation between observers if diastolic pressure is recorded at the point of complete disappearance of Korotkov sounds, or 'phase V'. It is good practice to record both the phase IV and phase V pressures: e.g. 150/98–92 where 150mm of mercury is the systolic pressure, 98 the phase IV diastolic and 92 the phase V diastolic pressure. In some normal subjects muffled sounds are still heard as the cuff pressure is reduced to zero, and this is recorded as, for example: 150/95–0. Allowing the pressure in the cuff to fall too rapidly prevents accurate measurement of the diastolic pressure.

There are many possible sources of observer-induced bias in blood pressure recording, and for accurate epidemiological work special apparatus may be needed.

When a difference in the pulse in the two arms is suspected, the blood pressure should be recorded on both sides. When a weak delayed femoral pulse is associated with hypertension in the arms (coarctation of the aorta, p. 111) the blood pressure in the legs should also be recorded, using a broad cuff round the thigh with the patient lying prone and the stethoscope applied to the popliteal artery. Casual records of blood pressure are less reproducible than repeated records with the patient at rest. Emotional factors may elevate the blood pressure remarkably in some patients, and the systolic pressure may be more than 50 mmHg, and the diastolic more than 30 mmHg higher than in subsequent records when the patient has become accustomed to the procedure. Such falls in pressure on repeated examination are often erroneously attributed to treatment provided for hypertension. Devices which record blood pressure continuously demonstrate the temporary hypertensive effect of doctors approaching the patient's bed. While it has been traditional to discount such 'stress induced' hypertension, epidemiological studies suggest it should not be regarded with complacency.

The Jugular Venous Pressure (JVP)

The central venous pressure (which is the same as right atrial pressure) is an important guide to cardiovascular function, and its elevation is an indication of cardiac failure or fluid overload. A useful estimate of central venous pressure can be made, without resort to instruments, by observing the jugular venous pulse.

The internal jugular veins are collapsible, relatively inelastic tubes in direct continuity with the right atrium. The 'normal' right atrial pressure seldom exceeds 5 mm of mercury, which is equivalent to a column of blood roughly 7 cm high. With a patient lying flat, the jugular veins are distended but not visibly pulsatile (Fig. 5.5). If a patient with a normal right atrial pressure sits upright, the upper part

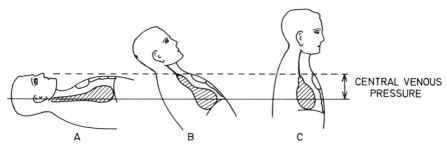

CENTRAL VENOUS PRESSURE

Fig. 5.5 Jugular venous pressure and pulse in normal subject. (A) Supine: jugular vein distended but invisible. (B) Reclining at 45 degrees: point of transition between distended and collapsed vein can usually be seen to pulsate just above the clavicle. (C) Upright: upper part of vein collapsed and transition point obscured by sternum.

of the vein collapses, but the lower part of the vein remains distended for a vertical height of some 7 cm above the middle of the right atrium. In the upright patient the point of transition between distended and collapsed vein is hidden behind the sternum and clavicles, but allowing the patient to recline at 45 degrees usually makes it visible just above the clavicle, where it can be recognised by its characteristic pulsation (Fig. 5.7).

The mean height of jugular venous pulsation above right atrial level is thus a measure of the central venous pressure. Because of the uncertainty which might be introduced by 'guessing' the position of the right atrium, it has become traditional to use the manubriosternal angle as a reference point for measuring the venous pressure. When this is done, it must be ensured that the patient always lies at the same angle, otherwise the measurements will not be comparable. The technique for measuring the JVP is shown in Figure 5.6

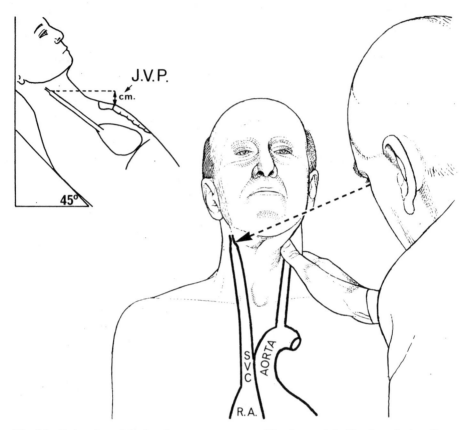

Fig. 5.6 Estimation of the jugular venous pressure. The observer is looking for pulsation of the skin transmitted from the uppermost point of distension of the right internal jugular vein and is feeling the left carotid pulse in order to identify the presystolic *a* wave. Alternatively the examiner may stand on the patient's right side with the left thumb on the patient's right carotid and inspect the pulsation of the skin on the left side of the neck. However the left internal jugular vein may be a less reliable manometer than the right.

A raised jugular venous pressure with visible pulsation may be due to right ventricular failure or overload, to right ventricular inflow obstruction as in constrictive pericarditis or pericardial tamponade, or to abnormalities of the tricuspid valve. Differences in the form of the pulse wave help to distinguish between these possibilities, as described below. Distended jugular veins without pulsation in the upright position may be due to obstruction of the superior vena cava or to a chronic and gross elevation of right atrial pressure sometimes seen in chronic constrictive pericarditis.

The jugular venous pressure normally falls during inspiration as the right atrium and ventricle dilate in response to a lowered intrathoracic pressure. Pressure with the examiner's hand in the right hypochondrium causes a transient rise in jugular venous pressure as the hepatic venous reservoir is compressed. In patients with constrictive pericarditis the jugular pressure may rise during inspiration (Kussmaul's sign) because the congested liver is compressed by the descending diaphragm and the right atrium and ventricle are prevented from distending by the rigid pericardium. This sign is also seen occasionally in severe right ventricular failure.

A low jugular venous pressure may result from haemorrhage or dehydration. An unexpectedly low venous pressure in patients with other signs of cardiac disease is commonly due to diuretic therapy.

It is important not to mistake arterial for venous pulsation in the neck. Points of distinction include:

1. Venous pulsation varies with posture and respiration, and venous pressure is transiently raised by abdominal compression; arterial pulsation is not affected.
2. When the venous pressure is elevated, the most rapid and therefore most prominent pulsatile movement is inward, whereas the most rapid movement in arterial pulsation is outward.
3. In sinus rhythm, there are two waves in the venous pulse to every one in the arterial pulse.
4. Venous pulsation can usually be abolished by gentle digital pressure above the clavicle, whereas arterial pulsation persists.
5. A very high jugular venous pressure may cause pulsatile displacement of the ear lobes, whereas arterial pulsation does not.

Although the external jugular veins are often distended when venous pressure is high, they are an unreliable guide since there is often a valve-like constriction where the external joins the internal jugular. A grossly elevated jugular venous pressure may sometimes be missed because the distended veins do not pulsate: pulsation may become apparent if the patient is placed in a more upright position, or it may be observed that the arm veins remains distended until the patient's hand is raised well above the head.

The Jugular Venous Pulse

Confusion is apt to arise in descriptions of the wave form of the jugular pulse, because jugular pulsation is often difficult to detect in subjects with normal hearts, and patients with readily-discernable jugular pulsation very commonly have some cardiac abnormality. Figure 5.7 shows a pressure tracing recorded from the internal jugular vein in a patient with a normal cardiac function. The a wave coincides with atrial systole, and the early part of the x descent following it is due to atrial relaxation. Continuation of the x descent is due to retraction of the tricuspid valve during early right ventricular systole. Continuing venous return while the tricuspid valve is closed causes right atrial pressure to rise again, and it reaches a second peak, called a v wave at the end of ventricular systole. Ventricular relaxation and tricuspid valve opening then cause a second fall in atrial pressure (the y descent) as the pent-up venous blood floods into the ventricle. The c wave, an extra wave transmitted from the carotid artery, is sometimes seen between a and v waves.

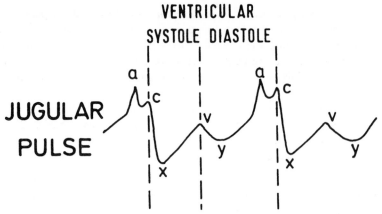

Fig. 5.7   Form of the venous pulse wave tracing from internal jugular vein. a = atrial systole; c = onset of ventricular systole; v = peak pressure in right atrium immediately prior to opening of tricuspid valve; a − x = x descent, due to atrial relaxation; v − y = y descent at commencement of ventricular filling.

Exaggerated *a* waves in the jugular pulse are a hallmark of right atrial hypertrophy. This may be due to tricuspid stenosis, or more commonly to right ventricular hypertrophy with an associated increase in ventricular 'stiffness'. They are readily recognised by being presystolic, especially when timed against the carotid pulse (Fig. 5.6). The prominence of the *x* descent is usually related to the size of the *a* wave. In cases of atrioventricular dissociation, for example complete heart block, atrial and ventricular systole sometimes coincide. Atrial contraction against a closed tricuspid valve then causes a strikingly large venous pulsation, called a cannon wave. Regular cannon waves may occur in patients with a ventricular pacemaker but intact retrograde conduction from ventricle to atrium, and are easily mistaken for a sign of tricuspid regurgitation (see below).

Tricuspid regurgitation, whether resulting from damage to the tricuspid valve or simply from dilatation of its annulus secondary to right ventricular failure, is characterised by exaggerated systolic venous pulsation (Fig. 5.8). Traditionally these waves are called *v* waves, which is unfortunate as their mechanism and timing are different from the physiological *v* waves described above. However to coin a new name for them would only add to confusion. The *v* waves of tricuspid regurgitation occur in mid-systole, are often accompanied by palpable venous pulsation, and in severe cases a tricuspid regurgitant murmur and a pulsatile liver can also be detached.

When the JVP is elevated, the *y* descent after tricuspid valve opening is usually the most prominent feature of the venous pulse, provided tricuspid regurgitation is absent. In the presence of right ventricular failure ventricular stiffness is increased and this tends to produce some 'damping' of the *y* descent. In constrictive pericarditis however initial ventricular filling is unimpeded, only to be brought to a sudden halt as the limits set by the pericardium are reached. The resulting combination of a raised venous pressure and a precipitous early phase of the *y* descent is often striking. Tricuspid stenosis on the other hand gives a slow *y* and *x* descent, together with large a waves.

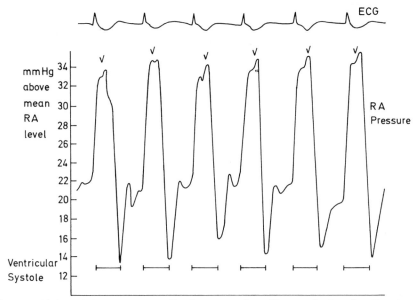

Fig. 5.8 Right atrial pressure recording in severe tricuspid regurgitation. Systolic pulse waves of large amplitude are present, and unlike the physiological *v* waves (Fig. 5.7) they start in early systole. The patient is in atrial fibrillation, so *a* waves are absent.

At first reading, some of the foregoing may appear to be formidable minutiae but their correct interpretation can provide valuable clinical evidence.

Cardiac and Vasomotor Reflexes

The normal function of the heart and vascular system is co-ordinated by a series of reflexes. Attempts to elicit these reflexes in patients with suspected disease may throw light on cardiovascular function on the one hand, and on that of the autonomic nervous system on the other.

The Carotid Sinus Reflex. Bradycardia produced by pressure on the carotid sinus has been described on page 109. In some patients this manoeuvre may also cause vasodilatation. The converse is tachycardia and vasoconstriction mediated via carotid sinus and aortic arch baroreceptors to compensate for circumstances such as a change in posture which might otherwise result in hypotension. There is normally an increase in pulse rate when a person stands up, but this is not seen in patients, e.g. diabetics, with autonomic neuropathy. The response is also reduced by beta-blockade. If the vasoconstrictor response is deficient, postural hypotension may occur; the commonest cause is medication with antihypertensive drugs, but sometimes postural hypotension may be due not to a deficient reflex, but to hypovolaemia.

The Valsalva Manoeuvre. This is a forced attempt at expiration when the mouth is shut and the nose held closed. It was originally devised as a method of inflating the eustachian tubes, but it is also a convenient way of stimulating certain cardiac reflexes. During the straining period the high intrathoracic pressure impedes venous return, and cardiac output falls. Reflex tachycardia occurs, and arteriolar constriction helps to limit the fall in blood pressure. When straining is relaxed, cardiac output increases rapidly, and in the presence of persisting vasoconstriction the blood pressure rises abruptly and may 'overshoot' the resting level. This in turn evokes the baroreceptor reflex and causes a final phase of relative bradycardia and vasodilatation (Fig. 5.9). The tachycardia during the Valsalva manoeuvre and the bradycardia afterwards are often detectable with the fingers on the radial pulse. In patients with cardiac failure, or with autonomic neuropathy, the tachycardia, 'overshoot' and bradycardia do not occur, and intra-arterial blood-pressure recordings show a characteristic 'square wave' response (Fig. 5.10).

The Valsalva manoeuvre can be used, in the absence of cardiac failure, to ascribe a murmur to the left or right side of the heart. Murmurs originating on either side tend to become quieter during the attempted expiration because venous return is reduced, but murmurs arising on the right side become louder immediately straining ceases, while those arising on the left regain their intensity about six beats later. An exception is the systolic murmur of hypertrophic obstructive cardiomyopathy which gets louder during the straining because reduced ventricular filling tends to increase the degree of obstruction.

EXAMINATION OF THE HEART

Inspection

Inspection of the chest with particular relevance to the heart includes the detection of deformity and both normal and abnormal pulsation.

Emphysema and severe kyphosis or scoliosis may be recognised by inspection alone; either of these conditions can lead to heart failure. Skeletal abnormalities such as pectus excavatum or kyphoscoliosis may be part of Marfan's syndrome in which congenital abnormalities of the heart and aorta are common. In those forms of congenital heart disease in which gross pulmonary arterial hypertension is a feature during the growing period, e.g. in some large ventricular septal defects, there may be prominence of the left chest over the hypertrophied right ventricle, and a bilateral Harrison's sulcus (p. 166) may be seen. The tense pulmonary arteries reduce lung compliance, the pull of the diaphragm is increased and the chest wall may be distorted at its attachment to the ribs just as in those who suffer from severe asthma during the growing period.

The forceful apical thrust of left ventricular hypertrophy, the diffuse left parasternal impulse of right ventricular hypertrophy, and the pulsation of an enlarged pulmonary artery in the second left intercostal space may all be detected on inspection. An aneurysm of the aorta may produce a pulsation in the second right intercostal space or of the upper sternum. When the heart is much enlarged the chest wall may be seen to move with each heart beat.

Epigastric pulsation transmitted from the abdominal aorta is a normal finding, particularly in thin people. Pulsation in this region may however also be abnormal due to enlargement of the right ventricle, abdominal aneurysm or to pulsation of the liver as a result of tricuspid regurgitation.

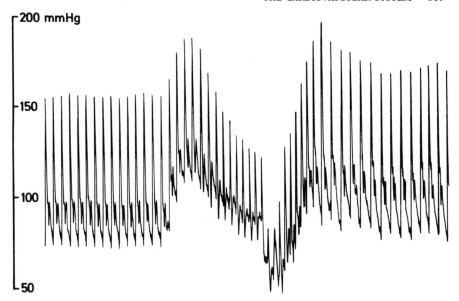

Fig. 5.9   Valsalva manoeuvre in a healthy subject. This shows (i) increase in arterial pressure at the onset of the rise of intra-thoracic pressure, (ii) the subsequent fall due to the obstruction of venous return and (iii) the reflex tachycardia and maintenance of mean arterial pressure by peripheral vasoconstriction during the straining period. When the straining period comes to an end, the arterial pressure temporarily drops to be followed by an increase in pressure and a reflex slowing in heart rate. In vasomotor paralysis there is no such rise in pressure or fall in rate (*courtesy of Dr L. Fananapazir*).

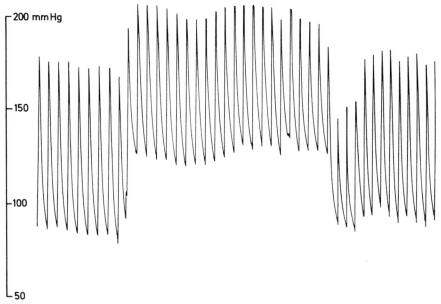

Fig. 5.10   Valsalva manoeuvre in cardiac failure. During the straining period, the venous return and the cardiac output are unaltered and the rise in arterial pressure reflects the increment due to the rise in intra-thoracic pressure. This is the typical 'square wave' response of cardiac failure (*courtesy of Dr L. Fananapazir*).

Palpation

Discriminating palpation of the chest is one of the most valuable methods in the examination of the heart, and can often enable prediction of some at least of the findings on auscultation. The right hand is first placed on the left chest wall with the middle finger lying in about the fifth intercostal space in the anterior axillary line. The position of the apex beat is then defined, if possible, and the quality of the apical impulse noted. Abnormal vibrations (see thrills below) are also sought. The hand is then placed to the left of the sternum and then on the manubrium and any pulsations and thrills again noted.

Apex Beat. The position of the apex beat is best defined as the furthest point downwards and outwards on the chest wall where the finger is lifted by the cardiac impulse. The patient should be semi-recumbent for the heart moves to a variable extent on standing or turning to one side. The normal apex beat is within the mid-clavicular line in the fifth interspace. The second costal cartilage is at the level of the manubriosternal angle whence the interspaces can readily be identified. When displaced, the site of the apex beat should be described in terms of intercostal space and with reference to mid-clavicular, anterior axillary and mid-axillary lines. Many students are puzzled by the fact that the finger is lifted during systole, when the ventricle is contracting. This due to the complex rotatory movement of the heart with systole, one effect of which is a forward movement of the apex. Sometimes the apex beat cannot be felt. The common causes of this are obesity or emphysema, and in the latter case the heart sounds may be faint or inaudible. A pericardial effusion may also make the heart beat impalpable. Very rarely as a congenital abnormality the heart lies on the right side (*dextrocardia*), but this should be revealed if due attention is paid to the site of maximum intensity of the heart sounds.

The apex beat may be displaced, or even impalpable, because of disease of the lung or pleura; then the trachea may be deviated (p. 164) and abnormalities found on examination of the chest. The apex beat may also be displaced because of cardiac enlargement. The apical impulse is abnormally forceful in left ventricular hypertrophy, and the terms heaving, thrusting or sustained are commonly used to describe it. In mitral stenosis, on the other hand, the abnormally increased shock of closure of the mitral valve may be palpable in which case the sensation is like that of an unusually hard knock on the other side of a closed door.

The best evidence of right ventricular hypertrophy is a diffuse impulse to the left of the sternum. As already described, these physical signs may be partially or completely obscured by obesity or emphysema. In emphysema there may be considerable right ventricular hypertrophy which cannot be detected in life, because the over-inflated lung intervenes between the heart and the chest wall.

Thrills. Murmurs (p. 128) may be so loud as to be palpable as thrills, the most common examples being the apical diastolic thrill of mitral stenosis and the basal systolic thrill of aortic stenosis (often accompanied by a suprasternal thrill and carotid 'shudder' p. 130). Thrills are best appreciated when the patient leans forward with the breath held in expiration, with the exception of the thrill of mitral stenosis which is most easily felt when the patient turns on to the left side. The back of a purring cat traditionally and accurately provides the nearest palpable equivalent to the diastolic thrill of mitral stenosis; systolic thrills are more nearly imitated by a bluebottle trapped in the hand. The upper left parasternal systolic thrill of pulmonary stenosis, and the lower left parasternal systolic thrill of a ventricular septal defect, are the most common examples among the congenital causes. A diastolic thrill over the sternum is very uncommon, occurring only with rupture or eversion of an aortic valve cusp causing gross aortic regurgitation. A suspected thrill is denied by the subsequent finding that there is either no murmur or only a very quiet one.

Other Palpable Abnormalities. When the semilunar valves close under an abnormally high pressure there may be a palpable shock at the upper end of the sternum. When this is due to closure of the pulmonary valves, it is often most readily appreciated to the left of the sternum. An aneurysm of the arch of the aorta may produce a pulsation which is generally maximal in the second right intercostal space, but which may also lift the sternum. Likewise, a dilated pulmonary artery may give a palpable pulse to the left of the sternum at about the second left intercostal space. Occasionally pericardial fraction (p. 135) is palpable.

Percussion

There is usually an area of dullness to percussion to the left of the sternum where the heart lies against the chest. This area is reduced or absent in many cases of emphysema. There may be abnormal dullness to percussion to the right of the sternum when a large pericardial effusion is present. Massive enlargement of the left atrium occurs occasionally in rheumatic disease of the mitral valve, usually with gross mitral regurgitation and the resultant dullness posteriorly has been mistaken for a pleural effusion. A large aneurysm of the aorta may produce an area of abnormal dullness to the right of the upper sternum. Percussion is usually employed only when these conditions are suspected. A radiograph of the chest provides more reliable evidence.

Auscultation

There is no need to put oneself at disadvantage by purchasing an inefficient stethoscope. The bell, with the chest piece lightly pressed against the skin, is best for conducting low pitched sounds and murmurs and the diaphragm, firmly applied, is used for detecting high pitched sounds or a very quiet early diastolic murmur; both are therefore required. The most popular stethoscope at the present time is the compact and lightweight Littman pattern (Fig. 5.11). The genuine

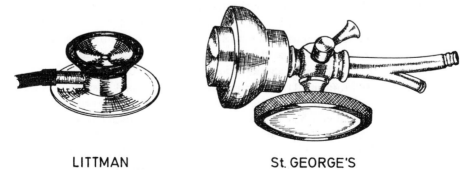

LITTMAN   St. GEORGE'S

Fig. 5.11 Stethoscope chest pieces. In the St George's model there is, in addition to a diaphragm, the choice of a small or a large bell. The latter slides forward to incorporate the former.

Littman stethoscope is efficient, but cheaper imitations vary greatly in quality. The St George's stethoscope is a more cumbersome but highly effective instrument preferred by many cardiologists: it has an extra-large bell for detecting low pitched murmurs and can be fitted with a steel diaphragm which accentuates high pitched sounds.

In all stethoscopes the ear pieces must fit comfortably and the spring must be strong enough to hold them in place. The tubing should be about 25 cm in length, thick enough to reduce external noise and of similar bore to the metal parts, i.e. about 3 mm.

Method in the Use of the Stethoscope. The novice is liable to be overwhelmed by the wealth of auscultatory phenomena described by cardiologists. Expertise comes with time and practice. In the first few months the student will be doing well if the first and second heart sounds can be identified, and murmurs accurately classified as systolic or diastolic. It is best in describing auscultatory findings to be modest but accurate rather than detailed but wrong.

Correct *timing* is essential, and it is good practice to feel the patient's carotid pulse with the thumb of one hand whilst the other hand holds the stethoscope to the precordium. The author starts auscultation at the cardiac apex, but others prefer to begin in the pulmonary area; students need to establish their own routine. Whatever the order, it is essential to listen at the apex, to the left and right of both upper and lower parts of the sternum, and beneath the clavicles. It is best to make a rapid survey of all these sites using the diaphragm of the stethoscope, and then to return for a longer period to those sites where an abnormality was heard, or to the best sites (see below) for detecting specific lesions suggested by the history and other parts of the examination.

Pulmonary valve closure and pulmonary ejection murmurs are usually best heard in the second or third intercostal spaces to the left of the sternum, and aortic ejection murmurs in a corresponding site to the right of the sternum. These sites are sometimes called the *pulmonary and aortic areas* respectively, but it must be appreciated that they are several centimetres away from the surface projection of the valves themselves (Fig. 5.12). At these sites most trained auscultators prefer to use the diaphragm of the stethoscope, since by filtering out low-pitched sounds it tends to accentuate the high-pitched sounds of aortic or pulmonary valve closure and of most ejection murmurs. At the apex, it is always necessary to listen with both the diaphragm and the bell of the stethoscope, as only the latter will detect low-pitched sounds such as the third heart sound or the mid-diastolic murmur of mitral stenosis. If heart sounds are not well heard at the apex, the patient should be asked to roll on to the left side. It is also essential to auscultate in this position if mitral stenosis is to be excluded. Conversely, the second heart sound and early diastolic murmurs are best heard if the patient sits up and leans forward.

Auscultatory Notation. Traditionally, the first and second heart sounds are said to sound like 'lub-dup'. This type of description, though evocative, is clumsy and lacking in precision when applied to more complex auscultatory findings. Phonocardiography, a technique for visually displaying heart sounds either on paper or on an oscilloscope screen, has provided the basis for a more flexible graphical notation for auscultation. Figure 5.13 shows a phonocardiogram recorded from a normal heart. The first and second heart sounds appear as vertical 'blips' on

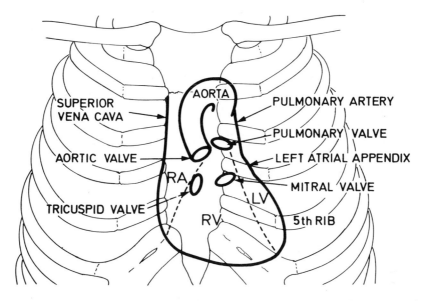

Fig. 5.12   The surface markings of the valves in relationship to the radiological outline of the heart. The directions in which sounds and murmurs are preferentially conducted from the valves are described on pages 128 to 135.

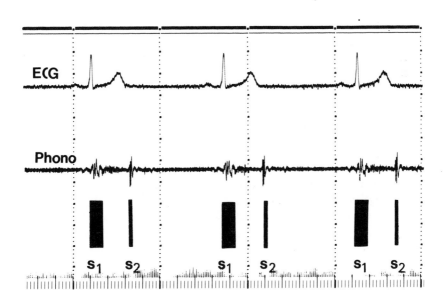

Fig. 5.13 Auscultatory notation. The relationship between a phonocardiogram (the graphic recording of the heart sounds) and the conventional 'shorthand' auscultatory notation.

either side of a baseline. The height of the blip depends on the loudness of the sound, and the width on its duration. The conventional shorthand auscultatory notation is simply a sketch of what might be seen on phonocardiography, using vertical lines or oblong blocks to represent the heart sounds, and shading to represent murmurs. By convention, systole is always represented by the space between the heart sounds, early diastole by the space after the second heart sound, and late diastole by the space before the first heart sound. These conventions will become clearer when the timing of individual murmurs and other sounds is discussed presently.

The Heart Sounds. Conventionally, there are first, second, third and fourth heart sounds. The first and second sounds (S_1 and S_2 in shorthand) are virtually always audible. The third and fourth (S_3 and S_4) become prominent only under special circumstances. Other sounds audible during the cardiac cycle but distinguished from murmurs by their short duration are sometimes grouped together as 'added sounds', although their causes are very diverse. They include the opening snap of mitral stenosis, ejection clicks arising in the aorta or pulmonary artery, mid-systolic clicks associated with mitral valve prolapse, and the sounds associated with mechanical prosthetic heart valves. The student will find that if attention is concentrated initially on the first and second heart sounds, identification of other heart sounds will come later.

THE FIRST HEART SOUND. This is principally the sound of mitral valve closure. Tricuspid valve closure is usually very quiet, but may be loud if right ventricular pressure is elevated. The loudness of the first heart sound varies with the position of the mitral valve cusps at the onset of systole. If the cusps are wide apart they are 'slammed' together to produce a loud S_1, but if they are close together at the onset of systole then S_1 tends to be quiet. The first sound thus tends to be prominent in patients with an increased cardiac output, and may be almost inaudible in severe cardiac failure. Beat to beat variation in intensity of S_1 occurs in atrial fibrillation, and also in atrio-ventricular dissociation, where the relation between atrial and ventricular systole is constantly changing. A loud S_1 is also characteristic of mitral stenosis, but the mechanism is different; here the abnormal valve acts as a rather stiff diaphragm which is suddenly tensed by the chordae tendiniae as the ventricle contracts. The resulting shock wave is not only heard as a loud S_1 but may also be felt on palpation of the precordium.

THE SECOND HEART SOUND. This is due to the closure of aortic and pulmonary valves at the end of ventricular systole. It is usually best heard at the upper left sternal edge using the diaphragm of the stethoscope. During quiet expiration the components of S_2 which are due to aortic valve closure (sometimes called A_2) and to pulmonary valve closure (P_2) are virtually inseparable. During inspiration P_2 tends to be delayed because of increased venous return, while A_2 occurs a little sooner because left ventricular filling is slightly reduced. The second heart sound may then become *split* — the earlier component is due to aortic and the latter to pulmonary valve closure (Fig. 5.14). This normal or physiological splitting of the second heart sound is easy to detect in children or young adults, but becomes much more difficult to hear in older patients. Like sinus arrhythmia, physiological splitting of the second heart sound disappears in the presence of heart failure.

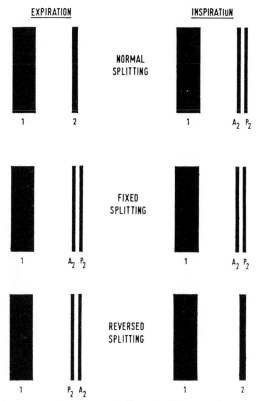

Fig. 5.14 Splitting of the second heart sound. Shown in diagrammatic representations of phonocardiograms.

Delayed closure of the pulmonary valve tends to occur when the right ventricle is dilated, when there is obstruction to right ventricular emptying as in pulmonary stenosis, or when there is delay in the electrical activation of the right ventricle as indicated by the appearance of right bundle branch block on the ECG. All these can lead to exaggerated splitting of the second heart sound, but the width of the split still tends to increase with inspiration and decrease with expiration.

In atrial septal defect the increase in right ventricular stroke volume as a consquence of a left to right shunt at atrial level causes wide splitting of the second heart sound, but because right and left atria are in free communication right and left ventricular stroke volumes vary in the same way during the respiratory cycle. The result is *fixed splitting* of the second heart sound which is pathognomic of atrial septal defect.

Chronic pulmonary hypertension does not in itself cause exaggerated splitting of the second sound, because, although the right ventricle is ejecting blood against a higher pressure, the actual ejection time of the hypertrophied ventricle is not appreciably prolonged. Both systemic and pulmonary hypertension may cause the second sound to be excessively loud, but the effect is more striking with pulmonary hypertension because the pulmonary valve lies closer to the chest wall. With severe pulmonary hypertension the shock of pulmonary valve closure may be palpable.

If left ventricular ejection is abnormally delayed, P_2 may occur before A_2, and the second sound splits in expiration and comes together in inspiration. This *reversed splitting* of the second sound is often striking in hypertrophic obstructive cardiomyopathy (p. 131). It may also occur in aortic stenosis, but here it can be difficult to detect because rigidity of the valve may make A_2 very quiet.

THE THIRD HEART SOUND (S_3). This sound coincides with the end of the rapid period of ventricular diastolic filling. It is analogous to the sound produced when a slack sail suddenly fills with wind. Usually S_3 is low-pitched and best heard at the apex with the stethoscope bell; it is sometimes palpable. Occasionally S_3 is loud and the casual auscultator mistakes it for S_2 (Fig. 5.15).

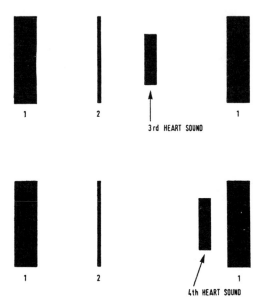

Fig. 5.15   Third and fourth heart sounds. The third sound coincides with the onset of ventricular filling, and the fourth sound with the ventricular filling which results from atrial contraction. The third and fourth sounds are heard at the cardiac apex when they arise in the left ventricle, and to the left of the lower sternum when their origin is in the right ventricle. (Diagrammatic representations of phonocardiograms.)

A third sound is 'physiological' in healthy young adults and particularly in athletes, with their slow resting pulse rate and large stroke volume. In older patients, and especially when it as associated with tachycardia and other signs of cardiac failure, its presence indicates imparied ventricular function, and specifically, a raised end-diastolic pressure. The combination of tachycardia and a loud S_3 gives a characteristic cadence to the heart sounds described as a *gallop rhythm*, or more prosaically, a *triple rhythm*. A third sound can originate from either ventricle, and the one responsible is usually deduced from the circumstances rather than the quality of the sound.

THE FOURTH HEART SOUND (S_4) This sound accompanies, and is due to, atrial systole. It can be heard only in the presence of sinus rhythm. Although phonocardiography can detect a quiet S_4 in many normal subjects, it tends to become particularly prominent when a hypertrophied left atrium pumps blood through an unobstructed mitral valve into a stiff left ventricle; these conditions are most often fulfilled in ischaemic heart disease or systemic hypertension. It is usually a rather low-pitched sound best heard at the apex with the bell of the stethoscope. Tachycardia with a fourth heart sound may also produce a triple or gallop rhythm. In patients with a sufficiently slow heart rate it is sometimes possible to make out fourth, first, second and third heart sounds, but as the heart rate increases third and fourth sounds tend to merge.

THE OPENING SNAP. This is a high-pitched sound which occurs in patients with mitral stenosis when the stenosed valve moves forward towards the left ventricle at the beginning of diastole. It is best heard with the diaphragm of the stethoscope, and is sometimes more obvious at the left sternal edge than at the apex. Occasionally it is mistaken for a widely split second sound. A loud opening snap implies that the valve, though stenosed, is still mobile. As the valve stiffens and calcifies the opening snap may become quieter or disappear. The interval between the second heart sound and the opening snap gets shorter with increasing left atrial pressure, and thus with more severe mitral stenosis.

EJECTION CLICKS. These are high-pitched sounds which closely follow the first heart sound. They originate from either the aortic valve and aorta or pulmonary valve and pulmonary artery. Aortic ejection clicks tend to be best heard in the 'aortic area' at the upper right sternal edge, and pulmonary ejection clicks in the 'pulmonary area' to the left of the upper sternum. Aortic ejection clicks are most commonly associated with congenitally bicuspid aortic valves or congenital aortic stenosis, and are probably due principally to the opening of the abnormal cusps. Ejection of blood into a dilated ascending aorta may also play a part. Similarly, pulmonary ejection clicks are most commonly due to valvular pulmonary stenosis, but can also be heard in patients with idiopathic dilatation of the pulmonary artery, or with pulmonary artery dilatation caused by pulmonary hypertension.

MID-SYSTOLIC CLICKS. It used to be taught that clicks occuring in the middle of systole were of extracardiac origin, but in fact mitral valve prolapse (p. 131) is the commonest cause of these added sounds. A small pneumothorax may also cause a regular systolic click (p. 180).

PROSTHETIC VALVE SOUNDS. Replacement heart valves may be grafts of suitably treated animal (usually porcine) tissue, or may be artificial mechanical valves such as the Starr-Edwards ball valve or the Bjork-Shiley disc valve. 'Biological' heart valves produce similar heart sounds to the natural valves they replace. Mechanical valves usually produce two sounds or clicks for each cardiac cycle: a quiet opening click and a louder closing sound. With a mitral prosthesis the loud closing sound accompanies (and largely constitutes) the first heart sound, and the opening click follows the second sound in a similar position to the opening snap of mitral stenosis. Conversely, with an aortic prosthesis the opening sound follows S_1 in a similar position to an ejection click, while the louder closing sound accompanies S_2. Careful recording of prosthetic sounds is important in reviewing patients after heart valve replacement, because disappearance or muffling of a previously-documented opening sound is an early indication of thrombosis in the valve.

The relationship of the normal and added sounds to the events and timing of the cardiac cycle is summarised in Table 5.1.

Table 5.1   Normal and added sounds related to events and timing of the cardiac cycle

Sound	Event	Timing
First sound	Closure of AV valves	
Ejection sound	Opening of semilunar valves	SYSTOLE
Second sound	Closure of semilunar valves	————
Opening snap	Opening of abnormal AV valves (e.g. in mitral stenosis)	
Third sound	Ventricular filling begins	DIASTOLE
Fourth sound	Ventricular filling increases with atrial contraction	

Murmurs

Attention must be paid to the intensity, quality and timing of a murmur. Murmurs arise from turbulent blood flow and they tend to be propagated in the same direction as the flow. Obviously, the louder a murmur is, the further it will be propagated, irrespective of its site of origin. In the analysis of a murmur its timing and quality are the most important distinguishing features; the latter has to be learned from experience, although recordings may be of help. In regard to timing, murmurs are classified, in the first instance, as systolic, diastolic or continuous.

The significance of a systolic murmur depends mainly on its intensity, for when quiet it may be due only to an increased blood flow. In pregnancy or anaemia, for example, a murmur ot this type is often heard in the pulmonary area. A diastolic murmur is almost invariably significant however quiet it may be.

The intensity of a murmur is often described in terms of grades, as follows:

GRADE 1. Just audible in a quiet room, with the patient's breath held and using a good stethoscope.

GRADE 2. Quiet.

GRADE 3. Moderately loud.

GRADE 4. Loud, and accompanied by a thrill.

GRADE 5. Very loud.

GRADE 6. Audible without a stethoscope and with the head away from the chest. Such a murmur may sometimes be heard with the stethoscope chest-piece on top of the patient's head, on the sacrum or at the wrists and even by the patient's spouse.

Murmurs of Grade 4 and louder are accompanied by a palpable thrill. It is unusual for competent observers to record more than one grade difference after listening to the same murmur. The record should state, for example, Grade 5/6 murmur, i.e. fifth out of six grades, so that the number of grades used is made clear.

Systolic Murmurs. These are divided into (1.) ejection systolic murmurs, (2.) pansystolic murmurs (sometimes called holosystolic in the United States) and (3.) late systolic murmurs.

1. EJECTION SYSTOLIC MURMURS. These result from turbulent blood flow through distorted or stenotic semilunar valves, or occasionally from turbulence

caused by increased bloodflow through normal semilunar valves. The murmur increases to a crescendo about the middle of systole, then diminishes and ceases just before the second heart sound. The murmur may be preceded by an ejection click (p. 127). The crescendo-decrescendo nature of the murmur gives a 'diamond shaped' pattern on the phonocardiograph (Fig. 5.17) and this is also used in the 'shorthand notation' for the murmur (Fig. 5.16). It is wrong however to speak of 'diamond shaped murmurs'.

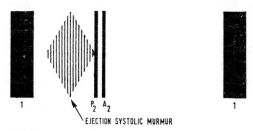

EJECTION SYSTOLIC MURMUR

Fig. 5.16 Ejection systolic murmur (aortic stenosis). The aortic element of the second heart sound is delayed and a split second heart sound results.

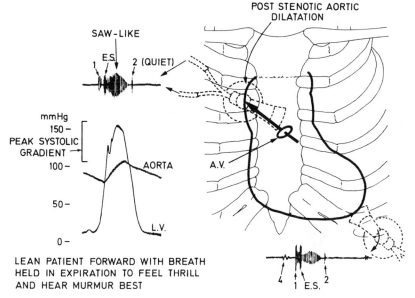

Fig. 5.17 Aortic stenosis. There is a systolic pressure gradient across the stenotic aortic valve (AV). The resultant high velocity jet (arrow) impinges on the wall of the aorta.and the diaphragm placed near to this on the chest detects the murmur best: alternatively the bell may be placed in the suprasternal notch. The phonocardiograms show the ejection systolic murmur preceded by an ejection sound (ES). A fourth heart sound may be heard at the apex.

EXAMPLES OF EJECTION SYSTOLIC MURMURS. The murmur of *aortic stenosis* (Figs. 5.16 and 5.17) was called a 'bruit de scie' (i.e. a saw-like murmur) by Laënnec, the founder of the stethoscopic art. The acoustic quality and the acceleration and deceleration of the saw provide a precise analogy. It is usually loudest·in the second right intercostal space or suprasternal notch, and radiates to the neck. With calcific aortic stenosis it sometimes has a mewing quality like the cry of a seagull. If the aortic stenosis is severe, and left ventricular function well preserved, there is usually an accompanying thrill, and in the carotid arteries the turbulence is felt as a carotid shudder. With the onset of cardiac failure the murmur may become surprisingly soft. The murmur is generally better heard at the apex than it is over the right ventricle, and occasionally may be louder at the apex than it is at the base. An ejection sound (p. 127) strongly favours valvular stenosis; in every other respect the murmur of the much rarer subvalvular stenosis is clinically similar.

Pulmonary Stenosis. This murmur is of similar quality to that of aortic stenosis, and at the same level, but loudest in the second left intercostal space. The murmur radiates towards the left shoulder.

Atrial Septal Defect. The increased pulmonary blood flow of an atrial septal defect also may produce a pulmonary ejection systolic murmur but this is not usually of more than grade 3/6 intensity. The flow of blood through the defect itself does not produce a murmur. The second sound may be split throughout the respiratory cycle in both pulmonary stenosis and atrial septal defects, due to delay in onset, or a prolongation, of right ventricular ejection, but fixed splitting is a characteristic of atrial septal defet (p. 125). A mid-diastolic murmur in the tricuspid area indicates turbulent flow at the tricuspid valve and strongly favours an atrial septal defect; it is the only diastolic murmur which sounds like a systolic murmur. It never rumbles like that of mitral stenosis.

2. PANSYSTOLIC MURMURS. These are so called because they extend throughout systole, and they are the result of escape of blood from a ventricle into an area of low pressure, as with a leaking atrio-ventricular valve, or a small ventricular septal defect. The murmur has little mid-systolic accentuation, and, unlike the ejection murmur, starts simultaneously with the first heart sound and may spill over into early diastole, for the pressure gradient responsible for the abnormal flow persists after closure of the semilunar valves (Fig. 5.18). The distincton between an ejection type systolic murmur and a pansystolic murmur can usually be made with the stethoscope, but occasionally may be impossible even with a phonocardiogram.

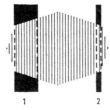 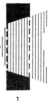

Fig. 5.18 **Pansystolic murmur** as with mitral regurgitation.

EXAMPLES OF PANSYSTOLIC MURMURS. *Mitral regurgitation* of significance usually produces an apical pansystolic murmur, radiating to the axilla and often heard over the lower left chest at the back. It may be as loud as grade 5/6. The increased forward flow through the valve in diastole often produces a low-pitched short mid-diastolic murmur of abrupt onset, or a third heart sound, but when some mitral stenosis coexists atrio-ventricular flow is throttled, and the murmur is longer and less abrupt in onset.

Tricuspid regurgitation usually produces a pansystolic murmur audible over the right ventricle to the left of the sternum in the fourth intercostal space. A much enlarged right ventricle may extend to the left anterior axillary line, and under these circumstancs the murmur is often mistaken for that of mitral regurgitation. The explanation already given for the diastolic murmur or third sound of mitral regurgitation applies to a similar murmur or sound at the left sternal edge in the fourth interspace accompanying tricuspid regurgitation. A tricuspid regurgitant murmur is usually accompanied by a systolic jugular venous pulse wave and often by systolic expansion of the liver. These are common findings in heart failure from rheumatic or ischaemic heart disease, or with chronic cor pulmonale.

Ventricular Septal Defect. A pansystolic murmur to the left of the sternum is the characteristic murmur of a jet of blood through this defect. It has a typical rough quality, like the tearing of fabric, and is usually accompanied by a thrill. When the defect is small this is the only physical sign. When it is larger the shunt is responsible also for an apical mid-diastolic murmur of increased flow through the mitral valve.

3. LATE SYSTOLIC MURMURS. These are systolic murmurs which do not start immediately after the first heart sound, but begin later in systole.

Hypertrophic obstructive cardiomyopathy is sometimes associated with a straightforward ejection systolic murmur, but in other patients the obstruction to left ventricular ejection develops only in mid-systole, and the result is a mid or late systolic murmur. The timing of the murmur, as well as its intensity, may vary with left ventricular volume, and can be affected by posture or the Valsalva manoeuvre. In addition to the murmur, there may be a loud S_4 and reversed splitting of S_2.

Mitral valve prolapse is another cause of a late systolic murmur. In this condition elongation or rupture of the chordae tendineae tethering the mitral valve to the left ventricular papillary muscles allows a portion of one of the mitral valve leaflets to prolapse into the left atrium during systole. The prolapse itself may be accompanied by a mid-systolic click (p. 127) and the mitral regurgitation which may result gives rise to a murmur. Sometimes the mid-systolic click (or clicks) is not associated with a murmur, and in other patients prolapse occurs at the onset of systole and the resulting pansystolic murmur is indistinguishable from that due to other causes of mitral regurgitation. Both the click and the murmur of mitral prolapse may vary strikingly with posture and phase of respiration; in some cases they can be heard only when the patient stands up. Echocardiography (p. 142) is very useful in confirming the diagnosis.

Diastolic Murmurs. The three main types of diastolic murmur are (1) those of leaking semi-lunar valves, which are loudest in early diastole when the pressure gradient is highest, and which are decrescendo; these are termed *early diastolic murmurs;* (2) the murmurs of turbulent blood flow at the atrio-ventricular valves, which start slightly later in diastole and are therefore sometimes called *mid-diastolic* or *delayed diastolic murmurs;* and (3) murmurs due to turbulence at one of the AV valves resulting from atrial contraction, so-called *presystolic,* or *atrial systolic* murmurs (Fig. 5.19).

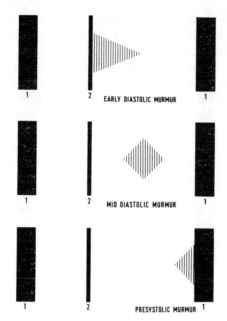

Fig. 5.19 Diastolic murmurs.

EXAMPLES OF DIASTOLIC MURMURS. *Aortic regurgitation* produces a blowing early diastolic murmur of all grades of intensity (Fig. 5.20). When very soft it resembles a breath sound, and can then be detected only when breathing is arrested

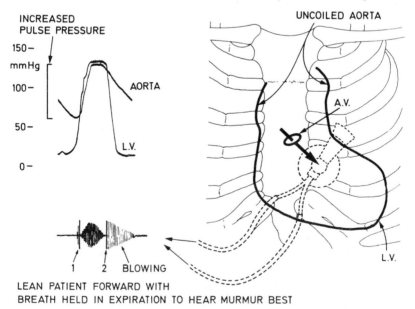

Fig. 5.20 Aortic regurgitation. The pulse pressure is usually increased; the jet from the aortic valve (AV) impinges on the interventricular septum (arrow) during diastole, producing a high pitched murmur which is best heard with the diaphragm. The phonocardiogram also shows the systolic murmur which is common because of the increased flow through the aortic valve in systole.

in expiration, and with the patient leaning forward. In aortic regurgitation of rheumatic origin the murmur is usually loudest to the left of the sternum in the fourth intercostal space; in syphilitic aortic regurgitation the murmur is often louder to the right of the sternum. Even the quietest aortic diastolic murmur cannot be ignored, and finding it may be of great clinical importance when infective endocarditis is suspected. In practice the murmur is often overlooked, and if the proper steps have been followed this is usually because the listener has not attuned his hearing to the necessary high pitch required.

Pulmonary regurgitation produces a murmur which is similar in quality and site to that of aortic regurgitation. A loud second heart sound to the left of the sternum or other features associated with pulmonary arterial hypertension favour pulmonary regurgitation as the cause of the murmur. Pulmonary regurgitation is much less common than aortic regurgitation. The murmur of pulmonary regurgitation is often called the *Graham Steell* murmur after the cardiologist who first described it; he called it the murmur of high pressure in the pulmonary artery long before it was possible to measure this pressure in man. It occurs with pulmonary arterial hypertension, e.g. in some cases of mitral stenosis or pulmonary arterial thromboembolism.

Mitral stenosis betrays itself to the stethoscope even when in all other respects the patient is normal (Fig. 5.21). The jet through the stenosed mitral valve impinges on the endocardium of the left ventricle at the apex, and the resulting turbulence shows itself as a murmur best heard at the site of the apical impulse. Duroziez described the auscultatory findings in mitral stenosis as FFOUT-TA-TA-ROU, where

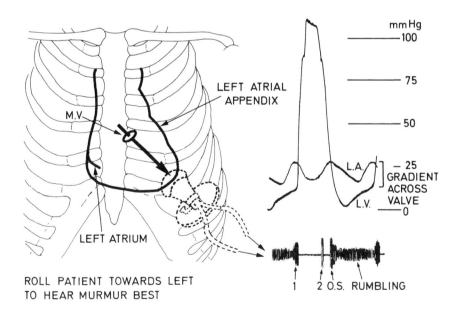

Fig. 5.21 Mitral stenosis. There is a pressure gradient across the mitral valve; in this example it continues throughout diastole. This causes a sharp movement of the tethered anterior cusp of the mitral valve at the time when flow commences and the opening snap (OS) results. The jet through the stenotic valve (arrow) strikes the endocardium at the cardiac apex. The murmur which results is best heard with the bell lightly applied there.

FFOUT represents the loud first sound (though LUP might be better), the first TA the second heart sound, the second one the opening snap, and the ROU the low-pitched rumbling mitral diastolic murmur which is reminiscent of the rumble of rocks in a mountain river in flood. The murmur is best heard, in most cases, when the patient is turned half on to the left side, thus bringing the apex a little nearer to the chest wall, and by increasing the turbulence of mitral valve blood flow by slight exertion. When the reduction of the mitral valve orifice is only slight, the characteristic rumbling murmur is heard only during the increased blood velocity of atrial systole — the so called presystolic murmur. The murmur of mitral stenosis causes a low-pitched vibration of the chest wall which can often be damped out by pressure with the bell of the stethoscope. It is not generally appreciated that two people can listen to the same area, in the same patient, with the same bell stethoscope, and yet disagree because one person presses the bell harder against the skin than the other.

A short rumbling apical presystolic murmur is often heard in patients with gross aortic regurgitation but without mitral stenosis, and is called after *Austin Flint,* who first described it. It is due the aortic regurgitant jet interfering with the normal opening of the antero-medial cusp of the mitral valve. The label is usually reserved for patients who have aortic regurgitation which is not due to rheumatic heart disease, for in the latter case mitral stenosis would be the more likely cause of the murmur.

Tricuspid stenosis produces a murmur which is similar in timing to that of mitral stenosis, loudest to the left of the lower sternum, and in quality is higher pitched and harsher, and hence more like a systolic murmur. Its intensity usually increases during inspiration.

Continuous Murmurs

1. ARTERIOVENOUS MURMURS. The characteristic murmur of an arteriovenous fistula is continuous throughout systole and diastole. A persistent ductus arteriosus, though not strictly an arteriovenous fistula as it joins the aorta to the pulmonary artery, provides a good example of this murmur, and in this case it is maximal in the second left intercostal space and generally accompanied by a thrill (Fig. 5.22).

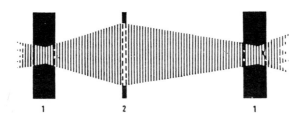

Fig. 5.22   Continuous murmur of persistent ductus arteriosus.

2. VENOUS HUM. A continuing roaring noise is often audible above either clavicle when the head and shoulders are higher than the heart (i.e. when the patient is sitting, standing or reclining against pillows). It is audible in most children when sitting. It is due to blood flow through the jugular veins, and is abolished by pressure with the hand against the side of the patient's neck above the stethoscope, or by the patient assuming a horizontal or head-down position. It alters in intensity with changes in position of the head, and when loud may be heard surprisingly far

away, e.g. to each side of the lower sternum. Its importance rests on the fact that it is extremely common, and often gives rise to a mistaken belief that there is a persistent ductus arteriosus. However, a venous hum lacks the late systolic accentuation charactersitic of the murmur of a persistent ductus (Fig. 5.22).

Exocardiac 'Noises'. Since murmurs are by definition sounds produced by turbulent bloodflow within the heart, it is best to use some other term for sounds recurring with each heartbeat but originating outside the heart. Pericardial rubs (p. 135) and the 'clicking' of a small pneumothorax (p. 180) are examples. Pneumomediastinum, which follows oesophageal rupture, may give rise to a spectacular exocardiac noise which sounds like a loud systolic murmur and is called a mediastinal crunch. Otherwise, exocardiac noises are seldom mistakeable for murmurs. Several bizarre murmurs formerly thought to be of exocardiac origin are now known to be due to mitral prolapse (p. 131).

Flow Murmurs. These are murmurs produced by increased blood flow through normal valves. Soft ejection systolic murmurs are common after vigorous exercise, in the presence of anaemia, or during pregnancy, and characteristically disappear when the cause of an increased cardiac output is removed. Echocardiographic demonstration of valvular normality adds to the confidence with which they can be diagnosed. Diastolic flow murmurs are much less common, but are sometimes heard in children with torrential mitral or tricuspid valve bloodflow resulting from an intracardiac shunt.

Pericardial Rub

The characteristic physical sign of acute pericarditis is a systolic and diastolic *pericardial rub* which is generally maximal to the left of the lower sternum, sounds like friction between rough surfaces and seems near to the stethoscope. It is accentuated when the patient leans forward, and by pressure with the stethoscope. Pleura overlies some of the heart and a pleural rub at this site may be indistinguishable from pericardial friction (p. 182).

EXAMINATION OF ARTERIES AND VEINS

THE ARTERIES

The symptoms of arterial disease arise from partial or complete occlusion, most commonly in the larger arteries as a result of atheroma or embolism. The clinical manifestations depend on the site and extent of the obstruction and the adequacy of the collateral vessels. For example, in children and young adults ligation of the femoral artery or the brachial will generally give rise to no serious symptoms, whereas in the elderly the collateral flow is less good and severe ischaemia and even gangrene are likely to result.

The History

Intermittent claudication (from the Latin, *claudicare* — to limp) is usually the first symptom of chronic arterial inadequacy in the legs. The complaint is of discomfort, cramp or pain in the calf provoked by exercise, and relieved by rest. The patient may be observed to limp if asked to exercise to the point of pain. The 'claudication distance' should be noted, i.e. how far the patient can walk on level ground at a steady pace before pain develops. This can be used as a basis for measuring progress. Claudication may also occur in the buttocks, from occlusion of the internal iliac artery, and in the thigh from occlusion of the common femoral artery; pain in the calf is much more common than these. Ischaemic pain in the forearm as a result of exercising the limb is rare but may follow occulsion of the axillary or brachial artery.

Rest pain may occur in a severely ischaemic limb and the patient may be forced to sleep in a chair or with the leg hanging over the side of the bed in an attempt to obtain relief. The change in position increases the perfusion pressure, but at the same time raises the venous pressure and may lead to oedema.

The Physical Examination

Inspection. (1) *Signs of Arterial Insufficiency.* If the blood supply is suddenly and critically reduced, the limb becomes cold, pale and later bluish, and gangrene may ensue. Power and sensation may be impaired or lost. Chronic ischaemia results in nutritional changes, such as failure of growth of nails and of hairs on the dorsum of the phalanges, and atrophy of the skin and subcutaneous tissues of the digits.

Arterial insufficiency in the lower limbs can be demonstrated in recumbency by elevating the legs to 90°. The blood drains away rapidly and if the distal arterial pressure is then too low to keep the vessels filled against gravity, pallor of varying degree develops within a few seconds. If there is considerable impairment of arterial flow, the foot may take on a cadaveric appearance. If the limbs are then lowered by changing the patient to the sitting position, as with the legs dangling over the side of the bed, colour returns slowly and irregularly with a patchy distribution of increasing intensity until the forefoot assumes a deep reddish colour (*reactive hyperaemia*). The rate at which these colour changes take place and their degree give an indication of the severity of the arterial insufficiency. They are most obvious when one limb is normal and can be used as a control. Similar changes can less commonly be demonstrated in the upper limbs. Normally the veins of the feet fill about five seconds after changing from an elevated to a dependent position. Poor arterial flow causes delay in venous filling in the reactive hyperaemia.

Raynaud's disease occurs most commonly in young women in whom the main arteries to the limb are apparently normal. The small arteries of the fingers may close from undue sensitivity to moderate cold. The fingers become white, cold and insensitive. This is followed by cyanosis from circulatory stasis and by painful rubor from increased blood flow with recovery. Similar changes may occur at any age in patients whose peripheral arteries have been damaged by trauma or by inflammatory changes as in the connective tissue disorders.

(2) *Visible Pulsation.* In the young, an obvious arterial pulse in the suprasternal notch or a very prominent carotid pulse should suggest coarctation of the aorta or aortic regurgitation. In elderly women, the pulsation of a tortuous or 'kinked' carotid artery may be seen, nearly always on the right side. This may be mistaken for an aneurysm, and has gained the (rather unkind) name of 'student's aneurysm'.

Pulsation of the brachial arteries may be visible as a result of sclerotic changes in the media and loss of elasticity. Aneurysms of the limb arteries are uncommon and are readily identified by their expansile pulsation. In coarctation of the aorta, arterial pulsation may be seen in the scapular areas and is best detected when the patient is leaning forward with the arms in front.

Palpation. When there are manifestations of arterial insufficiency in a limb, it is essential to determine whether there is any alteration in the pulses or of the temperature.

1. NORMAL PULSES. The pulse can be felt in most of the main arteries of the limbs and neck in normal subjects. Methods for palpating the radial, brachial, common carotid and femoral arteries have been described (p. 106). The *subclavian artery* (Fig. 6.2 p. 163) is felt from behind by pressing downward with the forefinger above the middle of the clavicle (first part of the artery) or from the front by feeling below the junction of the middle and lateral thirds of the clavicle (third part). The *ulnar artery* is palpable at the wrist where it crosses the distal end of the radius. Usually both the radial and the ulnar artery contribute to the blood supply of the hand. This can be demonstrated by asking the patient to make a fist, and then using the thumbs to compress both arteries simultaneously against the underlyking bone. When the fist is released the skin of the palm remains blanched, but colour should return quickly when either artery is released. If there is delay in the return of colour after release of the ulnary artery, then procedures such as arterial cannulation which might damage the radial artery should be avoided. The digital pulses are often palpable in a warm hand.

The *abdominal aorta* can be palpated in the epigastrium, and particularly easily in a thin elderly subject. An aortic aneurysm has to be distinguised from a redundant, tortuous loop of aorta: usually the width and expansile pulsation of an aneurysm are characteristic, but where there is doubt ultrasonic examination is helpful. The *popliteal artery* is felt by pressing with the fingertips in the middle of the popliteal fossa while the patient lies supine with the knee slightly flexed (Fig. 5.1). The artery lies immediately adjacent to the posterior aspect of the knee joint, and is thus one of the deeper structures in the fossa, but with practice it can nearly always be detected unless there is proximal obstruction. The *posterior tibial artery* is felt behind the medial malleolus, and the *dorsalis pedis artery* is palpable lateral to the extensor hallucis tendon on the dorsum of the foot. Often in the elderly one or both of these vessels will not be palpable. If the dorsalis pedis pulse is not palpable in a young person, there may be an enlarged perforating peroneal artery palpable in front of the lateral malleolus.

It is important to examine and record the pulses of each limb in a methodical manner when arterial disease is suspected; start centrally and work peripherally, or vice versa. In this way the anatomical site of any obstruction can readily be determined. In patients whose peripheral pulses are hard to feel, ultrasound flow probes working on the Doppler principle are often useful

2. TEMPERATURE. When the blood flow to a limb is suddenly impaired, the normal gradual decline in temperature towards the periphery becomes abrupt at the level where ischaemia begins. The opposite limb can be used for comparison. With chronic arterial insufficiency the affected limb commonly feels warmer, because it is being supplied through superficial arteries.

Auscultation. A systolic bruit is often audible over and distal to the site of an arterial stenosis. Disappearance of a bruit may be due to the complete occlusion of the vessel. Spurious bruits may be produced by excessive pressure with the stethoscope. It is sometimes difficult to decide whether a bruit heard over the carotid artery arises locally or is a transmitted sound originating from the aortc valve. It may help to 'walk' the stethoscope along the anterior margin of the sternomastoid muscle: carotid bruits are often heard only in a restricted area, while aortic bruits get steadily louder towards the base of the neck.

THE VEINS

The most important causes of impairment of the efficiency of the venous circulation are (1) obstruction to the flow by thrombosis, phlebitis or external pressure, and (2) incompetence of the valves in varicose veins. Evidence of these processes is sought by means of *inspection* and *palpation.* Thus the classical signs of inflammation may be detected, a thrombosed vein may be palpable or there may be evidence of venous obstruction.

The Manifestations of Venous Obstruction

As in the case of the arteries the clinical manifestations of venous obstruction depend on its site and extent together with the adequacy of the collateral vessels. Distal to the obstruction there may be distension of the veins, cyanosis and oedema.

When obstruction of a main vein occurs, an alternative route develops along collateral channels. These may become visible in the subcutaneous tissues at characteristic sites in relation to the primary lesion. Thus obvious veins may be established over the anterior chest wall when the superior vena cava is occluded (p. 161), and over the lower abdomen when the inferior vena cava is involved (p. 201). At the umbilicus, a caput Medusae (p. 201) may occasionally be seen in the presence of portal obstruction, and in the lower limbs the recognition of fullness of the superficial veins may direct attention to the presence of thrombosis of a deep vein of the leg (see below).

The direction of the blood flow can be demonstrated by emptying one of the anastomotic veins by running two fingers along it until they are a few centimetres apart and then releasing the pressure on each point in turn. When one finger is raised, inflow of blood into the occluded segment of vein is relatively slow, whereas lifting of the other finger will allow rapid and complete inflow of blood.

Thrombosis of the Deep Veins of the Leg. This is of great medical importance, mainly because of the risks of pulmonary embolism and pulmonary infarction, but also because organisation of the thrombus can damage the venous valves and result in chronic venous insufficiency. Although the clinical signs of deep vein thrombosis may be striking, far more often they are inapparent, and both post-mortem studies and in vivo studies with radioactive fibrinogen show that the majority of deep vein thromboses are undetected by the clinician.

Venous stasis is a common predisposing factor, and deep vein thrombosis is frequent in those confined to bed, particularly if this follows an operation or childbirth. Prolonged sitting in an aeroplane or car seat may also be responsible. Symptoms may be absent, or confined to slight calf discomfort or ankle swelling. In hospital patients a slight deterioration in well-being, a small rise in pulse rate, or an unexplained fever may alert the observant to the possibility of venous thrombosis.

Physical signs, when they are present, consist of swelling of the calf, slight duskiness of the skin of the leg and sole of the foot, and oedema of the ankle on the affected side. Dilatation of small veins passing over the shin of one leg is almost pathognomonic if it is of recent onset, and the dilated veins do not empty normally if the leg is elevated. The affected leg is warm to the touch, and the calf is often tense and tender on palpation. If thrombosis extends to the femoral or iliac veins, there may be increased discomfort and swelling, with tenderness on palpation along the course of the vein. It is possible however for extensive ilio-femoral venous thrombosis to occur with remarkably few physical signs.

Deep vein thrombosis may be closely mimicked by a haematoma or partial rupture of the gastrocnemius muscle or by rupture of a synovial cyst associated with an arthritic knee joint (Baker's cyst). The latter conditions tend to occur in active rather than bedridden patients, and there may be a history of minor trauma. Pain is common, and may be of sudden onset. Dilated superficial veins and a warm skin are less common, but swelling, tenderness and pain on dorsiflexion of the foot may be as prominent or more so than in venous thrombosis. Arthritis of the knee is usually obvious in patients with a Baker's cyst. Where there is any doubt about diagnosis, venography may be helpful.

The Assessment of Varicose Veins

Varicose veins are evidence of a progressive and often genetically determined condition in which there is dilatation and elongation of venous channels. The course of the vessels becomes tortuous and there is thickening of the walls together with some degree of fixation to the surrounding tissues. The nutrition of the part becomes impaired by venous stasis and hypoxia. Partly because of their length and partly because of an inherent weakness in their walls, the veins most commonly affected are the long saphenous, and, to a lesser extent, the short saphenous in the leg. At an early stage there is incompetence of the valves, both in the superficial veins and later in their communications with the deep system. Contrary to the normal, blood then flows from the deep to the superficial systems, and a further increase in the degree of dilatation and stasis results. The early symptoms of varicose veins are generally discomfort and fatigue in the leg, brought on by standing and relieved by elevation.

Examination. Gross varicosities, or the presence of secondary complications such as varicose eczema which is common and precedes ulceration, usually present no difficulty in diagnosis. Minor, or early dilatation, however, is often overlooked as a cause of symptoms and the examination must be capable of demonstrating this degree of abnormality.

The patient should be standing and the site and extent of the varicosities identified by inspection and palpation, the latter being of particular value in the fat leg. It is usual to see the maximal dilatation in the region of the inner side of the calf or above the ankle. This may well be the only evidence of varicosities affecting the entire vein. Dilated segments may also be seen at several sites on one or both of the major veins separated by apparently normal segments.

The competence of the valves, an assessment of which is essential for correct management may be demonstrated by the *Trendelenburg test*. The veins of the leg are 'emptied' by elevation of the limb. The long saphenous vein is then compressed by a finger or by a light tourniquet at the saphenous opening, and the patient stands. If the vein fills from below while the finger is in position the valves in the communicating veins are incompetent. If there is little or no filling within half a minute the finger should be removed and an immediate filling from above indicates incompetence at the sapheno-femoral junction. In the event of filling of the system from below, a more accurate estimate of the site of the incompetent communicating veins can be obtained by repeating the test using multiple points of compression, either with the fingers or several simultaneous tourniquets at various levels of the leg. Filling of any individual segment of vein indicates that this area is related to an incompetent deep communicating vein.

In those patients in whom there is difficulty in demonstrating the exact extent of the incompetence, or in whom there is some doubt as to the state of the deep venous system, it may be necessary to complete the investigation with a venogram.

FURTHER INVESTIGATION

The standard aids to the diagnosis of disorders of the cardiovascular system are radiography, electrocardiography and echocardiography. These can be supplemented with phonocardiography, ultrasonography, cardiac catheterisation, angiocardiography and radionuclide studies.

Radiography
A standard film of the chest, namely a postero-anterior exposure with at least six feet in distance between the X-ray tube and the film, provides valuable information, in particular about the size of the cardiac shadow, and of the main pulmonary artery and aorta. Enlargement of the left auricle (also called the left atrial appendix) appears as a bulge on the left border of the heart and is a usual feature of mitral stenosis; the left atrium may often be seen as a dense almost circular opacity within the cardiac outline and, in an oblique film, can be shown to indent the oesophagus outlined by barium. The shadow of an enlarged right atrium encroaches upon the right lung field. The relative contribution of each of the two ventricles to cardiomegaly is often impossible to determine in a posterior-anterior film and is unreliable even when lateral films are used. Both electrocardiography and clinical examination are usually better tools for this purpose.

A standard radiograph is valuable in indicating that a pericardial effusion has developed, particularly if a recent film is available for comparison. Pulmonary oedema, hydrothoraces and pulmonary infarction may be more certainly established by radiography than by clinical examination; radionuclides are used in the investigation of suspected pulmonary embolism (p. 185). Pulmonary arterial hypertension, and both increased and reduced pulmonary blood flow may also produce characteristic changes in the vascular shadows.

Fluoroscopy
Old-fashioned fluoroscopy, with the high radiation dose involved, has been

superseded by image-intensifier screening. The latter is more efficient than the plain radiograph in detecting valvular calcification, but the same information can also be obtained by echocardiography. Screening will also detect calcification in the coronary arteries, and is particularly useful in studying the movement of artificial heart valves, especially when these include a radio-opaque marker in the ball or disc.

Electrocardiography

The electrocardiograph amplifies and records electrical activity originating from the heart and detected via electrodes applied to the skin. Standard combinations of electrode positions are called leads, and it is conventional to record 12 leads which 'look at' the electrical activity of the heart from different directions (Fig. 5.23). The

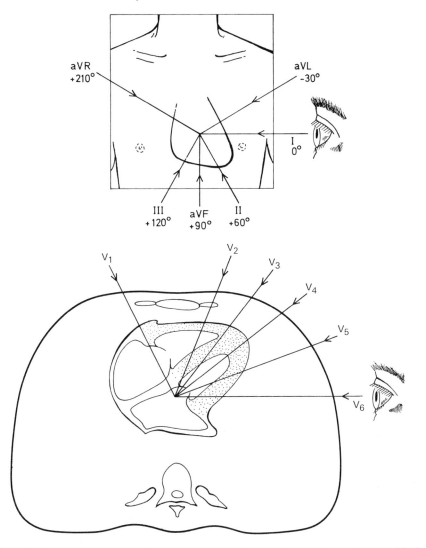

Fig. 5.23 Electrocardiography. Diagram to show the directions from which the 12 standard leads 'look at' the heart.

ECG is invaluable for elucidating arrhythmias, for detecting hypertrophy of each of the cardiac chambers, and above all for providing evidence of acute injury to heart muscle from ischaemia (including myocardial infarction) or metabolic disturbances. Full explanation of the ECG requires a monograph to itself (p. 149).

Echocardiography

This technique uses ultrasound to study the disposition and movement of valves and other structures within the heart and also the pericardium. It depends on the reflection of ultrasound waves at interfaces between liquid (e.g. blood) and more solid tissues. In 'M mode' echocardiography the ultrasound is focused into a narrow beam, and the output is a graph against time of the movement relative to the chest wall of those structures through which the beam passes (Fig. 5.24). By tilting the beam, the operator can study the movement of the anterior and posterior walls of the left ventricle, the mitral valve cusps, or the aorta and left atrium. Characteristic patterns of movement are produced in, for example, mitral stenosis, and pericardial effusions are easily recognised. Accurate measurements can be made of cardiac size.

In two-dimensional (2D) real time echocardiography, the ultrasound beam is swung rapidly back and fore over an arc or sector; this is done mechanically or, in some machines, electronically. The resulting information is synthesised into a two-dimensional map or picture of the position of reflecting structures in a sector-shaped 'slice' through the heart (Fig. 5.25). The structures shown in the 'slice' will of course depend on the position of the ultrasound crystal and the direction of oscillation of the beam. Because the beam oscillates very rapidly, the ultrasound picture accurately reproduces the movements of the structures in the living heart. This type of echocardiography is particularly good at detecting intracardiac masses, such as thrombi or tumours, or endocarditic vegetations. It is also very useful in sorting out complex structural abnormalities in congenital heart disease.

The advent of echocardiography has made it possible for information, previously accessible only by cardiac catheterization and angiocardiography, to be made available without an invasive procedure, and if necessary, without moving the patient from bed.

Radionuclide Studies

The availability of radioactive isotopes of short half-life emitting gamma rays, together with sophisticated equipment (the gamma camera) for detecting this radiation has made it possible to use radionuclides for studying cardiac function. Two basic types of technique are available:

1. Blood-pool Scanning. The radionuclide is injected into the bloodstream and mixes with the circulating blood. The gamma camera detects the amount of radionuclide in the heart at different phases of the cardiac cycle, and also the size and 'shape' of the cardiac chambers. By linking the gamma camera to the ECG it is possible to collect information over several cardiac cycles. Blood-pool scanning gives an accurate and reproducible measure of left ventricular function, and is also used for detecting left ventricular aneurysms. The main disadvantage is the high cost of the equipment.

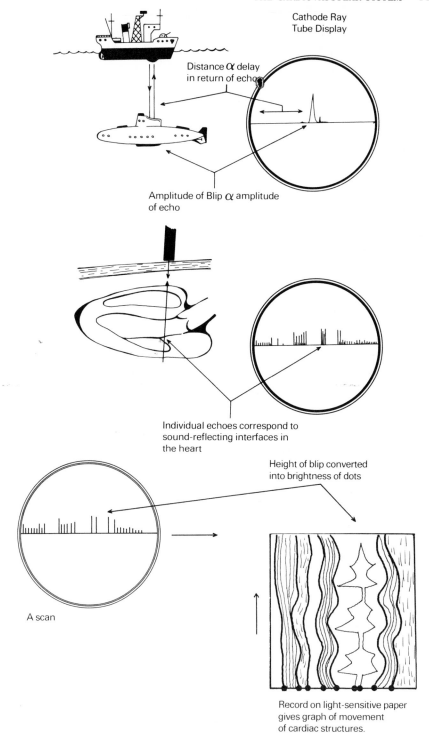

Cathode Ray
Tube Display

Distance α delay
in return of echo

Amplitude of Blip α amplitude
of echo

Individual echoes correspond to
sound-reflecting interfaces in
the heart

Height of blip converted
into brightness of dots

A scan

Record on light-sensitive paper
gives graph of movement
of cardiac structures.

Fig. 5.24   Principles of M-Mode Echocardiography. The reflected echoes of ultrasound are converted into blips of light on a cathode-ray tube. The blips can be used to plot a 'graph against time' of the position of cardiac structures on a moving strip of paper.

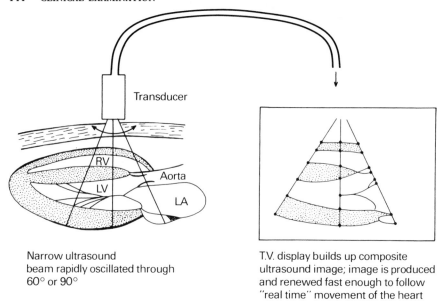

Narrow ultrasound
beam rapidly oscillated through
60° or 90°

T.V. display builds up composite
ultrasound image; image is produced
and renewed fast enough to follow
"real time" movement of the heart

Fig. 5.25 Principles of Two-Dimensional (2D) Real time Echocardiography. A moving, two-dimensional image of the echoes detected from a 'slice' of heart can be built up by swinging the ultrasound beam rapidly back and forth.

2. Myocardial Scanning. Although this uses the same gamma camera, both the isotopes and the concepts involved differ from those in blood-pool scanning. The object is usually to distinguish between ischaemic and non-ischaemic myocardium (using radioactive thallium) or between normal and damaged myocardium (using radioactive pyro-phosphate). Much care and attention to detail is needed if reliable results are to be obtained.

Cardiac Catheterisation and Angiocardiography

In contrast to the investigations described above, these are invasive techniques, which require the insertion of tubes or catheters into the patient's arteries or veins. This may be done percutaneously or after a surgical 'cut-down'. A catheter inserted into a vein can be advanced into the right atrium, and then manipulated into the right ventricle and pulmonary artery. In the presence of an atrial septal defect or patent foramen ovale, venous catheters can also enter the left atrium and left ventricle. If the atrial septum is intact, access to the left ventricle is usually by retrograde passage of a catheter across the aortic valve. Left atrial pressure can be measured directly by puncturing the interatrial septum with a special long, curved needle via a catheter passed up the femoral vein to the right atrium. For many purposes, however, a satisfactory approximation to left atrial pressure can be recorded by 'wedging' an end-hole venous catheter in a branch of the pulmonary artery. Cardiac catheters are usually manipulated under radiographic control using an image-intensifier, but if a venous catheter is provided at its distal end with a small balloon which can be inflated when the catheter is in the right atrium then the bloodstream itself will guide the catheter through the right ventricle and into the pulmonary artery. The balloon also makes it easy to 'wedge' the catheters so as to estimate left atrial pressure. These Swan-Ganz catheters are being used in increasing numbers in intensive and coronary care units, where they can be inserted without the need to transfer the patient to a radiology department.

Pressure measurements obtained through cardiac catheters can be used to assess the severity of valvular stenoses, and measurement of ventricular end-diastolic pressures gives an indication of ventricular compliance and indirectly of ventricular function. Measurement of oxygen saturation in samples withdrawn via the catheters at different sites in the heart allow the detection of intracardiac left to right or right to left shunts, and also allows calculation of pulmonary and systemic blood flow. Cardiac output can also be measured by dye-dilution or thermodilution techniques. Catheters also allow the injection of radio-opaque contrast medium into individual chambers of the heart, the aorta or pulmonary artery, or, using specially shaped catheters, into either coronary artery.

THE METHODS IN PRACTICE

So far, we have tended to consider points of history-taking or physical signs either in isolation or in the context of an orderly clinical examination. In practice, it is often clear from an early stage that the diagnosis will lie in a particular direction, and it is helpful to concentrate on certain specific points in the examination and subsequent investigation. Three common diagnostic problems have been selected to exemplify this approach, and also to demonstrate the integration which is often required between the physical examination and further investigation.

CARDIAC FAILURE

Cardiac failure is not a diagnosis, or at least, not a complete one. It is necessary to specify whether the failure affects the left or right 'side' of the heart, or both together (p. 98) and as far as possible to identify the underlying pathological process. Left heart failure characteristically presents with breathlessness and pulmonary oedema is an early manifestation. Pure left heart failure is seldom associated with much peripheral oedema, because pulmonary oedema develops so rapidly and causes symptoms before peripheral oedema has time to accumulate. Very commonly, however, left and right heart failure occur together, either because reflex pulmonary vasoconstriction in response to a raised pulmonary venous pressure causes secondary right heart failure, or because a process such as myocardial disease affects both the right and left ventricles simultaneously. In this situation pulmonary oedema, or at least pulmonary congestion, may co-exist with a raised jugular venous pressure and peripheral oedema. In contrast, peripheral oedema is often a prominent feature, together with a raised jugular venous pressure and hepatomegaly, of pure right heart failure. This is not because the mechanism of oedema is different in the different types of heart failure but because the relative absence of breathlessness often allows the insidious accumulation of considerable amounts of peripheral oedema before the patient complains.

Mechanisms of Cardiac Failure

There are a limited number of mechanisms which can be invoked as causes of cardiac failure. They are (1) volume overload, (2) inflow obstruction, (3) myocardial disease and (4) outflow obstruction. Some of these can involve either the left or right side of the heart.

1. Volume Overload. The simplest example of this is when a patient with a healthy heart is overtransfused with blood or plasma. As the venous pressure rises, cardiac output increases (a manifestation of Starling's law), and this is reflected in increased venous return. Until the excess fluid is excreted, the patient will have a raised venous pressure, a bounding pulse, tachycardia and an active or hyperkinetic apical cardiac impulse. If transfusion is continued, pulmonary oedema develops. The patient then begins to cough, becomes breathless and confused, and will rapidly die unless urgent measures are taken.

A less dramatic presentation occurs when there is an excessively low peripheral vascular resistance over a prolonged period. This may result from surgical or congenital arteriovenous fistulae, from anaemia, from Paget's disease of bone, or from various skin diseases causing cutaneous vasodilatation. It may also be due to vasodilating drugs. The kidneys interpret the low blood pressure as evidence of cardiac failure and retain salt and water. Blood volume is expanded, the jugular venous pressure rises, and there may be peripheral oedema. Occasionally the patient becomes breathless because of pulmonary congestion. There is tachycardia, the pulse volume is large, and there is a wide interval between systolic and diastolic blood pressure. The left and right vetricles respond by dilating, and the cardiac apex becomes displaced laterally and is hyperkinetic. Systolic flow murmurs are common. Sometimes, a continuous murmur can be heard over the site of an arteriovenous fistula. Echocardiography or nuclear angiography help to confirm the diagnosis by demonstrating an increased ventricular stroke volume and an increased cardiac output.

Atrial septal defect is a special case where the volume overload is confined to the right atrium and ventricle and in persistent ductus arteriosus the overload affects the left ventricle and left atrium. Aortic regurgitation is another special case where the 'run-off' from the arterial tree is back into the left ventricle itself. Mitral regurgitation is also characterised by the need for an increased left ventricular stroke volume to compensate for the leaking mitral valve, but here the clinical picture is modified by the increase in left atrial pressure caused by the leak.

2. Inflow Obstruction. The inflow of blood into the ventricles may be obstructed at the tricuspid or mitral valve. The resulting turbulence of the bloodflow causes characteristic murmurs (tricuspid stenosis p. 134, mitral stenosis p. 133). The chamber upstream of the obstruction (the left atrium in the case of mitral stenosis) is subjected to increased pressure and tends to enlarge, the chamber downstream remains of normal size. Left or right atrial enlargement may eventually lead to atrial fibrillation. Any rise in left atrial pressure is of course transmitted to the pulmonary veins, and pulmonary oedema may result; alternatively reflex pulmonary vasoconstriction causes secondary right heart failure. The radiographic appearances of left atrial enlargement are characteristic, but are sometimes absent even in severe cases of mitral stenosis. Echocardiography is of great value in the diagnosis of mitral or tricuspid stenosis, and also helps to elucidate less common causes of inflow obstruction such as left or right atrial myxomas or malfunctioning prosthetic valves.

A different form of inflow obstruction occurs when ventricular filling is limited either by excessive stiffness of the ventricle or by an external constraint, such as pericardial fluid in pericardial tamponade or a rigid peicardium in constrictive pericarditis. In the last two conditions signs such as pulsus paradoxus and Kussmaul's sign help to make the diagnosis, but when the restricting factor is 'built-in' to the ventricle, as in restrictive cardiomyopathy or endocardial fibrosis the diagnosis may be difficult. Echocardiography may again be helpful, by showing the chamber affected by the inflow obstruction to be of normal size, while the chamber upstream is dilated.

3. Myocardial Disease. This is by far the commonest cause of left heart failure, which in this instance can truly be called left ventricular failure. Impaired myocardial function may be secondary to coronary artery disease, may result from specific disease of the myocardium such as viral myocarditis, or may be caused by one of the many myocardial disorders of uncertain aetiology encompassed by the term cardiomyopathy. It may also follow long standing ventricular outflow obstruction (see below), probably as a consequence of diffuse myocardial ischaemia. Many of these processes can affect the right ventricle as well as the left.

There are few specific physical signs to indicate myocardial disease, and its diagnosis is often made by a process of exclusion. The heart sounds tend to be quiet when the cardiac output is low, and a gallop rhythm may result from the presence of a third heart sound. When the left ventricle is dilated and poorly contractile a diffuse apical impulse is often felt over a wide area. A history of angina or myocardial infarction may suggest the aetiology of the myocardial damage and the ECG helps to confirm ischaemia or infarction. Echocardiography and nuclear angiography are useful non-invasive methods of assessing ventricular function.

4. Outflow Obstruction. The afterload against which the ventricles have to work may be increased either because outflow of blood from the ventricles is 'throttled' as in pulmonary or aortic valve stenosis, or because the resistance in the pulmonary or systemic circulation is high, as in pulmonary or systemic hypertension. In either case the ventricle involved responds by undergoing hypertrophy, which may affect the character of the apical impulse. The hypertrophied myocardium demands an increased blood supply, and, if the coronary circulation is unable to provide this, the patient may suffer angina on exertion. The hypertrophied ventricle is less compliant, so left atrial pressure tends to rise, and left atrial hypertrophy causes an audible fourth heart sound. Characteristically, patients with ventricular outflow obstruction tolerate the condition with few symptoms for a prolonged period, but when symptoms appear deterioration is rapid. With left sided obstruction, pulmonary oedema is the usual result, and this frequently presents as paroxysmal nocturnal dyspnoea.

Increased pulmonary vascular resistance resulting from chronic lung disease is by far the commonest cause of chronic right heart failure in Northern industrial countries, and the combination is given the name of cor pulmonale. Two different mechanisms seem to be involved — pulmonary vasoconstriction resulting from hypoxia, and destruction of the vessels in the lung parenchyma in chronic emphysema. Right heart failure often develops for the first time during an infection of the respiratory tract. There is peripheral oedema, hepatomegaly and a raised jugular venous pressure. Arterial oxygen desaturation is common, but many patients have a depressed respiratory drive and may not complain of dyspnoea. Carbon dioxide retention is almost invariable and tends to cause peripheral vasodilatation; the warm hands and bounding pulse which result seem at first sight incompatible with cardiac failure.

Conclusion. Thinking along the above lines should complete the diagnosis of cardiac failure by determining which components of the heart are involved, and why.

SYSTEMIC HYPERTENSION

This common disease has no specific symptoms; it is recognised either on routine examination, or because of its complications, which include cardiac failure, renal failure and stroke. The clinical examination of a hypertensive patient has two main aims — to seek a specific cause for the hypertension, and to evaluate the extend of the damage done as the result of it.

A specific cause for hypertension is likely to be elicited only in a minority of patients, but is more commonly found in younger subjects. In the history, attention should be paid to a story of paroxysmal headaches, vomiting, sweating and other features of excessive sympathomimetic activity, as this may indicate the presence of a phaeochromocytoma. Rarely, such a tumour is so large as to be palpable in the abdomen. A history of recurrent urinary tract infections, or persistent enuresis in an adolescent, may give warning of renal disease. Specific enquiry should be made about chronic analgesic abuse, which may cause analgesic nephropathy.

General examination may reveal features of Cushing's disease, or abnormal virilisation resulting from an adrenal tumour or a congenital metabolic error. It is essential to palpate the femoral pulses and to check their synchrony with the radial pulses. Delayed femoral pulses indicate aortic coarctation, a diagnosis not infrequently missed in the adult. An abdominal bruit signals the presence of renal artery stenosis, but this is an unreliable sign. Renal polycystic disease commonly presents with hypertension, and the enlarged kidneys are frequently palpable.

The effects of hypertension on the heart are manifest initially as left ventricular hypertrophy, with a characteristic quality of the apex beat, and a fourth heart sound reflecting secondary atrial hypertrophy. Later, ventricular dilatation and cardiac failure may ensue. The optic fundi show characteristic changes with hypertension, and such changes may be a clue to intermittent hypertension even if the blood pressure is normal when the patient is seen. The urine must be tested for the presence of protein, and examined for cells and casts.

INFECTIVE ENDOCARDITIS

The clinical diagnosis of infective endocarditis is frequently overlooked until the condition is well advanced. Endocarditis may present as an obscure fever, as rapidly advancing cardiac failure, or as a cause of systemic arteral embolism. Virtually all patients have either valvular heart disease or a congenital lesion such as a ventricular septal defect or a persistent ductus arteriosus. Haemodynamically trivial lesions such as a bicuspid aortic valve may still be a cause of endocarditis. A murmur is therefore almost essential to the diagnosis, but even more important is the observation that a murmur changes in nature or intensity during the course of the illness. This is due either to the growth of endocarditic vegetations or to progressive destruction of the valve.

Extracardiac manifestations of infective endocarditis include splenomegaly and clubbing of the fingers which are usually, though not always, late signs. Splinter haemorrhages under the finger or toe nails are not diagnostic, but their presence in large numbers and recurrence in crops is highly suggestive. They were once thought to be due to minute emboli, but it now seems more likely they are a manifestation of a systemic vasculitis, induced by immune complexes. This vasculitis may also be responsible for petechial haemorrhages in the skin, mucous membranes and conjunctiva, for retinal haemorrhages, and for Osler's nodes. The same process in the kidney causes microscopic haematuria.

Conclusion

These three examples must suffice to illustrate the philosophy underlying the clinical examination of the cardiovascular system. At every stage, it is essential to think of the signs elicited in terms of their basic anatomy and physiology, and of their relevance to the suspected underlying disease. Once this is done, the examination will seldom be unrewarding.

REFERENCES

Hampton J R 1980 The ECG made easy, 2nd edn. Churchill Livingstone, Edinburgh — This is a basic and popular textbook.
Schamroth L 1982 An introduction to electrocardiography, 6th edn. Blackwells, London — This is a more detailed but very readable book.

6. The Respiratory System

Take care of the sense, and the sounds will take care of themselves.

Lewis Caroll, *Alice in Wonderland*

Many of the methods of physical examination we use today for the investigation of respiratory disease differ remarkably little from those described by Laënnec in his *Treatise on the Diseases of the Chest*, published in 1819. We still seek by means of inspection, palpation, percussion and auscultation to detect abnormalities in the bronchi, lungs and pleura and by analysis of the various physical signs to determine the gross pathology of the lesions. Advances in physiology, pathology, immunology, microbiology, radiology, endoscopy and thoracic surgery have, however, enabled us not only to diagnose respiratory disease with more precision but also to reappraise the value of clinical investigation in its various forms. Nowadays, for example, we place more weight on careful history-taking than on the elicitation of elegant, but possibly misleading, physical signs. We also realise that in many disorders the disease process may reach an advanced stage before any abnormal signs can be detected and that unless symptoms are promptly investigated by special techniques, such as radiology, serious delays in diagnosis and treatment may result. More is known, too, of the relationship between clinical findings and disturbances of respiratory function, and there is a better understanding of the significance of features such as dyspnoea and cyanosis.

The principal effects of these advances are threefold. Firstly, the technique of physical examination of the chest has been greatly simplified by emphasising the importance of those clinical findings which provide information of genuine diagnostic value. Secondly, the limitations of physical examination have been recognised and defined in relation to the diagnosis of conditions such as pulmonary tuberculosis and bronchial carcinoma, in which abnormal physical signs are a late development. Thirdly, the modern approach to clinical examination reflects the importance accorded to respiratory physiology and embodies acceptance of the principle that a morbid anatomical diagnosis can no longer be regarded as an end in itself. If, for example, a diagnosis of emphysema is made, the patient's investigation is considered incomplete until the effects of the disease on pulmonary function have been assessed.

THE HISTORY

The approach to history-taking in patients thought to have respiratory disease differs according to the nature of the illness, the main distinction being that between an acute or subacute illness and a chronic respiratory disorder. The methods used to obtain a coherent account of the patient's symptoms are, however, the same in the two types of case. Firstly, a narrative history is taken, the patient being encouraged to describe the symptoms in his or her own way, curbed only by restrictions on verbosity and irrelevance as outlined in Chapter 1. Specific enquiry is then made about any of the six principal respiratory symptoms (cough, sputum, haemoptysis, chest pain, dyspnoea and wheeze) not mentioned in the narrative history. At this stage the doctor may find it convenient to review the data so far obtained and make a mental note of all the conditions which might conceivably be responsible for the patient's symptoms. This will seldom be a formidable list, perhaps three or four items in an average case. The doctor should then ask a series of supplementary questions designed to provide evidence for and against each possible diagnosis. In the course of this interrogation the patient may have to be asked to confirm or expand some of the information previously given. This method of integrating and rationalising the history has an important place in the diagnosis of respiratory disease because it facilitates the recognition of certain characteristic symptom-patterns, such as those presented by chronic bronchitis and bronchial asthma, in which physical signs and even specialised investigations may be of limited diagnostic value.

In an *acute respiratory illness* history-taking usually presents no special difficulties, but one or two points are worthy of mention. It is always important to enquire carefully about the onset of the illness, which may provide a valuable clue to its nature. In pneumococcal pneumonia, for example, systemic disturbance (rigor, pyrexia, malaise) seldom precedes the first respiratory symptom (usually pleural pain) by more than a few hours, while in viral pneumonia the patient may be pyrexial and generally unwell for several days before there are any symptoms or signs to suggest pulmonary involvement. Acute dyspnoea is a presenting symptom of particular importance since it often demands urgent treatment, and an error in diagnosis between, say, tension pneumothorax, an acute attack of bronchial asthma and left heart failure may have catastrophic consequences. There, too, a carefully taken history, from a relative if the patient is too breathless to give a coherent account of the illness, may enable such a mistake to be avoided. The nature and effect of treatment prescribed before the patient is seen should also be carefully noted. If, for example, the symptoms are suggestive of an acute pulmonary infection but there has been no improvement after a few days of treatment with an antibiotic, consideration must be given to the possibility of the patient having a drug-resistant bacterial infection, a tuberculous or viral infection, an empyema or even a pulmonary infarct.

In *chronic respiratory disorders* history-taking is always a complex and time-consuming procedure. Care must be taken to record not only major incidents in the course of the illness but also to describe and assess the interval or background symptoms. In the case of acute episodes, such as exacerbations of chronic bronchitis, an enquiry should be made into the events which preceded them and the effects which they appeared to have on the course of the disease. Most chronic respiratory disorders pursue a fairly predictable course, and if a patient exhibits symptoms out of line with the established pattern of the illness, the development of another disease should be suspected. The influence of environmental factors, such as weather and time of year, changes of temperature and exposure to smoke and dust, should always be recorded. Such information, in addition to its diagnostic value, may be relevant to prevention and treatment. A clinical assessment of pulmonary function is an essential item in the history of every patient with chronic respiratory disease.

THE PRINCIPAL SYMPTOMS OF RESPIRATORY DISEASE

The six principal symptoms of respiratory disease are cough, sputum, haemoptysis, chest pain, dyspnoea and wheeze. It is important to remember that most of these symptoms may occur in the absence of primary respiratory disease. Certain types of central chest pain, for example, may be of cardiac, pericardial or oesophageal origin, dyspnoea may be due to pulmonary oedema secondary to left ventricular failure, and haemoptysis may occasionally be the presenting symptom in mitral stenosis or disorders of the blood clotting mechanism. Nevertheless, lateral chest pain and the other five principal symptoms are usually indicative of respiratory disease, and will be discussed in that context.

Cough

This is the most frequent symptom of respiratory disease. It may be caused by stimuli arising in the mucosa of any part of the respiratory tract from the pharynx to the smaller bronchi. Stimuli arising in the parietal pleura may, on rare occasions, also produce cough, for example in dry pleurisy or during pleural paracentesis. The frequency, severity and character of cough are dependent on several factors including (a) the situation and nature of the lesion responsible for the cough, (b) the presence or absence of sputum and (c) coexisting abnormalities such as vocal cord paralysis, impairment of ventilatory function and pleural pain.

Types of Cough. 1. Cough produced by stimuli arising in the *pharyngeal mucosa* occurs in pharyngitis or may be caused by secretions trickling down the posterior pharyngeal wall from the nasal sinuses. It is typically a persistent cough, but may be paroxysmal and explosive at times when the pharynx is coated with tenacious mucus or mucopus.

2. Cough arising in the *larynx* has a harsh, barking quality and may be painful, especially in acute laryngitis. If a vocal cord is paralysed, a cough, whatever its site of origin, will lose its normal explosive force and will cease to be effective in clearing the respiratory tract of secretion. Whooping-cough is characterised by prolonged severe paroxysms culminating in a long, stridulous, inspiratory whoop produced by laryngeal spasm.

3. Cough arising in the *trachea* is usually caused by tracheitis, in which it is harsh, dry and painful at first, becoming loose, productive and painless later. Cough

caused by a malignant tumour partially obstructing the trachea is persistent and at times severe and suffocating. Such patients may become deeply cyanosed and even unconscious during paroxysms of coughing.

4. Cough of several different types may be produced by stimulation of nerve endings in the *bronchial mucosa*.

Cough in *acute bronchitis* is similar in character to that which occurs in tracheitis but is often preceded or accompanied by transient wheeze and a feeling of diffuse tightness in the chest. In the early stages it sounds dry; later it becomes loose and productive usually of purulent sputum.

Cough in *chronic bronchitis* tends to occur in prolonged paroxysms, which usually culminate in the production of sputum. When the sputum is very tenacious, however, or if there is serious impairment of ventilatory function, the patient, exhausted by the effort of coughing, may abandon the attempt to clear the bronchi of secretions and the coughing comes to an indecisive stop. Bouts of coughing in these patients often produce severe dyspnoea, frequently accompanied by wheezing, and may be very distressing. Cough in chronic bronchitis has other typical features. It is particularly frequent and severe when the patient retires to bed at night and, even more so, on getting up in the morning, because of sudden changes in posture and in the temperature of the inspired air. Sleep is seldom disturbed by coughing, but most patients with chronic bronchitis waken in the morning with a slight wheeze and a sensation of tightness in the chest. These symptoms do not improve until sputum is brought up by a violent bout of coughing which may continue for several minutes. Cough in chronic bronchitis is stimulated not only by changes in atmospheric temperature but also by bronchial irritants such as smoke, fumes or dust, and by the sudden increase in the depth of ventilation which occurs with exertion and laughter. Some patients may experience cough syncope (p. 38) during bouts of prolonged and violent coughing. When patients with chronic bronchitis develop ventilatory failure, cough becomes progressively more feeble and ineffective, and eventually the accumulation of secretions in the larynx and trachea gives rise to a so-called death rattle.

Prolonged paroxysms of coughing may also occur in patients with *chronic asthma*. The cough, which invariably aggravates the dyspnoea and wheeze, is less directly related to atmospheric conditions than the cough of chronic bronchitis and often wakens the patient in the middle of the night. The dyspnoea and wheeze which follow may be wrongly attributed to left ventricular failure (p. 145).

In *bronchial carcinoma* cough may be and often is an early and persistent symptom. At first it is a frequent short dry cough, but later, when the tumour has caused bronchial obstruction with distal pulmonary infection, it becomes more severe and distressing. If the bronchus is not completely occluded, pus may be coughed up. The type of cough associated with interruption of the left recurrent laryngeal nerve, a common complication of tumour at the left pulmonary hilum, is described on page 264.

Cough in *bronchiectasis*, uncomplicated by chronic bronchitis or asthma, is characteristically loose and readily productive of sputum. It may be brought on by changes in posture, e.g. by stooping if the bronchiectasis affects the lower lobes. Patients with severe unilateral bronchiectasis prefer to sleep on the affected side in order to prevent cough being stimulated by the dislodgement of sputum. Cough in *pneumonia* and *lung abscess* is dry and irritable at first, later becoming loose and productive. When pleural pain is present, cough is typically short and half-suppressed. Cough in *acute pulmonary oedema* secondary to left heart failure is generally short, persistent and exhausting. A similar type of cough may occur in *allergic* and *fibrosing alveolitis*.

Sputum

When a patient has sputum, information should be obtained as to amount, character, viscosity and taste or odour.

AMOUNT. This can seldom be accurately estimated by the patient although statements that it is very large (e.g. a teacupful per day) or very small (one or two spits per day) are usually reliable. If it is important to obtain precise information about the amount of sputum, the patient should be given a graduated container and a 24-hour collection should be measured. It should be appreciated that some patients deny cough while admitting to the presence of sputum, saying that they bring it up merely by clearing the throat. A specific enquiry about sputum should, therefore, be made in every case. Most children swallow their sputum, even when it is being produced in large amounts. The character of the cough, if it is loose or moist, will, however, indicate that sputum is present.

CHARACTER. This is seldom described accurately by the patient and, wherever possible, a specimen should be inspected by the doctor. Apart from haemoptysis, there are four types of sputum — serous, mucoid, purulent and mucopurulent. *Serous* sputum, which is usually described by patients as clear and/or frothy, is seen in acute pulmonary oedema, in which it may acquire a pink colour through admixture with red blood cells, and in the rare condition of alveolar-cell carcinoma. *Mucoid* sputum, which is a characteristic feature of chronic bronchitis, is usually described by patients as grey, white, clear or sometimes black (when it contains soot particles). *Purulent* and *mucopurulent* sputum is usually described as yellow or green, but occasionally white sputum proves on inspection to be purulent. The term 'dirty spit' used by many patients is a misleading one, as it may refer either to purulent sputum or to mucoid sputum containing soot particles. Mucoid sputum may be copious and frothy in some cases of chronic bronchitis and asthma. Hysterical patients may spit out large amounts of saliva which they claim to be sputum.

VISCOSITY. Mucoid sputum is more viscous than purulent sputum and for that reason is often more difficult to cough up. Sputum is particularly viscous in the early stages of pneumococcal pneumonia and in severe asthma. Serous sputum is watery with a low viscosity.

TASTE OR ODOUR. When this is described as 'nasty' the patient may merely be referring to the normal taste of purulent sputum. Only when terms such as offensive, nauseating or putrid are used can it be assumed that the sputum is fetid (as in bronchiectasis or lung abscess with anerobic bacterial infection). The doctor's own sense of smell should be used to assess the odour.

Haemoptysis

This occurs in many respiratory diseases (e.g. bronchial carcinoma and adenoma, pulmonary tuberculosis, bronchiectasis, pulmonary infarction), in certain cardiovascular diseases (e.g. mitral stenosis) and occasionally in the absence of any demonstrable lesion in bronchi, lungs or heart. The blood in haemoptysis is bright red at first but may later become dark red. It is often frothy and may be mixed with sputum. Although most patients readily realise whether blood has been coughed up or vomited, haemoptysis is occasionally confused with haematemesis. Blood from the stomach can, however, usually be recognised by its consistently dark colour, by the absence of froth and sometimes by its admixture with food.

Whenever a history of haemoptysis is obtained, questions must be asked about its type, degree, frequency and duration. In some cases the events preceding it may be of importance in diagnosis, e.g. deep venous thrombosis in a lower limb or a respiratory infection.

TYPE AND DEGREE OF HAEMOPTYSIS. 1. *Frank haemoptysis*, in which the material coughed up consists wholly of blood, occurs most commonly in bronchiectasis, pulmonary infarction, tuberculosis and mitral stenosis. A rough estimate should be made of the amount of blood lost, bearing in mind that most patients tend to exaggerate this.

2. *Blood-stained sputum*, in which the blood and sputum are intimately mixed in various proportions, occurs most commonly in bronchial carcinoma.

3. *Blood-streaked sputum*, in which streaks of blood are present in mucoid or purulent sputum, is a fairly frequent symptom in chronic bronchitis but may also occur in bronchial carcinoma.

4. *Rusty sputum*, in which degradation products of haemoglobin give the sputum a colour varying between rust and golden-yellow, is a common feature of pneumococcal pneumonia and occurs in few other conditions.

FREQUENCY AND DURATION OF HAEMOPTYSIS. With frank haemoptysis it is usual for the blood in the sputum to become progressively darker for 24 to 48 hours at least after the bleeding ceases. When, however, small amounts of fresh blood are coughed up frequently, either as frank haemoptysis or blood-stained sputum, for example daily for a week, the symptom strongly suggests a diagnosis of bronchial carcinoma.

Chest Pain

Three types of chest pain are directly due to respiratory disease:

1. *Upper retrosternal pain* of the type experienced in acute tracheitis (p. 158)

2. *Retrosternal pain associated with lesions of the mediastinum*, e.g. tumours, acute mediastinitis and mediastinal emphysema. This type of pain, which is an uncommon but important symptom, has a constrictive or oppressive character similar to that of cardiac pain and may radiate into the arms or neck, but is seldom severe and is not related to exertion.

3. *Pleural pain*, caused by stretching of an inflamed parietal pleura, occurs in all forms of fibrinous (dry) pleurisy. Identical pain is produced by fractures of ribs. Pleural pain is recognised by its sharp, stabbing character and by its relationship to breathing and coughing. It may be present only at the end of a deep inspiration or during a cough; with more severe degrees even shallow breathing may produce

intense pain. Occasionally the pain is aggravated by exertion (which causes an increase in the depth of breathing) or by movements of the thoracic spine. Pleural pain often, but not invariably, subsides when an effusion develops, probably because the fluid limits expansion of the lung and thus reduces the range of movement of the chest wall.

In spontaneous pneumothorax typical pleural pain may be present, particularly if the amount of air in the pleural space is small. More often, however, after a brief initial episode of severe unilateral pain the patient complains mainly of tightness across the front of the chest, which may later become localised to the affected side. Rarely, there may be central retrosternal pain resembling that of cardiac infarction, with radiation into the neck and upper limbs. This type of pain may be due to mediastinal emphysema, with which spontaneous pneumothorax is occasionally associated.

Other intrathoracic diseases may produce central chest pain, e.g., lesions of the heart and great vessels (p. 100) or of the oesophagus (p. 192). Piercing unilateral chest pain may be due to involvement of a spinal nerve root by a vertebral lesion or by herpes zoster (p. 33). Pain caused by invasion of the chest wall by a malignant pulmonary tumour or by a metastatic deposit in a rib is constant, severe, aching and usually unrelated to breathing, while that produced by simple rib fractures resembles pleural pain. Chest pain in the absence of organic disease may be a manifestation of anxiety.

When a patient complains of chest pain the following information should be obtained about it as indicated on page 30; (1) Situation, (2) severity, (3) duration, (4) whether constant or intermittent, (5) nature and circumstances of onset, e.g. whether sudden or gradual; whether accompanied by other respiratory symptoms such as cough or dyspnoea, and (6) whether related to breathing, coughing, sneezing, spinal movements or exertion.

Dyspnoea

This has been analysed on pages 41 to 46.

Wheeze

When a patient complains of wheeze it is important first to discover what is meant by the term. Some patients use it merely to describe noisy and laboured breathing while others apply it to the rattling of secretions in the upper air passages. Wheeze should, however, be applied only to the musical sounds produced by the passage of air through narrowed bronchi. It is invariably louder during expiration and is often confined to that phase of the respiratory cycle. It is always more conspicuous during deep breathing and sometimes may become audible only when the depth of respiration is increased. Many patients become so accustomed to wheeze that they cease to be aware of its presence until a relative or friend draws attention to it. Patients with stridor (p. 158) may describe it as wheeze. Care must be taken to distinguish between these two sounds because stridor is usually caused by local obstruction of a major airway by a tumour or an inhaled foreign body, and thus demands urgent investigation and treatment.

SYMPTOMS INDICATIVE OF DISEASE OF THE UPPER RESPIRATORY TRACT

Nose and Nasopharynx. The most frequent symptoms of disease in the nose and nasopharynx are obstruction of the nasal airway, often described by patients as 'catarrh', and nasal discharge. Not uncommonly, these two symptoms co-exist.

It is necessary to enquire whether the *nasal obstruction* consistently affects the right or left nasal airway (or both), or whether it changes from one side to the other, according to the position of the head. This may be a relevant point since persistent obstruction is usually due to adenoids, to a deflected septum or to a collection of polypi, whereas intermittent obstruction is more often caused by mucosal oedema and excessive secretions. Bilateral nasal obstruction may lead to chronic mouth breathing, which, in children particularly, is often the reason for seeking medical advice.

The amount, nature and colour of any *nasal discharge* should normally be recorded in lay terms, e.g. profuse and watery, scanty, tenacious or green, unless a specimen is inspected by the doctor, and then technical terms, such as serous, mucoid or purulent, can be used. An attempt should be made to discover whether the discharge comes entirely from the nostrils or whether it drips into the back of the throat.

Factors which precipitate recurrent nasal obstruction and discharge, e.g. the inhalation of dust or grass pollens, should be identified whenever possible. An enquiry should also be made about excessive *sneezing,* a common feature of allergic rhinitis, and *headache* which may accompany acute infection of the nasal sinuses.

Epistaxis may give rise to haemoptysis if blood in the posterior nares is inhaled and then coughed up. This possibility should be kept in mind when a history is being taken from a patient with a complaint of haemoptysis.

Larynx. The two chief symptoms of laryngeal disease are hoarseness and stridor, but lesions of the larynx may also produce cough and pain.

Hoarseness may vary in degree from a slight harshness of the voice to aphonia. The voice may have a croaking quality in hypothyroidism. Enquiries should be made about the duration of hoarseness and about events which may have preceded its onset, such as a head cold, abuse of the voice, chronic cough or an operation on the neck or throat. The patient should be asked whether it is improving, worsening or remaining static.

Cough of a short, dry, barking character almost invariably accompanies hoarseness caused by an organic lesion within the larynx. The bovine cough of laryngeal paralysis is described on page 264.

Laryngeal stridor is a high-pitched crowing sound with each inspiration, and may be produced by a foreign body lodged between the cords, laryngeal spasm, exudate or oedema and bilateral vocal cord paralysis.

Laryngeal pain of mild degree occurs transiently in acute laryngitis; constant severe pain is a feature of advanced tuberculous laryngitis and laryngeal carcinoma.

All patients with stridor and those in whom a marked degree of hoarseness persists for more than a fortnight should have laryngoscopy (p. 164) carried out.

Trachea. Diseases of the trachea may produce pain, cough, stridor and dyspnoea.

Tracheal pain is referred to behind the sternal manubrium. In the early stages of acute tracheitis it may be quite severe and become momentarily intense on coughing but subsides as soon as the cough becomes productive.

Tracheal stridor is usually due to obstruction of the tracheal lumen by a malignant tumour and is always accompanied by dyspnoea. It is lower in pitch than laryngeal stridor, is heard best during inspiration and is accentuated by coughing. Stridor may also be present when a tumour partially obstructs one or both main bronchi.

History of Previous Illness

When the present illness appears to be involving the respiratory system, information of considerable value in diagnosis, prognosis, and treatment may be obtained from the past medical history. The following conditions are of particular importance in this respect:

Tuberculosis. Primary tuberculous infection in childhood may be responsible for lobar or segmental bronchiectasis in later life. Post-primary tuberculosis, if inadequately treated, may relapse. Extensive bilateral tuberculosis, even when no longer active, produces severe pulmonary fibrosis which may ultimately cause respiratory and heart failure. Bronchiectasis at the site of an inactive tuberculous lesion, or aspergillosis in a 'healed' tuberculous cavity, may give rise to severe haemoptysis. If a history of tuberculosis is given, full details of the nature and duration of treatment should be obtained, if necessary from the hospital or chest clinic which the patient attended.

Another point worthy of enquiry is a history of BCG vaccination which is offered to all tuberculin-negative British children at the age of 13 and in some countries is given to all new-born infants. Successful vaccination affords considerable protection against tuberculosis and this information may be of value in differential diagnosis.

Pneumonia and Pleurisy. Some chronic respiratory disorders, e.g. pulmonary fibrosis and bronchiectasis, date from an attack of pneumonia, sometimes described by patients as pleurisy or congestion. A history of recurrent pneumonia, particularly if it occurs on the same side each time, is suggestive of bronchiectasis, or, if the history is short (e.g less than a year), of bronchial carcinoma. Rarely, recurrent pneumonia may be a feature of myelomatosis or hypogamma-globulinaemia and it is common in children with cystic fibrosis. It may also be a complication of achalasia of the cardia.

Other Respiratory Illnesses. Severe attacks of measles or whooping cough in childhood used to be frequent causes of bronchiectasis. With the reduced incidence of these infections, bronchiectasis in children is now rare, but is still encountered in adults either as a sequel to such illnesses in childhood or as a complication of allergic bronchial aspergillosis.

Chest Injuries and Operations. It is necessary to enquire into the circumstances and nature of any chest injury or operation and to consider whether it might be related to the patient's current illness. For example, surgical or accidental trauma may produce deformities of the chest wall. A traumatic haemothorax, particularly if complicated by infection, may result in gross pleural thickening. A metallic foreign body lodged in the lung may cause recurrent haemoptysis or be responsible for the development of a chronic pulmonary abscess or bronchiectasis.

Other Surgical Procedures. The inhalation of septic material from the mouth or throat during dental extractions or tonsillectomy under general anaesthesia may result in the development of a pulmonary abscess. Any abdominal or thoracic operation, particularly an operation on the upper abdomen, may give rise to collapse of the lung; subsequent bacterial infection causes pneumonia and, at a later date, bronchiectasis if resolution is incomplete. Any major operation may also be complicated by pulmonary embolism and infarction.

Acute Abdominal Conditions. A perforated peptic ulcer or acute cholecystitis, may mimic pulmonary disease, and subphrenic abscess, amoebic liver abscess or pancreatitis may produce a pleural effusion.

Allergic Disorders. Patients who are believed to have an allergic disorder, such as bronchial asthma or allergic rhinitis, should be asked about previous manifestations of allergy, e.g. eczema, urticaria, and angio-oedema. A detailed enquiry should also be made regarding the effects of exposure to substances capable of producing allergic reactions, such as grass pollen, house dust, animal dander, foods and drugs.

Previous Radiological Examination. If an abnormality is present on the chest radiograph, such patients should be asked if they have been X-rayed in the past, and every effort made to obtain the earlier films, or at least the reports, since comparison with the current radiograph may be of considerable value in diagnosis.

Family and Social History

The *family history* of patients with respiratory disease may be significant in three ways:

1. Certain *infections*, notably tuberculosis, may be transmitted from one person to another. In such cases a history of contact with an infected person is, of course, more important than the family relationship.

2. In *allergic disorders*, such as bronchial asthma, there may be an inherited predisposition, and a family history is not uncommon. Routine enquiries into family circumstances may, however, reveal potential causes of anxiety, stress and domestic conflict, which may provoke attacks of asthma.

3. In *chronic bronchitis*, although an inherited predisposition cannot be excluded, the liability of several members of one family to develop the disease is more likely to be related to the conditions under which they all live, e.g. an overcrowded house situated in a district with a high level of atmospheric pollution.

Social problems, such as those of housing, finance and employment, loom large in the management of patients with all types of chronic respiratory disease and should be fully documented in every case. Information which should be obtained from all patients with chronic bronchitis must include the nature of their employment and the physical effort it involves. Should a man be advised to give up a well-paid job as an underground miner in favour of relatively poorly paid work in a less harmful atmospheric environment? Can anything be done to persuade a local authority or a landlord to exchange a top-floor flat without a lift for ground-level accommodation in the case of a patient too breathless to climb stairs?

Cigarette smoking is now accepted as the most important cause of bronchial carcinoma and chronic bronchitis. This fact is of some diagnostic relevance as bronchial carcinoma is rare in non-smokers. Tobacco smoking, especially of cigarettes, aggravates the symptoms of chronic bronchitis. A smoking history should include details such as the age when regular smoking started, the age when smoking was given up (where applicable), and the average consumption of tobacco (number of cigarettes or cigars per day, amount of pipe tobacco per week).

Overeating and overindulgence in alcohol may contribute to the development of obesity, which invariably causes an increase in exertional dyspnoea, whatever the basic pulmonary pathology. Extreme obesity may be directly responsible for respiratory and cardiac failure.

Occupational and Other Environmental Hazards

Since both acute and chronic respiratory disease may be caused by the inhalation of certain inorganic and organic dusts and chemical substances, it is important to record a complete occupational history, covering both present and previous employment. Such hazards may be encountered by workers in the coal, iron and steel, and pottery industries, by stonemasons and farmworkers, and by those who are liable to inhale asbestos dust and chemical substances, such as isocyanates, in the course of their work. Whenever such an occupational history is obtained, detailed information should be sought regarding the degree and duration of exposure, and its time relationship to the onset of symptoms.

In a separate but equally important category are dust hazards encountered in the patient's environment, but not necessarily at work. Persons in close contact with pigeons, parrots, budgerigars or canaries may develop extrinsic allergic alveolitis or psittacosis, while atopic subjects may develop allergic rhinitis or bronchial asthma when exposed to allergens such as pollen, house dust, feathers, animal dander or certain types of fungal spore. An enquiry should always be made about these and other environmental hazards when an occupational history is being taken.

THE PHYSICAL EXAMINATION

The External Features of Respiratory Disease

Initial Impression. There are a number of features which may have become evident during the course of history-taking and should immediately cause the observer to suspect respiratory disease. These are cough, wheeze or stridor, and laboured breathing.

The frequency, severity and type of cough should be noted. The character of wheeze and the degree of respiratory distress should also be observed. The speed with which a patient can dress or undress is often a useful index of respiratory disability. Attention should be paid to any abnormality of the voice and to fetor of the breath, for which an anaerobic infection of the lung may be responsible if a local cause in the mouth can be excluded. The state of nutrition should be roughly assessed (overweight, underweight, normal) pending precise measurements of height and weight. Finally, any suggestion of anaemia or polycythaemia should be noted, either of which may be a relevant finding in certain types of respiratory disease.

Cyanosis. Central cyanosis of respiratory origin is most frequently seen in chronic obstructive airways disease. In such cases peripheral vasodilatation due to carbon dioxide retention leads to warm blue hands, but the colour of the tongue is a more reliable indicator of central cyanosis. It may also occur in pneumonia, bronchial asthma and tension pneumothorax and in allergic and fibrosing alveolitis. The cardiac causes of central and peripheral cyanosis are described on page 105.

Peripheral cyanosis affecting the face and neck, and in some cases the upper limbs also, is one of the features of superior vena caval obstruction (see below). Severe chronic hypoxia of either pulmonary or cardiac origin is often associated with polycythaemia and an extreme degree of cyanosis, partly central and partly peripheral, may be seen in these conditions.

Oedema. The detection of peripheral oedema (p. 51) is especially important in patients with chronic obstructive airways disease which is often complicated by right ventricular failure. Oedema of a different distribution is seen in *obstruction of the superior vena cava*. In this condition, which is a fairly common complication of bronchial carcinoma, but may also be caused by a very large benign tumour or by chronic mediastinal fibrosis, the face and neck appear swollen and puffy — although the tissues seldom pit on pressure — and conjunctival oedema (chemosis) is often present. Because of more efficient collateral venous drainage the upper limbs are less frequently affected, but in some cases there is pitting oedema of the hands and forearms. When the superior vena cava is obstructed the external jugular veins become grossly distended but no venous pulsation is visible in the neck. After a week or two, dilated superficial veins and venules appear on the anterior and lateral aspects of the chest wall from the clavicles to below the costal margins. These veins convey blood from the tributaries of the subclavian and axillary veins to the drainage area of the inferior vena cava. The downward direction of blood flow can be demonstrated by the method described on page 138.

The Hands. Examination of the hands in patients with suspected respiratory disease, apart from the observation of cyanosis, is chiefly concerned with the recognition of *clubbing of the fingers*. This phenomenon occurs in a variety of respiratory, cardiovascular and alimentary diseases, including: (1) bronchial carcinoma and certain other intrathoracic tumours, some forms of pulmonary and pleural suppuration, e.g. bronchiectasis, pulmonary abscess and empyema, and most cases of fibrosing alveolitis, (2) cyanotic congenital heart disease and infective endocarditis, and (3) the malabsorption syndrome, Crohn's disease, ulcerative colitis and hepatic cirrhosis. It has also been observed as a familial trait and may occur unilaterally in association with an aneurysm of the subclavian artery. The swelling of the terminal phalanges in clubbing, which usually, but less obviously, affects the toes also, is due to interstitial oedema and dilatation of the arterioles and

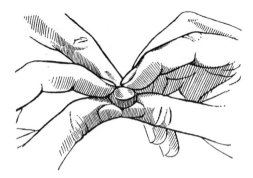

Fig. 6.1   Testing for fluctuation at the base of the nail.

capillaries. In the earlier stages there may be little or no visible swelling, but the test for abnormal fluctuation at the nail bases will be positive (Fig. 6.1).

The finger is placed on the pulp of the examiner's two thumbs and the dorsum of the finger is palpated over the base of the nail by the tips of the examiner's two index or middle fingers. If a sensation of fluctuation is elicited, the test is said to be positive, provided that this is greater than the very slight degree of fluctuation which can be detected in normal fingers. When fluctuation is marked, palpation of the nail itself may give the impression that it is floating free on its bed.

With more advanced degrees of clubbing, various visible changes develop progressively (Fig. 4.1):

1. Swelling of the subcutaneous tissues over the base of the nail, as illustrated, causes the overlying skin to become tense, shiny and red, with obliteration of the skin creases and loss of the normal angle between the nail and the nail base.
2. Later, as the swelling involves the nail bed, the curvature of the nail, especially in its long axis, increases.
3. Finally, swelling of the pulp of the finger in all its dimensions occurs in fully developed clubbing. In a few cases there may also be hypertrophic pulmonary osteoarthropathy causing pain and swelling of the hands, wrists, knees, feet and ankles, with radiographic evidence of subperiosteal bone formation.

Increased curvature of the finger nails is commonly seen in normal subjects and, as an isolated phenomenon without other evidence of clubbing, is of no significance.

The Eyes. The importance of examining the eyes in patients suspected of having respiratory disease is to recognise conditions such as phlyctenular keratoconjunctivitis, which may be a manifestation of primary tuberculosis, and iridocyclitis, which may be seen in tuberculosis or sarcoidosis. Ophthalmoscopy is essential whenever a diagnosis of acute miliary tuberculosis is suspected since choroidal tubercles are a pathognomonic feature of that condition. Chemosis and dilatation of the conjunctival and retinal veins are very common in patients with hypercapnia of long duration secondary to chronic obstructive airways disease, and a few of these patients may develop papilloedema.

The Neck. A systematic method of examining the neck has been described on page 80. The part of the examination which is of particular importance in patients believed to have respiratory disease is that concerned with the detection of enlarged scalene lymph nodes. These nodes are often involved when a pathological process, such as carcinoma, lymphoma, sarcoidosis or tuberculosis, affects the mediastinal nodes, and biopsy of an enlarged scalene node may yield information of conclusive diagnostic value. This group of nodes is within a pad of fat on the surface of the scalenus anterior muscle, just above its insertion into the scalene tubercle of the first rib (Fig. 6.2). To reach this situation the palpating finger must dip behind the clavicle through the clavicular origin of sternomastoid and for the examination to be adequate all the anterior cervical muscles must be completely relaxed. This is best achieved by having the patient sitting in a chair with the hands resting on the thighs and the cervical spine partially flexed. The examination should be carried out from behind, one side at a time, and the whole of the supraclavicular and retroclavicular regions of the neck from the trachea to the anterior border of trapezius should be carefully palpated for enlarged nodes, special attention being directed to the scalene regions (Fig. 6.3). When a node is found it should be assessed as indicated on page 46. Nodes which are greater than 0.5 cm in diameter, firm in consistence and round in shape are usually of pathological significance, many of them containing metastatic deposits from a bronchial carcinoma. Large, fixed masses are present in some of these cases. Hard, craggy nodes may, however, be caused by healed and calcified tuberculosis; in such cases calcification is always visible on radiographic examination.

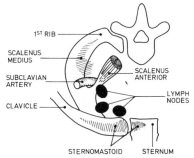

Fig. 6.2   Relation of lymph nodes to scalenus anterior.

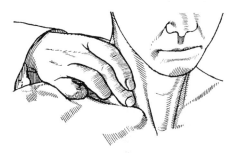

Fig. 6.3   Palpation of lymph nodes on scalenus anterior.

The Skin. Examination of the skin may, on occasion, yield information of considerable value in the diagnosis of respiratory disease. Some of the cutaneous and subcutaneous lesions which may be relevant in this connection are:

1. Erythema nodosum (p. 94), which may be the initial clinical manifestation of a primary tuberculous infection or of sarcoidosis.
2. Metastastic tumour nodules, which may be derived from a primary bronchial carcinoma.
3. Cutaneous sarcoids and lupus pernio, which may occur in association with sarcoidosis involving the intrathoracic lymph nodes or the lungs.
4. The rash of lupus erythematosus (p. 94), which may accompany systemic, including pulmonary or pleural, manifestations of this connective tissue disorder.
5. Herpetic vesicles, which may identify the cause of unilateral chest pain.

THE UPPER RESPIRATORY TRACT

The upper respiratory tract extends from external nares to the junction of the larynx with the trachea. It includes the nasal cavity, the nasopharynx, the nasal sinuses, the oropharynx and the larynx. Infective and allergic disorders of the upper respiratory tract are amongst the most common afflictions of mankind and infection in any part of it may produce or aggravate disease of the bronchi and lungs. Clinical examination of the nose and throat is therefore an essential part of the investigation of all patients with respiratory disease. Since oral sepsis, particularly suppurative gingivitis, may also cause pulmonary disease, such as lung abscess, the buccal cavity, the teeth and the gums should also be included in the examination. The procedure recommended for examination of the nose, mouth and throat is described on pages 76 to 80.

THE LARYNX

External examination of the larynx seldom yields any useful information, but swelling of the lips, the tongue, around the eyes and on the front of the neck caused by a hypersensitivity reaction (angio-oedema) is a relevant finding, since the oedema may involve the glottis and give rise to dyspnoea and stridor, which may be followed by complete respiratory obstruction.

Examination of the interior of the larynx by indirect or direct laryngoscopy is an essential step in the investigation of hoarseness. In indirect laryngoscopy, a small (demisted) mirror reflecting light from a head lamp, from a head mirror, or from the small electric bulb on the laryngoscopic attachment of a diagnostic set is placed just in front of the uvula and with a co-operative patient a clear view can be obtained of the epiglottis, the arytenoid region and the vocal cords (Fig. 6.4). The examination can often be facilitated by the use of an anaesthetic lozenge (benzocaine). Direct laryngoscopy, using a laryngoscope, is necessary in some cases, particularly if a biopsy has to be taken, but is an uncomfortable procedure which requires more extensive local anaesthesia. Lesions which can be detected by laryngoscopy include laryngeal tuberculosis, laryngeal tumours and vocal cord paralysis.

A paralysed vocal cord adopts a position midway between abduction and adduction and fails to adduct on phonation. Paralysis of abduction may precede complete paralysis of the cord.

THE TRACHEA

In normal subjects the upper 4 to 5 cm of the trachea can be felt in the neck between the cricoid cartilage and the suprasternal notch, but in thick-set or obese subjects it may be so deeply placed that is is difficult or impossible to feel.

The position of the trachea is determined by gently thrusting the tip of the index finger into the suprasternal notch, exactly in the midline (Fig. 6.5). By this manoeuvre any deviation of the trachea to either side can readily be detected. Thyroid enlargement may displace the trachea, and the thyroid gland should be examined before tracheal deviation is attributed to intrathoracic disease. In patients

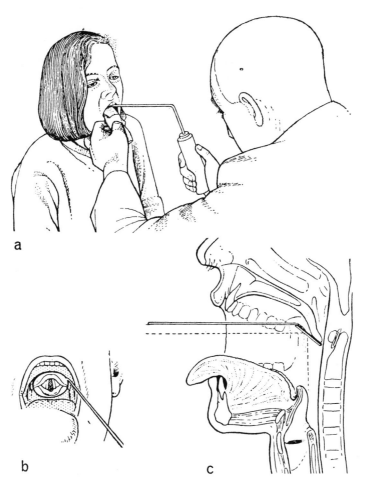

Fig. 6.4   Indirect laryngoscopy. (a) Positions of the patient and doctor. (b) View of larynx in mirror. (c) Position of mirror in relation to soft palate and larynx.

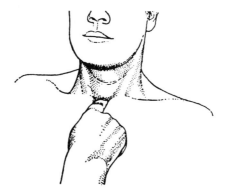

Fig. 6.5   Determining the position of the trachea.

with chronic airflow obstruction there is a downward movement of the trachea during inspiration. This can be detected by placing a finger below the cricoid cartilage, when the distance from the suprasternal notch may be greatly reduced and the cricoid cartilage may be tugged down with sufficient force to squeeze the finger.

THE CHEST

Physical examination of the chest, like examination of the heart and abdomen, makes use of the techniques of inspection, palpation, percussion and auscultation. It has three main purposes:

1. To detect abnormalities of the chest wall by inspection and palpation.
2. To observe and analyse respiratory movements primarily by inspection but also by palpation.
3. To elicit specific physical signs by means of which abnormalities in the structure and function of the bronchi, lungs and pleura can be recognised, using mainly percussion and auscultation.

1. The Examination of the Chest Wall

With the patient sitting erect in a good light and preferably stripped to the waist, the chest is inspected from the front, from the back and from each side. Abnormalities in the shape of the chest are observed, and by means of combined inspection and palpation a careful search is made for lesions of the chest wall.

Abnormalities in the Shape of the Chest. Those of clinical importance are as follows:

1. *The anteroposterior diameter may be increased* relative to the lateral diameter. In normal subjects the ratio is usually about 5 : 7, and in flat-chested patients without respiratory disease, it may be as low as 1 : 2. In some patients with emphysema, however, the two measurements may approximate (barrel-chest). It should be remembered that an increase in the anteroposterior diameter may be due to thoracic kyphosis unrelated to respiratory disease. Chest deformity in emphysema is not a reliable guide to the severity of the functional defect. It is seen most frequently in patients who have developed chronic respiratory disease (bronchitis or asthma) relatively early in life, i.e. before the age of 30 years. Those in whom the onset is delayed until after the age of 40 years may progress even to the stage of respiratory failure without exhibiting any increase in the anteroposterior diameter of the chest.

2. *Pectus carinatum* (pigeon chest) is a common sequel to chronic respiratory disease in childhood. It consists of a localised prominence of the sternum and adjacent costal cartilages, often accompanied by indrawing of the ribs to form symmetrical horizontal grooves (*Harrison's sulci*) above the costal margins, which are themselves usually everted. These deformities are thought to result from repeated strong contractions of the diaphragm while the bony thorax is still in a pliable state. Pectus carinatum deformity in undernourished populations may also be caused by rickets.

3. *Pectus excavatum* (funnel-chest) is a developmental defect in which there is either a localised depression of the lower end of the sternum, or, less commonly, depression of the whole length of the body of the sternum and of the costal cartilages attached to it. Pectus excavatum is usually asymptomatic, but, when there is a very marked degree of depression of the sternum, the heart may be compressed between it and the vertebral bodies. This produces displacement of the apex beat to the left, and the ventilatory capacity of the lungs may be restricted in severe cases.

4. *Thoracic kyphoscoliosis* (p. 339) ranges in degree from the minor changes in spinal curvature seen in many otherwise healthy subjects to grossly disfiguring and disabling deformities. Thoracic scoliosis may alter the position of the mediastinum in relation to the anterior chest wall, with the result that abnormalities in the position of the trachea and the cardiac apex beat may be mistakenly attributed to cardiac or pulmonary disease. Severe kyphoscoliosis may have profound effects on pulmonary function, as the chest deformity reduces the ventilatory capacity of the lungs and increases the work of breathing. Many such patients eventually develop hypoxia, hypercapnia and heart failure.

5. *Thoracic operations*, pacticularly thoracoplasty, may result in a considerable degree of chest deformity, of which scoliosis may be an important secondary feature.

Lesions of the Chest Wall. Combined inspection and palpation of the whole chest wall is essential for the detection of abnormalities which may include:

1. *Cutaneous lesions*, e.g. skin eruptions, sarcoid or other nodules, purpuric spots, bruises, scars, discharging sinuses.

2. *Subcutaneous lesions*, e.g. inflammatory swellings, metastatic tumour nodules, neurofibromas, lipomas. (The nature of certain cutaneous and subcutaneous lesions, e.g. sarcoid nodules and tumours, may require to be determined by biopsy.)

3. *Subcutaneous emphysema* (air in the subcutaneous tissues) may cause diffuse swelling of the chest wall, the neck and, in some cases, the face. The condition is recognised by the characteristic crackling sensation elicited by palpation of the air-containing tissues. When subcutaneous emphysema is localised to the chest wall, it is usually derived from a tension pneumothorax from which it has escaped along the track of a needle or intercostal catheter used to decompress the pleural space. In other cases air extruded from the lungs as a result of interstitial rupture of the alveoli tracks into the mediastinum (*mediastinal emphysema*). The air usually escapes innocuously into the neck and produces subcutaneous emphysema of the neck, face and chest wall which in severe cases may be very gross but is not in itself dangerous. When air is present in the mediastinum the heart sounds may be replaced by a churning noise, accentuated during systole.

4. *Vascular anomalies*, e.g. spider telangiectases (p. 92), enlarged vascular channels (arterial in coarctation of aorta; venous in superior vena caval obstruction).

5. *Localised prominences and deformities*, involving clavicles, scapulae, sternum, ribs, costochondral junctions and spinous processes.

6. *Localised tenderness on palpation*, e.g. from a fractured rib, from tumour invading the chest wall, from spinal injury or disease, or in association with pleural or nerve root pain.

7. *Lesions of the breasts* (p. 83) and *enlargement of the axillary lymph nodes* (p. 83).

2. The Observation of Respiratory Movements

(i) **Respiratory Frequency.** The number of breaths in a full minute is counted by surreptitiously observing the movements of the chest wall, with the fingers held on the pulse to avoid drawing the patient's attention to breathing. The normal frequency at rest in a healthy adult is about 14 respirations per minute. The rate is increased in a variety of pathological states, including pyrexia from any cause, acute pulmonary infections, particularly those accompanied by pleural pain, and conditions in which there is a sudden increase in the work of breathing, e.g. bronchial asthma and acute pulmonary oedema.

(ii) **Respiratory Depth.** This is difficult to estimate clinically as the movements of the chest and diaphragm, on which it is dependent, cannot be accurately measured. Furthermore, it is only too easy to confuse a dyspnoeic patient's strenuous but unavailing efforts to achieve an adequate tidal volume with a genuine increase in the depth of breathing. It is usually possible with practice, however, to recognise marked degrees of overventilation and underventilation. The latter may be of considerable clinical importance in the diagnosis of respiratory failure, while hysterical overventilation may cause tetany or epileptic fits.

In massive pulmonary embolism and in metabolic acidosis, usually due to diabetic ketosis or uraemia, pulmonary ventilation at rest may be considerably raised. This can be recognised clinically by an increase in the depth of respiration (*air hunger*) which may give rise to the subjective sensation of dyspnoea. In *periodic* or *Cheyne-Stokes breathing* there is a cyclical variation in the depth of respiration, with periods of overventilation alternating with complete apnoea. It is believed to be caused by a decrease in the sensitivity of the respiratory centre to carbon dioxide. This occurs in left ventricular failure and in certain neurological conditions, particularly those involving the medulla. The cycle usually lasts for less than two minutes and during the phase of overventilation the patient may experience respiratory distress.

Overventilation may also occur in patients who are unconscious as a result of severe brain damage caused by trauma, haemorrhage or infarction. In such patients laxity of the soft palate may cause *stertorous breathing*.

(iii) **Maximum Chest Expansion.** This is estimated by placing a tape measure round the chest at nipple level and recording the maximum inspiratory/expiratory difference in the chest circumference. There is a considerable degree of observer variation with this measurement and it does not correlate well with vital capacity, probably because in some subjects breathing is predominantly diaphragmatic. A figure of above 5 cm can, however, be regarded as normal and one of 2 cm or less as definitely abnormal. Chest expansion is diminished in almost every type of diffuse broncho-pulmonary disease, e.g. bronchial asthma, emphysema and pulmonary fibrosis, and in conditions which restrict movement of the ribs, such as ankylosing spondylitis.

(iv) **Mode of Breathing.** In normal subjects inspiration is effected by contraction of the intercostal muscles and the diaphragm, while expiration is a passive process dependent upon the elastic recoil of the lungs towards the hila. Women make more use of the intercostal muscles than of the diaphragm and their respiratory movements are predominantly thoracic. Men, on the other hand, rely more on the diaphragm and their respiratory movements at rest are mainly

abdominal. Babies of both sexes are also diaphragmatic breathers. Any departure from the normal mode of breathing should receive close attention. If respiratory movements are exclusively thoracic this may indicate that diaphragmatic movement is inhibited by pain caused, for example, by peritoneal irritation, or restricted by increased intra-abdominal pressure in conditions such as ascites, gaseous distension of the bowel, a large ovarian cyst or pregnancy. If respiratory movements are exclusively abdominal, ankylosing spondylitis, intercostal paralysis or pleural pain may be responsible for the lack of chest expansion.

Although dyspnoea is a subjective phenomenon it is usually accompanied by objective evidence of respiratory difficulty or distress. There is often an increase in respiratory frequency, which may be accompanied by dilatation of the alae nasi during inspiration, but as these features may be observed in the absence of dyspnoea they are not reliable indices of respiratory distress. A much more useful criterion is the presence of abnormal respiratory movements of the following types:

(a) *Abnormal inspiratory movements* produced by contraction of the cervical muscles (principally the sternomastoids, scaleni and trapezii), by which the whole thoracic cage is, in effect, lifted off the diaphragm with every inspiration. Patients breathe in this way if adequate pulmonary ventilation cannot be achieved by normal inspiratory efforts, for example, when there is gross overdistension of the lungs in conditions such as advanced emphysema and severe bronchial asthma. More violent inspiratory movements of a similar character are observed in patients with obstruction of the larynx or trachea. Indrawing of the suprasternal and supraclavicular fossae, the intercostal spaces and the epigastrium with each inspiration invariably accompanies airways obstruction of this type and may also be seen, although it is usually less conspicuous, in emphysema and asthma.

A much more striking degree of indrawing of the chest wall is seen in patients who have sustained double fractures of a series of ribs or of the sternum. The portion of the thoracic cage between the fractures becomes mobile and, with the overlying soft tissues, is sucked in with every inspiration. *Paradoxical movement* of this type interferes seriously with pulmonary ventilation and may cause grave respiratory distress and hypoxia.

(b) *Abnormal expiratory movements* produced by powerful contractions of the abdominal muscles and latissimus dorsi. These are observed if the elastic recoil of the lungs is insufficient to complete the expulsion of air from the alveoli, as in emphysema, or when expiratory airflow obstruction is present, as in bronchial asthma and some cases of chronic bronchitis. Patients with a severe degree of expiratory obstruction prefer to sit upright, grasping a bed table or the back of a chair. This enables them to fix the shoulder girdle so that the latissimus dorsi can be used to augment the expiratory efforts. Many patients who breathe in this way can be seen to purse their lips with every expiration. This manoeuvre keeps the intrabronchial pressure above that of the surrounding alveoli and prevents collapse of the bronchial walls which would otherwise result from the unopposed pressure of air trapped in the alveoli.

(c) *Localised impairment of respiratory movement* is usually caused by disease in the underlying lung or pleura, and is almost invariably associated with abnormal findings on percussion and auscultation.

3. The Elicitation of Specific Physical Signs of Pulmonary or Pleural Disease

In health the two sides of the chest are seen to move to an equal extent with respiration. The trachea is central and the apex beat is in the normal position. Percussion of the chest wall elicits a resonant note over both lungs. The breath sounds heard on auscultation are vesicular in type (p. 177). In diseases of the bronchi, lungs and pleura, various changes in these physical signs may be observed. For example, movement of one side of the chest may be reduced, the percussion note may lose its normal resonance, the breath sounds may alter in type or intensity and may be accompanied by added sounds, and there may be displacement of the trachea and cardiac apex beat to one or other side.

Certain groups of physical signs are typically associated with certain pathological changes in the lungs and pleura. Such changes are not necessarily specific for one particular disease. For example, the physical signs of consolidation may occur in pneumonia or tuberculosis and those of pleural effusion may be present in malignant disease, empyema or cardiac failure. Each group of physical signs therefore gives an indication only of the gross pathology of the lesion, and not of its precise nature, the diagnosis of which depends on an analysis of all the clinical and other evidence. The characteristic physical signs of the more common lesions are summarised on page 183.

The most convenient method of eliciting physical signs is to examine the front and sides of the chest and then the back. When the anterior and lateral aspects are being examined the patient should lie in a supine or semi-recumbent position on a bed or couch, with the chest and upper abdomen fully exposed and evenly illuminated down to the level of the umbilicus, and with the arms sufficiently abducted to allow access to the axillary regions. When the posterior aspect of the chest is being examined the patient should sit upright with arms folded across the chest. Some patients are too weak to maintain this position and have to be held forward by a third person standing at the foot of the bed and grasping the patient's outstretched hands. At this stage all pillows should be removed to allow unimpeded access to the whole length of the back.

Examination of the anterior and lateral aspects of the chest should begin with a comparison of the range of respiratory movement on the two sides during both normal and deep breathing. The position of the trachea (p. 164) and the cardiac apex beat (p. 120) should then be determined and vocal fremitus (p. 172) tested over equivalent areas of the right and left lung. Next, the percussion note on the two sides should be compared and any areas of dullness carefully delineated. Finally, by means of auscultation, the type and intensity of the breath sounds and voice sounds should be assessed and the nature of any added sounds identified. A similar procedure is adopted for examination of the back of the chest.

Inspection and Palpation

The object of these procedures is to detect differences in the range of movement on the two sides of the chest. Unless such differences are gross they are difficult to detect, especially by palpation. More reliance should therefore be placed on inspection. There are indeed some clinicians who believe that palpation is of such limited value that they do not take the trouble to perform it. Palpation is also used to elicit vocal fremitus and palpable accompaniments (p. 172).

Methods of Comparing Range of Movement of the Chest Wall. 1. *Respiratory movement in the infraclavicular* regions is compared by inspecting the chest with the patient supine and the head resting on a pillow. Care must be taken to ensure that the head and trunk are in a straight line and that the shoulders are relaxed and in a symmetrical position. The doctor crouches at the foot of the bed, views the infraclavicular regions tangentially (Fig. 6.6) and asks the patient to take steady deep breaths. By this technique slight unilateral impairment of chest wall movement can usually be recognised.

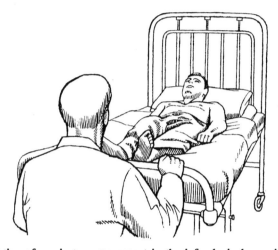

Fig. 6.6 Inspection of respiratory movement in the infraclavicular regions.

2. *Respiratory movement at the costal margins* can also be accurately gauged by inspection if the patient is thin. In other cases, however, palpation is the only technique available for this purpose. The sides of the chest are grasped firmly with the fingers in such a way as to approximate the tips of the outstretched thumbs in the region of the xiphoid process. The hands should be adjusted to ensure that there is a loose fold of skin between the two thumbs to that they can move apart as the chest expands. The movement of the two thumbs with deep breathing can then be used to estimate the relative degree of movement on the two sides.

3. *Respiratory movements of the lower ribs posteriorly*, where inspection is seldom helpful, have to be estimated by a similar technique (Fig. 6.7). With the patient sitting erect, the chest is grasped from behind with the two hands and the tips of the outstretched thumbs are brought together in the region of the tenth thoracic spine. Again it should be ensured that there is a loose fold of skin between the thumbs, the movement of which can then be used to estimate the relative degree of chest expansion on the two sides.

THE SIGNIFICANCE OF REDUCED MOVEMENT. Unilateral reduction of chest wall movement occurs in many types of respiratory disease. In pleural effusion and empyema, movement may be absent, and if the lesion has persisted for some weeks

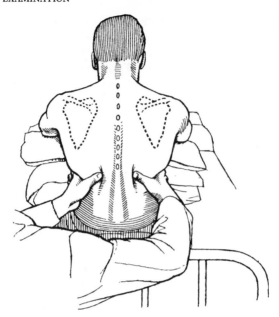

Fig. 6.7   Estimation of respiratory movements of the lower ribs posteriorly.

retraction of the ribs and intercostal spaces may produce flattening of the affected side of the chest, which is most obvious in the pectoral region. The term 'frozen chest' is sometimes applied to this condition. Less marked reduction of movement occurs in pulmonary consolidation and collapse, particularly if these conditions are accompanied by pleurisy. In pneumothorax the limitation of movement is related to the amount of air in the pleural space and thus to the degree of pulmonary collapse; in tension pneumothorax the affected side of the chest may be immobilised in a position of almost full inspiration. In pulmonary tuberculosis even extensive lesions may have little effect on chest wall movement during the early stages of the disease, but later, when fibrosis develops, there may be severe restriction of movement, with flattening of the affected side of the chest.

In bronchial asthma, emphysema and diffuse pulmonary fibrosis movements of the chest wall are symmetrically reduced. In the first two conditions this results from overinflation of the lungs. In diffuse pulmonary fibrosis, on the other hand, inspiratory movement is restricted by the reduced distensibility of the lungs. In severe cases this may bring each inspiration to an abrupt halt and produce the phenomenon of 'door stop' breathing.

Vocal Fremitus. This is tested by placing the palm of the hand on equivalent areas of the chest wall and asking the patient to say 'one, one, one'. This should be done at three levels anteriorly, at three levels posteriorly and at one level laterally. Vocal fremitus is a crude test and only when it is absent, e.g. over a large pleural effusion, is the test likely to provide useful information.

Palpable Accompaniments. The vibrations from a low-pitched rhonchus or a coarse pleural rub can occasionally be detected by a hand placed on the chest wall. In such cases an unusually loud rhonchus or rub is invariably present on auscultation and there is seldom any difficulty in distinguishing between the two. A palpable rhonchus generally has its origin in a large bronchus and, if persistent and unilateral suggests partial bronchial obstruction by a tumour or foreign body. A palpable pleural rub, which may be recognised by the patient as a grating sensation within the chest, has no specific significance, but a rub which can be detected by palpation is more often encountered in chronic than in acute pleurisy, and is not always accompanied by pain.

Percussion

The object of percussion is to compare the degree of resonance over equivalent areas on the two sides of the chest, and to map out any area in which the percussion note is abnormal. Resonance on percussion can be elicited wherever aerated lung tissue or a large air-containing space, such as a pneumothorax, a thin-walled pulmonary cavity or a hollow viscus, is in apposition to the chest wall. The percussion note loses its normal resonance whenever aerated lung tissue is separated from the chest wall by pleural fluid or thickening, or when lung tissue is rendered airless by consolidation, collapse or fibrosis. Over such lesions the percussion note is impaired or dull. The most marked degree of dullness on percussion is found over a large pleural effusion. Percussion over a solid viscus such as the heart or the liver will elicit a dull note, but the area of dullness is always less extensive than would be expected from anatomical surface marking, since aerated lung is interposed between part of the viscus and the chest wall.

A hyperresonant percussion note may be found over a pneumothorax, particularly if the pleural pressure is above atmospheric level, and also over lung which is markedly emphysematous. An apparent finding of generalised hyperresonance must, however, be accepted with reserve, since a change in the absolute pitch of a percussion note is always difficult to recognise and may depend mainly upon the thickness of the chest wall. For that reason it is not usually advisable to attempt to distinguish between normal resonance and hyperresonance when the percussion note is equally resonant on the two sides.

Anatomical Considerations. The regions of the thorax over which a resonant percussion note is normally found correspond approximately with the surface marking of the lungs (Fig. 6.8).

When an abnormality of the percussion note is due to pulmonary consolidation or collapse it is usually possible to identify the lobe or lobes involved by reference to the surface marking of the fissures but, unless a lobe is totally consolidated, the area over which the percussion note is impaired is often much smaller than would be expected from its surface marking. This is even more striking when a lobe is collapsed. With a pleural effusion the area of dullness on percussion is unrelated to the surface anatomy of the lobes. Except with localised effusions, it is situated over the lower part of the hemithorax and usually extends to a higher level posteriorly and laterally than at the front of the chest.

In localising the position of a pulmonary or pleural lesion the observer should make use of the breath sounds and voice sounds in addition to the percussion note. However, small lesions such as areas of segmental consolidation or collapse, may not produce any abnormal physical signs. Even with larger lesions the signs may be partly or completely obscured if the lungs are emphysematous.

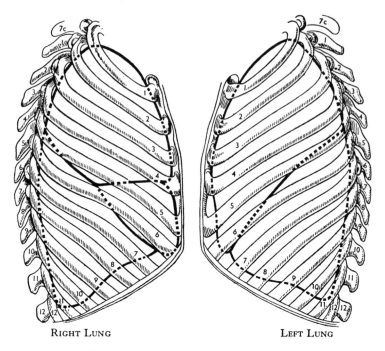

RIGHT LUNG   LEFT LUNG

Fig. 6.8 Surface markings of the lungs.

Technique of Percussion. The basic technique of percussion is as follows:

1. The left hand is placed on the chest wall, palm downwards and with the fingers slightly separated, so that the second phalanx of the middle finger is precisely over the area to be percussed.

2. The middle finger of the left hand is then pressed firmly against the chest wall and the centre of its second phalanx is struck sharply with the tip of the right middle finger. In order to produce a satisfactory percussion note the right middle finger must be held at a right angle (to produce a 'hammer' effect) and the entire movement must come from the wrist joint.

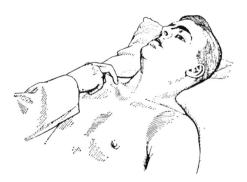

Fig. 6.9 Clavicular percussion.

The positions in which the percussion note on the two sides should be compared are as follows:

ANTERIOR CHEST WALL.

    (a) Clavicle (Fig. 6.9).

    (b) Infraclavicular region (Fig. 6.10).

    (c) Second to sixth intercostal spaces (Fig. 6.10).

LATERAL CHEST WALL. Fourth to seventh intercostal spaces (Fig. 6.10).

POSTERIOR CHEST WALL.

    (a) Trapezius, percussing downwards on lung apex (Fig. 6.12)

    (b) Above spine of scapula (Fig. 6.12).

    (c) At intervals of 4 to 5 cm from below spine of scapula down to eleventh rib (Fig. 6.12).

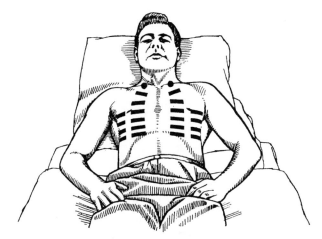

Fig. 6.10   Sites for percussion of anterior and lateral chest wall.

The technique of clavicular percussion (Fig. 6.9), which may be of considerable value in detecting lesions of the upper lobes, differs from that used elsewhere in that the clavicles are percussed directly with the right middle finger or, if preferred, with the right index, middle and ring fingers held closely together. The correct situation for percussion is within the medial third of the clavicle, just lateral to its expanded medial end. Percussion more laterally will merely elicit the dullness produced by the muscle masses of the shoulder. Clavicular percussion should be directed backwards and downwards. The lung apices are percussed by placing the left middle finger across the anterior border of the trapezius muscle, overlapping the supraclavicular fossa, and directing the percussion downwards (Fig. 6.11).

When an area of impaired resonance is discovered, its boundaries should be mapped out by percussing from a zone of normal resonance towards the suspected abnormality. The same technique should be used to determine the boundaries of cardiac dullness (p. 121) and hepatic dullness (p. 209).

A crude impression of the range of diaphragmatic movement can be obtained by measuring the distance between the lower borders of pulmonary resonance at the back of the chest in full inspiration and forced expiration, but this procedure (*tidal percussion*) is of little practical value.

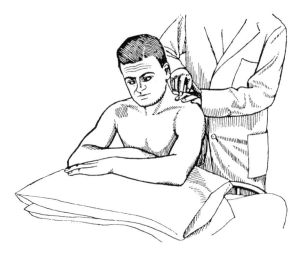

Fig. 6.11   Percussion of apex of lung.

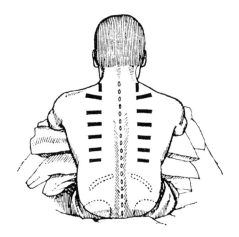

Fig. 6.12   Sites for percussion of posterior chest wall.

The terms used to describe different types of percussion note are shown on Table 6.1.

Auscultation

Auscultation of the lungs has an important place in the diagnosis of certain respiratory diseases, but is of little or no value in others. In bronchial asthma and 'dry' pleurisy, for example, the stethoscope provides information of positive diagnostic value which cannot be obtained in any other way. In contrast, auscultation is unhelpful in the early diagnosis of pulmonary tuberculosis, which may reach an advanced stage before any abnormality can be detected with the stethoscope.

Table 6.1 Percussion note

Type	Lesions by which produced
Tympanitic	Hollow viscus
Hyperresonant	Pneumothorax
Resonant	Normal lung
Impaired	Pulmonary fibrosis Pulmonary consolidation (some cases) Pulmonary collapse (some cases)
Dull	Pulmonary consolidation (some cases) Pulmonary collapse (some cases) Pleural thickening
Stony dull	Pleural effusion

Breath Sounds and Voice Sounds. Breath sounds are produced by vibrations of the vocal cords caused by the turbulent flow of air through the larynx during inspiration and expiration. The sounds so produced are transmitted along the trachea and bronchi and through the lungs to the chest wall. In their passage through normal lungs the intensity and frequency-pattern of the sounds are altered. When they are heard through a stethoscope on the chest wall they have a characteristic rustling quality to which the term *vesicular* is applied. The intensity of the sounds increases steadily during inspiration and then quickly fades away during the first one-third of expiration. Diseases of the bronchi, lungs and pleura may alter the breath sounds in several ways:

1. If the conduction of the breath sounds to the chest wall is attenuated by airflow limitation (either general, as in bronchial asthma, or local, as when a large bronchus is obstructed by a tumour) or by pneumothorax, pleural effusion or pleural thickening, they remain vesicular but are diminished in amplitude. This change in the breath sounds is invariably accompanied by a reduction in the amplitude of the conducted voice sounds.

2. If the lung tissue through which the breath sounds are transmitted from the air passages to the chest wall has lost its normal spongy consistence and has become firm or solid, e.g. in consolidation or fibrosis, the sounds picked up by the stethoscope resemble more closely those produced at the larynx than those heard over normal lung. They are usually louder during both inspiration and expiration, and the expiratory murmur is audible through the whole of expiration instead of only during the first one-third. The sounds have what is usually, but perhaps not accurately, described as a blowing quality derived from their origin in the larynx. The term *bronchial* is given to breath sounds of this type. Bronchial breath sounds, as would be expected, are similar in quality to those heard when the chest piece of a stethoscope is placed over the larynx or trachea, but they are, of course, less loud.

Voice sounds conducted through consolidated lung tissue also resemble more closely those produced at the larynx than those heard over normal lungs, in that they are louder and more distinct. In some cases the whispered voice may be transmitted almost without distortion, so that individual syllables can be clearly recognised (*whispering pectoriloquy*).

The pitch of bronchial breath sounds varies according to the nature of the pulmonary changes. As high-frequency sounds are selectively conducted through consolidated lung tissue, high-pitched bronchial breath sounds are heard in lobar or segmental pneumonia. Fibrotic lung tissue, on the other hand, transmits sounds of lower frequency and thus produces low-pitched bronchial breath sounds. With voice sounds, there is a similar selective conduction of certain frequencies. High-pitched bronchial breath sounds are associated with voice sounds of a bleating high-pitched quality, often described as *aegophony*, a phenomenon less often observed in the presence of low-pitched bronchial breath sounds.

3. When bronchial breath sounds traverse air-containing cavities in their passage to the chest wall, they may acquire a resonating *amphoric* quality, resembling the sound produced by blowing across the top of a bottle. Amphoric breath sounds are, however, present in only a small proportion of cases in which an abnormality of this type is present. In lung abscess and tuberculous cavitation, for example, they are heard only when the cavity is very large and superficial, and the draining bronchus or bronchi are patent, while in spontaneous pneumothorax the production of amphoric breath sounds is confined to those cases in which the intrapleural pressure is above atmospheric level (tension pneumothorax). When amphoric breath sounds are present the voice sounds are conducted more clearly and usually more loudly than normal, and whispering pectoriloquy can always be elicited.

The main importance of identifying breath sounds as bronchial in type lies in the fact that this indicates the presence of a pulmonary lesion. The criteria for their recognition must therefore be strict and unambiguous. Three conditions must be satisfied before breath sounds can be described as bronchial:

1. Both the inspiratory and expiratory sound must be blowing in character.
2. The expiratory sound must be as long and as loud as the inspiratory sound.
3. There must be a pause between the end of the inspiratory sound and the beginning of the expiratory sound.

Breath sounds may be intermediate in type between vesicular and bronchial, for example, vesicular with prolonged expiration. This type is heard commonly in the presence of diffuse pulmonary fibrosis, chronic bronchitis and emphysema. Other variants, such as bronchovesicular breath sounds, in which the inspiratory component is bronchial in type and the expiratory sound is vesicular, have no specific significance.

Added Sounds. For many years the terminology of added sounds has been confused by the ambiguity which has surrounded the use of the word râle. Translated literally from the French it means rattle, but Laënnec wrongly regarded it as equivalent to the Latin term 'rhonchus'. In fact, rhonchus is a latinised version of the Greek rhonchos, meaning wheezing, and its use should logically be restricted to the musical sounds produced in narrowed bronchi. The word crepitation, derived from the latin *crepitare*, to crack or rattle, is an unambiguous term which can be appropriately used to describe all non-musical crackling sounds. The adoption of the terms rhonchus and crepitation, as defined below, allows the term râle to be discarded and for the sake of clarity this policy has been followed in the description of added sounds originating in the bronchi and lungs.

Forgacs (1978) has suggested that the terms wheezes and crackles should replace rhonchi and crepitations. The word wheeze is, however, normally used to describe the sound heard without a stethoscope in patients with generalized expiratory airflow obstruction. The substitution of wheezes for rhonchi may thus give rise to confusion and the traditional terms are preferable.

Added sounds heard on auscultation of the chest are therefore of three types: rhonchi, crepitations and pleural sounds.

1. RHONCHI. These are musical sounds of high, medium or low pitch produced by the passage of air through narrowed bronchi in asthma and bronchitis. Rhonchi caused by mucosal oedema or spasm of the bronchial musculature are usually superimposed upon the expiratory phase of the respiratory murmur, which is always prolonged when rhonchi are present. Rhonchi heard during inspiration are more often due to secretion in the large bronchi and may disappear, or at least become less numerous, after coughing. It used to be assumed that the pitch of a rhonchus was related to the size of the bronchus in which it was produced, (the smaller the tube, the higher the pitch), but doubt has been cast on this hypothesis. A constant low-pitched rhonchus, however, usually indicates partial obstruction of a major bronchus by a local lesion in a large bronchus, such as a tumour or an inhaled foreign body.

2. CREPITATIONS. These are non-musical sounds of a crackling character, mainly audible during inspiration. At one time they were always attributed to the bubbling of air through secretions in the bronchi and alveoli, but that view is no longer tenable, except when the sounds originate in the major bronchi, dilated bronchi (bronchiectasis) and pulmonary cavities. In these circumstances the presence of secretions is confirmed by the observation that the crepitations either increase in number or disappear temporarily after coughing.

It is now recognised that a much more frequent cause of crepitations in parenchymal lung disease is the explosive reopening, during inspiration, of peripheral airways which have become occluded during expiration by viscid exudate in the bronchioles or by thickening of the alveolar septa by oedema, inflammatory cells or fibrous tissue. As would be expected, these crepitations are most numerous during the second half of inspiration, when they may be accompanied by rhonchi, and are completely uninfluenced by coughing. Such crepitations are more conspicuous over the lung bases, because small airway closure is more liable to occur there than in the upper lobes.

Another distinct type of crepitation may be heard over a pneumothorax when fluid is present in the pleural space. These sounds, which have a tinkling quality, seem to be related to the level of intrapleural pressure and their presence usually indicates that the air in the pneumothorax is under tension. Tinkling crepitations are often audible only during coughing, which creates the sounds by agitating the fluid in the pleural space.

3. PLEURAL SOUNDS. A *pleural rub* is a leathery or creaking sound produced by movement of the visceral pleura over the parietal pleura, when both surfaces are roughened by fibrinous exudate. It is usually heard at two separate stages in the respiratory cycle, towards the end of inspiration and just after the beginning of expiration. A pleural rub may be inaudible during normal breathing but can be easily heard when the patient is asked to breathe deeply.

It is sometimes difficult to distinguish between a low-pitched rhonchus, coarse crepitations and a pleural rub. If there is any doubt as to the nature of the sound, auscultation should be repeated after a forceful cough, when rhonchi or crepitations will usually alter in character or disappear, while a pleural rub will remain unchanged.

A *pneumothorax click* is a rhythmical sound, synchronous with cardiac systole, which may be heard with or without the aid of a stethoscope. It is produced by a shallow left pneumothorax between the two layers of pleura overlying the heart.

Technique of auscultation. The design of stethoscope recommended for routine clinical use is described on page 121. With this instrument the examiner has the choice of a bell or diaphragm. As most of the sounds reaching the chest wall from the bronchi and lungs are in the low-frequency range, the bell should normally be used in preference to the diaphragm. Another reason for selecting the bell for respiratory auscultation is that stretching of the skin under the diaphragm during deep breathing is apt to produce a scraping sound which may be difficult to distinguish from that of a pleural rub.

Auscultation should be carried out with the patient relaxed, breathing deeply and fairly rapidly. The mouth should be kept wide open and the patient should be specifically asked not to purse the lips during expiration. It should be borne in mind by the beginner that prolonged deep breathing may cause giddiness or even tetany.

The following information can be obtained from auscultation:

1. The type and amplitude of the breath sounds.
2. The type and number of any added sounds and their position in the respiratory cycle.
3. The quality and amplitude of the conducted voice sounds.

To ensure that small localised lesions are not overlooked, auscultation must be performed with the chest piece of the stethoscope placed in a large number of positions on the chest wall. It is important to compare the findings in equivalent positions on the two sides, anteriorly from just below the clavicle down to the sixth rib, laterally from the axilla down to the eighth rib, and posteriorly from above the level of the spine of the scapula down to the eleventh rib. Auscultation on the two sides alternately is particularly essential for comparing the amplitude of breath sounds and voice sounds. Auscultation within 2–3 cm of the midline, either anteriorly or posteriorly, may give misleading information in regard to the type of breath sounds and voice sounds, particularly in the upper half of the chest, where the stethoscope may pick up sounds transmitted directly from the trachea and main bronchi to the chest wall. Bronchial breath sounds heard in these situations should therefore be disregarded.

Auscultation should be carried out in two stages. In the first, attention should be directed to breath sounds and added sounds, and in the second to the voice sounds. A systematic method of listening to the breath sounds and added sounds is essential. With the patient breathing regularly and fairly deeply, the observer should concentrate separately on the inspiratory and expiratory phases, on their quality and amplitude, and also on the type, number and position of any added sounds. It should also be noted if there is any gap between the end of the inspiratory murmur and the beginning of the expiratory phase. Finally, it may be necessary to repeat auscultation during and after coughing.

The quality and amplitude of the voice sounds should be assessed and compared in the same positions as the breath sounds by asking the patient to say 'one, one,

one'. Where there is an increase in the amplitude and clarity of the voice sounds or an alteration in their quality (e.g. aegophony) the examiner should test for whispering pectoriloquy.

The technique of auscultation may have to be modified to meet the needs of individual cases. Examples of this are:

1. When abnormal breath sounds are heard, the extent of the lesion should be mapped out by moving the chest piece of the stethoscope with each breath from the normal towards the abnormal zone and noting the level at which the breath sounds change.

2. A patient with severe pleural pain should not be asked to take frequent deep breaths when an attempt is being made to elicit bronchial breath sounds or crepitations. It is preferable in such patients to test the voice sounds first. If an area is found in which the voice sounds are increased or aegophony is present, the patient should be asked to take one or two deep breaths and bronchial breath sounds will usually be elicited in the same area. Similarly, auscultation during a single breath after a short cough is often a more useful way of eliciting crepitations than auscultation during a series of deep, pain-producing breaths.

3. Auscultation after coughing is often a useful procedure in other circumstances. It may resolve doubt as to whether an added sound is a low-pitched rhonchus, a series of coarse crepitations or a pleural rub. When the breath sounds are diminished or absent over a lobe or segment thought to be involved in pneumonia, this may be due to bronchial obstruction by secretions, and bronchial breath sounds often become audible when these secretions are dislodged by coughing. When pulmonary cavitation is suspected, inspiration after a forceful cough may produce a low-pitched 'suction' sound as air re-enters the cavity.

4. Auscultation during expiration with the mouth wide open·is a valuable method of detecting rhonchi which may otherwise be inaudible, particularly if the patient is exhaling through pursed lips. This procedure should always be practised in suspected cases of chronic bronchitis or bronchial asthma, in which rhonchi elicited in this way may at times be the only clinical abnormality.

The Interpretation of Auscultatory Findings. 1. *High-pitched bronchial breath sounds* are heard over areas of pneumonic consolidation, over a collapsed lung or lobe when the large bronchi are patent but the peripheral bronchi are obstructed by secretions, and over a lung compressed by a large pleural effusion or a tension pneumothorax. In all these conditions the *voice sounds* have the quality of aegophony and are usually louder than normal. Whispering pectoriloquy is always present.

2. *Low-pitched bronchial breath sounds* are heard over localised areas of pulmonary fibrosis, e.g. in chronic pulmonary tuberculosis, chronic suppurative pneumonia or bronchiectasis. In all these conditions the *voice sounds* are louder and more distinct, and whispering pectoriloquy may be present.

3. *Amphoric bronchial breath sounds* are heard over large, superficial pulmonary cavities and occasionally over a pneumothorax. In these conditions *the voice sounds* are usually increased (but not with a pneumothorax) and whispering pectoriloquy is always present.

4. *Breath sounds* are *diminished* or *absent* over a pleural effusion, thickened pleura, a pneumothorax or a collapsed lung, lobe or segment where the major bronchus

supplying it is obstructed. The breath sounds are symmetrically diminished over both lungs in emphysema, this abnormality usually being accompanied by prolongation of the expiratory phase. In these conditions the *voice sounds* are decreased in amplitude to the same degree as the breath sounds are diminished.

5. *Rhonchi* are heard diffusely over both lungs in bronchial asthma and in most cases of acute and chronic bronchitis. In asthma the rhonchi are typically medium- or high-pitched and expiratory. In bronchitis they are usually low- or medium-pitched and both inspiratory and expiratory. A localised rhonchus may be heard over a partially obstructed large bronchus. If the obstruction is caused by a fixed lesion, such as a tumour or foreign body, the rhonchus is usually louder during inspiration, is not altered by coughing and is often accompanied by stridor. If due to secretions, the obstruction is immediately relieved by coughing, which causes the rhonchus to disappear.

6. *Crepitations* caused by secretions within the larger bronchi in acute or chronic bronchitis, or in resolving bronchopneumonia, are widespread and bilateral, while those audible over resolving lobar or segmental pneumonic consolidation, dilated bronchi (bronchiectasis), lung abscesses or tuberculous cavities are localised to the site of the lesions. In all these conditions they are audible throughout inspiration, and alter after coughing (p. 180). Crepitations in other forms of parenchymal lung disease, such as interstitial pulmonary oedema, allergic and fibrosing alveolitis, and perhaps early pneumonic consolidation and military tuberculosis, are in contrast audible mainly during the second half of inspiration, and are uninfluenced by coughing (p. 181). No useful purpose is served by trying to distinguish between moist and dry, and between fine, medium and coarse crepitations. It is much more important in diagnostic terms to note their timing in the respiratory cycle and how they are affected by coughing.

7. A *pleural rub* is heard over areas of dry pleurisy. It disappears as soon as the visceral and parietal pleura are separated by fluid, but often remains audible above an effusion. If dry pleurisy involves the pleura adjacent to the pericardium, a pleuro-pericardial rub may also be heard. This is a rather misleading term since the pericardial element in the sound is not due to pericarditis. It is caused merely by roughened pleural surfaces adjacent to the pericardium being moved across one another by cardiac pulsation. A pleuro-pericardial rub may, in some cases, be impossible to distinguish from a pericardial rub.

Other Physical Signs

Forced expiratory time (FET) is measured by placing the chest piece of a stethoscope over the trachea and timing the duration of forced expiration following a full inspiration. This is normally less than four seconds. A prolonged FET is indicative of diffuse airflow limitation, and is a feature of chronic bronchitis, emphysema and bronchial asthma.

The *coin test* may occasionally be of value in confirming the presence of a pneumothorax when the air pressure in the pleural space is above atmospheric level. It is carried out by placing a coin on the posterior chest wall and tapping it with a second coin while another observer listens with a stethoscope in front. When the test is positive, a ringing sound is heard; when negative, a dull thud.

Hippocratic succussion is the name given to the splashing sound which is produced by shaking the chest of a patient with both air and fluid in the pleural space. Care should be taken not to confuse gastric with pleural splashing.

Table 6.2 Summary of typical physical signs in the more common respiratory diseases

Pathological process	Movement of chest wall	Mediastinal displace-ment	Percussion note	Breath sounds	Voice sounds	Added sounds
Consolidation: as in lobar pneumonia	Reduced on side affected	None	Dull	High-pitched bronchial	Increased (with aegophony) Whispering pectoriloquy	Fine crepitations early Coarse crepitations later
Collapse due to obstruction of major bronchus	Reduced on side affected	Towards lesion	Dull	Diminished or absent	Reduced or absent	None
Collapse due to peripheral bronchial obstruction	Reduced on side affected	Towards lesion	Dull	High-pitched bronchial	Increased (with aegophony) Whispering pectoriloquy	None early — coarse crepitations later
Localised fibrosis and/or bronchiectasis	Slightly reduced on side affected	Towards lesion	Impaired	Low-pitched bronchial	Increased Whispering pectoriloquy	Coarse crepitations
Cavitation (typical signs only when cavity is large and linked with bronchus)	Slightly reduced on side affected	None, or towards lesion	Impaired	'Amphoric' bronchial	Increased Whispering pectoriloquy	Coarse crepitations
Pleural effusion Empyema	Reduced or absent (depending on size) on side affected	Towards opposite side	Stony dull	Diminished or absent (occasionally high-pitched bronchial	Reduced or absent (occasionally increased with aegophony)	Pleural rub in some cases (above effusion)
Pneumothorax	Reduced or absent (depending on size) on side affected	Towards opposite side	Normal or hyper-resonant	Diminished or absent (occasionally faint high-pitched bronchial)	Reduced or absent	Tinkling crepitations when fluid present
Bronchitis: Acute Chronic	Normal or symmetrically diminished	None	Normal	Vesicular with prolonged expiration	Normal	Rhonchi, usually with some coarse crepitations
Bronchial asthma	Symmetrically diminished	None	Normal	Vesicular with prolonged expiration	Normal or diminished	Rhonchi, mainly expiratory and high-pitched
Bronchopneumonia	Symmetrically diminished	None	May be impaired	Usually harsh vesicular with prolonged expiration	Normal	Rhonchi and coarse crepitations
Diffuse pulmonary emphysema	Symmetrically diminished	None	Normal or hyper-resonant	Diminished vesicular with prolonged expiration	Normal or reduced	Rhonchi and coarse crepitations from associated bronchitis
Interstitial lung disease	Symmetrically diminished	None	Normal	Harsh vesicular with prolonged expiration	Usually increased	Crackling crepitations uninfluenced by coughing

Integration of Physical Signs

The physical signs found in the more common respiratory diseases are shown in Table 6.2. It must be emphasised, however, that these signs are not necessarily present in every case. An area of consolidation or collapse may, for example, be too small to give rise to the classical pattern of physical signs. Furthermore, the picture may be confused by the coincidence of two groups of signs, as when consolidation or collapse is accompanied by pleural effusion. Difficulties are also apt to arise when the differential diagnosis rests on the observer's estimate of the position of the mediastinum. In patients with pulmonary collapse or pleural effusion mediastinal displacement of a sufficient degree to be recognised clinically is an inconstant feature and, even when present, may be difficult to detect with certanty since the trachea and cardiac apex beat are not always readily palpable.

FURTHER INVESTIGATION

From the history and clinical examination it is possible in many cases to make a reliable and reasonably complete diagnosis. This applies, for example, to conditions such as bronchial asthma, chronic obstructive airways disease and to some cases of pneumonia and pulmonary infarction. In many conditions, however, information required to expand and clarify the diagnosis must be obtained by other methods. By means of radiology the precise anatomical position of a lesion can be determined, and from this and other features its pathology may be deduced. Bacteriological and cytological examination of sputum and pleural fluid may provide even more reliable data, by means of which a clinical diagnosis can be elaborated into an aetiological diagnosis, for example by the identification of the organism responsible for an acute pneumonia or by the finding of malignant cells in sputum or in pleural fluid. In a few cases the diagnosis cannot be completed without more formidable investigations, such as bronchoscopy, bronchography, pleural biopsy and even thoracotomy.

In a rather different category are those cases in which clinical examination fails to reveal any abnormality and the diagnosis depends entirely on specialised investigations, particularly radiology. The two most important diseases in this group are pulmonary tuberculosis and bronchial carcinoma, which may not give rise to any clinical abnormality in the early stages. It is therefore essential to advise radiological examination of the chest whenever one of these conditions is suspected from the history.

Even when a precise diagnosis has been made, it is usually desirable to measure the effect the disease is having on respiratory function. This is useful for the assessment of fitness for work and suitability for certain forms of treatment, such as thoracotomy in bronchial carcinoma.

A full account of all the special methods of investigation cannot be given here, nor is it possible to indicate in any detail the information they can be expected to provide. The summary which follows is therefore intended to serve only as a guide to the value of each investigation and the indications for its use.

Radiological Examination. 1. *Radiographs* (postero-anterior and lateral of the chest) should be obtained whenever pulmonary or pleural disease is suspected. This examination may disclose a lesion or lesions undetected by physical examination. It will also show where a lesion is situated, and may suggest its possible cause. A comparison between current and previous films, if they can be obtained, may provide vital diagnostic information in three circumstances: (i) if a pulmonary opacity has not increased in size over a period of a year or longer, a diagnosis of bronchial carcinoma is highly improbable, (ii) if an opacity has become smaller or less dense in the course of a few weeks, pneumonia is its most likely cause; and (iii) if it was not present on an earlier film, or has become larger, the lesion is almost certainly a tumour or an active tuberculous infiltrate.

Radiographic examination of the nasal sinuses is an integral part of the investigation of chronic infection of the upper respiratory tract.

2. *Radioscopy* provides information about the movement of the diaphragm and position and outline of the oesophagus. It is indicated particularly in patients with bronchial carcinoma. Unilateral diaphragmatic paralysis or a localised displacement of the barium-filled oesophagus would, by demonstrating mediastinal invasion, contraindicate an attempt at surgical treatment.

3. *Tomography* is a special radiographic technique by means of which an opacity or part of an opacity lying in one particular plane can be visualised clearly, even when there are superimposed opacities in different planes. This technique is of value in the detection of pulmonary cavities and in demonstrating local variations in density (e.g. calcification) within a pulmonary lesion. It can thus be helpful in distinguishing between a tumour and a tuberculous lesion.

Computed tomography provides much more accurate information on the position and nature of localised pulmonary lesions.

4. *Pulmonary angiography* can be used to detect vascular abnormalities in the lungs. A series of chest radiographs is taken in rapid succession after the injection of contrast medium into the main pulmonary artery.

Radionuclide Scanning. Perfusion scanning of the lungs following the intravenous injection of isotope-labelled macro-aggregated albumin can be used to detect and delineate unperfused areas of lung. This technique is of value in the diagnosis of pulmonary embolism, particularly if combined with ventilation scanning following the inhalation of an isotope-labelled gas.

Examination of the Sputum. This examination, or that of laryngeal swabs if no sputum is available, is an important diagnostic measure in all suspected bronchopulmonary infections, particularly pneumonia and tuberculosis. In all such cases a direct film, appropriately stained, should be examined microscopically and suitable culture media inoculated. Sputum should also be examined for malignant cells if bronchial carcinoma is suspected.

Intradermal Tests. The *tuberculin test* is chiefly of value in excluding present or past tuberculous infection. A positive test is of diagnostic significance only in children. A positive *Kveim test* confirms a diagnosis of sarcoidosis. *Skin sensitivity tests* indicate the presence or absence of atopy, and may help to identify the cause of allergic rhinitis, asthma and pulmonary eosinophilia, thus assisting in the management of these conditions.

Examination of the Blood. *The total and differential white cell counts* may give guidance as to the nature of a radiographic abnormality, e.g. whether it is an area of acute pneumonic consolidation or an eosinophilic infiltrate. *Blood culture* and *examination of serum for viral and other antibodies* may be of value in determining the aetiology of a pneumonic illness.

Bronchoscopy. With a rigid bronchoscope the bronchi can be inspected as far as the segmental orifices. A flexible (fibreoptic) bronchoscope may be of value in the diagnosis of more peripheral lesions and can also be used to obtain specimens of lung tissue for histological examination in patients with diffuse pulmonary disease (transbronchial lung biopsy). Bronchoscopy is an essential investigation whenever bronchial carcinoma is suspected, and often the diagnosis can be confirmed histologically by biopsy. It is also a valuable method of investigating other causes of bronchial obstruction, e.g. inhaled foreign body, tuberculous lymph nodes.

Bronchography. In this examination radiographs are taken after the whole bronchial tree has been outlined by a contrast medium. Its main value is in the diagnosis of bronchiectasis and the precise determination of its degree and distribution.

Pleural Aspiration and Biopsy. Cytological and bacteriological examination of pleural fluid often provides information which reveals the cause of the effusion. Pleural biopsy taken from the site of aspiration is of particular value in the diagnosis of tuberculous and malignant effusions.

Thoracoscopy. The examination of the pleural surfaces with a telescope, after air has been introduced into the pleural space, may show pleural abnormalities from which tissue can be removed for histological examination. This technique need only be used when examination of pleural fluid and pleural biopsy by the ordinary method are unhelpful.

Lymph Node Biopsy. Removal or needle aspiration of a supraclavicular, particularly a scalene lymph node, or less frequently an axillary lymph node, may provide histological proof of the diagnosis in bronchial carcinoma, lymphoma sarcoidosis and, occasionally, tuberculosis. A lymph node can also be removed from the vicinity of the trachea and main bronchi by the technique of *mediastinoscopy*.

Lung Biopsy. If the nature of a diffuse pulmonary abnormality cannot be determined by other methods, a histological diagnosis can be made by transbronchial or transthoracic needle biopsy of lung. A similar technique can be used for the diagnosis of localised peripheral pulmonary lesions. Thoracotomy is occasionally required for the diagnosis of pulmonary or mediastinal lesions if the results of all other investigations are negative or inconclusive.

Tests of Respiratory Function. Disturbances of ventilation, distribution, diffusion and lung compliance can be measured, but many of these tests require complex facilities, which are not generally available. For practical purposes, respiratory function can be adequately investigated by the following procedures:

1. The measurement of the partial pressure of *oxygen* (PaO_2) and of *carbon dioxide* ($PaCO_2$) in a sample of arterial blood obtained from the radial, brachial or femoral artery. $PaCO_2$ is normally 4.8–6.0 kPa (36–45 mmHg), and is always increased when there is inadequate alveolar ventilation. The hydrogen ion concentration (normal range: 36–44 nmol/l) should be measured on the same sample to determine the patient's acid-base status.

2. The measurement of *forced expiratory volume* (FEV_1) and *forced vital capacity* (FVC). This requires either a recording spirometer, or a standard spirometer

incorporating an electronic timing device. The FEV_1 is the largest volume which can be expired, from full inspiration, in one second, and provides information about ventilatory capacity. In health the FEV_1 may be 3.5 litres or more, and amounts to at least 75% of the FVC. In diseases such as bronchial asthma and emphysema, which produce narrowing of the air passages during expiration, both FEV_1 and FVC are reduced but the reduction in FEV_1 is proportionately greater, i.e. the FEV_1/FVC ratio is reduced, perhaps to 40 per cent or less. In restrictive lung disease and ankylosing spondylitis, which render the lungs or chest wall more rigid, the FEV_1 and FVC are reduced proportionately and the normal FEV_1/FVC ratio is preserved. These simple measurements are thus of value in distinguishing between one type of respiratory disorder and another, as well as in providing an index of its severity. Serial measurements can be used to assess improvement or deterioration and also the response to bronchodilator drugs or corticosteroids in patients with asthma.

The *peak expiratory flow rate* (PEFR), which correlates closely with the FEV_1, can also be used to assess the degree of airflow obstruction. The device employed for this measurement (a peak flow meter) is portable and easy to operate, and is eminently suitable for use in general practice. The normal range of PEFR in healthy adults is 500–650 litres per minute.

THE METHODS IN PRACTICE

THE EXAMINATION OF THE INJURED CHEST

In patients suffering from severe multiple injuries in which there is damage to the chest, routine clinical methods of examination may be difficult to apply and their results may be misleading. Furthermore, the examination must be performed expeditiously since many of the patients urgently require resuscitation either because of respiratory insufficiency, blood loss, or injury to other systems.

Manifestations of respiratory inadequacy, such as dyspnoea or central cyanosis, may be the first indication that the chest has been injured. These may on occasions be misinterpreted as, for example, when panic causes hyperventilation, and the first object of the physical examination must therefore be to determine whether or not organic damage has occurred. If so, the next step is to discover whether the chest wall, the lungs or the air passages are involved and whether a pneumothorax or a haemothorax is present. Finally, it will be essential to assess the severity of respiratory insufficiency and decide how urgent is the need for resuscitation in this respect.

The Upper Respiratory Tract

The first part of the examination should be directed towards ensuring that the airway is adequate and that there is no obstruction to the oropharynx, larynx or trachea by the tongue, by damaged tissues or by blood.

The Chest

The examination of the chest follows the sequence that has been described, but must not be unnecessarily detailed or time consuming. Signs of particular importance should be sought, such as paradoxical movement of a segment of the chest wall or subcutaneous emphysema.

Inspection. Dyspnoea and central cyanosis must be assessed in the usual way. Paradoxical movement of the chest wall is seen in patients who have sustained double fractures of a series of ribs or of the sternum. The portion of the thoracic cage between the fractures becomes mobile and, with the overlying soft tissues, is sucked in with every inspiration. This seriously interferes with pulmonary ventilation. Subcutaneous emphysema develops when the trachea, bronchi or lungs have been damaged and air escapes into the adjacent tissues; in some cases, the resultant swelling may be visible. Haemopericardium causes tamponade which should be suspected when the jugular venous pressure is increased.

Palpation. The neck and chest should be palpated for the presence of subcutaneous emphysema. Deviation of the trachea from the mid-line, indicating displacement of the mediastinum by lesions such as haemothorax, pneumothorax or collapse, should be noted. The apex beat, which may also be displaced in these circumstances, is usually difficult to locate if there is tachycardia, subcutaneous emphysema or bruising of the chest wall. The extent of any paradoxical movement can be assessed by gently laying the palms on the injured and uninjured segments of the chest wall and observing how one hand moves inwards and the other one outwards with each respiration.

Percussion. This is of value only in helping to establish the presence of a gross pneumothorax or haemothorax. It should be carried out very gently.

Auscultation. This is also of little value when the chest is extensively injured, as the multiplicity of added sounds arising from lung, pleura and chest wall mitigates against their accurate interpretation.

Further Investigation

Radiographs taken in the erect position must be obtained at the earliest possible moment whenever a chest injury is suspected. In the severely injured a portable apparatus may have to be used at the bedside. Because of the technical difficulties with this method in dyspnoeic patients, radiographs are frequently of poor quality, but a pneumothorax, a haemothorax, severe lung damage or collapse and rupture of the diaphragm can usually be recognised.

Tests of Respiratory Function in the form of serial studies of arterial blood gas should be carried out whenever respiratory insufficiency is suspected. These measurements will indicate whether intermittent positive-pressure ventilation is required, and can also be used to monitor the patient's response to this form of treatment.

REFERENCE
Forgacs P 1978 Chest 73: 399

7. The Alimentary and Genito-Urinary Systems

> Every pain has its distinct and pregnant signification if we will but carefully search for it.
>
> John Hilton, *Rest and Pain,* 1863

The diagnosis of many abdominal diseases is often dependent more upon a careful analysis of the history than the presence of physical signs. Pain is particularly prominent among the symptoms that are encountered in both the alimentary and genito-urinary systems; a thorough interrogation about pain along the lines indicated on page 30 is essential before complicated investigations are initiated. If this is neglected, the clinician may arrange for unnecessary tests which may lead to discovery of a symptomless abnormality such as a hiatus hernia or gallstones to which the patient's complaint may be incorrectly attributed. This may result in inappropriate management and even unnecessary surgery. The history is therefore so important that considerable space is devoted to symptoms. However, after a careful history has been obtained, physical examination must not be neglected because inspection, palpation, percussion and auscultation may each provide essential information.

THE HISTORY

THE PRINCIPAL SYMPTOMS OF ALIMENTARY DISEASE

The principal complaints in alimentary disease include abdominal pain, difficulty in swallowing, indigestion, heartburn, loss of appetite, decrease in weight, vomiting, jaundice, abdominal distension, alteration in bowel habit and bleeding per rectum. Sometimes, organic disease may be suspected only from the development of a secondary feature such as anaemia. Occasionally patients may conceal important symptoms such as bleeding per rectum either because of a belief that the cause is trivial or because of a fear of serious disease. It follows that the clinician must not only listen carefully to the patient's presenting complaints but also enquire about the other principal symptoms of abdominal disease. It must also be remembered that the emotional state of a patient may produce symptoms in the absence of an organic cause often through the influence of the autonomic system on the gut.

Abdominal Pain. This is a very frequent symptom of disorders of the alimentary system. The pathophysiological bases are spasm or stretching of smooth muscle, inflammatory or neoplastic lesions and the effect of a high hydrogen iron concentration on the nerve endings in the base of a peptic ulcer. Pain may also be caused by ischaemia or congestion as a result of mesenteric vascular lesions. It must be borne in mind that the pain of visceral or somatic origin may be identical with respect to site, radiation, character and severity. A distinction can usually be made by taking other features into account. The diagnosis should be made if possible on the data provided by the history and by examination of the patient.

Questions should be framed in such a way as to analyse the complaint of pain in the manner described on page 30. A good guide to the source of the pain is often its main site. Pain from unpaired structures is usually central. Patients should be asked to demonstrate the exact site and also any area to which the pain may radiate. The type of pain should be elicited; 'stitch-like' pain seldom has an organic explanation. Frequency, duration and timing of attacks are also of diagnostic significance as are any associated factors and also those which may relieve or aggravate the condition. Analysis along these lines should distinguish pain due to causes such as perforated peptic ulceration, acute cholecystitis, pancreatitis or diverticulitis, intestinal obstruction or hepatic congestion. It should be borne in mind that abdominal pain, sometimes of great intensity, may result from disorders in which the alimentary system is not primarily at fault. These include diabetic ketoacidosis, acute intermittent porphyria, lead colic and tabes dorsalis. Likewise, abdominal pain may originate from structures outside the abdomen. Anterior abdominal pain may be caused by vertebral collapse or other diseases of the spine. Unilateral disease of a vertebra, prolapsed intravertebral disc or tumour affecting a nerve may give rise to pain on one side of the abdomen. Associated features such as aggravation by certain movements are usually present to indicate the source of the pain; there may be tenderness over the affected spine and segmental sensory and motor changes. In other instances, herpes zoster, epidemic myalgia, myocardial infarction or a dissecting aneurysm of the aorta may create difficulties by causing abdominal pain but a careful history and examination usually points to the correct diagnosis.

Difficulty in Swallowing (*Dysphagia*). Initiation of swallowing is a conscious action followed by reflex oesophageal peristalsis which is not normally felt. Difficulty in initiating swallowing may be due to a painful lesion of the mouth or throat or to a neurological or neuromuscular disorder such as pseudobulbar palsy or myasthenia gravis. Sticking of food is an important symptom of oesophageal disease for which an explanation must be sought. At the level of the cricoid cartilage this may be due to a growth, a stricture, a pharyngo-oesophageal pouch or as a reflex effect from some disorder farther down the gullet. Food felt to be held up behind the xiphisternum implies a lesion at the lower end of the oesophagus, either a tumour, achalasia of the cardia or a stricture resulting from peptic oesphagitis. The symptoms may be present intermittently and occur only with large lumps of food such as meat or potato. Later, any solid may be responsible and symptoms may become acute with its impaction at the area of narrowing. Discomfort may be relieved when food is regurgitated, usually in the same state in which it was swallowed, though the patient may describe this as vomiting. In patients with a pharyngo-oesophageal pouch or achalasia, when the oesophagus may greatly dilate, recognisable food may be brought back long after it was eaten. Patients with oesophageal obstruction may develop nocturnal coughing or dyspnoea due to spillage from the gullet into the trachea. Pneumonia and even death may follow.

Dysphagia should not be confused with globus hystericus, a psychogenic symptom in which there is a feeling of a lump in the throat which needs to be swallowed; the latter is present between meals and there is no difficulty in swallowing food.

Vomiting. Although vomiting suggests disease of the stomach, it can also be a symptom of a wide variety of local and systemic disorders, many of which are not associated with alimentary disease. Instances include functional and organic disorders of the nervous system, for example, vomiting due to nervous excitement, disgust or fear, motion sickness, labyrinthine disorders, migraine, meningitis or intracranial tumour. Vomiting may also result from any severe pain, as in renal colic or some cases of myocardial infarction. Amongst systemic conditions are renal failure, pregnancy, and endocrine disorders such as diabetic ketoacidosis, hyperparathyroidism or a thyrotoxic or addisonian crisis. Many drugs are also prone to cause vomiting, some such as digoxin or morphine due to a central action, and others such as aminophylline or potassium chloride as a result of gastric irritation.

In the alimentary system, vomiting may be induced by the patient to relieve the pain of peptic ulceration. Gastric outlet obstruction is associated with copious vomiting, sometimes amounting to several litres in the course of a day. More distal obstruction also leads to vomiting but the lower the level of the obstruction, the more marked are the accompanying symptoms of abdominal distension and intestinal colic. Vomiting also occurs in such diverse conditions as acute gastritis, acute cholecystitis, acute pancreatitis and hepatitis. Children are prone to vomit for trivial reasons such as a mild fever. In most instances, vomiting is preceded by nausea but in some cases of intracranial tumour, the vomiting may be without warning and may be projectile.

Enquiry should be made about the frequency of the vomiting, the time of day at which it occurs and also about its taste, colour, quantity and smell. If the taste and smell are inconspicuous, this suggests either the presence of achlorhydria or that the 'vomit' has been regurgitated from the oesophagus. Foul smelling vomitus occurs in ulcerating carcinoma of the stomach or in pyloric obstruction whereas faecal vomiting may occur in low intestinal obstruction. A yellow colour and bitter taste indicate the presence of bile and means that there has been regurgitation of duodenal content into the stomach. This has no serious significance.

Special attention should be paid to the presence of blood (*haematemesis*). Bright red blood usually arises from an oesophageal lesion. A dark red vomit, sometimes containing liver-like clots of blood, is due to profuse bleeding such as may occur from a peptic ulcer. Severe bleeding of this type is rarely due to a gastric carcinoma unless a malignant ulcer has eroded a large blood vessel. In less acute haematemesis the vomit is often blackish or dark brown and can contain sediment like 'coffee grounds', due to the conversion of the haemoglobin to acid haematin by the gastric acidity. In the presence of haematemesis, enquiry should be made about the recent ingestion of aspirin, other anti-inflammatory drugs or alcohol, and about symptoms suggestive of peptic ulceration.

Whenever possible, the patients description should be supplemented by inspection of the vomitus.

Heartburn refers to a burning retrosternal discomfort or pain. It is so common that most people have it at some time. It is particularly frequent during pregnancy and when a patient with a hiatus hernia is recumbent. The latter is its only diagnostic significance.

Jaundice. The clinical features are described on page 58.

Common causes of hepatocellular jaundice include viral infections of the liver and

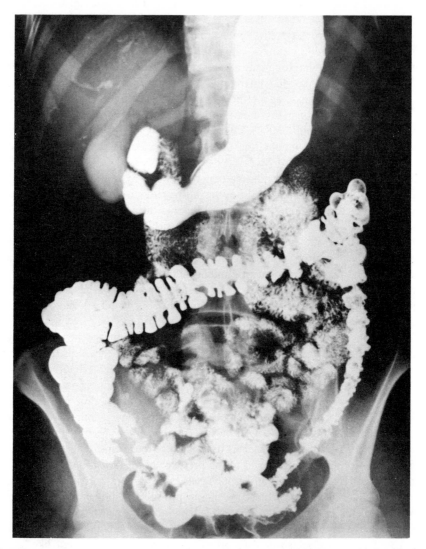

Fig. 7.1 Contents of abdomen demonstrated by cholecystogram and barium examination. Note the stomach with peristaltic waves most marked in the gastric antrum which is surmounted by the duodenal cap; the feathery jejunal pattern in the left hypochondrium and the ileum in the hypogastrium; the caecum, appendix and colon. Note the gall bladder alongside the duodenal cap and the calcification in the costal cartilages superimposed on the liver shadow. (*Courtesy of Dr W. A. Copland.*)

damage by alcohol. The outstanding complaints are anorexia and nausea even at the thought of food. The history should enquire about possible contacts and travel abroad (hepatitis A), consumption of alcohol and drugs, and any injections, blood transfusions or tattooing during the previous six months (hepatitis B). It should be borne in mind that hepatitis B is also common in male homosexuals and in drug addicts.

The two common causes of cholestatic jaundice due to large duct obstruction are gallstones and carcinoma of the head of the pancreas. There is usually, but not

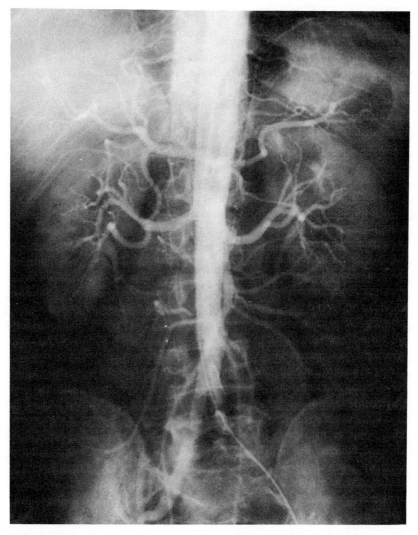

Fig. 7.2 Contents of abdomen demonstrated by aortography. Note on the left side from above downwards, the left phrenic artery immediately below the diaphragm; translucency from air in the splenic flexure overlying the splenic shadow; the splenic artery; the left renal artery; the left kidney and ureter; the superior mesenteric artery; the catheter in the left iliac artery passing into the aorta. Note on the right side, the liver; the hepatic artery; the right renal artery; the right kidney and ureter; the right psoas muscle; the right iliac artery. (*Courtesy of Professor Eric Samuel.*)

always, a history of one or more attacks of biliary colic if the cause is gallstones. There is often a persistent pain in the back made worse by recumbency when carcinoma of the pancreas is responsible and the gall bladder may be palpably enlarged (p. 206). Obstruction is frequently associated with fever, rigors and itching.

Important causes of jaundice due to widespread small duct obstruction are drugs or alcohol, or biliary cirrhosis which affects middle-aged women and is often preceded by months of itching.

Jaundice due to extensive metastases occurs occasionally, and the cause is usually obvious on abdominal palpation.

Fluid retention, encephalopathy and a bleeding tendency combined with jaundice are diagnostic of hepatocellular damage.

Alteration in Bowel Habit. Normal habit varies between several evacuations per day to one every three days or so. Changes in habit which are sufficient to bring a patient to a doctor should be taken seriously particularly in older persons. It is necessary not only to find out the frequency of stools but also if motions are occurring at special times of the day or night and if they are associated with abdominal discomfort or a feeling of urgency. The nature of any medication, prescribed or self-administered, should be established as some patients are unaware of the laxative properties of household remedies, and some drugs, such as mefenamic acid, may alter bowel habit. Diarrhoea may alternate with constipation, and faecal incontinence and constipation may coexist, especially from impacted faeces in the elderly.

A common cause of variability in bowel function is the irritable bowel syndrome in which periods of constipation and diarrhoea may alternate. At times the stool may be loose and at times pencil thin or round like pellets. Intermittent abdominal pain is another feature of this syndrome for which there is no organic explanation.

Tenesmus is the term used to describe a feeling of incomplete evacuation experienced by patients with a space occupying lesion in the rectum such as a carcinoma. Any pelvic mass pressing on the upper rectum may also cause this symptom.

APPEARANCE OF THE STOOL. The patient should be asked to describe the consistency and colour of the stool. Many patients do not normally inspect their faeces and therefore only positive observations can be accepted. If necessary, the clinician should confirm the description by observation.

A pale, bulky, soft, frothy and smelly stool is characteristic of steatorrhoea. Such stools tend to float and the patient may complain of difficulty in flushing the toilet after defecation. The stool is also pale in obstructive jaundice and pancreatic disease. It becomes black (*melaena*) following the sudden loss of more than 20 ml of blood into the upper gut while much larger quantities cause the stool to become loose and sticky like tar. Medicinal iron will also colour the faeces black.

A liquid stool of uniform consistency occurs with small intestinal diarrhoea. In the diarrhoea of colonic origin, the stool usually contains numerous small pieces of faeces.

Abnormalities such as threadworms, roundworms or segments of tapeworms may be present and special enquiry should be made about the presence of blood and about pus or mucus, often described by the patient as slime.

Bleeding per Rectum. The cause of this important symptom should always be determined. The commonest is haemorrhoids but these occur so frequently that their presence in a patient with bleeding should not lead to the assumption that they are responsible. The important differential diagnosis is from carcinoma of the colon. Other causes include inflammatory bowel disease, vascular anomalies and anal fissure.

Bleeding from the anal canal is bright red. It is often clearly separate from the stool and may be seen only on the toilet paper. Coming from haemorrhoids, it may also splash the toilet bowl or drip into the pan after a motion is passed, whereas an anal fissure may be associated with severe anal pain which persists after defaecation. When the site is more proximal, the blood may be altered and appear darker. In inflammatory bowel disease, blood is usually mixed within the stool which is often fluid and contains pus. Both polyps and carcinoma may also cause excessive production of mucus.

Loss of Weight and Loss of Appetite. A decrease in weight may be the first indication of serious organic disease or psychological disorder. In assessing its significance, the duration and extent of the weight loss should be established. It should be known whether it has been associated with loss of appetite (anorexia) or due to deliberate reduction in food intake. Weight loss accompanied by severe anorexia or other alimentary symptoms may not necessarily be due to intra-abdominal disease; such findings may occur, for example, in endogenous depression. Weight loss without anorexia may be due to diabetes mellitus or hyperthyroidism.

Abdominal Distension. Increasing abdominal girth is usually due to adiposity. Its development in a patient who is otherwise becoming thinner suggests intra-abdominal disease. Ascites, the accumulation of fluid in the peritoneal cavity, is usually due to liver disease or intra-abdominal malignancy. Abdominal distension may also be the presenting complaint with an ovarian cyst which sometimes achieves an enormous size. In younger women, unadmitted pregnancy is a possibility that must be remembered.

Intestinal obstruction will cause acute abdominal swelling, usually associated with intestinal colic. Chronic constipation may result in sufficient faecal retention to cause distension. In children, the possibility of Hirschsprung's disease must be considered and the history should determine if bowel habit has ever been normal and whether soiling occurs.

Fluctuating abdominal swelling which develops acutely or progressively during the day but resolves overnight is not uncommon, especially in women. This condition is caused by contraction of the diaphragm and lumbar muscles. It is often associated with evidence of psychopathology and is never due to organic disease.

Wind. To the patient this may mean repeated belching, excessive or offensive flatus per rectum, abdominal discomfort or even borborygmi. Belched wind may have been swallowed (aerophagy) without the patient being aware of it. Sometimes aerophagy occurs in an attempt to relieve abdominal pain or discomfort. Belching itself is of no significance as a principal complaint and is often a feature of anxiety.

The normal volume of flatus per rectum varies greatly from person to person in the range of 200 to 2000 ml per day. It consists of a mixture of gases mainly produced by bacterial action in the lower bowel. Offensive flatus is common but is persistent and particularly unpleasant in association with intestinal malabsorption from any cause. Absence of flatus occurs in intestinal obstruction.

Borborygmi are audible bowel sounds caused by peristalsis. They are often physiological but are especially obvious when there is subacute obstruction or in the rare carcinoid syndrome.

Dyspepsia and/or Indigestion. These vague terms are common complaints. Their usage is of value in obtaining a history but it is essential that the patient explains in detail what is meant. Thus 'indigestion' might describe nausea, heartburn, epigastric discomfort, abdominal pain or distension, or a feeling of postprandial bloating. It may even be used to describe alteration in bowel habit or angina pectoris.

THE PRINCIPAL SYMPTOMS OF DISEASE OF THE GENITO-URINARY SYSTEM

The principal symptoms of genito-urinary disease include dysuria, frequency, polyuria, nocturia, haematuria, alteration in the force of micturition, incontinence, pain, and changes in sexual function. The presence of renal disease may come to light only as the result of complaints of weakness or lethargy due to uraemia or of discovering arterial hypertension or its complications. All patients however, irrespective of the presenting complaint, should be asked about the principal symptoms of genito-urinary disease which they might otherwise fail to volunteer for a variety of reasons, including embarrassment.

Dysuria, Urgency and Frequency. Dysuria means pain on passing urine, often described as burning. Urgency is a sensation of constantly needing to urinate. Painful urgency is termed strangury. Dysuria with urgency is usually due to a bladder infection but may occur in prostatitis, tumours of the bladder or stone in the urethra. Dysuria alone suggests inflammation of the urethra as in gonorrhoea whereas urgency alone is a feature of neurological disease affecting the motor control of the bladder. Frequency of micturition involves the passage of small quantities of urine without an increase in total volume. It is a feature of bladder disease or anxiety.

Polyuria means an increase in urinary output and must be distinguished from frequency of micturition. It may be due to an increase in solute load as in uncontrolled diabetes mellitus. Other examples include the osmotic diuresis caused by urea in chronic renal failure and by sodium from the use of diuretics. Polyuria will also occur in diabetes insipidus where there is lack of anti-diuretic hormone (ADH) or if the renal tubules are non-responsive to ADH (nephrogenic diabetes insipidus). It may also result from psychogenic polydipsia. A patient's assessment of increased volume may be misleading and should be confirmed by performing a twenty-four hour urinary collection. Severe polyuria will cause thirst which may be the presenting symptom.

Oliguria and Anuria. Oliguria means a diminution in the quantity of urine excreted. It is a feature of renal failure and occurs when the urinary output is inadequate to maintain constancy of the 'milieu interieur'. The minimum quantity of urine which is necessary to achieve this objective varies with the diet, the amount of physical activity, the metabolic rate and the efficiency of the renal function. Thus about 200 ml might be sufficient for a healthy man at rest on a protein free diet, whereas 2000 ml might be insufficient when chronic renal failure is present. The patient should be questioned about possible aetiological factors such as a preceding sore throat in post-streptococcal glomerulo-nephritis.

Anuria means a complete cessation of urine production but occurs infrequently. More commonly the complaint of 'failure to make urine' arises from urinary retention within the bladder for which a mechanical, neurological or psychological explanation should be sought.

Haematuria. Like bleeding per rectum or haemoptysis, this symptom demands further examination and investigation. The history often indicates the probable source of bleeding. When haematuria is the sole symptom, the most likely causes include papilloma of the bladder, carcinoma of the kidney or bladder, schistosomiasis or bleeding from the prostate. Haematuria associated with severe loin pain indicates a renal or ureteric origin — commonly the passage of a calculus. When frequency or dysuria accompany the bleeding, its source is usually in the bladder. Haematuria that clears during micturition arises from the urethra. Sometimes other causes of urinary discolouration may be confused with haematuria. These include the ingestion of beetroot and of various drugs such as rifampicin.

Pneumaturia. This bizarre and rare symptom is usually accurately described as a sensation of passing bubbles in the urine. It is almost always caused by a vesico-colic fistula.

Alteration in the Force of Micturition. A poor urinary stream is particularly common in elderly men developing obstruction from prostatic hypertrophy. The force of the stream can be assessed roughly by asking the patient to demonstrate how near he has to stand to an imaginary toilet. Other features of obstructed micturition include hesitancy, urinary spray, post-micturition dribbling, and frequency with nocturia due to incomplete emptying of the bladder.

Nocturia. The need to pass urine during the sleeping hours may be a life-long habit. As a newly developing symptom, it may be due to insomnia or to a number of organic causes including polyuria or prostatic obstruction. Nocturia is also a common symptom of cardiac failure, the diuresis resulting from the excretion of oedema fluid due to the improved renal blood flow which occurs with rest in bed.

Incontinence of Urine. This is a deceptively difficult symptom to assess. A minor degree of incontinence may be a shaming disaster to one patient whereas another may not even consider it abnormal. The severity of the problem can be assessed by asking the patient what protection, if any, is required. Many females, especially the parous, suffer from urinary incontinence provoked by the stress of laughing, sneezing or lifting. This is due to the development of a cystocele, a weakness of the anterior wall of the vagina, often accompanied by some prolapse of the uterus. Incontinence may also arise from neurological disturbances of bladder function. With a primary sensory disturbance, dribbling incontinence will result from painless over-distension of the bladder. This occurs in tabes dorsalis and sometimes in diabetic autonomic neuropathy. The loss of motor control results in urgency and the desire to pass urine must be obeyed at once or incontinence will occur. Multiple sclerosis is the most common neurological cause of urgency in Britain. Combined motor and sensory damage occurs in spinal cord lesions. The bladder fills to a certain pressure and then empties reflexly. The patient may be able to control bladder emptying by raising the intravesical pressure at regular intervals by manual compression of the lower abdomen.

Urogenital Pain. The renal parenchyma is pain free and renal pain is associated with conditions affecting the pelvis of the kidney or causing stretching of the renal capsule. A dull aching discomfort in the renal angle may occur in such conditions as staghorn calculus and hydronephrosis. More severe and intermittent pain can occur in polycystic disease and may result from spontaneous bleeding into a cyst. In acute pyelonephritis the pain is more acute and is often accompanied by rigors and dysuria. A similar but more severe pain is caused by acute distension of the renal pelvis and kidney due to obstruction of the ureter by calculus or other causes such as blood clot. The pain may radiate to the hypochondrium or down to the groin and into the genitalia. Once a stone reaches the bladder, it is usually asymptomatic unless it enters the urethra to cause dysuria with strangury. Conditions causing urinary bladder pain also produce frequency.

Prostatic pain is felt in the perineum, may be caused by prostatitis and is usually associated with other features of bladder neck obstruction. Testicular and epididymal pain radiate into the groin and lower abdomen where the pain may be so intense that its testicular origin is obscured. Pain due to torsion of the testis usually occurs in pubertal boys or young men. It frequently develops at night and starts with pain in the iliac fossa. Tender swelling of the testis may require to be distinguished from a strangulated hernia or acute epididymo-orchitis. Ovarian pain is also felt in the iliac fossa and may be episodic as in endometriosis or more constant as in malignant tumours. Uterine pain is felt lower in the abdomen and may radiate through to the lumbosacral area, for example in labour pains and dysmenorrhoea.

Sexual Problems in the Male

The three principal symptoms are lack of libido, inability to achieve or maintain an erection and trouble with ejaculation. It is necessary to obtain precise information about such matters. Sexual problems are, however, difficult to assess for three main reasons: (1) the patient is often embarrassed and may not be forthcoming with a full history at the initial interview; (2) there may be a large psychiatric component to the complaint requiring expert analysis and help; (3) physical examination at the time the patient is sexually aroused is usually impossible.

One method of overcoming the patient's initial embarrassment is to use a sexual problems questionnaire which is sent to the patient for completion before attendance at the clinic. It contains the explicit questions that must be asked. It allows the doctor to identify the main problem and to achieve rapport quickly at the initial interview; then the individual's difficulties can be clearly defined. Examples are given on page 451 of the questions asked when the problem is concerned with erection or ejaculation and an illustrative case of impotence is described on page 225.

Sexual Problems in the Female

The menstrual history should include a note of the age of the menarche or the menopause and details of the menstrual cycle. These are the frequency, regularity and duration of menses and whether blood loss is small, normal or excessive. The presence of clots suggests heavy menstrual losses. The date of the last menstrual period should be noted. Secondary amenorrhoea is common and often psychological, but the possibility of an organic cause such as post-partum

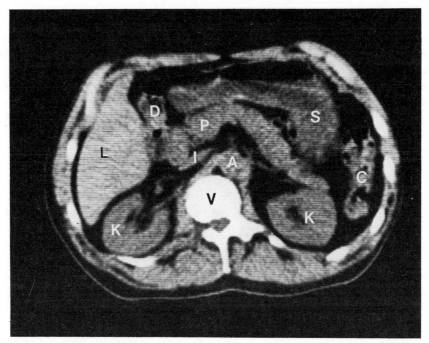

Fig. 7.3 Contents of abdomen as shown by CT scan; A: Aorta and renal arteries. C: Colon and faeces. D: Duodenum. I: Inferior vena cava. K: Kidney. L: Liver. P: Pancreas. S: Stomach. V: Vertebra, the apparent deformity of which is due to the scan passing through the pedicle and lamina on the left side and through the foramen on the right. (*Courtesy of Elscint (GB)Ltd.*)

hypopituitarism should be considered. Primary amenorrhoea demands a gynaecological or endocrinological explanation. The occurrence and the nature of any vaginal discharge must be assessed while a complaint of intermenstrual or postcoital bleeding should lead without delay to examination by a gynaecologist.

Dyspareunia (pain related to sexual intercourse) or failure to achieve an orgasm often occurs and is frequently due to, or may lead to, psychological difficulties. The longer these symptoms persist, the more difficult they are to eradicate. These topics may be avoided by the patient (or the doctor) because of embarrassment but if there is any indication of a difficulty, the patient should be encouraged to speak about it. Opportunity can be provided, once rapport has been established, by asking if sexual intercourse is satisfactory. Thereafter, any problem can be discussed frankly as indicated on pages 7 and 19. Questionnaires can also be helpful as, for example in cases of infertility; they can be answered at leisure and in privacy, in conjunction with the husband.

THE PHYSICAL EXAMINATION

Mouth and Throat

The examination of the mouth and throat is described on page 76. It is of particular relevance to the alimentary system to know whether the teeth provide an adequate chewing surface or, if the patient is edentulous, whether dentures are used for eating.

OESOPHAGUS

There is no bedside method of examination. However, when there is a complaint of dysphagia it can be helpful to watch the act of swallowing solids and liquids. The reproduction of the symptom may confirm the organic nature and the site of the lesion. If swallowing is immediately followed by a distressing bout of coughing, this suggests either a neuromuscular disturbance as in bulbar or pseudo-bulbar palsy, or rarely a fistula between the trachea and the oesophagus.

ABDOMEN

The contents of the abdomen are illustrated in Figures 7.1 to 7.3.

For purposes of description it has been customary to divide the abdomen into nine regions by the intersection of imaginary planes, two horizontal and two sagittal. The upper horizontal plane (transpyloric) lies at a level midway between the suprasternal notch and the symphysis pubis. The lower plane passes through the upper borders of the iliac crests. The sagittal planes are indicated on the surface by lines drawn vertically through points midway between the pubis and the anterior superior iliac spines (Fig. 7.4). The resultant regions are artificial and though useful guides are less satisfactory in localising border lesions. An alternative description is to refer to the right and left upper and low quadrants of the abdomen.

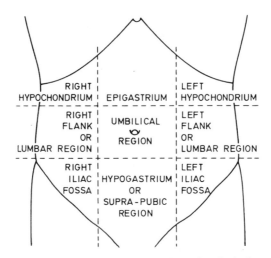

Fig. 7.4 Regions of the abdomen. Note also that MacBurney's point is situated one-third of the distance along a line from the anterior superior iliac spine to the umbilicus.

Whenever possible patients should be examined in a good light and in warm surroundings, warmth being particularly important as it facilitates muscle relaxation. The patient should lie comfortably supine with the head resting on one or two pillows in order to relax the muscles of the abdominal wall. Extra pillows may be necessary to prop up a patient with a kyphosis, or with severe breathlessness but the examination should be repeated in the optimum position once the dyspnoea has settled. Clothes must be removed so that there is complete exposure from the xiphisternum to the pubis. The chest and the legs should be suitably covered. For the examination of patients in bed, the bed-clothing except for the sheet should be pulled down. The sheet can then be folded back to the pubis and the night clothes drawn up to the chest. The examination then follows the routine sequence of inspection, palpation, percussion and auscultation.

Inspection

Skin Lesions. Any abnormality of the skin should be noted and the reasons for scars ascertained if these have not already been divulged. In elderly patients seborrhoeic warts, ranging from pink to brown or black, and haemangiomas (Campbell de Morgan spots) are so common that they could be considered as normal changes. The presence of striae requires a satisfactory explanation (p. 90).

Hair. Secondary sexual hair appears at puberty; its absence after this time should lead to a search for signs of hypopituitarism, or hypogonadism (p. 71). Adrenal virilism in the female leads to a male distribution of pubic hair, whereas hepatic cirrhosis in the male may produce a female distribution.

Veins. Collateral veins (p. 138) may be visible if the inferior vena cava is obstructed or if there is portal hypertension. These are usually tortuous dilatations of the superficial epigastric veins in which the blood flows upwards instead of down towards the groins. Rarely in the presence of hepatic cirrhosis, dilated collateral veins may also radiate from the umbilicus (caput Medusae) as a result of blood flowing from the portal vein through collateral vessels along the falciform ligament.

Movements and Contour. In males particularly, quiet respiration is predominantly diaphragmatic, so that the abdominal wall moves out during inspiration. Respiratory movements of the abdomen usually cease in the presence of acute peritonitis.

Pulsation in the epigastrium is usually transmitted from the abdominal aorta (p. 118). Much less frequently it is caused by the right ventricle, the liver or an abdominal aneurysm. It may sometimes be difficult to distinguish between pulsation of the aorta transmitted through an abdominal mass from an aneurysm. Expansile pulsation favours the latter but, by displacement of fluid, a pancreatic cyst may also produce expansile pulsation. The distinction can be made by ultrasonography (Fig. 7.16).

The shape and symmetry of the abdomen should be observed. A sunken abdomen may be due to starvation or wasting diseases. Protuberance may be due to obesity, gaseous distension, ascites, pregnancy or other swellings. In obesity the umbilicus is usually sunken, whereas in these other conditions it is flat or even projecting. Visible enlargement of the bladder, uterus or ovary shows a characteristic shape as these structures rise out of the pelvis, the swelling being predominantly central in contrast to the bulging of the flanks in ascites. Visible bulges may also be due to gross enlargement of the liver, spleen or kidneys, or to large tumours.

Distension of the stomach due to pyloric obstruction causes bulging of the upper part of the abdomen; tangential inspection is the best means of seeing the slow waves of gastric peristalsis passing from the rib margin on the left, across the midline, and subsiding beneath the right upper rectus. Activity may be stimulated by a drink, by massage or by flicking the skin over the area. Confirmation may be obtained by placing the observer's hands over the lower ribs, and giving the patient a quick shake from side to side, when a sound like that due to shaking a hot-water bottle which contains water and air is heard and is known as the succussion splash. This may also be evoked by quick dipping movements of the hand over the upper abdomen. Similar sounds can be produced from a normal stomach for an hour or two after food or drink.

Small intestinal peristalsis may normally be seen through a thin abdominal wall, especially if there is divarication of the recti abdominis or an incisional hernia. It may become unduly prominent in the presence of intestinal obstruction. It is recognised as writhing movements in the centre of the abdomen.

Hernias are frequent causes of local swellings. An *umbilical hernia* bulges through the fascia around the navel. It is very common in babies and usually disappears spontaneously. It is also frequently encountered in women who have borne many children. Divarication of the recti is also common in the multiparous and becomes evident immediately the supine patient attempts to sit; the intra-abdominal pressure rises and the region of the linea alba bulges between the recti abdominis.

An *epigastric hernia* is visible as a small swelling not usually more than 1 cm in diameter. It is due to a piece of extraperitoneal fat bulging through a defect in the linea alba. By gentle massage with the finger-tip it is often possible to reduce such a hernia and then the small defect in the tendon can be felt.

Incisional hernias may form at the site of any operation on the abdomen, especially if the wound has been complicated by sepsis.

Femoral and *inguinal hernias* and their examination are described on page 210.

Palpation

The examiner's hands must be warm. When they are cold, then the quickest method of warming them is by immersion in hot water. If there are no facilities for warming, the hands should be rubbed together vigorously and the temperature of the skin of the patient's abdominal wall should be brought into equilibrium with that of the examining hand by light palpation all over. It may help to prepare the patient and to reduce the shock of a cold examining hand if it is first placed upon the patient's forearm. An assessment of obesity can be made by grasping a double thickness of skin and subcutaneous tissue between the fingers and thumb. The elasticity of the skin provides a rough index of the degree of hydration and redundant skin folds are evidence of weight loss.

The patient should be asked to place the arms alongside the body, as this helps to relax the abdomen, and to report any tenderness that may be elicited during the examination. In addition, the patient's face should be observed for any grimace indicative of local discomfort.

Palpation can be conveniently divided into three phases; light palpation, deep palpation and bimanual palpation of those organs which move on respiration.

Light Palpation. During initial light palpation, the examiner's hand should remain in continuous contact with the patient's abdomen. Muscle tone should be tested by light dipping movements over symmetrical areas commencing at the point most remote from the site of any pain. Resistance due to increased muscle tone commonly accompanies organic lesions, particularly when pain is present, and it may be restricted to one side or to any region of the abdomen according to the organ affected or the area over which the peritoneum is involved e.g. at MacBurney's point (p. 200) in acute appendicitis (p. 33). *Rebound pain* indicates inflammation of some part of the peritoneum. It is elicited by the sudden release of pressure of the hand which has been applied firmly over an area of the abdomen which may even be remote from the pain.

Generalised rigidity of the abdominal muscles is commonly due to the inability of an anxious patient to relax. This cause can usually be suspected by the circumstances, and confirmed by variability in the resistance and transient relaxation during the earliest phase of expiration. The tendency can be reduced by ensuring that the patient is warm and comfortable and that the examiner's hand is not cold, and by gaining the patient's confidence by very light palpation at first. Generalised rigidity due to acute peritonitis is persistent and is accompanied by tenderness; the abdomen does not move with respiration and bowel sounds cease.

Deep Palpation. The abdomen should now be palpated more deeply. The predominant use of the finger-tips is apt to induce muscular resistance and lead to inefficient results. Using the flat of the hand, the gut can be displaced and abnormal masses may be felt. The liver edge and the lower pole of the right kidney are often palpable in normal persons.

Enlargement of the bladder, ovary or uterus, often already suspected from inspection, may be confirmed as a dome-shaped swelling rising above the pubis (Fig. 7.5). It should be possible to identify the normal colon in the left iliac fossa; the caecum and sometimes the transverse colon may also be palpable particularly if

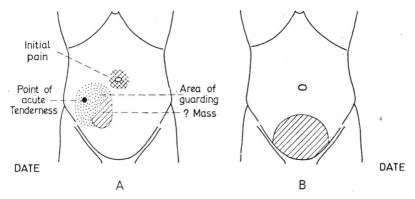

Fig. 7.5 The use of diagrams in case recording. (A) Pain, tenderness, guarding and mass in patient with acute appendicitis and appendix abscess. (B) Tumour arising from the pelvis. This could be a bladder, uterine or ovarian swelling.

they contain faeces. The massaging effect of feeling for these structures often causes them to contract and to become more readily palpable. The aorta is often palpable and it may be slightly tender. These and other normal findings which are often misinterpreted are shown in Figure 7.6.

If any mass is present, then its characteristics should be identified so that all the points mentioned on page 46 have been observed. It must be borne in mind that a hard craggy lump, indistinguishable at first from a malignant tumour, may be due to faeces in a constipated patient in which case the lump disappears or changes its position after the next bowel action. Faeces are commonly palpable in the sigmoid

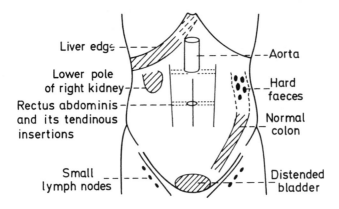

Fig. 7.6 Palpation of the abdomen. Diagrammatic representation of some findings which are often misinterpreted.

colon; in severe constipation, irrespective of whether it is due to bad habit or to organic obstruction, faecal masses may be palpable throughout the colon or in any part of it. Indentation of a lump by finger pressure is evidence that it is faecal.

An upper abdominal mass which does not move with respiration either arises from or has become attached to the abdominal wall. Masses which are superficially situated in the abdominal wall continue to be palpable when the muscles are contracted by raising the head off the pillow or by blowing against resistance. Tightening the muscles in this way identifies the intersections of the recti abdominis (Fig. 7.6). An intersection frequently misleads the unwary beginner into believing that a tumour or the liver edge has been felt. Parietal masses situated deep to the abdominal wall, and also swellings in the abdominal cavity, are less easily felt when the muscles are contracted.

Bimanual Palpation. A bimanual technique should be used for palpating the liver, kidneys, spleen and intra-abdominal masses. Examinaton couches are generally made at a convenient height. When the patient is in a low bed it may be necessary in the interests of comfort and efficiency to sit on or kneel beside the bed, especially while examining the nearside of the abdomen. One hand should be placed posteriorly in the gap between the twelfth rib and the iliac crest, with the finger-tips lateral to the erector spinae. There is usually space enough for one to three fingers which should be pressed firmly over this area and kept still. This pushes forwards and steadies the structures to be felt by the other hand. Bimanual palpation should now easily detect any solid mass between the hands. If a mass is felt, the front hand should then be moved in all directions to define its limits, attachments and other characteristics (p. 46). It is often useful to remind the patient from time to time to relax. If there is difficulty in complying, suggestions such as 'lie heavily on the bed' or 'relax as if going to sleep' may achieve the desired result; if not, it is helpful to press down the front hand firmly immediately after the height of inspiration, for at this moment the abdominal muscles will be relaxed.

The liver, spleen and kidneys should be examined in turn by a bimanual technique. The secret of success is to keep the hands still and wait for the diaphragm to push down the organ onto the hands waiting to receive it.

Palpation of the Liver. The front hand should be placed flat with the fingers pointing upwards and positioned so that the sensing fingers (index and middle) are lateral to the rectus muscle (Fig. 7.7). The hand should be firmly pressed inwards and upwards and it should be kept steady while the patient takes a deep breath through the mouth. At the height of inspiration the inward pressure on the front

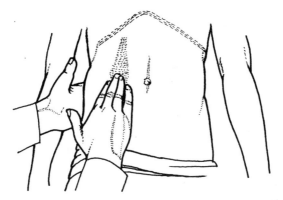

Fig. 7.7 Palpation of the liver.

hand is released while the upward pressure is maintained. With this movement the tips of the fingers should slip over the edge of a palpable liver. It should be noted whether the edge is sharp and flexible as is normal, or whether it is rounded, firm, irregular or tender. The surface and edge of a palpable liver should then be felt for irregularities using the finger-tips and keeping them steady in a new position each time the patient takes a deep breath. Irregularities may be felt as the liver slides under the finger-tips with each respiration. Two common errors should be avoided. One is to feel for the liver with the hand placed horizontally. In this position the palm of the hand is pressing backwards the edge which it is desired to feel. This is particularly the case in those people in whom the right lobe of the liver lies almost vertically. The second error is to start feeling too high up with the front hand.

In the presence of ascites, enlargement of the liver may be detected by the dipping technique (p. 209).

As the liver descends 1–3 cm on inspiration, it can normally be palpated in adults below the right costal margin during deep inspiration. Common causes of enlargement of the liver in the adult in Britain are cardiac failure, cirrhosis and metastatic carcinomatosis. In chronic congestive cardiac failure the liver is firm and the edge is sharp, while in acute failure it is also tender but may be less easily defined. Carcinomatosis commonly causes the liver to feel hard, with a rounded edge and a nodular surface (Fig. 7.8), and there may be tenderness. If a cirrhotic liver is palpable, the edge is rounded and perhaps slightly irregular, but the striking feature is its very hard consistency. In advanced cirrhosis, the spleen is usually palpable but the liver may contract and become impalpable.

Palpation of the Gall Bladder. Gallstones occur very commonly with advancing years, especially in women. These are not palpable. Stones, however,

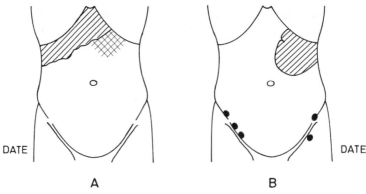

Fig. 7.8   The use of diagrams in case recording. (A) Abdominal mass and enlarged liver in patient with gastric carcinoma and hepatic metastases. (B) Splenomegaly and lymphadenopathy in a patient with Hodgkin's lymphoma.

may be associated with attacks of acute cholecystitis, with tenderness below the right costal margin midway between the xiphisternum and the flank. If the examiner's fingers are placed over this point and the patient is asked to take a deep breath, inspiration may be sharply arrested due to a sudden accentuation of pain (sometimes described as *Murphy's sign*).

A palpable gall bladder implies its enlargement. In the absence of jaundice this is due to obstruction of the cystic duct leading to mucocele or empyema. Obstruction of the common bile duct produces jaundice; if the gall bladder is also enlarged, the obstruction will usually be due to causes other than gallstones since in most cases of cholelithiasis the wall of the gall bladder is thickened and toughened by changes due to chronic cholecystitis and it cannot stretch (*Courvoisier's law*). Carcinoma of the head of the pancreas is the most common cause of palpable enlargement of the gall bladder in the presence of obstructive jaundice.

Palpation of the Spleen. This should be done bimanually with one hand supporting the tissues in the left renal angle. The front hand should be firmly placed flat over the left hypochondrium. A palpable spleen is always pathological. Common causes of splenomegaly are various infections including glandular fever and malaria, hepatic cirrhosis, the leukaemias and the myeloproliferative disorders. A very large spleen can be detected immediately, as a slight quick movement forwards with the back hand will bump the spleen against the other hand. When the tip of the spleen is just beneath, at, or just below the costal margin, the front hand should be placed an inch or two below the ribs and then pressed upwards towards the left axilla, so that the fingers either touch the spleen or come to lie beneath the costal margin (Fig. 7.9). When the patient takes a deep breath through the open mouth, an enlarged spleen will bump against the tips of the index and middle fingers. At the height of inspiration, the pressure on the hand should be released so that the finger-tips slip over the pole of the spleen, confirming its presence and feeling its surface and consistency. An enlarged spleen retains its shape. Therefore if a lump is felt below the left costal margin which is not smooth and rounded, it should be regarded as something other than the lower pole of the spleen. On rare occasions it is easier to feel the tip of the spleen with the patient lying on the right side and with the left hip and knee flexed at a right angle. Alternatively, a spleen

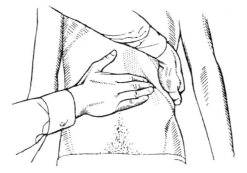

Fig. 7.9. Palpation of the spleen.

which is just palpable may be more easily felt by standing to the left of the patient chest, placing the left hand on the lower chest and 'hooking' the examining fingers round the costal margin while the patient breathes in deeply.

Even when the spleen is large enough to be felt in the groin, it should not be mistaken for a large kidney. The examining fingers can usually be pushed deep to the lower pole and anterior edge of the spleen and one or two notches may be felt on the edge (Fig. 7.8). It will not be possible to insert the fingers between the spleen and the costal margin. In addition, a very large spleen tends to point towards the right iliac fossa and may cross the mid-line. In contrast, an enlarged kidney rarely crosses the mid-line; it fills the loin diffusely, and unless a lump projects from it, the fingers cannot be inserted deep to the mass at any point, but can usually be inserted between the kidney and the costal margin. In addition, the kidney is much more readily appreciated bimanually than the spleen.

Palpation of the Kidneys. A bimanual technique should be employed. The front hand should be laid lightly over the abdomen in a position suitable for deep palpation just lateral to the rectus abdominis and immediately overlying the posterior hand placed with the fingers in the renal angle (Figs. 7.10 and 7.11). The two are firmly but gently pushed together as the patient breathes out. During deep inspiration, the lower pole of the descending kidney may now be felt to bump into the hands. Sometimes if the pressure is postponed until the end of inspiration, it may be possible to trap the kidney between the two hands. Then when the pressure is reduced on expiration, the kidney can be felt to slide back above the hands thereby providing an excellent idea of its size and consistency.

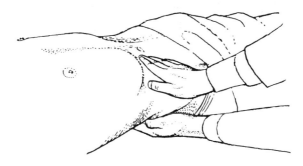

Fig. 7.10. Palpation of the kidney from the same side.

A normal kidney has a very firm consistency and the surface is smooth. The lower half of the normal right kidney is often palpable, especially in slim women. The normal left kidney is less often palpable. Owing to the varying thickness of the parietes, enlargement of a kidney, unless it is gross, is difficult to judge without a good deal of practice. Irregularity of the surface or an abnormally hard consistency may be appreciated quite easily. When the liver is readily palpable, it may be difficult to decide whether the right kidney can also be felt. Tenderness of the kidney is usually greatest posteriorly and is readily elicited by tapping the renal angle with the patient sitting forward.

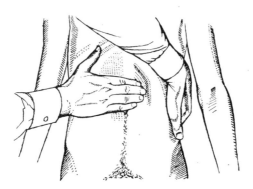

Fig. 7.11   Palpation of the kidney from the opposite side.

Percussion of the Abdomen

The basic technique has been described (p. 174). Three additional principles can be applied to abdominal percussion:

(i)   percuss from resonant to dull;
(ii) place the finger used for percussion on the abdomen parallel to the direction of the anticipated note change;
(iii) percuss softly for superficial structure, such as the lower border of the liver and more firmly for deeper structures.

The main value of abdominal percussion is to find out whether distension is due to gas, ascites, a fluid filled cyst or solid tumour. Gaseous distension is resonant. A large ovarian cyst causes dullness in the centre of the abdomen and resonance due to any gas in the gut is arranged around it.

Ascites. In the presence of ascites the gas-containing gut floats uppermost. The liquid flows to the dependent part of the peritoneal cavity, to the lower part on standing, to both flanks on lying supine and to one side when reclining. This *shifting dullness* should be sought in confirmation of ascites. It is usually simplest to detect it by examining the patient supine and by percussing from the centre of the abdomen into the left flank until a dull note is obtained. The finger is kept in place while the patient rolls on to the right side. After pausing for a few seconds, the presence of ascites is suggested if the note has become resonant and established by obtaining a dull note while percussing back towards the umbilicus. The presence of small quantities of free fluid in the peritoneal cavity cannot be determined with certainty, for slight changes in percussion note may be due to gravitational shift of normal bowel.

A moderate accumulation of ascites should be suspected from inspection and palpation. If the abdominal muscles are well relaxed, a characteristic wobbly sensation similar to that of handling a partly filled rubber water-bottle, may be noted.

Very large accumulations of ascites or large liquid-containing cysts may give a *palpable thrill*. In order to detect this, one of the examiner's hands is placed flat on the patient's flank. The other flank is then flicked or tapped, and a shock wave is transmitted to the palpating hand. A third person, or the active participation of the patient, is required, for a hand should also be placed in the midline of the abdomen to prevent any ripple from passing through the fat of the anterior abdominal wall. In a thin patient this is not necessary.

An additional useful sign in ascites is *dipping* over the liver or spleen if either of these organs is enlarged. The examiner's hand is laid over the abdomen, and quick dipping movements are made. The sudden displacement of liquid gives a tapping sensation over the surface of the liver or spleen comparable to the patellar tap (p. 354). By this manoeuvre it may also be possible to detect and to map the outlines of enlarged organs or of tumours which cannot be felt in the ordinary way because the abdomen is so distended.

Percussion of the Spleen. Percussion is a poor method of seeking for enlargement of the spleen, but its employment may be necessary when adequate relaxation of the abdominal muscles cannot be achieved or if it is doubtful whether the tip can be felt. Normally the spleen lies against the posterolateral wall of the abdominal cavity beneath the ninth, tenth and eleventh ribs. As it enlarges, it remains closely applied to this wall, expanding forwards, downwards and eventually medially, the tip emerging somewhere beneath the left costal margin. The patient should therefore be asked to take in a deep breath and hold it while the area below and then just above the costal margin is percussed. The position of the underlying spleen may be detected by impairment of the percussion note.

Percussion of the Liver. Heavy percussion from above and a light percussion from below in the mid clavicular line can give only a rough estimate of the size of the liver. The range of observer error (p. 12) is wide when compared with the findings on radionuclide scanning particularly in regard to the upper border. Although this may be raised above the level of the fifth rib by a greatly enlarged liver, the percussion note is largely dependent upon the state of the lung and pleura.

The apparent level of the lower border of the liver varies with the amount of gas in the colon and a palpable lower border may be 3 or 4 cm below the edge detected by percussion. However, a positive finding on percussion implies that the borders of the liver extend at least as far as the level of impairment. Absence of liver dullness may be of contributory diagnostic value when gas has leaked from a perforated peptic ulcer.

Auscultation of the Abdomen

Movement of the bowel contents by peristaltic activity of the gut creates characteristic gurgling sounds which may be heard from time to time by the unaided ear. Through the stethoscope they can be heard every 5 to 10 seconds, though the interval varies greatly in relationship to meals. Bowel sounds disappear in paralytic ileus (obstruction) which is usually secondary to peritonitis. They increase in frequency and intensity in association with malabsorptive disorders of the small intestine, and when there is much blood in the bowel from upper alimentary haemorrhage; the noise may be so loud in the rare carcinoid syndrome as to cause social embarrassment. When mechanical obstruction is present, not only are sounds increased in frequency and intensity, but gaseous distension of the gut adds a tinkling quality to the sounds.

Most arterial bruits in the abdomen arise from the aorta. Systolic murmurs due to stenoses of mesenteric or renal arteries may be audible but owing to the distracting effects of the bowel sounds, a conscious effort must be made to listen for them. An arterial bruit may be heard over a hepatoma. A venous hum is occasionally audible between the xiphisternum and the umbilicus due to turbulence in a well-developed collateral circulation from portal hypertension. Friction sounds resembling those of pleurisy may be present over an area of perisplenitis or perihepatitis.

Examination of the Groins

Now is a convenient time to examine the groins for the femoral pulses (p. 107) and for abnormal lymph nodes. The normal variation in size and consistency of the latter can be appreciated only by making this a routine practice. At the same time, hernias may be observed but their presence cannot be excluded unless the groins are examined while the patient is standing.

The Examination of Hernias. The principles described on page 46 for the examination of swellings apply to hernias but emphasis has to be placed on certain anatomical features. Hernias occur at the site of operation scars and at points of anatomical weakness. All hernias bulge more when the pressure within them is raised. Hernias of the abdominal wall are therefore more prominent in the erect position, and an impulse can be felt in the hernia when the patient coughs. It must be remembered, however, that both of these features also apply to a saphenous varix. After the identification of a hernia, an attempt should be made to replace the contents by the application of a gentle sustained pressure. An obstructed hernia cannot be reduced and a strangulated hernia is tense and tender and shows no impulse on coughing.

A *femoral hernia* lies in the femoral canal below the inguinal ligament and is therefore below and lateral to the pubic tubercle.

An *inguinal hernia* emerges from the abdominal wall through the external inguinal ring and is therefore above and medial to the pubic tubercle.

It is customary to attempt to differentiate direct from indirect (oblique) inguinal hernias. An indirect inguinal hernia occurs into a persistent remnant of the processus vaginalis. It therefore occurs in young men and may extend to the testes. Following reduction, control will be obtained by pressure over the internal inguinal ring, just above the mid-point of the inguinal ligament.

Direct inguinal hernia occurs directly through the weakened posterior wall of the inguinal canal medial to the inferior epigastric artery and lateral to the rectus muscle. It is more common in older men and does not reach the testes. It will not be controlled by pressure over the internal inguinal ring.

Examination of the Male Genitalia

In the male, examination of the genitalia conveniently follows palpation of the groins. The penis and scrotum are inspected and the testes, epididymes and vasa deferentia palpated. Minor degrees of hypospadias (p. 395) occur once in every 300 boys. Other conditions which should be borne in mind include the sexually transmitted diseases, and enlargement of the groin lymph nodes should lead to careful search for a chancre or a urethral discharge. Both testes are atrophic in hypogonadism and one may atrophy after orchitis due to mumps. An empty scrotum on one or both sides should lead to a search for incompletely descended testes in the inguinal canal or for ectopic testes in sites such as the groin.

Examination of a scrotal swelling should follow the principles laid down on page 46. The first objective must be to confirm that the swelling is of the scrotum and its contents rather than an inguinal hernia. Since the scrotum contains paired structures, the two sides should be compared; its accessibility enables the exact site of origin of a swelling or other change to be accurately determined by careful palpation. Finally an indication of the pathology will be provided by the consistency of the swelling and by the presence or absence of signs of inflammation.

Swellings within the scrotum commonly contain a clear liquid, a finding which can be confirmed by transillumination (p. 50). A hydrocele, a spermatocele and a cyst of the epididymis are differentiated by their relationships to the testis (Figure 7.12). The possibility that a hydrocele may obscure a testicular tumour must not be overlooked and in each case the testis must be palpated with care. Infections other than syphilis and mumps affect primarily the epididymis and tuberculosis produces a characteristic nodular change within the epididymis accompanied by thickening of the cord. Shortening of the cord is a characteristic of torsion of the testis.

Examination of the genital organs in the female is described on page 214. It is not a routine procedure.

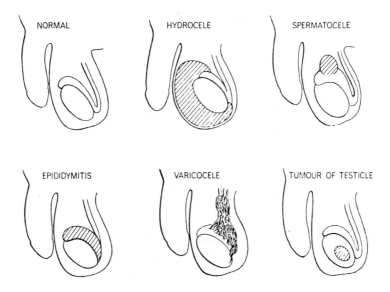

Fig. 7.12 Swellings of the scrotum.

Examination of the Rectum

Because digital examination of the rectum is slightly disagreeable to the patient and a little extra trouble for the doctor it is often omitted. There is no doubt that many have suffered from the consequences of the neglect of this simple procedure. It is very important that the student should become familiar with the feel of the normal structures. Male students must ask a nurse or a female colleague to be in attendance when the patient is female. Digital examination of the rectum should be performed in the following circumstances:

1. *Alimentary problems*
   Suspected appendicitis, pelvic abscess, peritonitis.
   Lower abdominal pain in which the cause is obscure.
   Diarrhoea or constipation; mucus or blood in the stools.
   Anal irritation or pain; tenesmus or rectal pain.
   Bimanual examination of a lower abdominal mass.
   In the search for tumours or transperitoneal metastases either diagnostically or in making a decision about treatment.

2. *Genito-urinary problems*
   Dysuria; haematuria; haematospermia; epididymo-orchitis.
   In lieu of gynaecological examination in virgins.

3. *Miscellaneous problems*
   In the search for a cause of backache, root pains in the legs or unexplained bone pain.
   In all cases of pyrexia of unknown origin.

Digital Examination. The patient should be informed that it is necessary to examine the back passage. If the examiner is right-handed, the patient should lie in the left lateral position with a maximal degree of flexion of the spine and legs consistent with comfort. The buttocks should be at the edge of the couch or bed. The patient should be encouraged to relax and be reassured that the examination should not be painful. The examiner's right forefinger, protected by a fingerstall or a suitable glove, should be smeared with a lubricant. In a good light the perianal skin should be examined for intertrigo or for evidence of scratching, thrombosed external piles fissure or fistulae. The last should lead to a search for tuberculosis or inflammatory bowel disease. The possibility of a chancre or of gonorrhoea must also be borne in mind.

The forefinger tip is placed on the anterior anal margin and with steady pressure on the sphincter is moved backwards. The finger then slides gently through the anal canal into the rectum (Fig. 7.13). Resistance at the anus is commonly due to spasm induced by anxiety, and this can sometimes be overcome by asking the patient to strain down in an attempt to defaecate. If spasm is associated with local pain, the presence of an anal fissure should be suspected; a local anaesthetic suppository may be required before a satisfactory examination can be made. Rarely, tightness is due to a fibrous stricture or a growth or to Hirschsprung's disease in the infant (p. 395). The upper end of the anal canal is marked by the pubo-rectalis muscle which should be easily palpable and which will be felt to contract reflexly on coughing or on conscious contraction by the patient. Any weakness of the sphincter should be noted.

Beyond the anal canal, the direction of the rectum is upwards and backwards along the curve of the coccyx and the sacrum. The exploring finger should then feel round the whole extent of the rectum. The normal rectum should be empty and the wall should be smooth and soft. In cases of habitual constipation the rectum is full of firm faeces. An obstructing carcinoma of the upper rectum will produce a ballooning of the empty cavity below. Posteriorly the coccyx and sacrum can be felt through the rectal wall, while anteriorly from below upwards, the membranous urethra, the prostate and often the base of the bladder may be felt in the male, while the firm round cervix uteri can be felt projecting backwards in the female (Fig. 7.13). The normal prostate is smooth and has a fairly firm consistency with the contours of miniature buttocks represented by the lateral lobes and a median groove between them. Prostatic hyperplasia in the adult, which is a common cause of urinary obstruction, often produces a palpable enlargement but may not do so if the

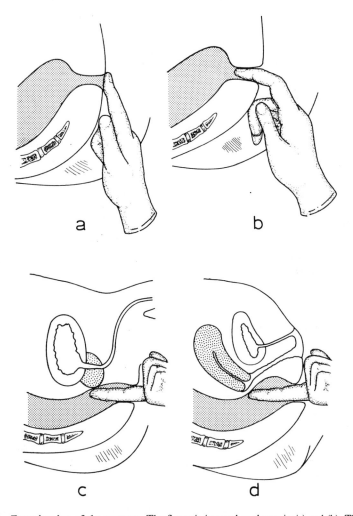

Fig. 7.13 Examination of the rectum. The finger is inserted as shown in (a) and (b). The hand is then rotated and the most prominent features are the prostate in the male (c) and the cervix in the female (d).

hyperplasia is confined to the median lobe. The prostate is abnormally small in hypogonadism. Tenderness, accompanied by other local and systemic symptoms and by a change in the consistency of the gland, may be due to prostatitis or an abscess. A hard, irregular gland, which may be fixed to the mucosa or the surrounding structures, and usually without a detectable median groove, is characteristic of carcinoma. Piles which are not thrombosed and normal seminal vesicles cannot be felt.

Any deviation from normal should be noted, and lumps in particular should be examined by the systematic method described on page 46. For this purpose it is sometimes helpful to palpate bimanually with the other hand laid flat over the abdomen. A faecal mass is commonly palpable and this should be movable and may be indented. If several masses are present, the examination should be repeated after the patient has defaecated. Metastases or a tumour in a loop of colon lying in the lower part of the peritoneal cavity may otherwise be mistaken for faeces. In lesions palpable within the rectum the percentage of the rectal circumference involved and the distance of the upper and lower edges from the anal margin should be recorded.

The finger after withdrawal should be examined for blood, and the colour of the faeces should be noted. A sample of faeces from the finger-stall can be tested chemically for occult blood (p. 217).

Proctoscopy. Visual examination of the rectum and anal canal is an extension of the digital method. It is essential for the diagnosis of inflammatory lesions and of piles. Through the proctoscope it is also possible to inspect any palpable lesions, to remove polypi and to take specimens for biopsy. Proctoscopy should always be preceded by digital examination. With the patient in the left lateral position the forefinger and thumb of one hand separate the buttocks, while with the other, a warmed and well-lubricated proctoscope is gently inserted in the same directions as described for digital examination. The surface of the normal rectum can be closely compared to the appearance of the buccal mucosa — clean, shiny, smooth, reddish pink with clearly visible submucosal veins. For the detection of piles the patient should be asked to strain down as the proctoscope is gradually withdrawn. Under these conditions the piles will be distended with blood and their extent can be fully appreciated.

Gynaecological Examination

The contents of the female pelvis are illustrated in Figure 7.14.

The intimate nature of a gynaecological examination not only makes it difficult to combine with routine abdominal examination, but also renders it more likely to raise medico-legal problems than any other form of medical examination. The patient's consent must be obtained, and a third person should be present during the examination.

For the comfort of the patient and for ease of interpretation of the examination, the bowel and bladder should be empty. The patient should lie comfortably on her back with her head on a pillow to relax the abdominal muscles. The trunk is covered with a sheet. The hips and knees should be flexed, the thighs abducted, and illumination arranged so that a good light falls upon the vulva. The examiner is advised to wear gloves. The labia minora should be separated by the forefinger and

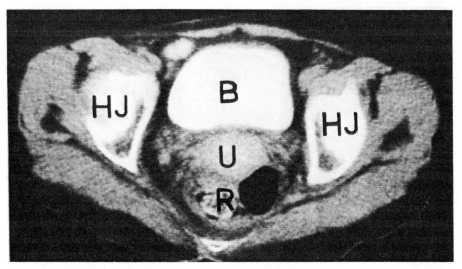

Fig. 7.14 Contents of pelvis as shown by CT scan. B: Bladder outlined by contrast medium.
H J: Hip joint. R: Rectum. U: Uterus. (*Courtesy of Professor Ian Isherwood.*)

thumb of the left hand, bringing into view the clitoris anteriorly, then the urethra, the vagina and finally the anus posteriorly. Any discharge from the urethra or vagina should be swabbed; one specimen should be sent for culture and another smeared on to a glass slide for microscopical examination. Direct microscopy of a smear is particularly useful in the confirmation of infection due to *Trichomonas vaginalis*; a smear, promptly stained, may also give conclusive evidence of gonorrhoea or thrush.

The lateral walls of the vulva on either side of the lower third of the vagina should be palpated with the right hand for abnormalities of Bartholin's glands. In parous women two fingers should then be turned palmar surface down and spread, to test for laxity of the superficial muscles, and to allow inspection of the vaginal walls for prolapse when the patient is asked to strain down. The index finger of the right hand smeared with a lubricant and in most cases the middle finger too should then be inserted into the vagina (Fig. 7.15). The cervix uteri is readily felt, being circular, with a small central os in the nulliparous patient. The normal cervix points downwards and slightly backwards. In parous women, the cervix is usually larger and the os a good deal bigger and often palpable as a transverse slit.

Bimanual palpation is now made. With the middle finger of the right hand at the os and the forefinger in the anterior fornix, the left hand is placed flat on the abdomen and worked down towards the pubis. The position and other characteristics of the uterus can then be identified between the hands. Each fornix should now be palpated in turn with particular regard to tenderness and swellings of the Fallopian tubes and ovaries. The bladder lies immediately anteriorly. In the posterior fornix, abnormalities may be appreciated in the pouch of Douglas, and faecal masses may be identified by the fact that they become indented.

Digital examination should be supplemented by inspection of the vagina and uterine cervix through a vaginal speculum. Using an Ayre spatula a smear is taken from the cervix for cytological examination. This important screening procedure in

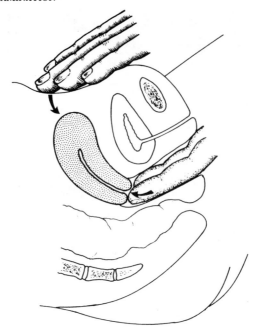

Fig. 7.15   Vaginal examination.

the early detection of cancer of the cervix should be carried out at least every five years after the age of 35.

Vaginal examination of virgins should if possible be avoided, and minors should not be examined without the consent of a parent or guardian. In these circumstances adequate information can often be obtained by digital examination of the rectum.

FURTHER INVESTIGATION

In many cases it will be possible to make a satisfactory diagnosis by clinical examination alone. Further investigation will then be required only for confirmation. When the diagnosis is uncertain, the clinician must decide which investigations should be performed and in which order because an indiscrimate series of tests is a burden on the patient, costly and time consuming.

General Assessment. This must not be neglected in a rush to perform specific investigations. Testing of the urine is an essential part of every clinical examination and is described in Chapter 12. In all but the most trivial cases, additional investigations will include a full blood count and estimation of the blood urea and electrolytes. Most patients over the age of forty will require a chest radiograph because the discovery of a primary or secondary tumour in the lung will alter the requirements for more detailed investigation. A chest radiograph may also show medistinal widening and the absence of air in the gastric fundus due to achalasia of the cardia, or a fluid level seen through the heart shadow may be caused by a paraoesophageal hernia. A raised right diaphragm with pleural effusion may contribute to the diagnosis of liver abscess.

ALIMENTARY TRACT

Examination of the Faeces. Inspection of the consistency and colour of the faeces is often of diagnostic value (p. 194). Supplementary investigations include stool culture, microscopic examination and testing for occult blood.

MICROSCOPIC EXAMINATION. A film is prepared by emulsifying a small portion of faeces with a drop of isotonic saline on a glass slide and applying a cover-slip. Most information is obtained from an examination with the low-power objective of the microscope, and under illumination suitably reduced by lowering the substage condenser. The principal values of this examination are 1) in the finding of pus cells, red blood cells and macrophages, all of which are usually present in large numbers in ulcerative diseases of the large intestine, and 2) in the finding of parasitic protozoa and their cysts and metazoal ova. The presence of undigested meat fibres is a useful pointer to pancreatic steatorrhoea.

OCCULT BLOOD IN THE FAECES. The chemical detection of occult blood in the stools is frequently important in the investigation of gastro-intestinal and haematological problems. It may be an early, and the only, clinical manifestation of carcinoma of the colon or the rectum. Since bleeding may be intermittent, two samples should be tested from each of three stools over several days. If one is positive, further investigation is indicated. When difficulty is encountered in obtaining specimens, sufficient material for testing can usually be obtained on the gloved finger at rectal examination. In patients with haemorrhoids it may be necessary to obtain the stool samples through a proctoscope above the pile-bearing area if bleeding from the upper gastrointestinal tract is suspected. The test employed should not be too sensitive because there is a 'normal' faecal blood loss of about 2.5 ml daily as measured by radiochromium.

The *Haemoccult test* is recommended. In this commercial preparation guaiac is oxidised to a blue colour by the peroxidase-like activity of haemoglobin. Neither barium nor medicinal iron interferes with the test.

Gastrointestinal Radiology. A plain film should be taken before contrast radiography as it may give information which would be obscured by the barium. A good quality radiograph will show the outline of the kidneys, the lateral borders of the psoas muscles and, sometimes, the spleen. Radio-opaque stones may be present in the renal or, less frequently, in the biliary tract. Calcification may often be seen in lymph nodes in the right iliac fossa, in phleboliths in the pelvis and, in older patients, in the abdominal aorta and its major branches. Pathological calcification may also occur within the kidneys, adrenal glands or pancreas. Faeces are seen as a stippled pattern within the colon. Large amounts of faeces in the right side of colon are an indication of delayed intestinal transit and although this may be caused by disease in the distal large bowel, it is often due to constipation.

Plain radiographs of the whole abdomen can be taken in both the erect and supine positions. Both views are often required in the assessment of the acute abdomen. The erect view will show any fluid level and the supine view gives a better impression of the distribution of gas within the gastrointestinal tract. A small air/fluid level is normal in the gastric fundus but fluid levels elsewhere may indicate an obstruction or an ileus. The presence of gas beneath the diaphragm in acute perforation of a hollow viscus is often best seen on the erect chest film.

Contrast radiography can outline the whole of the gastrointestinal tract (Fig. 7.1). A barium swallow delineates the oesophagus. Hold-up of barium can be due to a failure of the lower oesophageal sphincter to relax in achalasia of the cardia or to oesophageal narrowing due to either a benign or malignant stricture. Other lesions that can be identified include mucosal ulceration and oesophageal varices. Barium swallow is usually combined with barium meal. As the barium passes through the stomach to the duodenum, the radiologist looks for lesions such as peptic ulceration and carcinoma. Displacement of the stomach or widening of the duodenal loop may be seen in disease within the pancreas. The further progress of barium through the small bowel may be studied in the course of a 'follow through' examination. Better quality pictures are obtained when this investigation is performed without prior examination of the stomach; then the duodenum is intubated and a 'small bowel enema' is performed. An abnormal small bowel pattern may be due to malabsorption or to an inflammatory lesion such as Crohn's disease.

The colon is examined by barium enema in which the contrast medium is run in through an anal catheter and which will outline tumours, polyps, diverticula and inflammatory disease of the colon. Preparation for a barium enema consists of complete evacuation of faeces by purgation and/or enemas. Sometimes this is inadvisable, for example in ulcerative colitis, and an unprepared examination may have to be performed. In all cases, the radiologist must be given adequate details to understand the clinical problems so that the best examination can be undertaken for the particular patient. Digital examination of the rectum, supplemented if necessary by proctoscopy, must always be done before proceeding to a barium enema.

When both barium meal and enema examinations are required, the enema should be performed first as the barium should be evacuated quite quickly and enable the meal to be performed without undue delay. Both examinations may be enhanced by the double contrast technique of introducing air as well as contrast medium.

Endoscopic Examination. The development of flexible fibreoptic instruments has made it possible to diagnose lesions of the oesophagus, stomach and duodenum by visual inspection supplemented where necessary with small but adequate biopsies. The rectum and lower sigmoid colon are visualised during rigid sigmoidoscopy. Particular attention must be paid to passing the sigmoidoscope around the rectosigmoid junction as this is where lesions are missed during a barium enema. The colon may also be examined by flexible fibreoptic endoscopy. During this procedure not only can biopsies be taken from any point in the colon but also polyps of quite large size can be removed by snaring them with a diathermy loop. thereby avoiding the need for laparotomy.

CHOICE OF INVESTIGATION: ENDOSCOPY OR CONTRAST RADIOLOGY. Barium examination and upper alimentary endoscopy should be regarded as complementary. When an adequate diagnosis has been made by one method, it is often unnecessary to proceed to the other. Both may be required if the diagnosis is elusive and are often indicated in the investigation of dysphagia. In most other circumstances, the choice will depend upon the urgency of the investigation and the availability of the facilities. In general, a radiograph is cheaper but in some situations, for example, acute upper gastrointestinal bleeding, an early endoscopy may give information that radiology cannot provide.

Sigmoidoscopy usually precedes barium enema examination. The latter should be avoided for a day after sigmoidoscopy and for several days if a biopsy has been taken. A repeat sigmoidoscopy may be impossible until the barium has been completely evacuated and these factors must be considered when planning colonic investigations. Fibreoptic colonoscopy is time consuming and is undertaken only if there remains an indications for it after barium enema and rigid endoscopy examinations.

Ultrasonography. Ultrasound examination provides a two-dimensional picture which is built up to give the impression of a 'cut' through the body. Transverse cuts are usually viewed, like CT scans, as though looking up from the patient's feet. Examination is non-invasive, and requires no special preparation other than ensuring that the patient has an empty stomach and bladder. The investigation is useful in assessing abdominal and pelvic masses and in distinguishing between solid and cystic lesions (Fig. 7.16). Aspiration of cysts may be performed under ultrasound guidance and biopsy of solid tumours directed by ultrasound control.

Computed Tomography (CT Scan). This provides an alternative non-invasive method of investigation. It is particularly of value in assessing the presence or absence of intra-abdominal malignancy in such conditions as seminoma of the testis and in those subjects in whom the value of ultrasound imaging is restricted by factors such as obesity.

Tests of Gastrointestinal Function. The pentagastrin secretion test is of value in the assessment of the patient with peptic ulceration. In the investigation of intestinal absorption, several tests are usually employed in conjunction thus: (1) stools are examined, e.g. for evidence of failure to absorb food, especially fat; (2) blood may be tested for a rise in the concentration of a substance, such as glucose, given by mouth; (3) urine may be collected for the estimation of substances which, after absorption are largely excreted by the kidneys, e.g. xylose. Folic acid and vitamin B_{12} absorption tests may help to differentiate between disease of the jejunum and ileum as hydroxocobalamin is absorbed solely in the ileum.

Tests of Motility. Intra-oesophageal pressure and motility studies occasionally supply diagnostic information in difficult problems such as the differentiation of atypical chest pain of oesophageal origin from myocardial ischaemia. It is also a straightforward procedure to insert catheters into the anus and rectum to measure pressures but the clinical application is confined to those few patients with sphincter problems in which some form of surgery is contemplated.

THE LIVER AND BILIARY TRACT

General Assessment. The commonest problem is to distinguish between hepatocellular and obstructive jaundice. This is established partly by chemical investigations based on the excretory and synthetic functions of the liver and on enzymes released by cell damage. None of these tests is specific so that several are done in conjunction and the results must be interpreted in the light of the clinical features. Other tests and investigative procedures are indicated for specific reasons.

Hepatitis B Surface Antigen. In any case in which viral hepatitis could be implicated, this antigen should be looked for as soon as possible, and preferably before performing any other blood tests. A positive result is not only of diagnostic value but should also alert to the danger of infection those dealing with the patient or handling the blood in the laboratory.

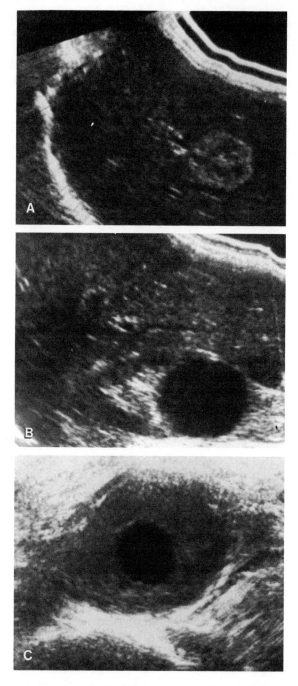

Fig. 7.16 Ultrasonography as a diagnostic aid. (A) Solid tumour in liver (longitudinal scan through right lobe of liver towards diaphragm which is seen as a curved white line). (B) Renal cyst (anterior longitudinal scan of right kidney through liver). (C) Aneurysm of aorta the lumen of which is reduced by mural thrombus. The vertebral body is seen as the curved white area towards the lower left (transverse scan). *Note:* (1)A, B and C are at different magnification. (2) Best results are obtained if the abdomen is not obese, scarred or flatulent. (*Courtesy of Dr S. R. Wild.*)

Biochemical Tests. BILIRUBIN. Clinical jaundice is not evident until the serum level has risen to about 50 μmol/l (normal range 5–17 μmol/l). A rise in conjugated bilirubin occurs in obstructive jaundice or hepatitis. Unconjugated hyperbilirubinaemia indicates haemolysis or an abnormality of bilirubin transport or metabolism such as Gilbert's disease. Some increase in unconjugated bilirubin in the plasma also occurs in the early and recovery stages of acute hepatitis in which the jaundice is largely due to conjugated bilirubin.

ALKALINE PHOSPHATASE. This is increased much more in obstructive than in hepatocellular jaundice. As the enzyme occurs in most tissues an isolated rise is usually not due to liver disease; electrophoretic separation of the isoenzymes can distinguish that derived from bone which is the other common source.

PLASMA PROTEINS. Albumin is synthetised solely in the liver. In chronic liver disease its concentration is frequently below normal and electrophoresis may show a concomitant rise in the gammaglobulin peak.

PROTHROMBIN TIME. The concentration of coagulation factors II, VII and X of liver origin falls in a matter of days in severe hepatitis, and the one stage prothrombin time gives a good guide to prognosis. In obstructive jaundice there is malabsorption of vitamin K which results in prolongation of the prothrombin time.

SERUM TRANSFERASES. The principal value in estimating the activity of these enzymes is to test the integrity of liver cells, this helping to distinguish obstructive from hepatocellular jaundice. Aspartate and Alanine amino transferases (AST and ALT) are the most important, and increased activity is a very sensitive index of hepatic damage. Neither enzyme is specific to the liver and results must be interpreted in the clinical context. As ALT occurs in much higher concentration in the liver than in other organs, an increase in its activity is a more specific indication of hepatic damage.

Other Tests of Liver Disease. AUTOANTIBODIES. Nuclear, smooth muscle or mitochondrial antibodies may be of diagnostic value in chronic liver disease; for example the last is positive in primary biliary cirrhosis.

ALPHA-FETOPROTEIN. The reappearance of this fetal alpha-globulin in adult life is almost always due to a hepatoma, although the test is often negative in the presence of a hepatoma.

Investigative Procedures in Liver and Biliary Disease.

SCANNING. Ultrasonography may show the presence of diffuse liver disease such as cirrhosis or focal lesions within the liver exceeding 2 cm in diameter. Radionuclide scanning is complementary to ultrasound as each may detect lesions missed by the other. Ultrasound is the ideal initial investigation for the patient with jaundice because it shows the presence or absence of features such as dilated ducts, stones or pancreatic masses.

RADIOLOGICAL EXAMINATION. Gallstones may be seen on routine radiography but many are radiotranslucent and the contrast technique of cholecystography or cholangiography is necessary. If the patient is jaundiced, the bile ducts can be demonstrated by percutaneous transhepatic cholangiography (PTC) provided ultrasonography shows dilated ducts. If the ducts are not dilated, they may be filled from below by catheterisation via the flexible endoscope — endoscopic retrograde cholangio-pancreatography (ERCP).

A barium swallow may give evidence of portal venous hypertension by showing evidence of oesophageal varices. Selective angiography via the hepatic artery, hepatic vein or portal vein can define the site of local lesions and portal pressures can be measured.

BIOPSY. The pathological diagnosis of focal lesions can be established by local aspiration but percutaneous liver biopsy is usually of greatest value in providing information in diffuse liver disease.

PARACENTESIS ABDOMINIS. Diagnostic paracentesis allows examination for protein and cell count and cytology for malignant cells.

PANCREAS

Tests of exocrine secretion can be made by collecting pancreatic juice through a tube passed via the mouth or nose into the duodenum. The pancreas can be stimulated either indirectly by a test meal containing carbohydrate, protein and fat or directly by secretin and/or pancreozymin. Following stimulation the duodenal aspirate is collected for 30 min and the volume of aspirate and the concentrations of bicarbonate, amylase, trypsin and lipase are estimated.

Extensive disease of the pancreas may damage its endocrine function with the development of overt or latent diabetes. A glucose tolerance test is particularly useful in distinguishing between malabsorption due to pancreatic disease, in which there is a diabetic type of curve, and that due to diffuse disease of the small intestine in which there may be an abnormally small and sustained rise in the blood sugar.

Acute pancreatitis is accompanied by a transient but often marked increase in serum amylase, although this may also rise in other abdominal crises such as a perforated duodenal ulcer.

Radiological examination may indicate that the pancreas is swollen by showing displacement of the stomach and duodenum and absence of gas in the middle of the transverse colon. Hypotonic duodenography may demonstrate that the duodenal loop is distorted by a pancreatic neoplasm.

The pancreatic ductal system can be visualised by endoscopic retrograde cholangiopancreatography and changes indicative of neoplasm or chronic pancreatitis may be demonstrated.

Ultrasonography and computed tomography (CT scan) are both non-invasive methods of detecting otherwise elusive pancreatic tumours.

URINARY SYSTEM

In renal disease accurate collection of the urine, biochemical testing and microscopic and bacteriological examination are essential if diagnosis is to be achieved. These procedures and simple tests of tubular function are described in Chapter 12.

Estimation of blood urea and creatinine will indicate the degree of renal failure and a creatinine clearance determination will give an estimation of the glomerular filtration rate.

An excretion urogram is always preceded by a plain radiograph of the abdomen which may show the presence of renal calculi or indicate renal size. Following intravenous injection of a radio-opaque dye a nephrogram appears first. This will allow measurement of the size of the kidneys and definition of the renal outlines. Asymmetry may be due to enlargement from obstruction or to a small kidney from congenital causes or renal artery stenosis. Symmetrically small kidneys suggest chronic parenchymal disease. A pyelogram next appears and delineates the pelvicalyceal system. This can be distorted in chronic pyelonephritis to cause a clubbed appearance or destruction of papillae can take place in analgesic abuse and in diabetes mellitus. After the pyelogram the ureters and bladder will also be shown.

The urethra can be inspected through a urethroscope and the bladder and ureteric orifices can be examined by means of a cystoscope. Retrograde pyelography can demonstrate ureteric obstruction and give a more precise definition of the renal pelvis if there is doubt about the excretion urogram.

Ultrasonography is non-invasive and can distinguish solid from cystic lesions (Fig. 7.16). Radionuclide studies provide renal scans and renography. The former give information about renal structure and function. Renography helps in determining the function of each kidney and is most useful in assessing urinary tract obstruction.

The renal arteries may be outlined by aortography. In this way stenosis of a renal artery or the abnormal circulation in a tumour can be demonstrated.

Histological examination of the kidney can be carried out by percutaneous renal biopsy. Specimens are examined under the light microscope, electron microscope and also by immunofluorescent techniques.

GENITAL SYSTEM

Comparatively few investigations of the genital system are available or are indeed necessary, as for most purposes the structures concerned are reasonably accessible to clinical examination. In either sex appropriate specimens may be required to confirm the diagnosis of sexually transmitted infection or to identify the cause of discharges.

The investigations of infertility may require seminal analysis or testicular biopsy in the male, and laparoscopy in the female. Pregnancy can be confirmed by immunological and other tests whereby the presence of chorionic gonadotrophin in the patient's urine is demonstrated. The diagnosis can be made in this way at a much earlier stage than is possible by clinical means but it must be borne in mind that positive results are also obtained when a hydatidiform mole or a chorionepithelioma is present. Ultrasonic examination can be very helpful in this clinical dilemma.

Microscopical examination of the lining of the uterus after dilatation of the cervix and curettage (D. & C.) is a routine procedure in the investigation of abnormal vaginal bleeding, and the cytological examination of cervical smears, supplemented if necessary by biopsy of the cervix, is invaluable in the early detection of carcinoma (p. 215). The laparoscope is particularly useful in the elucidation of the cause of lower abdominal pain of gynaecological origin.

THE METHODS IN PRACTICE

Two contrasting examples have been chosen. In the 'acute abdomen' the facts must be obtained directly and immediately to contend with an emergency. In sexual problems explicit and highly personal questions must be asked but this can be done at leisure and prefaced by the use of a questionnaire. A case of impotence has been selected to illustrate the methods involved.

THE EXAMINATION OF THE ACUTE ABDOMEN

The term 'acute abdomen' is applied to disorders of sudden onset which may involve surgical intervention and thus require a prompt decision about appropriate action. Correct diagnosis may be lifesaving and will depend primarily upon an accurate history and careful physical examination.

The History. Pain is often the presenting feature and care should be taken to obtain a full description (p. 30). Pain of sudden onset in a patient who was well a few moments before may indicate a free perforation of a hollow viscus whereas pain of more gradual onset may suggest an inflammatory lesion such as appendicitis, salpingitis or diverticular disease. Changes in the character of the pain should be sought. Thus, the pain of appendicitis may start in the periumbilical area and later move to the right iliac fossa as the local peritoneal inflammation develops. Similarly the onset of a constant pain in a patient who has been experiencing small bowel colic implies the development of an ischaemic loop. During the general interrogation of the patient it is important to enquire about drug treatment. For example, systemic corticosteroid therapy may not only increase the risk of a perforation but also mask the clinical features.

The Physical Examination. A full general assessment must be made as abdominal symptoms may be prominent in disorders such as myocardial infarction, pneumonia or even diabetic ketoacidosis. Examination commences while the patient recounts the symptoms and includes recording the temperature, pulse and respiratory rates and blood pressure. Some patients will be very ill, and a prolonged history and examination will be displaced by the need for resuscitation. Shock may be due to concealed haemorrhage as in a leaking aortic aneurysm or ruptured ectopic pregnancy. It can also be associated with septicaemia due to infection in the biliary or urinary systems and may also be a feature of pancreatitis.

Examination of the abdomen follows the usual pattern of inspection, palpation, percussion and auscultation. On inspection all abdominal scars should be accounted for and the patient's story should be verified by referral to the original operation notes when possible. Palpation may reveal the special features found in the acute abdomen: tenderness, rebound tenderness, guarding and rigidity. Generalised board-like rigidity implies peritonitis and attempts to elicit other signs such as rebound tenderness are then unnecessary. Guarding, the reflex spasm of the abdominal wall muscles over an area of peritonitis, must be differentiated from contraction of the abdominal muscles due to the patient's anxiety or the examiner's cold hands. Deep seated inflammation not causing localised guarding may be revealed by rebound tenderness. Pelvic peritonitis may be advanced before signs are apparent on abdominal palpation and a rectal examination must never be omitted. The groins should be carefully examined for small hernias and the external genitalia palpated in the male.

Percussion of the abdomen is useful in localising an area of tenderness and the presence of free gas may be suspected by the absence of normal liver dullness.

Auscultation may reveal the active bowel sounds of intestinal obstruction and these may develop a 'tinkling' quality when bowel is distended. A 'silent' abdomen is ominous and implies paralysis of the intestines (ileus).

Further Investigation. A urinary specimen should be routinely tested for blood, glucose, ketones and bile. A faecal sample obtained during the rectal examination should be inspected and tested for occult blood.

Laboratory studies of value include a white cell count; a leucocytosis supports a diagnosis of an inflammatory lesion. If pancreatitis is a possibility, the serum amylase should be estimated.

Routine radiographs of the abdomen are not required to diagnose such disorders as appendicitis; the need for any films should always be questioned in women of child-bearing age. Erect and supine views are required in assessing patients with suspected perforation or obstruction of the bowel, in confirming the presence of radio-opaque calculi in the biliary or renal tracts and in some cases where the diagnosis remains obscure.

Management. Further treatment may involve surgery and the patient's discomfort may then be relieved by analgesics. If an operation is not required, suitable medication including analgesia should be given but it must be borne in mind that the initial diagnosis may be wrong; the patient will need continued observation and reassessment before further doses of analgesics are prescribed.

IMPOTENCE

An Illustrative Case

A 50-year-old barman was referred with a history of impotence which had not responded to an empirical course of mesterolone — a synthetic androgen which does not depress the pituitary. The sexual problem questionnaire (p. 451) revealed no suggestion of neurological disease, diabetes or hypertension and the man was on no medication. There was however a history of regular drinking with episodic heavy drinking. The sexual history was of partial erections not enough to allow intercourse although morning erections were present. He had stopped trying to have intercourse because of worry about further failure.

Physical examination showed a normal male physique with no evidence of gynaecomastia and the penis and both testes were normal. Gentle pressure on the testes produced normal testicular pain — a simple test to help to exclude autonomic neuropathy. General neurological examination was normal and in particular, sensation around the anus was unimpaired and the tone of the anal sphincter was normal on rectal examination. The prostate gland was slightly enlarged but was not hard or tender. The blood pressure was normal.

A urine sample was tested for glucose and protein with negative results. Blood estimations of urea, haemoglobin, testosterone, follicular stimulating hormone and liver function tests were all normal. If there had been gynaecomastia or uraemia a prolactin estimation would also have been performed as male hyperprolactinaemia is associated with impotence and sometimes renal failure.

The history of full erections in the morning suggested that there was nothing wrong with the vascular or neurological mechanisms of erection and it was concluded that the patient's libido and performance were simply diminished by his excessive consumption of alcohol. Initial advice from the clinical psychologist attached to the psychosexual clinic had to be followed by further guidance from an alcoholism unit before the drinking problem was brought under control. Libido then returned to normal.

8. The Nervous System

> Discard in the first instance all attempts to identify or to name, and try instead
> to read the malady, tracing the symptoms to the seat of their cause, and
> discerning the nature of the morbid process by their character and course.

Gowers, 1892

After a period of study of modern neurophysiological concepts, students often approach clinical neurology with an exaggerated idea of its difficulties. This is confirmed and compounded if their initial explorations are confused and misdirected by the use of polysyllabic and eponymous signs and the division of neurological disorders into rigidly labelled compartments.

The study of neurology is founded on those principles of clinical medicine which are outlined in Chapter 1 of this book. No other clinical discipline offers so exemplary an illustration of the logical and scientific foundations on which medicine is based. Deviations from normal neural function are observed. The nerve pathways and tracts whose interruption would cause such functional disturbances are inferred. Where possible the precise anatomical sites of lesions are then determined. In the light of the distribution of lesions, the history of the patient's illness and collateral evidence of disease in other systems, the causal pathological process is deduced. This diagnostic process constitutes a logical sequence which should always be followed. Though increasing facility will enable the steps to be made more rapidly, there are no short cuts; no signs are pathognomonic of disease processes.

The nervous system is organised functionally in a hierarchical fashion. Hughlings Jackson introduced the concept of different roles subserved by different levels of the nervous system. Peripheral effectors and receptors are supplied by nerves whose function is restricted, which originate from the spinal cord and dorsal root ganglia and which are arranged in a segmental fashion. Connections within a spinal cord segment between afferent and efferent nerve fibres enable reflex motor responses to occur as a result of certain sensory stimuli. Activities within the spinal cord are modified by influences deriving from 'higher' levels such as the basal ganglia or cerebellum which function as co-ordinating centres. The highest level of activity is represented in the cerebral cortex which is concerned with the elaboration of ideas, with the complex patterns of learned movements and with the integration and interpretation of sensory information. This organisational pattern is of fundamental clinical importance. Dissolution of neural activity at different levels produces different patterns of disability as is illustrated in the section on the motor system.

Neurological lesions may produce deviations from normal function in three ways:

(1) they may give rise to positive phenomena, i.e. there may be overaction of part of the nervous system, as for instance in Jacksonian epilepsy where convulsive movements of a limb result from an irritative lesion affecting the motor cortex; (2) abnormal function may occur because of a 'release' of lower levels of nervous activity from restraints or inhibitions which in normal circumstances are imposed by the functions of higher levels. A common example of this is the increased tone seen in limbs after damage to the pyramidal pathway; (3) 'negative' features result from the loss of normal neural functions as, for example, the muscle paralysis and impaired sensation which follow damage to a peripheral nerve. Sometimes damage to nerve pathways will concurrently cause patterns of positive, release and negative phenomena which are distinctive, as, for example, the tremor, rigidity and hypokinesis of the parkinsonian syndrome.

The significance of some signs may cause difficulty during the neurological examination. The results of examination often depend on the patient's cooperation and subjective responses to stimuli as well as on the examiner's interpretation based on an experience of normality. It should be recognised at the outset that with the most careful and meticulous examination, some signs are less reliable and more difficult of interpretation than others. There are 'soft' and 'hard' neurological signs, using these terms to denote reliability by analogy with currencies. An extensor plantar response denotes a lesion of the corticospinal pathways. This is the paradigm of a 'hard' neurological sign. The assessment of deep pain sensation by pinching the patient's calf depends on the patient's reaction and personality and, unless deviation from the normal response is marked, little reliance can be placed on this sign in isolation. Such difficulties are obviated to some extent since it is rarely necessary to base one's pathophysiological interpretation on single signs. Several abnormalities elicited during the examination will add weight to each other. A lesion in the posterior lobe of the cerebellum is more certainly diagnosed if intention tremor in the limbs on one side of the body is accompanied by a jerking type of nystagmus on looking to the same side. It is important, however, that this process of assessing signs in combination in order to localise lesions should not lead to a false importance being given to indeterminate observations. It is even more dangerous to attribute significance to findings in order to complete a pattern which is 'typical' of a disease. It sometimes occurs that an immediate prejudice is formed in favour of a diagnosis and thereafter signs are elucidated which support this diagnosis. When a young patient presents with paralysis of the legs (paraparesis), it may be immediately assumed that the diagnosis is multiple sclerosis. Examination of the optic discs in such a case reveals pallor of the temporal halves of the discs relative to their nasal halves which is a normal phenomenon. If, however, this normal variation is recorded as 'bitemporal pallor', putatively a sign of multiple sclerosis, then a spurious significance is given to a normal finding and the diagnosis of multiple sclerosis is made on flimsy grounds and a potentially remediable lesion such as a spinal cord tumour may be missed. This type of thinking is tautological. Signs are invented to fit the intuitions of the observer who then adduces such counterfeits as confirmation of the diagnosis to which he or she is already committed. This is the antithesis of good medical practice.

Clinicians must appraise each of their observations in the light of their knowledge of normal variations and then decide whether a given finding is abnormal. There is little point in saying that a patient's optic discs look pale; the observer must decide whether the discs are abnormally pale or not. The statement that tendon reflexes are brisk says little more than that they are present and enables no useful inferences to be drawn. A decision that tendon reflexes are pathologically brisk implies a lesion of the upper motor neurone. It is legitimate sometimes to say that one does not know whether a finding is beyond normal limits but in such instances the indeterminate findings should not be given undue weight when evaluating the sites of lesions. Throughout the neurological examination, there is a need for the constant exercise of judgement regarding the significance of signs.

THE HISTORY

Taking a history from a patient with neurological disease follows those principles outlined in Chapter 1. Many neurological symptoms are both frightening and mysterious to the patient who will often find them difficult to describe and may use words which are inappropriate and even misleading. For example, most physicians equate a complaint of 'numbness' with a disturbance of sensation, whereas many patients use this term to describe weakness; therefore in an individual case the precise meaning of this complaint must be determined. The nature of an altered sensation is hard to communicate to a listener who has not experienced it. Terms like 'pins and needles' are generally understood only because everyone has occasionally felt them. More complex sensory disturbances lead to profound difficulties of description, particularly if the patient is relatively inarticulate. The physician should allow patients time to elaborate their descriptions, encouraging them to try alternative phrases until they find one which they think most apt. It is often better in these circumstances to record the patient's actual words rather than to translate them into potentially misleading jargon.

Some words are thought by laymen to have a precise meaning. Thus pain is considered by many to be self-explanatory and indeed patients may be confused and even resentful if asked to elaborate on the nature of their pain. It is sometimes helpful to offer several adjectives such as 'stabbing', 'throbbing', 'pressing', 'burning', giving each word similar emphasis and then asking the patient to choose one which most closely fits. The distribution of the pain, its time relationships and precipitants should also be delineated (p. 30). Dizziness is a term in common usage but of varying implication. It will sometimes describe a hallucination of movement which we call vertigo, but it is also used for such varying conditions as syncope, hypoglycaemia, epilepsy and episodes of anxiety. It is thus of little diagnostic value to record that a patient suffers from dizziness without considerable amplification. Likewise complaints of 'blackouts' or 'fits' need to be critically assessed (p. 37).

In contrast, double vision is a phenomenon easily understood by both patients and doctors. However this complaint becomes much more informative if the directions of displacement of the two images, the direction of gaze in which they are maximally separated, and the variation, if any, of the diplopia are established (p. 245). Each symptom must therefore be carefully analysed in order that the maximum amount of diagnostic information can be gathered; this can sometimes be a time consuming process needing patience on the part of the physician and of the patient.

The object of taking a neurological history should be to plot in the mind's eye the course of the patient's illness in terms of its severity and time relationships; the process of interpretation by the clinician should be applied while doing so in terms of the possible physiological and anatomical implications of previous or present symptoms. Thus the process of eliciting a history is an active one, in the course of which hypotheses are formulated, and not merely the passive narrative of an illness.

Physical examination will often enable lesions of the nervous system to be localised with precision, but the nature of the pathology of the lesion can be intelligently surmised only in the light of the development of the illness. In general, lesions which suddenly affect the nervous system, cause maximal disability within a few hours and after a static period of days or weeks then show a tendency to improve, are due to vascular disturbances. Lesions of insidious onset and slow but inexorable progression are often due to degenerative disorders or to tumours of the central nervous system. A remittent history, wherein episodes of disability are followed by periods of marked improvement and well being, with later recurrence of symptoms elsewhere in the nervous system, suggests a diagnosis of multiple sclerosis.

INTERROGATION. After evaluation and recording of the patient's history, specific questions should routinely be asked about headache, fits, visual difficulties, weakness, tingling or numbness of the limbs and disturbances of micturition or defaecation.

THE PHYSICAL EXAMINATION

The technique and the order of the physical examination is highly variable. An individual clinician's method is as characteristic as that person's golf swing. Many neurologists begin at the head and work down to the feet. In this way the examination of the central nervous system can be interspersed with that of other systems. Though the order in which the examination is carried out may be varied, the findings should be recorded in a systematic way (p. 454).

GENERAL OBSERVATIONS

Whilst a patient is giving the history, observation should be made of those features which are outlined in Chapter 4. Signs of disease of other systems may be relevant to a patient's neurological disorder. During the course of listening to the history, observation of the patient's face will often suggest the nature of neurological disabilities or may lead to relevant direct questioning of the patient and augmentation or expansion of the history. There may be cranial nerve palsies such as ptosis, squint or facial weakness. The cheeks may show the typical pigmented papules of adenoma sebaceum and hence point to tuberous sclerosis as the cause of epilepsy in a child. Poverty of facial expression observed during the diagnostic interview may be due to depression or to the hypokinesis of parkinsonism. Facial grimacing may point to a diagnosis of chorea. A facial weakness which develops during the course of the patient's history may be a direct diagnostic pointer to myasthenia gravis. The pouting lips and transverse smile of myopathic weakness may indicate the presence of one of the primary diseases of muscle.

During this period of observation an estimate will be made of the patient's intellectual and speech function as well as of mood and personality. The detailed examination of specific nerve functions should be preceded by assessment of the patient's intellectual function, speech and gait.

INTELLECTUAL FUNCTION

Usually the coherence and circumstantial detail volunteered by the patient during the history will indicate whether intellectual function is within normal limits and in many cases a formal clinical assessment is unnecessary. However when the patient's narrative or conduct, or evidence from relatives suggests that there may be intellectual deterioration, an assessment should be made as described in the examination of the mental state (p. 22). Attention should therefore be paid to the patient's orientation, memory, attention and concentration, fund of general information and powers of abstraction. The examiner's approach must be flexible and tailored to the patient's previous level of intellectual function and educational background, as a patient whose professional achievements were high may still be functioning competently even when there has been some deterioration in capability. A mathematician, although demented, may still possess a facility for calculation which is greater than the examiner's. In contrast, a man whose inherent intellectual gifts were poor should not be expected to perform as well during testing as his more talented fellow.

SPEECH

In the assessment of speech it is first necessary to determine whether the patient suffers from a defect of language or of speech production. Impairment of language functions is manifest by inappropriate usage of words or by a disturbance of the appreciation of the symbolic value of words. This may occur as part of a generalised intellectual disturbance; incoherence of thought processes is mirrored in incoherence of speech (p. 22). Such a defect should be perceived when taking the history and the associated widespread intellectual defect would become more apparent during the testing of general intellectual function. Specific difficulty with language function is called dysphasia. It may be that words are used appropriately but that speech production is impaired either because of a defect in articulation (dysarthria) or because of alteration in the quality or reduction of volume of speech (dysphonia). A total inability to fulfil these functions is denoted by the prefix 'a' — (Gr. *a* = without) hence aphasia, anarthria and aphonia respectively.

Dysphasia

This specific language difficulty results from a lesion affecting the speech area in the dominant hemisphere. The examination of speech function should therefore be preceded by an assessment of the likely side of the dominant hemisphere. When a patient is right handed, the decision is usually easy. In the vast majority of right-handed people language function is represented in the left hemisphere. Occasional exceptions to the rule occur in those people who claim to be right handed because they have been trained in early childhood preferentially to use the right hand though their natural inclinations are left handed. This will usually become apparent on questioning the patient. However, the situation is more complicated in those who preferentially use the left hand, in at least half of whom language functions are served by the left hemisphere. The remaining half comprise genetically determined left handers and the right hemisphere is concerned with language. Patients are asked which hand they use for writing, though this perhaps is one of the more misleading indices of hand preference since many left-handed people, particularly those now of middle age, were forced to write with the right hand at school. One needs to know which hand the patient uses for cutting bread; which hand would be used to catch a ball; and which foot would normally be used for kicking a ball. Since hand preference, in most instances, is congruous with the side of the dominant eye, one should ask the patient which eye would be used for sighting a rifle. One may ask a patient to look through a rolled-up newspaper as if it were a telescope. This will almost always be put to the dominant eye. This eye dominance test is invalidated if there be a marked discrepancy of visual acuity in the two eyes. In many clinical circumstances, these problems of dominance are largely irrelevant. If the patient has a dysphasic defect accompanied by a right hemiplegia, it is clear that the left hemisphere is affected and that it is dominant for speech. Sometimes, however, it may be a matter of importance to determine which is the hemisphere concerned with speech if surgical removal of part of a hemisphere is contemplated.

Those areas which are principally concerned with speech function are shown in Figure 8.1 and include the inferior frontal, superior temporal, and inferior parietal regions of the dominant hemisphere. The simplest clinical classification divides dysphasia into motor (expressive) and sensory (receptive) categories. In *motor or expressive dysphasia* internal speech is preserved intact and patients comprehend language satisfactorily. They know what they wish to say but are unable to say it, in the absence of any affection of the peripheral speech apparatus. This type of disturbance arises from discrete lesions in the inferior part of the frontal lobe.

Sensory or Receptive Dysphasia. This is the term used when comprehension of speech is impaired. It is always accompanied by derangement of the patient's own

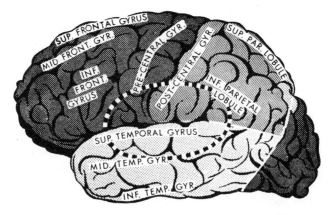

Fig. 8.1   The cerebrum. The dotted line indicates the approximate extent of the 'speech area' in the dominant hemisphere.

use of language since the learned conventions of verbal symbolism and syntax are disturbed. Sensory dysphasia arises from lesions in the temporal and temporo-parietal areas.

Global Dysphasia. Very commonly in clinical circumstances there is a combination of both motor and sensory dysphasic difficulties which is referred to as global or central dysphasia.

Examination of Language Function. This should include careful attention to the patient's speech when giving the history and responding to questions during the course of examination. Inappropriate usage of words, the use of nonsense words or the formulation of sentences in which the word order is unconventional betray an underlying defect of language function. It should be remembered during the appraisal of dysphasia that very well known or automatic speech is often surprisingly well preserved in the presence of severe dysphasia. Patients may be able to count fairly well, may be able to say 'yes' and 'no' quickly and confidently and they may be able to swear with fluency.

Comprehension of spoken speech should be tested by asking patients to carry out commands. The level of difficulty of these commands can gradually be raised. One may start by asking the patient to close the eyes or raise an arm and go on to make the command more difficult by asking the patient consecutively to touch the nose with the left thumb and thereafter to bow the head. Patients are commonly thought to suffer from a purely motor dysphasia when in fact they have a global dysphasia. The responses to these simple commands will often reveal that in addition to impaired production of speech there is impaired comprehension thereof.

During the assessment of language function the ability to speak and to comprehend the spoken language is supplemented by tests of the patient's ability to read. Impaired ability to read (*dyslexia*) often results from a lesion in the dominant parietal lobe. This may be associated with an inability to write (*dysgraphia*) which may result from lesions of the frontal or parietal lobes.

Dysarthria

Speech may be normal in its use of language but may still be difficult to comprehend because of defective articulation (dysarthria). The impaired intelligibility produced by dysarthria is largely due to the imprecise enunciation of consonants. In the English language vowel sounds, though important, vary markedly in duration and character in different dialects. Speech may remain intelligible despite quite marked alterations in vowel sounds but becomes very difficult to understand if consonants are imperfectly formed. The production of clearly defined consonants requires precise, co-ordinated movements of the lips, tongue and palate. Before seeking the origin of dysarthria in terms of neural dysfunction the mechanical integrity of all these structures should be established. Ill-fitting false teeth commonly cause slurring of consonants; a cleft palate will give rise to a nasal speech quality similar to that produced by a palatal palsy.

It is sometimes possible to define which of the executive speech organs is primarily affected. A rapidly vibrating tongue is required to produce the rolled 'R' and impairment of tongue movements cause a lisp due to imperfect pronunciation of 'R'. The enunciation of 'P', 'B' and 'M' demands finely co-ordinated movements of the lips.

Dysarthric difficulties vary in severity from complete inability to articulate (*anarthria*) to very minor slurring of consonants. In the latter case attention to the patient's spontaneous speech may leave the examiner in doubt as to whether dysarthria is present. The patient should then be asked to repeat such well known tongue-twisters as 'Royal Irish Constabulary', 'The Leith police dismisseth us', 'Red leather, yellow leather' to emphasise the problem. Slurring of speech, even when of minor degree, is easily recognised by lay, as well as professional observers. The patient is often unaware of the dysarthria even when the speech is badly affected.

Having established the presence of dysarthria the clinician must then determine the site of the neural lesions which may underlie it. This requires the same sort of analysis of motor function as outlined on page 276. Dysarthria may occasionally arise from intrinsic weakness of the articulating muscles due to myopathy; it may occur as a result of lesions at the myoneural junction in myasthenia gravis where characteristically the dysarthria becomes more marked as the patient continues to speak. Diffuse lesions of the lower brain stem leading to bulbar palsy and bilateral upper motor neurone lesions causing supranuclear bulbar palsy give rise to dysarthria. In parkinsonism, impairment of voluntary movements may affect speech as it does other motor functions. Cerebellar defects may cause a distinctive type of dysarthria in which the slurring of consonants is accompanied by a staccato, interrupted cadence of speech referred to as 'scanning' dysarthria.

Dysphonia

Normal speech not only involves the articulation of learned language but also requires a method of sound production or phonation. Phonation depends on an adequate flow of air passing from the lungs through the glottis, causing vibration of the vocal cords. Impairment of phonation (dysphonia) may result from disordered function of the vocal cords or from respiratory dysfunction leading to inadequate expiratory air flow. Lesions of both vocal cords and respiratory musculature may be combined. Dysphonia is characterised by an alteration in quality (often a hoarseness) of the voice or by a loss of voice volume or both features may be evident.

Dysphonia is the result of neurological disease in only a minority of cases; other more common causes are described on page 59. Dysphonia may rarely result from primary diseases of muscles or may be due to myasthenia gravis when it tends to be variable. More often it results from damage to neural structures, such as bilateral lesions of the vagus nerve in bulbar palsy or bilateral upper motor neurone lesions above the level of origin of the vagus nerves causing supranuclear bulbar palsy. Dysphonia may be a manifestation of impaired movements in parkinsonism wherein speech tends to be low in volume and monotonous.

Miscellaneous Disorders of Speech

Though most speech disorders will fit into the broad categories outlined above, the examination should also include a detailed analysis of the rhythm and cadence of speech.

Stammering or Stuttering. This comprises an abrupt halt to the flow of speech together with repetitive utterance of sounds or syllables or of the initial consonants of words. This disorder usually arises in childhood and is more common in boys. It is not associated with organic neurological disease but can be mimicked occasionally by patients with expressive dysphasia and sometimes the delayed initiation of speech seen in parkinsonism may superficially resemble a stammer.

Bradilalia. Undue slowness of speech occurs in some patients with depression, parkinsonism or myxoedema. It should be emphasised that the rate of verbal utterance varies greatly from individual to individual and only profound slowness of speech should be regarded as of pathological significance. Likewise a rapid delivery of speech is a manifestation of temperament rather than of any organic disease. It may be particularly noticeable in some patients with hypomania.

Echolalia. Echolalia is a term used to describe the automatic repetition by the patient of the examiner's utterances. This imitative repetition is a normal stage of development of language in childhood. When it occurs in adults, it is usually a manifestation of widespread cortical disease.

Palilalia. This rare disorder of speech differs from echolalia in that patients here repeat the terminal parts of their own utterances. Either the last sentence, the last phrase, or even the last word may be reiterated again and again, often at an increasing rate. It is best exemplified, rather flippantly, in 'My father was a gramophone maker but it hasn't affected me, affected me, affected me'. The disorders of neural function which produce this speech phenomenon are ill understood. It tends to occur in widespread cerebrovascular disease but is also found in patients suffering from post-encephalitic parkinsonism.

Summary of Assessment of Speech

Spontaneous speech should be listened to attentively and, if necessary, language or articulatory function should be tested. The appraisal of speech defects should first determine the type of disturbance, whether it be due to dysphasia, dysarthria or dysphonia or to one of the miscellaneous disorders discussed above. It should also be emphasised that these categories are not exclusive. Some patients may exhibit several types of speech disturbance concurrently. Patients suffering from diffuse cerebrovascular disease may exhibit generalised intellectual deterioration as well as dysphasia and may also be dysarthric. Patients with parkinsonism are frequently dysphonic, often dysarthric and they may show the features of bradylalia or palilalia.

Having assessed the type of speech disturbance, the clinician should then determine the level in the central nervous system at which a lesion might cause such a disorder.

GAIT

Inspection of a patient's gait is an integral part of the neurological examination and should never be omitted if the patient is fit enough to walk. It is appropriately considered during the general examination of the nervous system rather than under a specific heading such as the motor system, since normal walking depends also on intact proprioception and normally functioning higher centres such as the cerebellum and the extrapyramidal system. A careful examination of gait will often lead to an accurate deduction of the nature of a patient's neurological deficit.

A patient with a hemiparesis will often exhibit a characteristic gait. The affected leg is stiff and swings forward and outward in a circular fashion rather than being lifted from the ground. Paraparetic patients, i.e. patients with upper motor neurone lesions of both legs, show a slow, stiff movement of each leg in turn with the feet remaining in contact with the ground.

Foot drop due to a lower motor neurone lesion will often be detected as readily by the ear as by the eye, for patients so affected tend to lift the foot high to clear the toes from the ground and, as it is returned, there is often a loud slapping noise. Unilateral foot drop may be due to compression of the common peroneal nerve or to a prolapsed intervertebral disc. Bilateral foot drop may be due to a generalised polyneuropathy and can cause a high-stepping gait affecting both legs; a similar gait is produced by loss of postural sensation in the feet in tabes dorsalis. Instability of a knee joint, or wasting and weakness of the muscles around the knee joint leading to hypotonia, may cause the patient to fling the leg forward in a flail-like manner when walking. Such lesions may be seen in patients suffering from the after-effects of poliomyelitis. A waddling gait like that seen in congenital dislocation of the hips (p. 321) also results from a weakness of the gluteal muscles in primary diseases of muscles (myopathies); it is occasionally also seen in lesions of anterior horn cells.

A patient who walks unsteadily on a wide base or in a drunken, reeling manner may have a disease of the cerebellar hemispheres. Lesions confined to one posterior lobe of the cerebellum cause the patient to stagger or drift towards the affected side when trying to walk in a straight line, or this may become apparent as the patient turns. Lesions at the lower end of the vermis are uncommon and cause a jerky rocking of the trunk from side to side, akin to a tightrope walker. Various combinations of gait disturbances may occur, a common example being unsteadiness due to a cerebellar lesion combined with spastic stiffness of the legs in multiple sclerosis.

A patient suffering from parkinsonism will usually exhibit a slow shuffling gait, each step being smaller than normal. One of the earlier signs of this disease is an absence of arm swinging on walking. Some patients with parkinsonism tend to take increasingly rapid, small steps forward in an attempt to maintain an upright posture. This type of gait is called festinant. Some patients with encephalitis lethargica or post-encephalitic parkinsonism show odd interruptions of their forward progression; they may halt, spin round on their axis and then continue forward.

Bizarre gaits may be due to hysteria (p. 28) and walking may be disturbed by diseases of the locomotor system (p. 319).

THE EXAMINATION OF THE CRANIAL NERVES

After general inspection of the patient and assessment of intellectual function, speech and gait, the clinician should proceed to examine the cranial nerves. The junior student may find the understanding of this section is facilitated by reading first about the examination of the motor system, the sensory functions and the reflexes.

Cranial nerves should be examined individually and systematically in consecutive order. Some carry special afferent fibres like the distance receptors of the optic, olfactory and auditory nerves. Others are concerned with exteroceptive sensation (pain, temperature and touch) and proprioceptive sensation (muscle and joint sense and deep pressure). Some cranial nerves contain efferent fibres to voluntary muscles and resemble spinal nerves in this regard. Others also contain visceral efferent fibres which, being part of the autonomic system, innervate smooth muscle and regulate glandular secretion. In order to test cranial nerves effectively a knowledge of their functions and their anatomy as well as their connections with higher levels of the central nervous system is essential. These features will be outlined for each cranial nerve, the tests of function described and then an interpretation given of the findings.

THE OLFACTORY (FIRST CRANIAL) NERVE

The olfactory nerve subserves the sense of smell. Its receptors are situated high in the nasal cavity from whence thin filaments pass centrally, through the cribriform plate, where they are extremely vulnerable to injury, to the olfactory bulbs. Second order neurones arise here, run through the olfactory tract and divide into the medial and lateral olfactory striae. Some of the medial group cross to the opposite side; the remainder pass to the medial surface of the cerebral hemisphere. The lateral striae pass to the temporal lobe. The sense of smell is essential for the appreciation of flavours and hence a patient whose sense of smell is impaired may complain of a loss of taste.

Testing the Sense of Smell

Loss of sense of smell is much more commonly due to nasal disease than to neurological causes and hence before examining the sense of smell the patient should be questioned about nasal disorders such as hay fever, sinusitis and catarrh and the nasal passageways should be inspected.

The sense of smell should be tested separately in each nostril, the other being occluded by finger pressure. The patient, with the eyes closed, is asked to sniff test substances through each nostril in turn and to name the odours. Irritating, pungent substances should be avoided since these stimulate the trigeminal nerve rather than the olfactory nerve. Ammonia, vinegar and menthol are, therefore, inappropriate. Easily recognised substances such as coffee, cocoa, oil of almonds or vanilla are suitable. If bottles of these are not available, an orange, toothpaste or soap from the patient's bedside locker will serve.

Interpretation

Loss of the sense of smell (anosmia), if due to a neurological lesion, is most commonly the result of trauma. Head injuries, even of minor degree, accelerate the brain differentially from the skull. The thin olfactory filaments are thus subjected to shearing strain and are readily torn. Less common causes of anosmia are lesions within the anterior cranial fossa. Tumours in this area may arise from the frontal lobe or in the olfactory groove itself and usually involve the optic as well as the olfactory nerve. Tumours arising near to the pituitary gland may cause bilateral anosmia at an early stage. Chronic basal meningitis of tuberculous, syphilitic or neoplastic origin may also involve the olfactory pathways.

Increased olfactory acuity is rarely due to organic disease though it is occasionally a feature of the premonitory phase of migraine. Perversion of smell (parosmia) is nearly always of psychological origin though it occasionally occurs from the ingestion of certain drugs such as phenytoin.

Olfactory hallucinations, usually of an unpleasant nature, are characteristic of fits arising in the uncinate gyrus of the temporal lobe and then are often accompanied by smacking gustatory movements of the lips.

Disturbances of function of the first cranial nerve are uncommon, but the sense of smell should be meticulously examined whenever a patient's history suggests a lesion in the anterior cranial fossa.

THE OPTIC (SECOND CRANIAL) NERVE

The basic anatomy of the visual pathways is shown in Figure 8.2. The examination consists of inspecting the optic nerve head and fundus by opthalmoscopy as described in Chapter 11, and the testing of visual acuity and the visual fields.

Inspection of the Optic Nerve Head

Alteration in the colour of the disc may be very important. There is a wide normal colour variation and there will be a small group of patients in whom the colour changes will not be extreme enough to enable diagnoses to be made with certainty. Pathological pallor when present indicates *optic atrophy.* Pallor is due to gliosis in the optic nerve head together with an associated loss of some small blood vessels. There is confusion in the terminology which is applied to optic atrophy. Primary optic atrophy is a term generally used to describe a pathologically pale disc with well defined margins. Secondary optic atrophy usually refers to a pathologically pale disc with irregular or blurred margins. Some people, however, subdivide this latter group into 'secondary' and 'consecutive' categories. Consecutive optic atrophy is then the label given to pale discs of irregular outline associated with disease of the retina or choroid; secondary optic atrophy is applied to these changes when they are the sequel to a period of raised intracranial pressure. Unfortunately these two terms are used in directly contrary ways by other authorities, one man's 'secondary' is another's 'consecutive' and vice versa. It is best to describe the disc's appearance and then deduce from the history or other features the likely nature of any antecedent condition. There is usually some loss of visual acuity associated with optic atrophy. This is not necessarily of severe degree. When there is marked loss in visual acuity due to optic atrophy, this is reflected in an impaired direct pupillary response to light on the affected side (p. 248).

A heightened pink colouration of the disc (often referred to as hyperaemia) makes the disc less easily distinguished from the surrounding retina and hence is accompanied by difficulty in defining the edges of the disc. Hyperaemia of the disc is a sign of swelling of the optic nerve head and will usually be attended by obliteration of the optic cup, congestion of the veins and, if the changes be of recent, acute occurrence, by haemorrhages radiating out from the disc. Swelling of the optic nerve head may be a manifestation of raised intracranial pressure when it is called *papilloedema* (Plate III); it may arise from an intrinsic lesion of the optic nerve when it is known as *papillitis*. The ophthalmoscopic appearances of these two conditions are indistinguishable. They are differentiated by associated changes in visual acuity and in the visual fields. Papilloedema of recent onset usually produces little or no change in visual acuity, but the visual field of the affected eye will reveal enlargement of the blind spot. With more profound and prolonged papilloedema there is often concentric constriction of the whole visual field. On the other hand papillitis due to intrinsic lesions of the optic nerve, such as a retrobulbar neuritis, is attended by severe diminution in visual acuity; if the visual fields can be delineated, a central gap (scotoma) will be demonstrated.

Examination of Visual Acuity

Visual acuity should be measured for both near and distant vision. The latter should be estimated by the ability of the patient, with each eye in turn, to read standard Snellen types at a distance of six metres. The results are recorded as 6/6, 6/18, etc., the latter meaning that at 6 m, the patient can just read what should be read at 18 m. Near vision is tested by using standard reading charts such as the Jaeger card. Each of the patient's eyes is covered in turn and spectacles can be worn if required. Patients should be asked, with each eye, to read the smallest print possible. The result is recorded by noting the chart number of the passage read.

Examination of Visual Fields

During examination of the second cranial nerve it is customary to assess visual function throughout the visual pathways from the retina to the occipital cortex. The defects in the visual fields resulting from lesions of the visual pathways are shown in Figure 8.2. At the bedside it is possible to obtain a rough assessment of the visual fields by the technique of *confrontation* (Fig. 8.3). This is based on a direct comparison of the patient's visual field with the examiner's, presumed normal, field. The patient sits upright and directly faces the examiner whose eyes should be about 1 metre away from the patient. The patient is then instructed to close or cover one eye and to look directly into the opposite eye of the examiner. Thereby the patient's left visual field will correspond to the examiner's right visual field. The examiner, throughout the test, monitors the fixation of the patient's gaze since if the patient looks away from the examiner's eye the test is invalidated. The clinician then proceeds to test the outer limits by bringing a target into the field of vision from the periphery at several points on the circumference. The direction of approach should be distributed over upper and lower quadrants and nasal and temporal aspects of the visual fields. The test object should be moved on a plane mid-way between the patient and the examiner. A finger is a satisfactory target but a more accurate assessment may be made by using a pin with a large head (e.g. a hat

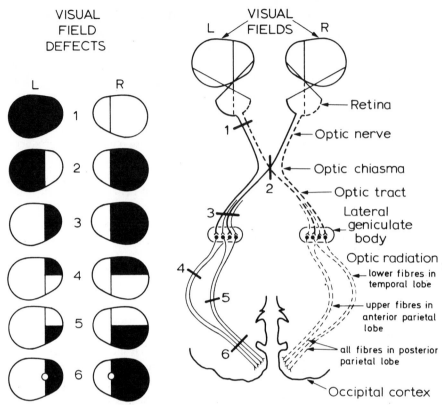

Fig. 8.2   Visual field defects. (1) Total loss of vision in one eye due to a lesion of the optic nerve. (2) Bitemporal hemianopia due to compression of the optic chiasma. The upper quadrants are usually first affected. (3) Right homonymous hemianopia from a lesion of the optic tract. (4) Upper right quadrantic hemianopia from a lesion of the lower fibres of the optic radiation in the temporal lobe. (5) Less commonly a lower quadrantic hemianopia occurs from a lesion of the upper fibres of the optic radiation in the anterior part of the parietal lobe. (6) Right homonymous hemianopia with sparing of the macula from a lesion of the optic radiation in the posterior part of the parietal lobe.

pin). This has the advantage of enabling an estimate to be made of the extent of the visual fields to different coloured objects by using pins with white, red and green heads. The visual fields for coloured objects are concentric with, but smaller than, those for white objects. When using a pin the distraction caused by movement of the examiner's hand is minimised if the pin is stuck into the end of a pencil. A pin can also be used to plot gaps in the central areas of the fields (scotomas). While temporal defects can be detected, the method does not define the full extent of the lateral aspects of the normal visual fields.

If the patient is unable to cooperate by fixing on the examiner's eye, other techniques may be used roughly to map out hemianopic or quadrantic field defects. The patient may be asked to look at the examiner's nose with both eyes open. The examiner then stretches out both arms and moves the fingers asking the patient to point to the moving hand. When the patient, as the result of disturbed consciousness or because of a dysphasic defect is unable to cooperate at all, it is possible to demonstrate gross defects in the visual fields by rapidly moving one hand towards the patient's face from the side. This menacing stimulus will usually

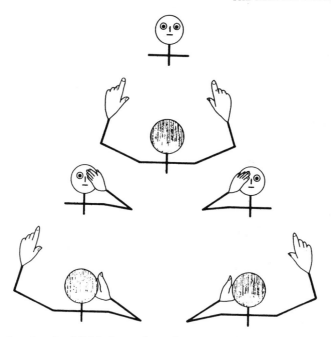

Fig. 8.3   Testing the visual fields by confrontation.

evoke reflex blinking when it is perceived from a normal visual field but the patient will not blink when menaced from a hemianopic side.

A patient suffering from a lesion in a parietal lobe may see the test object perfectly well when presented in isolation in each visual half field but will consistently fail to perceive an object in one half of his visual field when stimuli are presented simultaneously and bilaterally. This is called an inattention hemianopia.

In most cases confrontation will map out visual defects with sufficient precision for clinical purposes but, when minor defects are present or when the shape of the visual defect is important in localisation, the visual fields should be mapped out more accurately by using a tangent (Bjerrum) screen and a perimeter.

THE OCULOMOTOR, TROCHLEAR AND ABDUCENT (THIRD, FOURTH AND SIXTH CRANIAL) NERVES

During the close inspection of the eyes and their movements which examination of the third, fourth and sixth cranial nerves requires there should be concurrent observation of local abnormalities of the eye (pp. 72–75). The examination of the functions of these three nerves requires a fairly detailed knowledge of the anatomy and physiology of the nerves and of the muscles they supply. There are interconnections between the nuclei of the three nerves and pathways to them from higher centres of control. As with every other motor activity the clinical examination is designed to establish the sites of lesions. Some basic considerations are an essential preliminary to an understanding of the techniques employed in the examination and the interpretation of signs.

Ocular Muscles. The principal voluntary muscle of the upper eyelid is the levator palpebrae superioris. Fibres of the orbicularis oculi and involuntary (tarsal) muscles are also found in the network of muscle fibres in the eyelids.

The involuntary muscle fibres in the iris subserve two functions. Concentric fibres form the sphincter pupillae which constricts the pupil; radial fibres within the iris dilate the pupil. The ciliary muscle, when contracted, causes an increase in convexity of the lens.

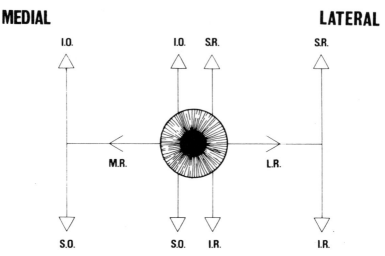

Fig. 8.4   Testing of ocular movements. Medial and lateral rectus (MR and LR) move the eyes medially and laterally respectively. With the eyes in the mid position inferior oblique (IO) and superior rectus (SR) elevate the eye and superior oblique (SO) and inferior rectus (IR) depress the eye. When the eye is turned medially inferior oblique moves the eye upwards and superior oblique moves it downwards. When the eye is turned laterally superior rectus elevates the eye and inferior rectus depresses it.

Six external ocular muscles supply and move the eye-ball. Whenever movement of the eye occurs there is participation to a greater or lesser extent of all the external ocular muscles but individual muscles are particularly responsible for individual movements of the eyes and a knowledge of these is important in testing eye movements. It can be seen from Figure 8.4 that the lateral rectus is almost solely responsible for turning the eye outwards (abduction) and the medial rectus for adduction of the eye-ball. When the eye lies in the mid position the movement of the eye in the vertical plane is a function of four muscles. The inferior oblique and superior rectus are responsible for upward movement, the superior oblique and inferior rectus for downward movement. Upward and downward movements of the eyes in the mid position do not separate the actions of these muscles. The actions of the four muscles are easily elucidated if Figure 8.5 is studied. Here it can be seen from the planes of action of the oblique muscles that when the eye is adducted the superior oblique is a pure depressor of the eye and the inferior oblique is almost solely responsible for elevation of the eye. When the eye is turned outwards, or abducted, the superior rectus bears the main responsibility for upward movement and the inferior rectus for downward movement.

Nerve Supply. The *oculomotor* or *third cranial nerve* originates in a series of nuclei in the mid-brain whence fibres run anteriorly in close relationship to the red

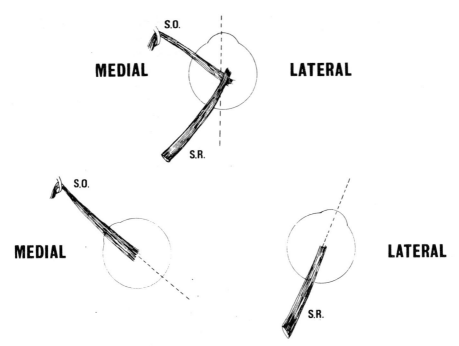

Fig. 8.5   Testing of ocular movements. To show the actions of the superior oblique (SO) and superior rectus (SR) muscles. The dotted line represents the optical axis. It will be seen that when the eye is turned medially, superior oblique is a depressor of the eye. When the eye is turned laterally superior rectus elevates the eye. The actions of inferior oblique and inferior rectus are similar.

nucleus, the substantia nigra and the pyramidal pathways in the cerebral peduncle (Fig. 8.34, p. 307). After leaving the mid-brain the third nerve enters the cavernous sinus on its lateral wall, there lying lateral to the internal carotid artery. It then enters the orbit through the superior orbital fissure and separates into branches which supply the levator palpebrae superioris, the superior, medial and inferior recti and the inferior oblique muscles.

The *trochlear* or *fourth cranial nerve* arises from its nucleus anterior to the aqueduct of Sylvius in the mid-brain just below the third nerve nuclei. The fourth nerve passes posteriorly and is the only cranial nerve which leaves the brain stem on its posterior aspect. It too passes through the cavernous sinus, lying immediately below the third nerve and enters the orbit through the superior orbital fissure. It supplies only the superior oblique muscle.

The *abducent* or *sixth cranial nerve* arises in the lower pons anterior to the fourth ventricle (Fig. 8.35, p. 307). The fibres of the seventh cranial nerve loop around the abducent nucleus. The sixth nerve fibres leave the brain stem at the junction between pons and medulla and then run a very long intracranial course. As it passes forward and laterally the nerve lies over the petrous part of the temporal bone. It then pierces the dura near the dorsum sellae to enter the cavernous sinus, passing along the lateral aspect of the sinus to enter the orbit through the superior orbital fissures and supply the lateral rectus muscle.

Parasympathetic fibres take origin from cells within the nuclear complex of the third nerve. Preganglionic fibres pass with the fibres of the third nerve. Most run to the ciliary ganglion whence postganglionic fibres arise to supply the ciliary muscle and sphincter of the pupil. A smaller number of parasympathetic fibres bypass the ciliary ganglion to end in episcleral ganglia. It is thought that these latter fibres are responsible for the reaction of accommodation.

Sympathetic fibres arise in centres in the hypothalamus and run through the midbrain, pons, medulla and cervical cord and emerge through the ventral roots of the first two or three segments of the thoracic spinal cord. These fibres then ascend through the sympathetic chain to the superior cervical ganglion. From here postganglionic fibres arise and ascend in the carotid plexus and enter the orbit with the ophthalmic artery to terminate on the radial (dilator) muscle of the iris. Sympathetic fibres also supply the tarsal muscles and the orbital muscle, the latter tending to hold the eye forward in the orbit.

Internuclear Connections. The medial longitudinal bundle coordinates the activity of the motor nerves to the eye. It connects the nuclei of the three ocular nerves to each other and to other nuclear masses, particularly the vestibular nuclei. A diagram of this system is shown in Figure 8.6. Near to the sixth nerve nucleus in the pons is a centre, the parabducens nucleus, which co-ordinates conjugate lateral movements of the eyes. Fibres from this centre run to the sixth nerve nucleus on the same side. Other fibres cross the mid line and run in the medial longitudinal bundle to that part of the contralateral third nerve nucleus which supplies the medial rectus. This provides a mechanism which ensures that the optical axes remain parallel when the eyes are turned conjugately to the side.

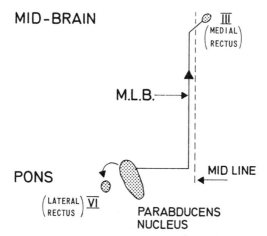

Fig. 8.6   Co-ordination of lateral gaze. Fibres from the parabducens nucleus run to the immediately adjacent sixth nerve nucleus. Other fibres run in the medial longitudinal bundle (MLB) to that part of the third nerve nucleus on the opposite side which activates the medial rectus. Thus the lateral movements of the abducting eye and medial movements of the adducting eye can be synchronised.

Supranuclear Connections. There lies in the cortex of the frontal lobe at the posterior end of the second frontal convolution an area which when stimulated causes conjugate deviation of the eyes away from the stimulated side. Fibres from this area probably run through the anterior part of the internal capsule, through the basal ganglia to terminate in the pontine centres co-ordinating lateral gaze. Damage to these frontal centres, paralysing or weakening their function leads to an inability to turn the eyes away from the side of the lesion.

There are also centres in the occipital cortex concerned with conjugate eye movements but these are much less well defined than are those in the frontal area and their clinical role is not clear.

Examination

Inspection. The examination should be prefaced by a detailed inspection of the eyes commencing with the *eyelids*. The size of the palpebral fissures and any asymmetry between the two should be noted. Minor degrees of asymmetry often are seen in normal people. Drooping of one or other eyelid should be observed and any variation in the degree of the ptosis should be noted; it may be accompanied by compensatory overactivity of the frontalis muscle. Conversely any widening of the palpebral fissures should be observed. Involuntary movements of the eyelid, particularly spasms which also usually involve the orbicularis oculi, may be seen. The rate of blinking should be estimated. The patient should be asked fully to open and forcibly to close the eyes.

The *pupils* should be inspected. Pupils normally are round, regular in outline and equal in size. The size of the pupils varies with the amount of ambient lighting but is usually between 3 and 5 mm in diameter. Pupils which are less than 3 mm in diameter in average conditions of illumination are called meiotic and dilatation of the pupils above 5 mm is referred to as mydriasis. The size of the pupils on the two sides should be compared.

Pupillary Reflexes. If a light is shone on the retina, the pupil on the same side, as well as that on the opposite side, constricts. The reaction of the pupil on the side stimulated is called the *direct light reflex* and the constriction of the other pupil is the *consensual light reflex*. The speed and extent of constriction should be assessed in each eye separately, shielding the other from the light while doing so in order to test both direct and consensual reflexes. The light should approach from the side in order to avoid an accommodation response. Occasionally an initial constriction is followed rapidly by alternating dilatation and constriction. This is called hippus and is a normal variation.

The *reaction of accommodation* refers to the constriction of the pupils which accompanies convergence of the eyes when the patient looks at a near object. The patient should be asked to relax accommodation by gazing into the distance at, say the ceiling and then asked to shift the gaze to fix on the observer's finger, held near the patient's nose. Alternatively the patient may be asked to keep the gaze fixed on the clinician's finger which at first is held several feet away and is then brought nearer and nearer to the patient's face. The significance of abnormal pupillary reflexes is discussed on page 248.

Ocular Movements. During inspection of the eyes the direction of any deviation of the optical axes of the eyes from parallel should be noted. The patient should be asked to move the eyes upwards, downwards, medially and laterally and then also to look upwards and laterally, upwards and medially, downwards and medially, and downwards and laterally. The patient should first perform these movements on request and then be asked to follow with the eyes a target held by the examiner who moves it in the directions listed. The patient should first make conjugate movements with both eyes open. In some instances each eye should then separately be tested, the other being covered by the examiner's hand. Patients should be asked specifically whether they see double when the eyes are deviated into the positions outlined above. If double vision is present, they should be asked in what direction of gaze the objects seem to be most widely separated. In the position of maximal separation of the images the more peripheral of the two images is the false image and is attributable to the eye whose movement is impaired. By covering the eyes alternately and asking the patient to say when the outer image disappears it is possible to establish which eye is at fault. The weakened muscle is that which normally moves the affected eye in the direction in which maximal double vision occurs. These principles are illustrated in Figure 8.7. If diplopia has been present for more than a few months it may be difficult to obtain clear cut answers about the direction of gaze in which maximal separation of images occurs because the patient has learned to suppress the false image. Occasionally double vision is absent despite obvious ocular paresis; this is particularly common when *strabismus* (squint) has been present for many years. The differentiation of paralytic squint from the non-paralytic (concomitant) squint, common in children, is described on page 396.

Nystagmus. Whilst ocular movements are being tested the presence of nystagmus, i.e. involuntary oscillations of the eyes, should be observed. Nystagmus is described as 'pendular' when the oscillations about a central point are equal in rate and amplitude like the swing of a pendulum. Nystagmus is said to be 'jerking' when there are quick and slow phases of unequal duration. The quicker phase is arbitrarily used to define the direction of nystagmus. If one talks of 'nystagmus to the right' one is referring not to the direction of gaze in which nystagmus occurs but to the direction of the quick phase. Jerking nystagmus may be graded. If nystagmus is present only on lateral deviation of the eyes it is of first degree. Nystagmus which is present on looking straight ahead as well as on looking to one side is of second degree. Third degree nystagmus is present if it occurs when the patient looks in the direction opposite to that of the fast phase.

Note should be made of the directions of gaze which evoke nystagmus, whether nystagmus occurs on vertical movement or on lateral movement, whether it is equal in amplitude and rate in all directions of gaze, or whether rate and amplitude vary with direction of eye movements. Nystagmus usually comprises a to and fro oscillating movement but sometimes there is a rotary component; the eyes turn around their axes. This too should be noted. When attempting to elicit nystagmus the finger or target, which the patient's eyes are following, should be held at least two feet away from the patient. Normal people may occasionally exhibit jerking movements of the eyes at the extremes of gaze and particularly so when the test object is held close to the subject's eyes.

Interpretation

Ptosis. This may be due to a lesion of the levator palpebrae muscle itself, of its neuromuscular junction, of the third nerve or of the cervical sympathetic pathways. Damage to the sympathetic supply rarely causes more than slight drooping of the

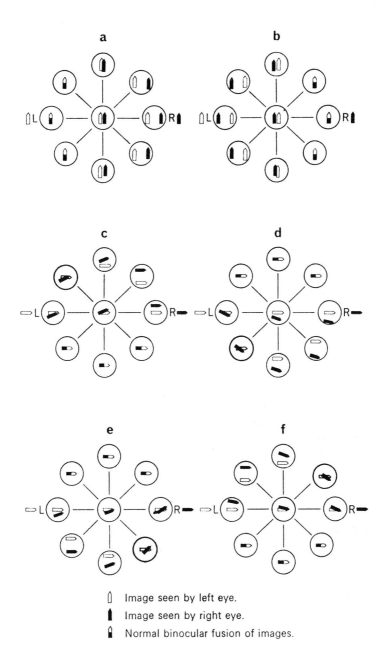

⬭ Image seen by left eye.

❚ Image seen by right eye.

❚ Normal binocular fusion of images.

Fig. 8.7 Diplopia. The diagram shows the direction of diplopia, from the patient's viewpoint, in paralysis of the individual external ocular muscles of the *right* eye. The muscles involved are: (a) lateral rectus; (b) medial rectus; (c) superior rectus; (d) inferior rectus; (e) superior oblique; (f) inferior oblique.

eyelid and sympathetic involvement can easily be differentiated from weakness of the levator palpebrae superioris by asking the patient to elevate the eye voluntarily. If the levator muscle is weak the patient will be unable to elevate the lid completely, but will be able to do so if the cervical sympathetic is involved since this results only in weakness of the superior tarsal muscle.

Ptosis may accompany some myopathies and is commonly present, often bilaterally but unequal and usually variable in myasthenia gravis (Fig. 10.3). If this condition is suspected and there is little spontaneous variation during the period of observation it may be helpful to ask the patient to look at an object held above the head whilst holding the head still. This causes continued elevation of the eyelids and after a period the ptosis will become more marked in patients with myasthenic weakness.

When ptosis is an accompaniment of a third nerve palsy there will usually also be dilatation of the pupil and a pattern of defective ocular movements attributable to a third nerve lesion (p. 249).

Widening of the palpebral fissure or fissures may occur because of lid retraction in thyrotoxicosis. Unilateral widening may indicate a paresis of the orbicularis oculi on that side caused by a seventh nerve lesion.

Spasmodic closure of the lids is often a psychogenic phenomenon but may occasionally occur in parkinsonism. In the latter condition blinking is infrequent.

Constriction of the Pupils. This may be due either to paralysis of the sympathetic system or to stimulation of the parasympathetic system. Some drugs such as neostigmine, by inhibiting the action of cholinesterase, cause constriction of the pupil. Constriction of a pupil may be due to a lesion of the cervical sympathetic when it will usually be accompanied by a degree of ptosis and with enophthalmos and impaired sweating on the same side, comprising *Horner's syndrome* (Fig. 10.3). A reduction in pupillary size is a normal manifestation of ageing sometimes called senile meiosis.

Dilatation of the Pupils. This is often a manifestation of anxiety. It can also result from stimulation of the sympathetic system or paralysis of parasympathetic nerves. Drugs such as atropine and homatropine paralyse cholinergic nerves and therefore give rise to mydriasis whilst amphetamine and similar drugs dilate the pupil by sympathetic stimulation. Enlargement of the pupil may result from blindness due to damage to the optic nerve.

Abnormal Pupillary Reflexes. Impairment or absence of the pupillary reaction to light may be due to interruption of afferent or efferent sides of the reflex arc. Since both pupils constrict in response to light shone into one eye afferent lesions can easily be distinguished from damage to efferent pathways. If a pupil constricts when light is shone into the opposite eye, (i.e. the consensual light reflex is preserved), the motor pathway for constriction to that eye is intact and the damage must lie on the sensory side of the reflex arc. Lesions of the optic nerve such as acute retrobulbar neuritis, damage the afferent side of the arc. In such cases there will be no direct light reaction but the consensual light reaction will be observed. This is the '*amblyopic light reaction*'. The afferent side of the reflex arc is impaired also in the *Argyll Robertson pupil* where the affected pupils tend to be small and characteristically the two pupils are unequal and irregular. Here there is loss of the light reaction but preservation of the reaction to accommodation. A lesion in the pretectal area explains most of the phenomena of the Argyll Robertson pupil (Fig. 8.8). Isolated loss of reaction to accommodation with preservation of the light reflex is uncommon but may occasionally occur in some cases of brain stem encephalitis involving parasympathetic fibres (p. 244). Loss of reaction to both light and accommodation may be due to structural damage to the iris itself, occasioned by trauma or by inflammatory lesions, which prevent the pupil from changing size. The motor pathway serving pupillary reflexes may be damaged by a complete third nerve palsy when both reactions to light and to accommodation will be lost.

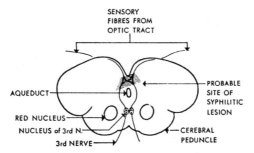

SENSORY FIBRES FROM OPTIC TRACT

AQUEDUCT

PROBABLE SITE OF SYPHILITIC LESION

RED NUCLEUS

NUCLEUS of 3rd N.

3rd NERVE

CEREBRAL PEDUNCLE

Fig. 8.8   The light reflex pathway in the midbrain and the probable site of the lesion in the Argyll Robertson pupil. The pupillary reflex to accommodation involves a different pathway through the lateral geniculate body and the occipital cortex.

A relatively common abnormality of pupillary reflexes, usually seen in adult women, is the *tonic pupillary reaction (Holmes-Adie syndrome)*. In this condition the reaction to light appears absent and the reaction to accommodation is delayed and sustained in a tonic fashion after convergence ceases. In some instances the light reaction is present but is delayed and sustained. This is a benign condition due to a lesion in the ciliary ganglion, but it needs to be differentiated from the Argyll Robertson pupil. Absence of ankle jerks and other tendon reflexes may accompany these tonic pupillary reactions.

Disorders of Ocular Movements. Disordered ocular movements may result from lesions of ocular muscles (myopathies), neuromuscular junctions, ocular nerves and their nuclei, or from interruption of internuclear and supranuclear connections. Analysis of the defects in ocular movements will help to decide whether they fit a pattern of muscular or neural involvement, and if neural, which nerves are implicated. *Myopathies* tend in the early stages to affect all the muscles equally and partially, presenting a generalised restriction of eye movements. Ptosis accompanies this general impairment in the rare condition of ocular myopathy and a similar picture may be manifest in myotonic dystrophy.

Myasthenia gravis usually effects ocular muscles variably. Characteristically the ocular paresis associated with myasthenia gravis is associated with ptosis but there are no pupillary abnormalities.

Lesions of the third cranial nerve, if complete, cause ptosis, weakness of superior, medial and inferior recti and inferior oblique muscles, as well as pupillary dilatation and absent pupillary reflexes. Third nerve lesions may be incomplete and the pupillary reflex abnormalities and ptosis may be absent. Bilateral third nerve palsies are usually incomplete and most commonly arise from lesions within the mid-brain where the two third nerve nuclei lie very close together (anterior internuclear ophthalmoplegia, Fig. 8.34 p. 307). A lesion of one third nerve in the mid-brain will often be associated with upper motor neurone signs on the side opposite the lesion (Fig. 8.34). Third nerve damage within the cavernous sinus is almost always accompanied by lesions of the fourth and sixth nerves and impaired sensation over the distribution of the ophthalmic division of the fifth nerve (p. 351).

Lesions of the fourth cranial nerve are rare in isolation but affection of the superior oblique muscle commonly results from trauma to the orbit causing dislocation of the trochlea through which the tendon of the superior oblique muscle runs. The fourth nerve may be involved, together with the third and sixth nerves in diffuse lesions of the brain stem such as multiple sclerosis and acute vitamin B_1 deficiency (Wernicke's encephalopathy). The fourth nerve is also involved together with the third and sixth nerves in lesions within the cavernous sinus.

Lesions of the Sixth Cranial Nerve. Paralysis of the lateral rectus may be due to a lesion affecting the muscle itself, its neuromuscular junction or the sixth nerve, the last being a common accompaniment of raised intracranial pressure whatever the cause. In such instances the sixth nerve palsy constitutes a false localising sign. If the sixth nerve is involved in the brain stem it is usually associated with a seventh nerve palsy on the same side and upper motor neurone signs on the other.

Internuclear Disturbances. A lesion of the medial longitudinal bundle (Fig. 8.6) anywhere along its course between the pons and mid-brain will obviously cause a weakness of adduction on attempted lateral conjugate gaze and this is the characteristic clinical phenomenon of internuclear ophthalmoplegia. Such lesions may be unilateral or bilateral. If the medial longitudinal bundle is damaged in the mid-brain, impaired convergence will accompany the defect of lateral conjugate gaze (anterior internuclear ophthalmoplegia, Fig. 8.34 p. 307). When a lesion lies in the lower part of this tract, in the pons, fibres to the adjacent sixth nerve may also be interrupted so there will be defective abduction as well as restricted adduction on lateral deviation. The weakness of abduction may be reflected by nystagmus in the abducting eye (posterior internuclear ophthalmoplegia, Fig. 8.34). This type of nystagmus confined to, or more marked in the abducting eye on attempted lateral gaze, is known as ataxic nystagmus and denotes a pontine lesion.

Supranuclear Disturbances. Irritative lesions of the frontal lobe, such as occur when an epileptic discharge arises there, cause conjugate deviation of the eyes away from the side of the lesion. An infarct in this area may not only cause hemiplegia but in the early stages also function as an irritative lesion. Thus, immediately after a stroke it may be observed that the patient's head and eyes are turned towards the paralysed limbs. Later there is often a paralysis of function and the patient will find difficulty in conjugate deviation of the eyes towards the paralysed side.

Nystagmus. A full discussion of the nature and significance of nystagmus can be found in *Davidson's Principles and Practice of Medicine* (p. 314). Nystagmus may be caused by visual disturbances, by lesions of the labyrinth or of the central vestibular connections or by brain stem or cerebellar lesions. Pendular nystagmus is usually due to a loss of macular vision but is occasionally seen in diffuse brain stem lesions. Jerking nystagmus which is of constant direction regardless of the direction of gaze suggests a labyrinthine lesion or a cerebellar disturbance. Nystagmus which changes direction with the direction of gaze suggests a widespread central involvement of the vestibular nuclei. Jerking nystagmus absent with the eyes in the mid position but which develops only on lateral gaze and whose fast component is in the direction of gaze indicates a lesion of the brain stem or cerebellum. Nystagmus which is confined to one eye suggests a peripheral lesion of the nerve or muscle responsible for movement in the appropriate direction or it may be due to a lesion of the medial longitudinal bundle. Nystagmus which is restricted to the abducting eye on lateral gaze, ataxic nystagmus, is due to a lesion of the medial longitudinal bundle between the pons and mid-brain as in multiple sclerosis. Nystagmus which occurs on upward gaze, with the fast component upwards, (upbeat nystagmus) may be due to a lesion in the mid brain at the level of the superior colliculi. Downbeat nystagmus (fast phase downwards) suggests a lesion in the lower part of the medulla.

THE TRIGEMINAL (FIFTH CRANIAL) NERVE

The trigeminal nerve carries both motor and sensory fibres. The motor nucleus is situated near the floor of the fourth ventricle in the lateral part of the pons from whence the motor root emerges near to the sensory root and passes below the trigeminal (Gasserian) ganglion to leave the skull through the foramen ovale. After joining the mandibular division of the sensory nerve it supplies the muscles concerned with mastication, the masseters, temporals and pterygoids. The masseters elevate the jaw as, to a lesser extent, does the temporal muscle. The pterygoid muscles depress and protrude the jaw when acting together and when one acts alone it causes the jaw to move laterally away from the side of the contracting muscle.

The sensory part of the trigeminal nerve carries exteroceptive sensation from the face, the anterior part of the head and inside the mouth via:

1. *The ophthalmic division* which supplies the skin of the forehead, the root of the nose and the scalp as far back as a line joining the ears. It also supplies the cornea, conjunctiva and the intraocular structures as well as the mucosae of the frontal, sphenoidal and ethmoidal sinuses and of the upper part of the nasal cavity. It lies on the lateral wall of the cavernous sinus as it passes from the orbit to join the trigeminal ganglion.

2. *The maxillary division* supplies the skin of the nose, cheek and upper lip, the mucosae of the maxillary sinus, posterior part of the nasal septum and the lower part of the nasal cavity. The upper teeth and gums, the hard and soft palate receive sensory fibres from this division.

3. *The mandibular division* supplies the skin of most of the jaw, other than its angle, the mucosae of the cheek, jaw, floor of the mouth and the tongue. It also supplies the lower teeth and gums.

The cells of origin of the sensory part of the nerve lie in the trigeminal ganglion. *Tactile impulses* conveyed in the central processes of these cells pass into the substance of the pons to terminate in the principal sensory nucleus of the fifth nerve. After synapsing here fibres carrying tactile sensation proceed to the thalamus in the ascending tracts of the fifth nerve which lies near the medial lemniscus. *Impulses concerned with pain, temperature and some concerned with tactile sensation* terminate in the nucleus of the spinal tract which extends downwards from the principal sensory nucleus, through the pons and medulla into the spinal cord where it reaches the third cervical segment. Here nerve fibres from different parts of the face are grouped in the following manner. The area around the mouth is supplied by fibres which synapse with second order neurones lying in the highest part of the spinal tract. Concentric areas spreading outwards from the mouth are supplied by fibres which synapse at progressively lower levels in the spinal tract. The outermost segment of the face is represented by fibres which descend to the lowest part of the tract. These arrangements give rise to the so called 'onion-skin' distribution of facial sensory representation (Fig. 8.9). The fibres arising from the neurones in the spinal tract, cross to the opposite side and pass upwards to the thalamus and thence with those from the body, to the sensory cortex.

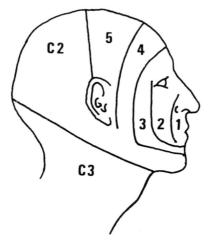

Fig. 8.9   Pain fibres to the head. Areas marked 1 to 5 indicate the central distribution within the spinal tract of the fifth cranial nerve. 1 is represented in the pons, 2 the pontomedullary region, 3 the lower medulla, 4 and 5 the upper cérvical cord. The areas labelled C.2 and C.3 derive from the spinal segments directly.

Examination

Sensory Functions. Light touch and pain sensation is tested in the territory of the three sensory divisions using cotton wool and pin prick respectively. Temperature sense can also be tested. The methods of examination conform to those for sensory testing in general (p. 280). The two sides of the forehead, of the cheeks, and of the jaw should be compared.

Sensory deficits occasionally may involve the periphery of the face whilst sparing the central area, or the converse may occur. In addition to testing sensation in the major divisions some comparison should be made between the sensation in the 'snout' area around the nose and mouth, and sensitivity at the periphery of the cheek.

Motor Functions. This starts with inspection of the muscles of mastication. Muscle wasting may be revealed by a flattening of the face above and below the zygoma. In some instances fasciculation may be seen in the masseters and temporal muscles. If there is bilateral weakness of the muscles of mastication the jaw will hang loosely open.

The patient should be asked to open and close the jaw against resistance. As the patient clenches the teeth hard the masseters should be palpated and an estimate made of their bulk and symmetry. When the patient opens the jaw against resistance, if there is unilateral weakness of the pterygoids, the jaw will deviate towards the weakened muscle. If weakness of the pterygoid muscles is suspected patients should be asked to move the jaw laterally against resistance; it may then be found that the jaw can be moved towards the affected muscle but cannot deviate it towards the normal side. Facial asymmetry, resulting from a seventh nerve palsy, may give rise to a misapprehension that the jaw is deviated.

Reflexes. The *corneal reflex* comprises a brisk contraction of the orbicularis oculi evoked by touching the cornea. The afferent part of the reflex arc is the first division of the trigeminal nerve; the motor limb lies in the facial nerve. Each fifth nerve communicates with both seventh nerves and therefore both eyes close when each cornea is stimulated.

The corneal reflex is elicited by touching the cornea, not the conjunctiva, with a wisp of cotton wool. The cornea is extremely sensitive and is vulnerable to injury, so that the touch must be light. The wool should approach the eye from the side, as an object jabbed at the patient from directly in front will elicit a reflex closure of the eyes which is a response to menace and is not dependent on fifth nerve stimulation. The patient should be asked whether the stimulus to the cornea is felt equally on the two sides and the contraction on both sides should be observed. This will enable lesions of the fifth cranial nerve to be differentiated from damage to the efferent pathway of the reflex. If there is a seventh nerve palsy on the side stimulated there will be no direct response of the orbicularis oculi on that side but the patient will feel the touch on the cornea and there will be a brisk closure of the other eye. The briskness of the direct response on each side should be compared. Impairment of the corneal reflex may be`the earliest sign of a lesion affecting the ophthalmic division of the trigeminal nerve and may be observable before cutaneous sensation is demonstrably impaired.

The *jaw jerk* is analogous to the tendon reflexes in the limbs. The afferent and

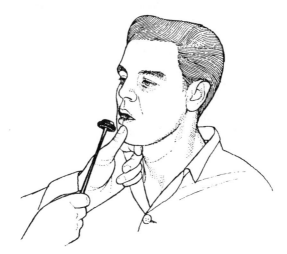

Fig. 8.10   Eliciting the jaw jerk.

efferent pathways are subserved by the fifth cranial nerve. The effective stimulus is a brisk downward stretch of the masseter muscles which is best evoked by placing the thumb or forefinger over the tip of the patient's mandible and then tapping the examiner's finger downwards with a tendon hammer (Fig. 8.10). This manoeuvre should be performed with the patient's jaw hanging open. The reflex response comprises a brisk closure of the jaw. Measured by electrophysiological methods the jaw jerk is always present. It is usually not visible in young people but is commonly seen above the age of 50; the decision as to whether a jaw jerk is merely present or is pathologically exaggerated is sometimes difficult.

Interpretation

Peripheral Lesions. Trigeminal neuralgia gives rise to no signs. If sensory changes are present, it is likely that there is a structural lesion of the fifth nerve. Multiple sclerosis in young people, or tumours invading the fifth nerve may give rise to episodic trigeminal pain which mimics trigeminal neuralgia. Much commoner than pains caused by neural lesions are those which arise from the structures supplied by the fifth nerve such as dental abscesses or caries, inflammation of the sinuses and abnormalities of the temporomandibular joints.

Herpes zoster (p. 73) often affects the ophthalmic division of the fifth cranial nerve and in elderly people is liable to cause persistent burning pain in the distribution of the nerve. Post-herpetic neuralgia is usually accompanied by scars and by slight impairment of sensation over the forehead in the distribution of the affected ophthalmic division.

Peripheral divisions of the fifth cranial nerve may be damaged by trauma, or may be involved in neoplastic processes at the base of the skull. Tumours arising in the nasopharynx may erode the base of the skull and cause pain and diminished sensation in one or more divisions of the fifth cranial nerve.

Central Lesions. When the fifth cranial nerve is affected more proximally in its course, it is often associated with other cranial nerve signs which indicate the site of the lesion. The first division of the trigeminal nerve may be implicated in lesions within the cavernous sinus, in company with the third, fourth and sixth nerves. Tumours lying in the cerebello-pontine angle often impinge on the trigeminal sensory nerve root, giving rise to paraesthesiae and numbness affecting almost all the face of the appropriate side. Lesions here are frequently associated with deafness, cerebellar signs and seventh nerve signs and the combination suggests the site of the affection.

Motor lesions of the trigeminal nerve are much less common. Bilateral involvement of the masticatory muscles may occur as part of a bulbar palsy in motor neurone disease, when wasting and fasciculation may be observed. In bilateral lesions of the upper motor neurones above the level of the pons the jaw jerk is markedly exaggerated.

THE FACIAL (SEVENTH CRANIAL) NERVE

The facial nerve consist of two parts. The larger motor component supplies all the muscles of facial expression. The smaller part (nervus intermedius) comprises sensory and parasympathetic constituents which carry taste fibres from the anterior two thirds of the tongue and visceral efferent fibres to the lacrimal, submaxillary and sublingual glands. There are a few somatic sensory fibres which carry cutaneous sensation from a small area of the external ear.

The motor nucleus of the facial nerve is found in the pons medial to the descending nucleus of the fifth nerve. Efferent fibres loop round the nucleus of the sixth cranial nerve before leaving the pons on its lateral aspect (Fig. 8.35 p. 307). It is there joined by the nervus intermedius in the cerebello-pontine angle near the sixth and eighth nerves. Motor fibres and the nervus intermedius then enter the facial canal. The afferent fibres of the nervus intermedius have their cells of origin in the geniculate ganglion and terminate in the upper medulla. From the geniculate ganglion secretory fibres pass via the petrosal nerves to the lacrimal glands. The facial nerve then runs through the facial canal, gives off two branches and leaves the skull at the stylomastoid foramen. The first branch is the nerve which supplies the stapedius muscle, which limits the movement of the ear drum and ossicles in response to high tone noise. The more distal branch is the chorda tympani (Fig. 8.11) which joins the lingual nerve (a branch of the mandibular nerve) and carries taste fibres from the anterior two-thirds of the tongue as well as parasympathetic fibres to the submandibular and sublingual salivary glands.

After leaving the stylomastoid foramen the facial nerve passes anteriorly through the substance of the parotid gland and is then distributed via a number of branches to all the musculature of the face. Among the more important muscles of facial expression are the frontalis which raises the eyebrows, the orbicularis oculi which causes closure of the eyes and the corrugator which draws the eyebrows downwards to produce a frown. The nares may be constricted or dilated by muscles supplied by

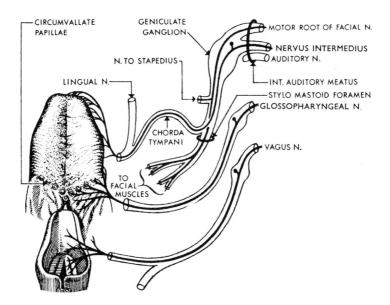

Fig. 8.11   To show (1) taste pathways from the tongue in the facial and glossopharyngeal nerves, (2) the essential components of the facial nerve as it passes through the skull and (3) the vagus nerve and the larynx.

the seventh nerve. The orbicularis oris closes and purses the mouth whose angles are raised by the levator anguli oris. The platysma draws down the lower lip and depresses the chin.

Examination

Motor Functions. This is the most important part of the assessment of the seventh cranial nerve and should be preceded by careful inspection of the face. Any involuntary movements should be noted. These may take the form of tics or habit spasms (p. 269) which are stereotyped but may comprise very complex movements in certain individuals. In elderly patients spasms may affect one side of the facial musculature.

Alteration of facial expression during conversation may be indicative of emotionally charged topics. Furthermore, emotional expression may be preserved while voluntary movement is impaired. Signs of facial palsy may be obvious on inspection; there may be a widened palpebral fissure on the affected side; there may be absence of wrinkling on one side of the face causing drooping of the corner of the mouth with dribbling of saliva and flattening of the nasolabial fold. The two sides of the face should be compared. Bilateral weakness of the facial muscles may be manifest in pouting of the lips and a transverse smile. Movements of the upper part of the face should be compared with activity in the lower face.

Voluntary contractions of facial muscles should be examined. The patient should be asked to frown, raise the eyebrows, wrinkle the forehead and to close the eyes as strongly as possible. The examiner should attempt to open the eyes when the patient is forcibly closing them. The patient should be asked to show the teeth but should not be asked to smile since in most patients this request evokes an emotional response (p. 257). The patient should be required to blow out the cheeks, to purse the mouth and to whistle.

Sensory Functions. The exteroceptive sensation supplied by the seventh nerve is unimportant and cannot effectively be tested since the small area of the auditory canal supplied by sensory fibres from the seventh cranial nerve also receives an overlapping supply from the fifth and ninth cranial nerves and the upper cervical nerves. The sensory examination should include testing of taste over the anterior two thirds of the tongue. The primary tastes, sweet, salt, bitter and sour, should be tested using sugar or saccharin, salt, quinine and vinegar respectively. When testing taste the tongue should be protruded, the examiner holding it gently with a swab. The test substances are placed on each side in turn and the patient, whose eyes should be closed, is asked to identify the tastes. The patient should be instructed not speak, since when the tongue is retracted into the mouth to speak, saliva flows over the tongue carrying taste to both sides, and to the posterior third, of the tongue. The patient should, therefore, be required to open the eyes and point to the apposite word sweet, salt, sour or bitter, written on a card.

Secretory Functions. These are usually not tested formally. If lacrimation is excessive, it will be observed during the taking of the history; it is often due to obstruction of a tear duct. The patient will complain if there is increase or decrease of salivation.

Reflexes. The *glabella or nasopalpebral* reflex is elicited by percussion with the finger over the root of the nose. It is important that the tap is light and that the patient is not visually menaced by a direct stab of the fingers from in front. The reflex response to a tap over the glabella is a brisk bilateral closure of the eyes. In most normal people repeated percussion evokes three or four contractions and then the response ceases.

Tapping the upper lip or stroking it with the edge of a wooden tongue depressor normally produces no visible response but may, in bilateral upper motor neurone lesions, give rise to puckering and protrusion of the lips. This response is called the *snout reflex.*

Interpretation

Impaired facial movements may be due to disturbance of supranuclear motor pathways which influence the activity of the facial nerves, to affections of the seventh cranial nerve itself or to lesions within the facial muscles. The first stage of interpretation involves the assessment and differentiation of lesions at these various levels.

The paucity of spontaneous facial movements and of pliant emotional expressiveness in *parkinsonism* may at first suggest bilateral weakness of the facial musculature. But the parkinsonian patient will exhibit no weakness when performing voluntary facial movements on request. A sustained glabellar reflex may help to support the diagnosis of parkinsonism, but it alone is insufficient evidence on which to base a diagnosis. Some anxious, normal people continue blinking as long as the tapping is repeated and in some patients with parkinsonism the sustained response is absent.

Upper Motor Neurone. *Unilateral lesions* (above the level of the pons) characteristically weaken movements of the lower part of the face more than those of the upper face. This discrepant affection is due to innervation of the upper facial structures from both hemispheres whilst lower facial movements are represented largely in the contralateral motor cortex. This pattern of weakness is the rule in upper motor neurone lesions but there are occasional exceptions. A patient who has recently and suddenly sustained a hemiplegia may initially suffer from paresis equally affecting both upper and lower face.

Patients with *bilateral upper motor neurone lesions* may exhibit an obvious snout reflex. Such patients may also show a lability of emotional expression. Their faces sadden and they weep without adequate cause and conversely they brighten and laugh in inappropriate circumstances. In patients with upper motor neurone lesions a dissociation between emotional and voluntary movements may be observed, for example some patients with a marked lower facial weakness may yet move the paralysed side normally when they smile. The reason for this dissociation is not known but presumably there are alternative pathways subserving emotional movement.

Lower Motor Neurone. The facial nerves may be affected anywhere along their pathways from the pons to peripheral branches to give a lower motor neurone palsy.

Unilateral affection of a seventh nerve is a common clinical presentation, most frequently arising without known cause in the condition called *Bell's palsy.* It is often possible to localise the site of damage in the nerve with some precision. Interruption of the facial nerve after its emergence from the stylomastoid foramen may be due to trauma or to lesions of the parotid gland. Characteristically these distal lesions involve only some of the muscles of facial expression on the appropriate side. Involvement of the facial nerve proximal to its exit from the facial canal causes a paresis of all the muscles on the corresponding side of the face. Facial asymmetry will be apparent on inspection. Widening of the palpebral fissure and flattening of the facial groove are quickly recognised. It should be emphasised however, that where a facial palsy has been present for some time the muscles undergo shortening and contracture and in such instances the nasolabial fold and other facial markings may be more deeply etched than on the normal side. Therefore, when ascertaining the presence of facial nerve palsy the diagnosis should not be made on facial appearance alone but should be confirmed by asking the patient to move the facial muscles.

One of the most diagnostically useful accompaniments of a lower motor neurone facial palsy is an exaggeration of a normal reflex; when the patient attempts to close the eye on the affected side there will be restricted movement of the orbicularis oculi but there is a brisk upward movement of the eyeball, often to such an extent that the pupil becomes completely hidden under the eyelid. This phenomenon occurs only in lesions of the seventh nerve and is not a feature of upper motor neurone facial weakness.

The site of lesions within the facial canal can be assessed by the presence of features other than the facial palsy which is common to all of them and which is the only finding in the most distal affections below the chorda tympani (Fig. 8.11). Lesions above the chorda tympani are accompanied by loss of taste over the anterior two thirds of the tongue and by diminished salivation. Proximal to the nerve to stapedius, hyperacusis in the ear on the same side is added to the other features; such is the picture presented by lesions of the geniculate ganglion. Affection of the geniculate ganglion is rare and in nearly all cases is due to herpes zoster. Damage to the facial nerve in the most proximal part of the facial canal is uncommon. When it occurs defective lacrimation is added to the manifestations of more distal lesions.

Within the *cerebello-pontine angle* lesions of the motor part of the seventh nerve, together with the sensory and secretory changes due to interruption of the nervus intermedius, are often accompanied by signs of damage to some or all of the eighth, fifth and sixth nerves as well as by cerebellar disturbance. *Pontine lesions* of the seventh nerve affect only its motor component and usually cause a concurrent sixth nerve palsy on the same side together with contralateral upper motor neurone signs (Fig. 8.35 p. 307).

Bilateral facial weakness due to neural lesions is much less common than affection of one seventh nerve. Both motor nuclei may be implicated in motor neurone disease causing a bulbar palsy and a few generalised polyneuropathies may extend to involve both seventh nerves. The immunologically-precipitated, demyelinating polyneuropathy, called the Guillain-Barré syndrome, has a particular predilection for the facial nerves.

Facial Muscles. *Myasthenic lesions* tend to affect facial muscles variably with facial weakness and the attendant dysarthria becoming more apparent as the patient uses the facial muscles and as the day wears on. *Myopathic weakness* of the face is always bilateral and symmetrical; pouting of the lips, a transverse smile, and flattening of the facial creases on both sides present a characteristic picture. In almost all instances muscles other than the facial muscles will also be affected by the myopathic process.

THE VESTIBULOCOCHLEAR (EIGHTH CRANIAL) NERVE

The eighth cranial nerve comprises two components. There are auditory fibres which arise from the cochlea and vestibular fibres which arise from the otolith organs (saccule and utricle) and semicircular canals; the functions of these two elements are distinct so that they need to be considered separately.

The Cochlear (Auditory) Division. Sound waves are normally conducted by air to the ear but they may also be transmitted through bone if a vibrating object is in contact with the skull. Central processes from the cochlea within the inner ear enter the skull through the internal auditory meatus near to the facial nerve, pass through the cerebello-pontine angle to enter the brain stem, eventually to synapse in the cochlear nuclei in the lower pons. Second order fibres ascend in the lateral lemnisci of both sides. There are side connections to cell groups such as the superior olive but most fibres pass to the medial geniculate body. Thence the final sensory relay is conveyed in the auditory radiations to the anterior transverse temporal gyrus which is the auditory receptive area; each receptive area receives impulses from both ears.

The Vestibular Division. The end organs of the vestibular nerves are situated in the semicircular canals and in the utricle and saccule. Fibres are thence carried to the cells of origin in the vestibular ganglia in the internal auditory meatus whose central processes form the vestibular nerve. This passes through the internal auditory meatus in company with the cochlear nerve to enter the upper medulla. The vestibular fibres terminate on the vestibular nuclei whence a new relay of fibres runs to the medial longitudinal bundles of both sides, establishing communications with the third, fourth and sixth nerve nuclei. There is a major connection from the vestibular nuclei to the vermis of the cerebellum. Some fibres pass from the nuclei downwards into the spinal cord to form the vestibulospinal pathway. The vestibular system coordinates the motor reflexes which maintain equilibrium and make the postural adjustments occasioned by movements of the eyes, head and body.

Examination

The Cochlear Component. This should be tested as part of the routine neurological examination. Assessment of the patient's auditory acuity should be preceded by auriscopic examination of the external ear passages and of the drums (p. 75).

Hearing should be tested in each ear in turn by whispering to the patient whose eyes are closed and whose other ear is occluded by finger pressure on the tragus. Normally a whisper can be heard at a distance of three metres. A wristwatch may also be used and rubbing of the forefinger and thumb together beside the patient's ear provides an alternative stimulus.

If there is some impairment of hearing the next step is to determine whether this results from a lesion within the external auditory meatus or middle ear, i.e. conduction deafness, or whether it is due to a defect of the cochlea or its nerve, i.e. perceptive or nerve deafness. Normally air conduction of sound is more efficient than bone conduction, but when there is conduction deafness, the reverse is the case. A *tuning fork* may be used to make the differentiation, (*Rinne's test*). A vibrating fork (256 or 512 cycles per second) is held close to the external auditory meatus. Its base is then pressed against the mastoid bone. The patient is asked which of these two stimuli seems to be the louder.

The tuning fork test of hearing should be supplemented by *Weber's lateralising test;* the vibrating tuning fork is applied to the midline of the forehead and the patient is asked whether the sound is heard in the midline or whether it seems to come from one or other ear. If hearing is normal the sound appears to arise in the midline. If there is damage to the cochlea or its neural connections the sound will be perceived less well on the affected side and will appear to arise on the healthy side. If there is a lesion in the middle ear or blockage of the meatus, the sound sometimes is referred to the affected ear.

These rules are generally applicable but they are not conclusive because some patients with nerve deafness may have better bone conduction than air conduction. Patients with defective hearing should be assessed by *audiometry* which measures the degree of hearing loss at different sound frequencies. Pure tone audiometry combined with speech discrimination audiometry will differentiate neural deafness from conductive deafness.

Vestibular Function. This cannot effectively be evaluated at the bedside, but *positional nystagmus* may be sought. The patient is asked to lie on the back, with the shoulders at the end of the couch (Fig. 8.12). The head, projecting beyond the couch, is supported by the examiner's hands; the head is then fully extended and turned to one side. The patient's eyes should remain open; nystagmus may appear some ten seconds after the head has been positioned and may disappear spontaneously after about a minute. Nystagmus which appears after this manoeuvre and subsides spontaneously indicates a lesion of the otolith organs in the ear which lies inferiorly. Nystagmus which is persistent in this situation usually indicates a lesion affecting the brain stem or cerebellum. After a short interval the test should be repeated with the head extended and rotated to the other side. Nystagmus does not appear in normal people as a result of this manipulation.

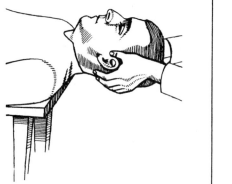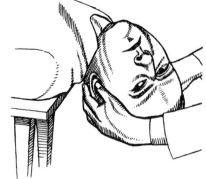

Fig. 8.12 **Testing for positional nystagmus.**

Interpretation

Damage to the cochlear part of the eighth nerve results in diminished hearing and tinnitus. *Tinnitus* is defined as a subjective awareness of noise, such as a hissing sound, in the absence of an external stimulus. The noise may be high pitched or low pitched and often seems to be originating in the affected ear. Lesions of the vestibular pathways give rise to an abnormal sensation of movement — vertigo. In many instances both components of the eighth nerve are affected together, as in Ménière's syndrome characterised by a combination of tinnitus, deafness and vertigo associated with a progressive dilatation and oedema of the cochlea and the vestibular parts of the labyrinth.

Deafness. Conduction deafness most frequently results from blockage of the external meatus by wax or from chronic otitis media. Perceptive deafness most often has its origin in the cochlea in association with advancing years or as a result of damage from measles, from antibiotics such as kanamycin, or from trauma. A blow, blast injury or noise of high intensity may cause deafness which is particularly marked for high frequency sounds.

Vertigo. This may result from a large number of conditions of which the vast majority affect the labyrinth itself or the most peripheral part of the vestibular nerve. In almost all cases these peripheral lesions also involve the cochlea or its nerve; a notable exception to this rule is vestibular neuronitis in which a viral infection causes intense vertigo without deafness or tinnitus.

Vertigo may be due to lesions of the cerebellum and is then usually not associated with auditory loss or with tinnitus. In general, bouts of vertigo, separated by periods of normality, are due to labyrinthine lesions. If paroxysms of vertigo are accompanied by ataxia which persists between the vertiginous episodes the lesion probably lies centrally, in the brain stem or cerebellum. In labyrinthine lesions nystagmus is often prominent only during attacks of vertigo and in general the degree of nystagmus is proportional to the vertiginous disturbance. In central lesions affecting the brain stem or cerebellum there is often persistent nystagmus with relatively slight vertigo.

Peripheral Lesions. Assessment of lesions of the cochlear and vestibular divisions of the eighth nerve in its peripheral path requires specialised knowledge and apparatus and includes audiometry, caloric testing and nystagmography.

Central Lesions. In the cerebello-pontine angle the commonest lesion is a neuroma of the eighth nerve itself causing tinnitus followed by deafness and occasionally vertigo. Neoplasms of the fifth nerve, meningiomas and tumours arising from the cerebellum may also affect structures in the cerebello-pontine angle where space occupying lesions are often accompanied by cerebellar ataxia, facial palsy, or sensory disturbances of the fifth nerve and, later, raised intracranial pressure.

Perceptive deafness on the same side as the lesion may result from damage to the brain stem by such conditions as infarcts of the pons or plaques of multiple sclerosis. In most instances intrinsic lesions of the brain stem will be accompanied by other cranial nerve disturbances as well as by long tract signs.

Since auditory impulses are relayed to both temporal lobes unilateral damage to the auditory receptive area usually produces only very transient impairment of hearing.

THE GLOSSOPHARYNGEAL (NINTH CRANIAL) NERVE

The motor part of this nerve arises in the nucleus ambiguus in the medulla and in company with the tenth and eleventh cranial nerves leaves the skull through the jugular foramen. The ninth nerve supplies the stylopharyngeus muscle which elevates the upper pharynx, in combination with the palatopharyngeal muscle which is supplied by the tenth nerve.

The glossopharyngeal nerve contains a large sensory component which transmits common sensation from part of the lining of the tympanic cavity and the Eustachian tube. It also carries pain fibres from the pharynx and the tonsillar region and general afferent sensation from the posterior third of the tongue, the soft palate and the uvula. These sensory fibres run back through the medulla; those subserving touch terminate in the solitary nucleus in the medulla and pain fibres end in the nuclei of the fifth nerve. The glossopharyngeal nerve conveys taste from the posterior third of the tongue and these fibres terminate in the solitary nucleus. The ninth nerve also transmits impulses from chemoreceptors and baroreceptors in the carotid body and sinus. It conveys parasympathetic fibres to the parotid gland and partially supplies the submaxillary and sublingual salivary glands.

Examination

Sensory Functions. Many of the functions of the glossopharyngeal nerve are intermingled with those of the tenth cranial nerve. One aspect of the ninth nerve function which can be tested in isolation is taste on the posterior third of the tongue but it is difficult to do so in the manner outlined for the seventh cranial nerve (p. 256) as precise placement of test substances on the back of the tongue is hard to accomplish. Taste in this area is most conveniently, though rarely, tested by applying a weak electric current to the back of the tongue. This normally evokes an acid taste if sensation is intact.

The sensory supply to the posterior third of the tongue and the pharynx can be tested by touching these areas with the point of a long pin or a wooden stick. The procedure is unpleasant and should be performed only when it is important to define ninth function exactly.

Reflexes. Touching the posterior wall of the pharynx evokes its constriction and elevation. This is the *'gag' reflex* whose afferent arm is the glossopharyngeal nerve and whose efferent path is the vagus nerve. It may occasionally be absent in normal people. When there is no reflex response to this manoeuvre the patient should be asked if the pharyngeal stimulus is felt, in order to differentiate interruptions of the reflex arc on its afferent side from those affecting the vagal efferent limb. A reflex arc of similar constitution supplies the *palatal reflex*. When the soft palate is touched it moves upwards. When testing these reflexes the stimulus should be applied to each side in turn.

Motor Functions. These cannot be tested satisfactorily since paralysis of the stylopharyngeus muscle is not manifest clinically if tenth nerve function is intact.

Interpretation

Lesions of the ninth nerve are extremely rare in isolation. It may be implicated by lesions at the base of the skull such as fractures or invasive tumours but usually the tenth nerve and some of the lower cranial nerves will be simultaneously involved. Glossopharyngeal neuralgia is the most important condition solely affecting the ninth nerve. This is felt in the back of the throat and resembles trigeminal neuralgia in its lancinating character, in its episodic occurrence and in the absence of any detectable disturbance of ninth nerve function.

THE VAGUS (TENTH CRANIAL) NERVE

The motor part of the vagus nerve originates in the nucleus ambiguus of the medulla which it leaves in a series of rootlets adjacent to the glossopharyngeal nerve. It passes through the jugular foramen to the neck, chest and abdomen, supplying motor fibres to the soft palate, the pharynx and, via its recurrent laryngeal branch, to all the intrinsic muscles of the larynx.

The tenth nerve conveys sensory impulses from the dura mater of the floor of the posterior cranial fossa and from part of the external auditory meatus. These sensory fibres, after they enter the medulla, pass to the fifth nerve nucleus. Tactile impulses from the pharynx are also conveyed in the vagus to the fifth nerve nucleus. The vagus has extensive afferent and efferent connections with the heart, lungs and gut.

Examination

Clinical examination of the tenth cranial nerves includes close attention to the patient's *speech*. Lesions of the vagus nerve or its recurrent laryngeal branch may give rise to dysphonia; interruption of its motor fibres, by paralysing the palate, will give a nasal quality to the voice.

The *soft palate* should be inspected. In bilateral lesions of the tenth nerves the whole soft palate droops; in a unilateral palsy there will be drooping of one side of the soft palate, the uvula being deviated to the normal side. The patient should be asked to sustain phonation by uttering a prolonged 'Ah' and palatal movements should be observed whilst doing so. In bilateral palsies the palate will not elevate and in unilateral lesions one side of the palate remains immobile, and the uvula moves towards the normal side. Movement of the posterior pharyngeal wall should be observed during phonation. If one side is paralysed it tends to move laterally, like a curtain, towards the normal side. The palatal and pharyngeal reflexes should be examined (p. 262).

In the presence of dysphonia or whenever a lesion of the tenth nerve is suspected, the *vocal cords* should be inspected (p. 164).

Interpretation

Unilateral lesions of the tenth cranial nerve occur at the base of the skull as a result of fractures, tumours or chronic basal meningitis, and the adjacent ninth and eleventh nerves are usually also implicated. Isolated lesions of the vagus nerve are uncommon but its *laryngeal branch* may be damaged in the neck by trauma or by malignant tumours. Abductor vocal cord palsy is often the earliest sign of recurrent laryngeal nerve palsy. Later the adductors are also affected and the cord lies in the midway position between abduction and adduction. In a unilateral palsy the voice is usually hoarse but the degree of dysphonia is variable since compensatory movements by the unaffected cord across the midline mitigate the disability. If the palsy is bilateral and partial the cords do not abduct on inspiration so giving rise to inspiratory stridor. When there is complete interruption of both recurrent laryngeal nerves, the cords rest in the cadaveric position and cannot abduct or adduct. Phonation is thus impossible; if asked to cough, the patient cannot build up intrathoracic pressure by closing the cords and thus produces a 'bovine' cough which is a prolonged, low-pitched noise, without the explosive quality of a normal cough. Isolated paralysis of the adductors of the cords is usually bilateral and of hysterical origin. The patient loses voice volume but can talk in a whisper. There is no respiratory disturbance and the cough has its normal explosive quality, indicating that the adductors can in fact function normally.

Bilateral tenth nerve lesions are seen as part of true bulbar palsy and bilateral supranuclear affection of the structures innervated by the tenth nerve contribute to the picture of supranuclear bulbar palsy (p. 266).

THE SPINAL ACCESSORY (ELEVENTH CRANIAL) NERVE

The major part of the eleventh cranial nerve derives from the anterior horn cells of the first to the fourth cervical segments. Fibres leave the lateral aspect of the cord and ascend, uniting as they course upwards with fibres from higher cervical segments. Eventually the spinal part of the nerve enters the skull through the foramen magnum. Within the skull the nerve is joined by its smaller cranial component which arises in the medulla. The two constituents separate as they leave the skull through the jugular foramen. The spinal accessory nerve again descends into the neck where it supplies the sternomastoid and the upper half of the trapezius muscles. The lower half of trapezius obtains its nerve supply directly from the third and fourth cervical segments.

Examination

The eleventh cranial nerve is tested by examining the bulk and power of *the sternomastoid and trapezius muscles*. When testing the former it is useful, in the first instance, to examine both sides together by asking the patient to press the chin downwards against the resistance of the examiner's hand. Both sternomastoids will, in normal circumstances, then stand out and can be inspected and palpated. Differences in bulk can quickly be recognised by this technique. Each sternomastoid should afterwards be tested by asking the patient to turn the chin against resistance to each side; there will be weakness on turning the head away from the side of a muscle whose strength is impaired.

When examining the upper fibres of the trapezius the patient, standing upright, should be inspected from behind. If there is wasting of the upper trapezius a flattening of the muscle on the side affected will be apparent. The vertebral border of the scapula will be displaced away from the spine in its upper part and towards the spine at its lower end. The whole arm droops and hence the finger tips on the involved side reach nearer the ground than do those on the normal side. The power of the trapezius should then be tested by asking the patient to shrug the shoulders against resistance.

Interpretation

Involuntary movements frequently implicate the sternomastoid muscles. Turning movements of the head due to contraction of one sternomastoid may occur as part of the picture of chorea or dystonia. Spasm of the sternomastoid may be a feature of spasmodic torticollis (p. 269) but usually other nearby muscles also are involved in this condition which sometimes is due to disease of the basal ganglia and sometimes is a psychiatric manifestation.

Upper motor neurone lesions produce only slight weakness of the sternomastoid muscles and cause little disability.

Bilateral lower motor neurone affections of the spinal accessory nerves may occur as part of the picture of true bulbar palsy. Marked weakness on the two sides is manifest by the head falling backwards. Bilateral wasting of the sternomastoid muscles is more often due to a myopathy rather than a neural lesion but the former is itself rare. Myasthenia may cause intermittent weakness of both sternomastoids.

Unilateral lower neurone lesions of the eleventh nerve are uncommon and, in isolation, are rare. Lesions of the nerve at the jugular foramen by fractures of the skull, basal meningitis or tumours usually also implicate the ninth, tenth and twelfth nerves. Within the neck, trauma, particularly missile wounds, may damage the nerve.

THE HYPOGLOSSAL (TWELFTH CRANIAL) NERVE

The hypoglossal nerve arises from its nucleus in the medulla which it leaves medial to the ninth, tenth and eleventh nerves. It then passes through the hypoglossal canal into the neck and on via the angle of the mandible to supply all the muscles of the tongue. Each twelfth nerve receives an upper motor neurone supply from the precentral gyri of both cerebral hemispheres.

Examination

Inspection is the most important aspect of the examination of the tongue which should first be scrutinised as it lies on the floor of the widely opened mouth; it should then be protruded and again carefully inspected. Atrophy is usually easily recognised since it causes the tongue to become wrinkled and thinner. Spontaneous contractions (fasciculation) of the muscles may be apparent (p. 268). They persist when the tongue is at rest and may also be seen on its underside. Tremors usually are prominent when the tongue is protruded and are much less evident when the tongue lies relaxed in the mouth.

If there is unilateral weakness of the tongue, it deviates, on protrusion, towards the paralysed side, because of the action of the normal genioglossus. The patient should be asked to move the tongue in and out and from side to side, slowly and rapidly in turn and then should press the tongue against the cheek whilst the examiner's finger resists the movement by pressure on the outside of the cheek. If there is unilateral paresis there will be an impairment of the ability to move the tongue towards the normal side.

Interpretation

Involuntary movements of the tongue may occur. Rapid protrusion and retraction, called a 'trombone' tremor may be seen in parkinsonism and occasionally in general paresis of the insane. Choreiform movements of the tongue may be a feature of Sydenham's or Huntington's chorea. Irregular and continual rotatory movements of the tongue may be induced by drugs, such as levodopa and the phenothiazines.

Bilateral upper motor neurone lesions cause the tongue to assume a more conical form and its voluntary movements are sluggish. Bilateral supranuclear lesions are sometimes due to vascular lesions in both internal capsules and they may also result from the generalised degeneration of motor neurone disease. Such supranuclear lesions invariably affect others of the lower cranial nerves and usually also implicate the fifth nerves. This produces the picture of *supranuclear or pseudobulbar palsy,* where dysarthria, dysphonia and dysphagia are accompanied by a spastic, immobile tongue and an abnormally brisk jaw jerk.

A *lesion of one upper motor neurone* above the medulla causes the protruded tongue to be deviated slightly towards the paralysed side. There is no accompanying weakness or fasciculation nor does the slight weakness produce any significant disability.

Bilateral lower motor neurone lesions are most commonly part of *a true bulbar palsy* and will be found in association with weakness of the other motor cranial nerves. Severe disability with dysarthria, dysphagia and dysphonia results. Bilateral wasting of the tongue accompanied by fasciculation is often observed in motor neurone disease and much less frequently may result from poliomyelitis, from tumours or vascular lesions in the medulla, or from syphilis.

Unilateral lower motor neurone lesions of the twelfth nerve are uncommon but may arise occasionally from vascular disease in the medulla or from lesions at the base of the brain such as chronic syphilitic or tuberculous basal meningitis. Tumours arising in the post-nasal space may erode the skull base and implicate the twelfth nerve. Trauma may also damage the nerve and is particularly liable to do so after its exit from the hypoglossal canal. When the twelfth nerve is unilaterally involved by these processes there are usually attendant lesions of ninth, tenth and eleventh cranial nerves.

SUMMARY OF EXAMINATION OF CRANIAL NERVES

Incomplete examination of the cranial nerves can lead to clinical disaster. It is not necessary, however, routinely to test the sense of smell unless there is a suspicion of a lesion in the anterior cranial fossa.

The testing of taste is difficult and time consuming; it should be performed only if it is important to localise a lesion of the seventh nerve. As indicated on page 00, it is rarely necessary and barely feasible to test taste over the posterior third of the tongue.

Eliciting the gag reflex is unpleasant and need be performed only if the clinical picture, as in bulbar palsy, makes it worthwhile. Though hearing should always be assessed there is no need routinely to look for positional nystagmus (p. 260).

With these exceptions the usual clinical examination of the cranial nerves should follow the outline given on page 456.

THE MOTOR SYSTEM

At the bedside it is convenient to consider motor and sensory functions separately but precise, skilled, willed movements require an intact sensory system as well as a properly functioning motor apparatus. Normal motor activity may be disturbed by:

1. A loss of learned movement patterns. The organised sequences of motor activation which underlie voluntary actions may be impaired in the absence of paralysis. This is called dyspraxia or apraxia.
2. Paralysis or weakness.
3. Impairment of coordination.
4. Changes in tone.
5. Involuntary movements.
6. Hypokinesis.

The examination of the motor system seeks to define which of these defects are present and, in conjunction with other signs such as the patient's gait and changes in reflexes, will enable the examiner to localise lesions of the motor system to the various pathways and levels of the central nervous system. The motor pathways are shown in Figure 8.13. Assessment of motor function includes detailed inspection, and examination of tone, power, coordination and fine movements. In some cases more specialised tests designed to reveal dyspraxia may also be employed.

Inspection

The ability accurately to observe requires more than just seeing. It involves knowledge of likely deviations and awareness of changes derived from previous experience. If the gait and other motor functions are carefully scrutinised by an informed clinician it is often possible, on inspection alone, to diagnose the nature of a patient's disabilities.

Posture. The posture of the patient should be noted. The distinctive hemiplegic picture resulting from intracranial lesions of the pyramidal pathways is the posture of *decorticate rigidity;* the affected arm is flexed and adducted across the chest with the leg on the same side stiffly extended. The features of *decerebrate rigidity* are extension of the neck, back and legs; the arms are internally rotated, adducted and extended except at the wrist where they are flexed. Such a posture immediately suggests the presence of a lesion of the motor pathways in the mid-brain. Flexion at neck, hip, knee and elbow presents a posture characteristic of parkinsonism. A patient suffering from this disease may, when lying, hold the head above the pillow for long periods.

Muscle Wasting. After an overall examination of posture the examiner should inspect the shape and bulk of the patient's musculature. Differences in bulk between corresponding muscle on the two sides of the body are valuable clues to the presence of wasting or atrophy but it is important to remember that in patients who do heavy manual work the dominant arm and hand often show disproportionate muscle hypertrophy. This is illustrated by the marked increase in size of muscles in the racket arms of professional tennis players. The assessment of wasting should include comparisons of the relative affection of proximal and distal parts of limbs.

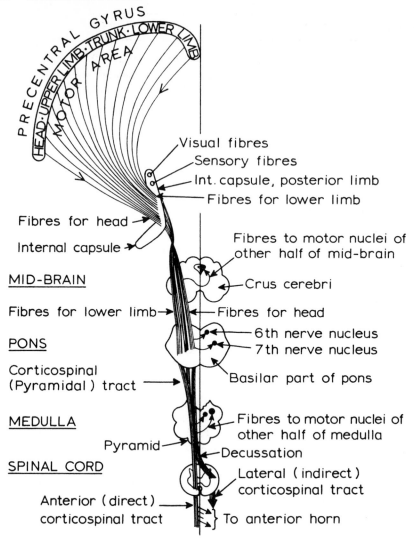

Fig. 8.13 The motor pathways.

In most instances muscle wasting is more easily and more certainly detected by inspection than with a tape measure.

Fasciculation. In wasting muscles it is often possible to see fasciculation. This is produced by the spontaneous contractions of large groups of muscle fibres or of whole motor units. It is usually visible through the skin. The contractions commonly occur sporadically and successively involve different parts of the muscle. The movements are usually of fine amplitude. When seen it suggests a lower motor neurone lesion lying proximally near the anterior horn cells as in progressive muscular atrophy (motor neurone disease). It is not always present when there is denervation.

Sometimes fasciculations are seen in normal people. In such instances the movements are usually rather coarser and tend continually to affect the same area of muscle in the thighs or the thenar eminences after unwonted exercise. A similar phenomenon (myokymia) may cause spasmodic contractions of the orbicularis oculi, levator palpebrae superioris or other facial muscles. This is a benign condition commonly produced by fatigue and anxiety. Benign fasciculation and myokymia are particularly liable to arouse fears in medical students and doctors who may interpret them as having sinister significance. Their distribution, the absence of associated muscle wasting and their usually transient nature point to the absence of an organic lesion.

Voluntary Movements. Inspection will also reveal something of the precision, speed and quality of movements. Clumsy movements of the hands may imply incoordination or dyspraxia. Delay in initiation of movements and reduction in their amplitude once initiated will suggest extrapyramidal hypokinesis. The complete lack of use of one limb or of one side of the body may indicate the presence of a monoplegia or a hemiplegia respectively.

Involuntary Movements. There should be a careful inspection and analysis of any involuntary movements, of which tremors are the commonest.

Tremors are defined as rhythmic movements resulting from alternating contraction and relaxation of groups of muscles. In the limbs, where they are usually seen, tremors produce oscillations about a joint or group of joints. When a tremor is observed its rate and amplitude should be estimated and the directions of movements analysed. The tremor most frequently seen is rapid and fine in amplitude and is an exaggeration of normal physiological tremor. All apparently smooth movements are underlain by a tremor whose rate is 10 per second in adults. In normal circumstances this oscillation can be demonstrated only by utilising some form of amplification. If a large sheet of paper is laid over the out-stretched hand of a healthy subject it will be seen that the edges of the paper are in continuous fine movement. If normal physiological tremor is increased in amplitude it becomes visible to the naked eye. This is the mode of production of the tremor seen so often in anxious patients, in hyperthyroidism, in alcoholics and in those who over-indulge in tea, coffee, tobacco and other drugs. A slow, coarse tremor is a cardinal feature of parkinsonism and characteristically involves a beating of the thumb towards the index finger. In its fully developed form it is of 'pill-rolling' type when the thumb runs across the tips of all the fingers. Parkinsonian tremor may be reduced during a voluntary movement. Intention tremor is described on page 274 and flapping tremor on page 59.

Myoclonus is a term used to describe sudden shock-like contractions which involve one or more muscles or a whole limb. Myoclonic jerks may occur singly or repetitively. They are common in grand mal epilepsy but also are an uncommon manifestation of some widespread degenerative diseases of the brain.

Choreiform movements are irregular, jerky, semi-purposive and ill sustained. These involuntary movements tend to move from one part of the musculature to another in quick succession. This latter observation is important since it distinguishes choreiform movements from the much commoner *tic* or *habit spasm*. Tics are common and their forms vary widely in different individuals. Facial grimaces are frequently encountered. The tic of an individual is a repetitive, stereotyped movement; the same movement, even if complex, is repeated over and over again.

Spasmodic torticollis is a common type of involuntary movement, resembles a tic and usually comprises repetitive, rotatory movements of the head and neck to one side, sometimes accompanied by extension of the neck.

Hemiballismus is similar to choreiform movement but is much greater in amplitude and more forceful. There are violent flail-like, throwing movements of the limbs which, as the name implies, are usually unilateral. These tend to occur acutely as the result of vascular damage to the sub-thalamic nucleus.

Athetoid spasms are slow writhing movements principally affecting the distal parts of limbs. Many extrapyramidal diseases lead to involuntary movements which are both choreiform and athetoid in type.

Dystonic movements (sometimes called *torsion spasms*) are similar to athetoid movements but tend to affect the proximal part of the limb or the trunk so that turning, twisting movements of the trunk or limbs occur.

Palpation

Palpation of muscles is not of primary importance in the examination of the motor system but may sometimes give information of value. Muscles may be tender in inflammatory conditions (myositis). Palpation of the apparently large muscles in the Duchenne type of dystrophy reveals the doughy consistency of fatty infiltration (pseudo-hypertrophy) rather than the elastic feel of normal muscle tissue. Palpation is sometimes useful in confirming minor degrees of wasting suspected on inspection. If the bulk of a fully contracted muscle belly is palpated and compared to its fellow on the opposite side slight differences may be detected.

Examination of Tone

Tone, for clinical purposes, may be defined as the resistance felt when a joint is moved passively. In normal people who are relaxed the manipulation of a joint evokes a slight, elastic resistance from the adjacent muscles. The degree of this tension can be gauged only by repeated examination of normal people.

There are certain essential prerequisites for the accurate assessment of muscle tone. The patient should lie supine with the head and neck resting in the neutral position, comfortably upon a pillow. Time must be spent, if necessary, in achieving the cooperation and relaxation of the patient. The elbow joint and the wrist, hip, knee and ankle should then be put through a full range of passive movements. The knee, for instance, should always be put into a position of full extension before it is flexed. Each of these joints should first be manipulated rapidly and then more slowly. It is a useful preliminary, having got the patient relaxed, to grasp the forearm and shake the upper limb gently. The resulting passive movements at the wrist joints can then be observed. This is a valuable way of checking that the patient is relaxed as well as providing information about the muscle tone around the wrist. A similar manoeuvre can be employed in the legs. The patient's leg, supported on the bed, should be grasped below the knee and the leg gently rocked from side to side. The evoked passive movements of the ankle are observed. Any local lesion such as arthritis should be excluded before ascribing neurological significance to increased resistance to joint movements. Tone may be increased (hypertonia) or decreased (hypotonia).

Hypertonia. There are two distinct types, spasticity and rigidity. The increase in tone which accompanies lesions of the upper motor neurones is called *spasticity.*

It is characterised by a rapid build-up in resistance during the first few degrees of passive movement and then, as the movement continues, there is a sudden lessening of resistance. This phenomenon is likened to the sensations encountered when opening a clasp knife and in shorthand terms is called 'clasp-knife spasticity'. This phenomenon is much more commonly and more easily detected in passive movements of the knee joint in upper motor neurone lesions than it is in the upper limbs.

Rigidity is the term used to describe a resistance to passive movement which is sustained throughout the range of the movement. This phenomenon gives rise to sensations reminiscent of those produced by bending a lead pipe and occurs in diseases of the basal ganglia. It is variously referred to as lead-pipe, plastic or extrapyramidal rigidity. When tremor is superimposed on rigidity the resistance to passive movement is jerkily increased as if a ratchet were slipping over the teeth of a cog. This is called cogwheel rigidity and is commonly felt in parkinsonism. Extrapyramidal and cogwheel rigidity are most easily detected at the wrist when relatively slow manipulation is employed.

Hypotonia. This is usually harder to assess than an increase in tone. Decreased resistance to passive movement is difficult to distinguish from good relaxation. A more useful sign of hypotonia in the arms is a change in posture. When a patient suffering from rheumatic chorea (which is attended by hypotonia) is asked to stretch out the hands and spread the fingers it will be found that the wrists are flexed and the metacarpophalangeal joints are hyperextended giving rise to the so-called 'dinner fork' deformity.

Associated Features. Tone can often be difficult to evaluate. Some help in its assessment may be obtained by comparing one side with the other. In many cases alterations in tone achieve clinical significance only because there are associated features such as clonus and increased tendon reflexes.

CLONUS. This is the term applied to a rhythmic series of involuntary muscular contractions evoked by a sudden stretch of muscle. A few beats of clonus are commonly elicited in nervous patients, especially in the calf, and such a finding may or may not be significant. Sustained clonus, i.e. contractions which continue as long as stretch is applied, reflects exaggerated tendon reflexes as a result of damage to the upper motor neurones and is a 'hard' neurological sign. Clonus is most commonly evoked at the knee and ankle joints. Patellar clonus is elicited by sharply pushing the patella towards the foot whilst the patient lies supine and relaxed with his knee extended and supported by the bed as illustrated in Figure 8.14. Clonus at the ankle is produced by a brisk dorsiflexion of the foot with the leg in the position shown in Figure 8.15.

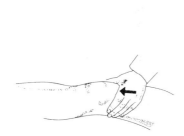

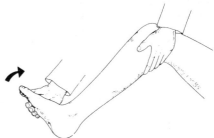

Fig. 8.14 Testing for knee clonus.   Fig. 8.15 Testing for ankle clonus.

Testing of Power

There are two methods by which muscle power can be tested. The patient may be asked to contract a group of muscles as powerfully as possible, and thus move a joint and then maintain the deviated position of the joint whilst the examiner tries to restore the part to its original position. This is called *isometric testing*. Alternatively the patient may be asked to put a joint through a full range of movement using maximal power whilst the examiner opposes the movement trying to prevent its accomplishment. This is *isotonic testing*. Both methods are effective; many clinicians employ either technique at will. To detect minor degrees of weakness isotonic testing is more sensitive than the isometric method. Any variability and undue fatiguability of muscle power should be noted.

The testing of power should not degenerate into an unseemly trial of strength between the patient and the examiner. The temptation to display one's virility by using excessive force should be resisted. Clinicians should be aware of similar irrational ambitions on the part of patients, some of whom may take pleasure attempting to hurt or humiliate them by pushing them off balance. The alert examiner will be aware of this and easily avoid it by suddenly withdrawing the resistance.

Major Movements. In most instances it is necessary only to test the power of movements of major joints. It is recommended that a regular routine be followed; thus first the power of flexion and extension of the neck should be tested; abduction and adduction, flexion and extension of the shoulders should be examined. Flexion and extension at the elbow, flexion and extension of the wrist, pronation of the forearm, abduction and adduction of the fingers, the power of opposition of thumb and little finger and the power of the hand grip should be assessed.

Trunk muscles should be tested by examining the power of flexion and extension and of lateral flexion of the trunk against gravity and against resistance. The muscles of the anterior abdominal wall may best be examined by asking the supine patient to raise the head from the pillow against resistance. Whilst the patient performs this manoeuvre the abdominal muscles should be observed and palpated. If upper or lower segments of the rectus abdominis are weak, the umbilicus will be drawn away from the weakened muscles.

In the lower limbs, flexion, extension, abduction and adduction of the hips, flexion and extension of the knees, dorsiflexion and plantar flexion, inversion and eversion of the ankles and flexion and extension of all the toes should be tested.

Individual Muscles. If there is localised weakness or wasting a more detailed examination of appropriate individual muscles should be made. The evaluation of muscle power should be recorded quantitatively using the grading recommended by the Medical Research Council, viz:

0 — No active contraction
1 — Visible palpable contraction without active movement
2 — Movement which is possible with gravity eliminated
3 — Movement which is possible against gravity
4 — Movement which is possible against gravity plus resistance but which is
   weaker than normal
5 — Normal power.

The methods by which the actions of individual muscles are tested, details of motor nerve distribution and the segmental derivation of nerves needs to be known. These details are graphically set out in the Medical Research Council publication *Aids to the Examination of the Peripheral Nervous System* (HMSO, London), and it is recommended that this booklet be purchased and until familiarity is achieved it should be constantly available for reference. Examples of the testing of individual muscles are given on page 330.

Significance of Loss of Power. Weakness may result from generalised loss of muscle tissue associated with some systemic or metabolic disease. Myopathic weakness is often most evident in the proximal limb musculature. Myasthenia gravis produces loss of power which fluctuates in severity and which can be improved transiently by the intravenous injection of edrophonium. Weakness due to lower motor neurone lesions is attended by wasting of muscles. The pattern of weakness produced by lower motor neurone lesions may conform to the distribution of one or more peripheral nerves or of motor roots. Systematised affection of lower motor neurones as in motor neurone disease tends to produce weakness which is initially distal and is usually symmetrical.

Damage to upper motor neurones causes weakness of movements not of individual muscles and tends to affect whole limbs. Paresis of one limb (monoplegia) results from a lesion affecting upper motor neurones near the motor cortex since they are here spread over a wide area (Fig. 8.13). A hemiplegia is commonly caused by interruption of the upper motor neurones in the opposite internal capsule where the fibres are closely packed together and all are damaged by quite a small lesion. Paraparesis, weakness of both legs, is usually caused by lesions of both upper motor neurones in the spinal cord. Tetraplegia refers to paralysis of all four limbs and is produced by high spinal cord lesions.

The examination of motor power should assess the presence and severity of weakness but it is equally important to define its distribution as this provides clues to the site of the causative lesion.

Coordination

The smooth and accurate performance of purposeful movements requires intact sensory and motor functions as well as efficient control by higher centres. Any lesion which causes weakness may be accompanied by clumsiness but incoordination is particularly prominent in sensory and cerebellar ataxia.

Sensory Ataxia. This results from defective proprioception and can to some extent be mitigated by visual control of movements. It is, therefore, exacerbated when the eyes are closed.

Cerebellar Ataxia. The posterior lobe of the cerebellum functions as a feedback centre. The progress of a limb in motion is monitored by proprioceptive information fed to the cerebellum. Through its connections with the motor cortex the cerebellum causes adjustments to be made in patterns of motor activation so that the limb's movements are accurately and smoothly aimed. When this guidance system is disturbed movements err in direction and velocity. The inco-ordination thus produced, cerebellar ataxia, is not susceptible to visual compensation.

Testing Coordination. A most useful test of coordination in the arm is the *finger-nose test*. The patient is asked to hold an arm outstretched and then to touch the tip of the nose with the tip of the index finger. A variation on this test which renders it more sensitive requires the patient to touch first the tip of their own nose and then the end of the examiner's index finger held at arm's length away from the patient. The sensitivity of this test may still further be increased if the examiner moves the index finger from place to place whilst the patient's finger is en route to it. An alternative manoeuvre is the *finger-to-finger test* in which the patient is asked to extend and abduct the arms fully and then to bring the tips of the index fingers through a wide circle to the midline where they are brought into approximation with each other. They should not touch but should be held separated by about a quarter of an inch. Whilst the patient performs these various actions the smoothness and accuracy of movements are observed. The patient with sensory ataxia may perform these acts smoothly when the eyes are open but performance will markedly deteriorate when the eyes are closed due to loss of awareness of the position of the limbs in space. If cerebellar ataxia is present movements are clumsy and jerky (dyssynergia). The patient may overshoot the target (dysmetria). *Intention tremor* is most characteristic of damage to the posterior lobe of the cerebellum. Here the patient's hand is steady at rest but develops a tremor of increasing amplitude as it approaches its target.

In the lower limb the patient is asked to perform the *heel-knee test* by placing one heel on the opposite knee and then sliding the heel accurately down the front of the shin to the ankle and back again. This test too can be made more sensitive by first making the patient raise a leg to touch the examiner's index finger with the great toe before proceeding to perform the heel-knee test as outlined above.

Rapid alternating movements are rendered irregular in force and rhythm by cerebellar disorders. They may be tested by asking the patient quickly to pronate and supinate the forearms or to slap the palm of the examiner's hand repeatedly with the front and back of the hand. This sequence is performed several times in quick succession. Impairment of rapid alternating movements is called *dysdiadochokinesis*. Patients vary widely in their abilities to perform such movements. Labourers tend to perform less well than those whose jobs require manual dexterity. Most people perform the tests more precisely and rapidly with the dominant hand and some are very clumsy indeed when using the other hand.

Assessment of Fine Movements

The examination of the motor system should include an assessment of the patient's capacity to carry out small, precise, coordinated finger movements. Such movements are usually the earliest to be affected by lesions of upper motor neurones and are the last to recover therefrom. The hypokinesis associated with diseases of the basal ganglia is often most easily and earliest detected by slowing and poverty of fine finger movements; as already outlined one of the signs of cerebellar defect is the inability to make rapid movements of the hands.

The most useful and the simplest of the various tests of fine movements is to ask patients, as rapidly as possible, with each hand in turn to make 'piano-playing' individual finger movements. A supplementary test consists of rapidly touching the tips of the little, ring, middle and index fingers successively with the tip of the thumb of the same hand.

In addition to these formal tests one should always observe the patient carrying out those mundane, everyday activities which demand precise coordination of finger movements, such as fastening buttons, tying ties and shoe laces.

Testing for Dyspraxia and Apraxia

Difficulty in the performance of fine movements may have been noted despite the fact that formal examination has revealed no evidence of incoordination or weakness or sensory defect. This would suggest that the patient has difficulty in formulating and synthesising movement patterns, i.e. suffers from dyspraxia. If this suspicion is aroused it should be explored by specific tasks. The patient should be asked to pick up small objects from a table, to wind a watch, and to simulate throwing a ball, combing the hair and putting on spectacles. Cutting paper with scissors, tying a knot in a piece of string and folding paper and placing it in an envelope are other examples.

These simple tests may be supplemented by asking the patient to draw geometrical figures such as a square or a triangle and to construct similar figures from matchsticks.

The patient's writing should be examined. Dyspractic patients write slowly and with difficulty. The formation of letters may be incomplete and their size variable; what is written rarely keeps to the horizontal.

Suspected dyspraxia may sometimes be confirmed as patients dress for they may attempt to put their coat on back to front or in extreme instances try to put their trousers on their arms. Bilateral dyspraxia may arise from a lesion in the parietal lobe of the dominant hemisphere. A lesion in the non-dominant parietal lobe may give rise to dyspraxia confined to the non-dominant arm and hand. Very often dyspraxia will be associated with other signs of cortical disturbance such as agnosia (p. 306) or dysphasia (p. 231) which will aid in the localisation of the lesion. The bizarre nature of dyspractic disturbances may sometimes lead the unwary to make a diagnosis of hysteria.

SUMMARY OF EXAMINATION OF THE MOTOR SYSTEM

The examiner should develop an approach which will enable the information outlined above to be elicited with economy of effort and the minimum of duplication of tests. A useful preliminary to the examination of the motor system is to ask the patient to hold the arms out straight with the fingers spread, first with the eyes open and then maintain this position with the eyes closed. Observation of this very simple manoeuvre will often give information which will direct the emphasis of the rest of the examination. Involuntary movements of the arms will be apparent. Abnormal postures may be seen. If one arm tends slowly to drift downwards this will be an indication of paresis of that arm. Intention tremor revealed during the initial examination of the arms may indicate the need to examine other cerebellar functions with care.

In general the scheme for examination of motor function will be applied first to the upper limbs and then repeated in the lower limbs.

Inspection should take note of posture, of wasting and its distribution, of the presence or absence of fasciculation and of voluntary and involuntary movements. Tone should be assessed by passive movement of all joints of the relaxed patient. Attempts should be made to elicit clonus at knee and ankle. Power in muscle groups should be tested and if necessary it should be evaluated in individual muscles. Coordination and fine movements should be examined and in appropriate instances the patient should be set specialised tests to explore the possibility of dyspraxia.

Interpretation of Abnormalities of Motor Function

Examination of motor functions will determine which of the six modes of disturbance considered on page 267 are operative. The next stage in analysis is to decide where the lesion is situated. Motor function may be disrupted at any of seven levels, viz.:

1. The Highest Level. Here ideas of movement are formulated and movement patterns are elaborated and stored so that they can be placed at the disposal of the executive motor system. Parts of the cortex of the frontal and parietal lobes are especially concerned with this level of motor activity whose derangement causes apraxia or dyspraxia.

2. The Level of the Upper Motor Neurone. This comprises a motor system which originates in cortical neurones whose axonal prolongations run downwards to establish connections with the contralateral motor cranial nerves and through the pyramidal tracts with the lower motor neurones on the opposite side of the spinal cord (Fig. 8.13). Interruption of this system anywhere along its extensive course causes paralysis of movement and an increase of tone accompanied by clonus. Attendant reflex changes are discussed on pages 288 to 295.

3. The Level of the Lower Motor Neurone. This provides a link between the higher motor pathways and the final effector apparatus where axons of the anterior horn cells terminate as part of the neuromuscular junctions. Dissolution at this level causes weakness and wasting of those muscles innervated by the damaged lower motor neurones. If there is widespread wasting of muscles in a limb or around a joint then tone may be decreased.

4. The Level of the Neuromuscular Junction. This constitutes a communication between the neural motor pathway and the muscle. The electrical impulses carried along the lower motor neurone evoke the release from the neural termination of a transmitting substance, acetylcholine, which causes depolarisation of the muscle membrane. Interference with the chemical transmitter's role causes a variable weakness of muscles, usually unaccompanied by wasting.

5. The Muscular Level. This is the terminal and effector part of the motor pathway. Depolarisation of muscle, biochemically initiated, spreads electrically and causes the muscle fibres to shorten or contract. Impairment of this process leads to weakness which is usually attended by loss and atrophy of fibres.

6. The Cerebellar Level. This influences the direct motor circuit. The cerebellum takes part in a feedback system, processing information about the state of motor activity and by modifying cortical activity adjusts the rate and direction of movements and provides a stable postural base for movements. Disruption at this level does not lead to weakness but to incoordinate, imprecise movements which sometimes are associated with hypotonia.

7. The Extrapyramidal Level. This comprises a complex lattice work of fibres and interspersed nuclear masses running from the cortex to the brain stem whence descending motor fibres pass downwards into the cord to influence lower motor neurone activity. Impairment at this level causes not paralysis but a delay in initiation and a poverty of movement, attended by involuntary movements and alterations in tone.

To localise the level of motor dysfunction supplementary evidence about, particularly, reflex functions may be required and the process of final synthesis occurs when the whole examination of the nervous system is completed (p. 303).

THE SENSORY SYSTEM

The testing df sensation is considerably simplified if the clinician pays attention to the patient's symptoms and is aware of the basic physiological and anatomical substrates of the sensory pathways. For clinical purposes sensation is divided into:

1. *Exteroception* — Superficial modalities comprising touch, pain and temperature.
2. *Proprioception* — Deep sensations concerned with muscle and joint (or position) sense.
3. *Interoception* — Visceral sensations largely served by the autonomic nervous system.
4. *Distance reception* — Senses such as smell, sound, sight and taste providing information about the distant environment.

Information from all the active sensory pathways is correlated, integrated and interpreted in the cerebral cortex.

There is still a divergence of opinion as to whether the different modalities of sensation are subserved by specialised end organs or by end organs which are flexible and which respond to different types of energy. Touch end organs are distributed in a punctate manner over the skin and are activated by pressure which distorts or deforms them. Pain may arise superficially in the skin, from deep structures such as muscles or tendons or from viscera. Pain endings have the capacity to respond to high intensity stimuli of any nature, such as extremes of heat and cold which, in common, are potentially damaging to the tissues. Sherrington referred to pain as a nociceptive mechanism, sensitive to noxious agents. Deep pressure and deep pain are probably subserved by end organs similar to those of pain in the skin.

Clinically it is customary to refer to temperature sensation but it seems clear that there are discrete receptors distributed in a punctate manner over the skin, some of which respond to heat and others which respond to a fall in temperature.

Proprioceptive function comprises two components. The first concerns the appreciation of passive movement, and the second an apprehension of the position of body parts after movement.

Vibration sense is a term in common usage but it refers not to specific sensory modality but rather to discernment of repeated patterns of pressure mediated by end organs in the skin as well as in deeper structures. Vibration is felt particularly well through bone which probably serves merely to amplify the stimulus. Vibration sense is the perception of a temporal dispersion of touch and pressure and is analogous to the appreciation of flicker by the visual system.

Sensations of touch, pressure and position are carried in the peripheral nerve in relatively large, fast-conducting afferent fibres. Pain is conducted in two types of fibre, transmitting impulses at different speeds and serving different types of pain sensation.

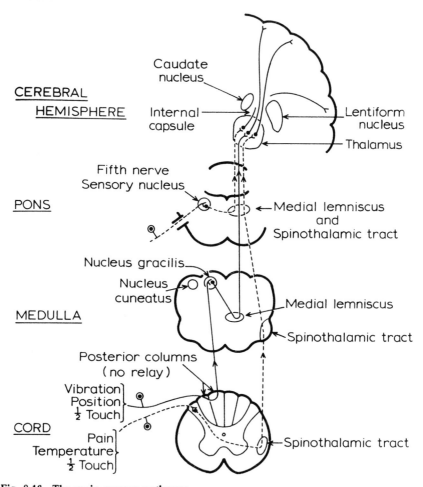

Fig. 8.16 The main sensory pathways.

Sensory Pathways. The cells of origin of peripheral sensory fibres lie in the dorsal root ganglia whence proximal processes enter the spinal cord via the posterior spinal nerve roots. On entering the cord the fibres separate into two groups which then travel in the spinal cord by two distinct pathways (Fig. 8.16). Some of the fibres which subserve the sensations of touch and light pressure and all of those subserving joint position sense and perhaps all concerned with vibration sense, ascend in the posterior columns to the gracile and cuneate nuclei at the lower end of the medulla. Here second order neurones arise; their fibres decussate and pass upwards through the medial lemniscus to the ventral nucleus of the thalamus.

Fibres which transmit pain and temperature sensation and some of those subserving touch, synapse in the posterior horn, in the cord, near to their point of entry. Thence fibres from second order neurones, cross to the opposite side and ascend in the lateral spinothalamic tract. This tract preserves its laminated structure in its passage upwards through the cord. Those fibres from the lowest segments lie outermost in the tract whilst those arising from more proximal segments lie nearer the centre of the cord (Fig. 8.17). Those fibres concerned with touch which cross within the cord lie anteriorly in the anterior spinothalamic tract. The spinothalamic pathways run to the ventral nucleus of the thalamus. From the thalamus third order neurones, transmitting all forms of sensation, pass to the sensory cortex.

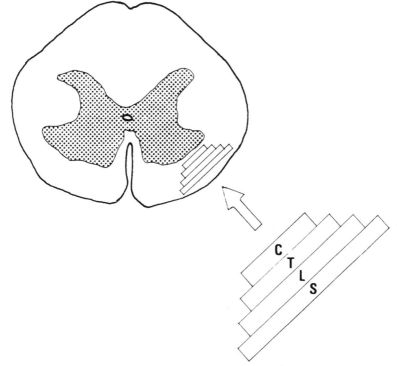

Fig. 8.17 Spinothalamic tract. To show layering of the lateral spinothalamic tract in the cervical region: C represents fibres from cervical segments which lie centrally; fibres from thoracic lumbar and sacral segments (labelled T, L, and S respectively) lie progressively more laterally. Extrinsic compression (represented by the arrow) will first affect fibres from lower segmental levels.

Symptoms. The most frequent sensory symptoms are pain, numbness and altered sensation or paraesthesiae. Pain due to neural lesions is often described as burning or stabbing. Patients usually describe impairment or loss of sensation as numbness. Paraesthesiae may also be referred to as numbness or as 'pins and needles' by the patient but sometimes the altered or perverted sensation may be more imaginatively interpreted as a feeling of, for instance, wet sand on the limbs or a feeling of hot water running down the skin. In many instances patients who complain of pain or paraesthesiae or numbness will be able to delineate the distribution of their sensory symptoms fairly precisely and hence guide the examiner to the areas which need careful examination.

Patients usually are aware of any significant reduction of temperature sensation. They may know that they can grasp hot objects without discomfort or realise that they burn themselves, or scald themselves in their baths without being alerted by a painful warning.

Examination of Sensation

The object of sensory testing is to delineate the extent of sensory impairment and to determine which modalities are involved. It is important to evolve efficient yet time-saving methods of examination. Duplication of tests of sensory function do not increase the amount of information obtained and indeed as one loses the patient's cooperation, repetition becomes less and less informative. The clinician who first examines a patient's sensory system, if competent, is much more likely to get accurate information than are those who follow. Routine testing of cutaneous sensation is relatively easy if the anatomical distribution of sensory nerves be used to determine those points which must be surveyed in order to cover the territories of peripheral nerves as well as posterior nerve roots. These are indicated in Figures 8.18 and 8.19. On the trunk the effects of root lesions are easily identified by the orderly arrangement of dermatomes.

Touch. This is usually tested using a small point of cotton wool which should be laid directly on the skin and not moved over it since moving the wool produces a tickling sensation which is mediated by the pathways for pain rather than those for touch. A light camel hair brush, or failing this, a piece of paper can also effectively be used to test touch. Should an area of altered sensation be found its border should be determined by moving the point of wool to different points on the skin. Mapping out areas of altered sensation depends on the patient's responses and it is easier for a patient quickly to detect enhancement of a sensation rather than its diminution. The stimulus should, therefore, be moved from a region of diminished sensation towards normally sensitive areas. The boundaries of the abnormality should be plotted and if necessary marked on the skin. In the less common circumstance when sensation in an affected area is abnormally heightened, the stimulus should be moved from the normal into the hypersensitive area.

Pain and Temperature Sensations. These are tested respectively by pin prick and by hot and cold water contained in tubes. The pin should be used gently. Transmission of infection, notably of type B hepatitis, is a danger if the same pin is used repeatedly to test sensation in patients. Disposable, sterile, hypodermic needles, discarded after one examination, obviate this danger but their sharp edges easily penetrate and lacerate the skin. It is best to use a new, cheap, steel, dressmaker's pin for the sensory testing of each patient.

Patients should be asked what they feel when pricked. They should not be asked directly if they feel the pin because they may well feel the touch of the pin point even when pain sensation is impaired. It should, therefore, be established that they feel the sharp or painful sensation of the pin point. They should be asked, with the eyes closed, to distinguish between stimulation with the point and the head of the pin answering respectively 'sharp' or 'blunt'. Patients should also be asked to comment on any heightening or lessening of pain felt as the pin is moved along the limb or along the trunk at the points indicated in Figures 8.18 and 8.19.

It is necessary to preface the testing of temperature sensation by a careful explanation of what is required. In practice it is tested only in special circumstances as, for example, if there is reason to suspect dissociated anaesthesia (p. 288). Then hot and cold tubes should be applied in random sequence to the skin; the patient with the eyes closed attempts to distinguish between them.

Deep Pain. This is tested by firm squeezing over the muscles and tendons. The patient is asked to indicate when the pressure becomes painful and the examiner gauges whether the force applied would be painful in normal people.

Position Sense. This is tested by passive movements. When it is impaired the distal part of the limbs are almost always first affected hence it is customary to test position sense first at the terminal interphalangeal joint of the great toe. The proximal phalanx is fixed by grasping it firmly in the finger and thumb of the examiner's left hand. The thumb and forefinger of the right hand grip the terminal phalanx on its lateral borders. The distal phalanx is then extended or flexed gently and the patient is asked to close the eyes and then indicate the direction of movement. It is important that several random movements be made before assuming that the patient's sensation is intact. Many patients even when they are unaware of the direction of movement will guess and answer 'up' or 'down' and obviously on any given occasion the patient has a 50% chance of being right. The test, therefore, should be meticulously appraised. If the sensation of passive movement is only moderately impaired, the patient may be aware that movement has taken place but will be unable correctly to assess the direction of movement. When there is gross diminution the movement itself may be undetected. If position sense is normal at the periphery of a limb it is unnecessary to test more proximal joints. However, if there is impairment of joint position sense peripherally then similar tests should be employed at the ankle and knee. A similar process of testing may be adopted in the upper limbs. The terminal interphalangeal joint of the index finger is first examined and if indicated the proximal joints are studied. It is rare for gross impairment of position sense to be manifest at the hip or shoulder joints.

Concomitant signs of diminished position sense should be assessed. A deterioration in the performance of the finger-nose test (p. 274) when the patient's eyes are closed indicates impaired postural sensibility in the arms. When position sense in an arm is markedly impaired involuntary movements occur in the limb when the patient holds it outstretched with the eyes closed. The movements thus produced may closely resemble athetosis but may be differentiated therefrom by their amelioration when the patient opens the eyes and can then visually control the arm's posture.

Rombergism may be observed. To demonstrate this phenomenon the patient stands upright with the feet together, arms outstretched and eyes closed. If there is loss of postural sensation the patient rocks and sways. Unfortunately many normal people who are suggestible and apprehensive may exhibit similar instability under the test conditions and importance should not be attached to Romberg's sign unless it be accompanied by demonstrable loss of joint position sense in the limbs. In

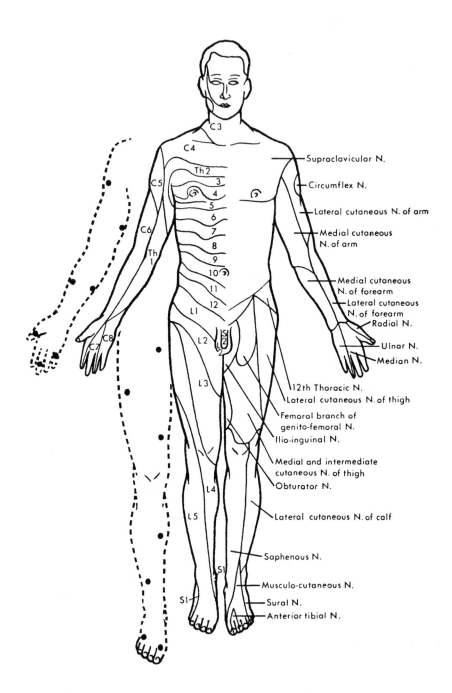

Fig. 8.18 Segmental and peripheral nerve innervation and points for testing cutaneous sensation of limbs (anterior). By applying stimuli at the points marked within the dotted outline both the dermatomal and main peripheral nerve distribution are covered simultaneously.

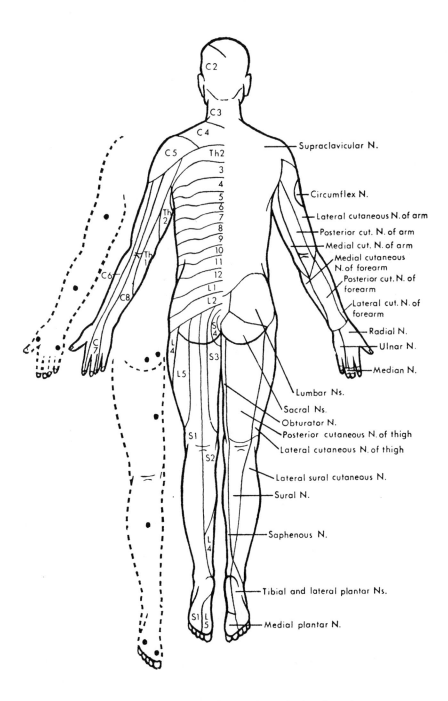

Fig. 8.19 Segmental and peripheral nerve innervation and points for testing cutaneous sensation of limbs (posterior). By applying stimuli at the points marked within the dotted outline, both the dermatomal and main peripheral nerve distribution are covered simultaneously.

contrast it is significant if symptoms suggestive of Rombergism are volunteered by patients. They may state that when they close their eyes whilst washing the face they pitch forward against the washbasin or that they are very unsteady when walking in the dark. Such symptoms strongly suggest marked diminution of position sense.

Vibration Sense. This also is usually first impaired at the periphery of limbs. The base of a vibrating tuning fork, ideally a weighty one, with a frequency of 128 cycles per second, is placed on the dorsum of the terminal phalanx. It should be explained to the patient that it is the sensation of vibration not cold or touch which is being detected. The test may be made more objective and sensitive; a careful explanation and a demonstration of the vibratory sensation is given to the patient. The patient is then asked to close the eyes and the tuning fork, sometimes vibrating and sometimes still, is placed against the dorsum of the toe. The reliability of the patient's responses can thus be gauged. Minor degrees of impairment may then be detected if the examiner's own appreciation of the fork's vibration is used as a yardstick against which to measure the patient's response. Should vibration sense be lost or impaired distally then the tuning fork should be moved proximally in order to establish the level at which it is normally appreciated. Because of the amplification of the vibrating stimulus afforded by bone it is customary to apply the form to bony prominences; after the dorsum of the terminal phalanx it is placed successively over lateral malleolus, the upper part of the tibia, the iliac crests and if necessary over the costal margin. Similarly in the arm one may proceed from the terminal parts of the fingers to the wrist and the elbow.

Barber's Chair Sign. A distinctive sensory sign may sometimes be provoked by flexing the patient's neck. The patient should be asked rapidly to touch the chest with the chin and to relate any sensations thus evoked. Patients may describe an intense tingling, commonly likened to an electric shock, radiating down the arms, along the spine or down the legs when the head is bent forward. An account of this phenomenon may be volunteered by the patient in the history. This idiosyncratic feature was first described by Babinski who correctly attributed it to disruption of the sensory pathways in the mid-cervical region of the spinal cord. Later Lhermitte ascribed it to multiple sclerosis. It most commonly occurs in sufferers from multiple sclerosis but it is sometimes a feature of cervical spondylosis, syringomyelia or vitamin B_{12} deficiency or indeed of any lesion in the cervical cord. This sign thus has fairly precise anatomical, not pathological, significance.

Examination of Cortical Sensory Functions

Lesions of the sensory cortex impair the discriminative aspects of sensation. Accurate localisation of stimuli, and the assessment of shape, weight, size and texture of objects are the functions of this highest sensory level. The cortex receives information transmitted by the afferent pathways, integrates and correlates the several sensory impressions and interprets them in the light of previous experience. If there is peripheral disruption of the conducting pathways then the tests of the highest sensory level are invalidated. Patients must be able to understand what is required of them during testing and be able to communicate their responses. Intact basic sensations and adequate intellectual and language functions are therefore essential prerequisites for the study of cortical sensory performance. The following tests are employed:

Two Point Discrimination. This tests the ability to distinguish the contact of two separate points applied simultaneously to the skin. Special dividers, calibrated to show the amount of separation of their blunted points, are used for this test. The object is to determine the minimum distance of separation at which two points are identified as two distinct stimuli. Over the finger pulps two points separated by only 2 to 3 mm are normally so recognised. In the legs a separation of 50 to 100 mm is required before two discrete stimuli are appreciated and the test is seldom employed there. One or both points of a pair of dividers, opened to varying widths, should be applied randomly over the skin of the fingers, the patient, whose eyes are closed, being asked to say if one or two points is felt after each stimulation. It is abnormal if the two points need to be separated by more than 5 mm before they are distinguished over the finger pulps.

Point Localisation. This tests the ability of the patient accurately to localise the point touched with the head of a pin or orange stick when the eyes are closed. The eyes are then opened and a finger placed on the stimulated site. Localisation is more precise at the periphery of limbs than in the proximal parts thereof.

Stereognosis. This tests the ability to identify objects by palpation and requires not only intact peripheral sensation but the evocation in the cortex of the constellation of ideas and memories necessary for recognition. Suitable common objects such as a coin, a key, a pen, or a wallet are placed in the patient's hand whilst the eyes are closed. After careful palpation the patient is asked to identify the object.

Identification of Textures. This depends on the same mechanism as does stereognosis. A piece of paper, cloth, wood or metal is placed in the hand of the patient who is then asked to identify the nature of the substance from its feel.

Graphaesthesia. This tests the ability to recognise numbers traced by a blunt object on the palm of the hand and, although normally accurate to a surprising degree, is impaired or lost in lesions of the sensory cortex.

Sensory Extinction. This tests perception of stimuli at corresponding sites on both sides of the body. It is first necessary to demonstrate that a stimulus, either touch or pin prick, is felt when separately applied to an appropriate point on each side. If like stimuli are delivered, bilaterally and simultaneously, the stimulus may be perceived by the patient only on one side. The test should be repeated several times, the patient's eyes being closed throughout, in order to confirm that the responses are consistent. The stimulus is extinguished, or suppressed on the side opposite that of a lesion in the sensory cortex. This phenomenon is also known as *perceptual rivalry*. It must be re-emphasised that this test is applicable only if cutaneous sensations are preserved on both sides of the body.

SUMMARY OF EXAMINATION OF THE SENSORY SYSTEM

During routine sensory examination it is not essential to test cortical functions. However, these tests are often omitted in circumstances in which they would be most informative and one must be alert to recognise the situations which demand their performance. Temperature sensation need be tested only if dissociated anaesthesia (p. 288) is suspected. Touch, superficial and deep pain, position and vibration sense should always be examined and particular attention paid to areas of subjective sensory disturbances delineated by patients.

Interpretation of Sensory Abnormalities

It may sometimes be difficult to decide whether there is significant sensory loss. The intensity of successive stimuli such as pinprick will vary slightly since they are applied by the examiner who cannot deliver identical pressures repeatedly. Some meticulous and obsessional patients will detect and report such minimal variations and thus tend to confuse the examiner. Superficial sensation tends to be blunted over the thickened, hard skin of the hands of manual workers, and may appear to be heightened over the face or trunk. Some patients can easily be conditioned to recognise altered sensation in various areas. One half of the body or the distal parts of limbs are particularly liable to be implicated in this spurious sensory diminution which sometimes results from previous inept examinations of sensation.

Diminution of vibration sense at and below the ankles is a frequent finding in normal elderly people. The perception of deep pain sensation depends partly on the pressure applied to deep tissues by the examiner and partly on the readiness of the patient to interpret the feelings as painful. Evaluation of abnormalities of this modality is, therefore, difficult. Marked diminution or absence of deep pain, as in tabes dorsalis, can usually be recognised. Excessively tender calf muscles in vitamin B deficiency can also usually be validated by comparison with the patient's responses to similar degrees of pressure applied over the thighs or upper arms. Apparent diminution or heightening of deep pain sensation when of minor degree should not be given undue significance.

There are no easy rules whose application will enable the examiner infallibly to distinguish significant from spurious sensory signs but, in general, organic alterations of sensation are consistent and reproducible in their nature, degree and extent if they are diligently and competently sought. The history will help to avoid some of the difficulties. Virtually all patients of normal intelligence who have any considerable alteration of superficial sensation will volunteer an account of sensory symptoms. The finding of extensive or severe sensory loss in the absence of such symptoms should always cause the examiner sceptically to review the signs. Close observation of patients' reactions will often help to confirm their spoken interpretations. When the pricking of a pin crosses the boundary between a cutaneous area wherein pain is diminished to one of normal pain appreciation the transition is usually accompanied by a facial grimace or a withdrawal movement of a limb. Such involuntary responses are strong evidence of organic sensory affection.

Once the extent and nature of sensory loss has been determined with confidence the localisation of lesions is comparatively simple.

Peripheral Nerves. Lesions of individual peripheral nerves or sensory nerve roots commonly give rise to subjective feelings of numbness and to diminution of all sensory modalities in their defined areas of distribution (Figs. 8.18 and 8.19). Less commonly, partial lesions of peripheral nerves give rise to pain of a burning, exquisitely unpleasant quality. It is thought that this type of pain is mediated through the slower conducting, smaller pain fibres (p. 278). It is called 'delayed' or 'second' pain to distinguish it from the 'normal', 'first' or 'bright' pain which is conducted at faster rates in the larger pain fibres. This peculiarly unpleasant pain (causalgia) is liable to occur in the region supplied by nerves which have been damaged, but not completely disrupted, by trauma. The median and sciatic nerves are vulnerable to this type of reaction. Causalgia is accompanied by diminished sensation in the cutaneous area of the nerve involved and the skin itself may become thin, red and hairless.

Generalised polyneuropathies uncommonly give rise to similarly unpleasant pain in those few instances when smaller pain fibres are relatively spared by pathological processes which damage the larger ones as in the 'burning feet syndrome' sometimes caused by prolonged vitamin B deficiencies. Much more commonly generalised polyneuropathies cause numbness or paraesthesiae. The subjective and objective sensory features then affect the distal parts of limbs and usually involve the legs before the arms. Superficial sensory loss in a polyneuropathy is found over the distal parts of the extremities and extends along the limbs to a level which is uniform around their whole circumference. This is the 'stocking' and 'glove' type of sensory disturbance. Deep sensation, such as proprioception and vibration are usually little affected in polyneuropathy. If they are significantly impaired in association with glove and stocking anaesthesia it suggests that the causal lesion is diffusely damaging the cells in the dorsal root ganglia, or that there is a concurrent affection of the dorsal columns.

Spinal Cord. Sensation may be disturbed in several ways by lesions involving the spinal cord. Tumours which compress the cord may also impinge on an adjacent sensory root and hence give rise to diminution of all modalities in the corresponding dermatome. Sensory fibres may be damaged in the dorsal root entry zone, and lesions here also cause sensory loss in segmental dermatomes. The spinal sensory tracts may be interrupted and the level reflected in a loss of sensation at and below the segmental level of the lesion in the cord.

When the spinothalamic pathway is disrupted there will be a diminution of pain and temperature sensation below the level of the lesion on the opposite side of the body. The upper border of this impairment will not necessarily correspond to the segmental level of the lesion because of the laminated structure of the tract (p. 279). In the cervical region, for instance, the fibres from cervical segments lie in the innermost part of the lateral spinothalamic tract. Fibres from thoracic, lumbar and sacral segments lie in bands, successively more laterally (Fig. 8.17). An extrinsic lesion such as a tumour which compresses the cord first affects the outermost layer of fibres, i.e. those from the sacral region and then progressively damages fibres from higher segments. Thus the upper level of sensory loss may correspond to a segmental dermatome lying well below the cord segment which is the site of damage. Intrinsic lesions often initially damage those fibres which have just entered the tract and spare, for a time at least, fibres from lower levels. The 'saddle' area of the buttocks, comprising the lower sacral dermatomes would be the last to be affected by a central cord lesion spreading centrifugally in the cervical region. Such topographical considerations help in the clinical differentiation between intramedullary tumours, which are rarely removable, and extramedullary tumours which may be curable with surgery.

Spinal cord lesions may cause loss of one modality of sensation in an area wherein other modalities are preserved. This is called 'dissociated' sensory loss. Most commonly pain and temperature sensations are lost whilst touch, vibration and position senses are intact. This pattern results from lesions which interrupt the lateral spinothalamic system but do not impinge on the dorsal columns. Dissociated anaesthesia is found in cases of syringomyelia but may also result from other processes, such as a tumour, damaging the central or lateral parts of the spinal cord.

Intracranial Lesions. Within the *lower brain stem* lesions may give rise to impairment of pain and temperature on the ipsilateral side of the face and on the contralateral side of the body (sometimes called alternating analgesia).

Above the pontine level the spinothalamic tract and the medial lemniscus lie close together and are often damaged together. Lesions here which cause sensory impairment affect all modalities on the face, as well as on the body, on the side opposite the lesion. A hemianaesthesia involving the face and body is often due to interruption of the closely-packed sensory radiations in the contralateral *internal capsule.*

Lesions of the *thalamus* may give rise to spontaneous, intense, burning pain on the contralateral side, associated with diminution to touch over the same area. Pain can be provoked on the affected side of the body only by a painful stimulus of greater than normal intensity, i.e. the threshold of painful stimuli is raised. Pain, when thus evoked, has an ill-localised, particularly unpleasant quality.

Damage to the *sensory cortex* does not impair perception of pain, temperature and touch but causes a loss of discriminatory and correlative sensory appreciation.

EXAMINATION OF THE REFLEXES

A neurological reflex depends on an arc which consists of an afferent pathway triggered by stimulating a receptor, an efferent system which activates an effector organ and a communication between these two components. Since a reflex response to an appropriate stimulus is involuntary, disturbances of reflexes afford objective signs of neural function. Some of the reflexes subserved by cranial nerves such as the corneal reflex and jaw jerk are described on page 253. The routine neurological examination should include elicitation of tendon (deep) reflexes in the limbs and of some superficial (cutaneous) reflexes, including the plantar responses.

TENDON REFLEXES

The tendon reflexes are phasic stretch reflexes, which involve only two neurones, one afferent and one efferent with one synapse between them. Tendon reflexes depend on a sudden brief stretch of muscle spindles which evokes from them a synchronous afferent discharge. A volley of sensory impulses is conducted to the spinal cord wherein they activate motor neurones whose axons run back to the stretched muscles causing them to contract. Each reflex is subserved by its own spinal cord segments. During routine clinical examination the biceps jerk, the jerk from brachio-radialis (earlier called the supinator longus and hence by long established custom referred to as the supinator jerk) and the triceps jerk are tested in each upper limb; the knee and ankle jerks in the lower limbs. The segmental innervation of these reflexes is illustrated in Figures 8.20–8.25. There are suprasegmental influences which modify the function of the tendon reflex arc.

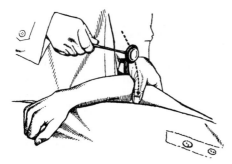

Fig. 8.20   Eliciting the biceps jerk, C.5 (C.6).

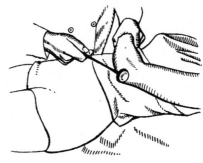

Fig. 8.21   Eliciting the triceps jerk, C.6, C.7.

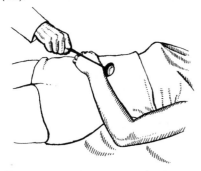

Fig. 8.22   Eliciting the supinator jerk, (C.5), C.6.

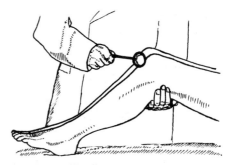

Fig. 8.23   Eliciting the knee jerk *(N.B.* the legs must not be in contact with each other), L.3, L.4

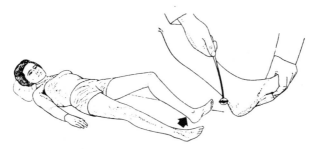

Fig. 8.24   Eliciting the ankle jerk of recumbent patient, L.5, S.1.

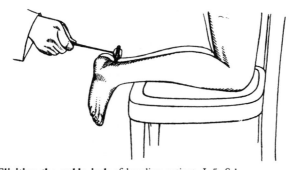

Fig. 8.25   Eliciting the ankle jerk of kneeling patient, L.5, S.1.

Elicitation of Tendon Reflexes

These reflexes are evoked by a brisk stretch of the tendons of appropriate muscles, and this is most efficiently done by a tap from a tendon hammer. This instrument should have a firm but flexible shaft and should contain most of its weight in its head which should preferably be made of metal and well padded with soft rubber. The tendon, not the muscle, should be struck by the hammer as mechanical stimulation of a muscle belly produces a contraction of the muscle which is not dependent on the reflex arc.

The patient should be placed in a comfortable, relaxed position which allows the examiner easily to reach the limbs. The muscle being tested should be visible. When the tendon jerks are tested, the one side should immediately be compared with its fellow on the opposite side. Convenient positions and methods are illustrated in Figures 8.20–8.25.

Interpretation of Tendon Reflexes

A normal tendon reflex results in a sudden displacement of part of a limb which then rapidly returns to its original position. The normal amplitude of such movements may be increased or decreased or there may be no movement.

Increased Tendon Reflexes. Many patients, particularly when they are paying their first visit to a doctor or hospital, are anxious. This tension is reflected in slight contractions of their muscles which facilitate tendon reflexes which become brisker than usual. A decision about whether reflexes are abnormally brisk is not always easy and may depend upon other evidence such as asymmetry or the plantar responses. When assessing a reflex response other muscles in the limb, as well as the one stimulated, should be observed. When tendon reflexes are pathologically exaggerated there is often a spread of the evoked contractions beyond the muscle stimulated, as, for example, the finger flexion which often accompanies biceps and supinator jerks when they are pathologically exaggerated.

The finger flexion jerk may help to confirm the presence of significant hyperreflexia. The tips of the examiner's middle and index fingers are placed across the palmar surfaces of the proximal phalanges of the patient's relaxed fingers; the examiner's own fingers are then tapped lightly. A slight flexion of the patient's fingers often occurs normally but a very brisk contraction suggests hyperreflexia.

Hoffman's sign is another manifestation of hyperreflexia. It is elicited by first flexing the distal interphalangeal joint of the patient's middle finger and then flicking the terminal phalanx into extension. When tendon reflexes are hyperactive the thumb quickly flexes in response to this manoeuvre. Minimal flexion of the thumb may sometimes be evoked in normal people, particularly if they are apprehensive. If Hoffman's sign is unilaterally positive, it is a very strong indication of a significant increase in tendon reflexes on that side.

Diminished or Absent Tendon Reflexes. It should be emphasised that a few normal people have tendon reflexes which are difficult to obtain. Some patients who regularly take hypnotic or anticonvulsant drugs show a generalised reduction in the amplitude of their tendon reflexes. The significance of depressed tendon reflexes needs to be appraised by a comparison between the responses obtained on the two sides and between the amplitude of the jerks in the arms and those in the legs. If normally brisk contractions are seen in the arms and very poor responses are evoked at knee and ankles then it is probable that the latter findings are pathological.

In rare instances all the tendon reflexes may be absent in people who have no neurological disease. Usually, however, absence of one or more tendon jerks denotes a neural lesion. When no response is obtained after a routine tendon tap, the absence of the reflex should be confirmed by *'reinforcing'* the jerk. Tendon reflexes are increased in amplitude (i.e. potentiated or reinforced) by forcible contraction of muscles remote from those being tested. To reinforce the knee and ankle jerks the patient may be asked forcibly to clench the hands. An alternative procedure requires the patient to hook the fingers of the hands together and then forcibly to attempt to pull one away from the other without disengaging the fingers (Fig. 8.26).

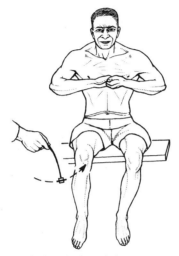

Fig. 8.26 Reinforcement in eliciting the knee jerk.

Reinforcement of the reflexes in the upper limbs may best be obtained by asking the patient to clench the jaws or to push the knees hard together. It is important to remember that the phenomenon of reinforcement lasts for less than a second. The patient should, therefore, be told to perform the appropriate manoeuvre (previously demonstrated) almost synchronously with the examiner's tap of the tendon.

SITE OF LESION. When tendon reflexes are absent or pathologically diminished the next stage of the interpretation is to localise where the reflex arcs are damaged or interrupted. Lesions of muscle, myoneural junction, peripheral nerve or spinal cord might cause loss of reflexes. It is an important clinical observation that tendon reflexes disappear very late in the course of diseases which primarily affect muscle (i.e. myopathies). Whilst there are muscle spindles to respond to stretch and whilst the neural arc is intact, surviving muscle fibres continue to contract even when there is marked muscle wasting and weakness. By contrast lesions which damage peripheral nerves cause very early loss of tendon reflexes. As outlined above the reflex response depends on a synchronous volley of afferent impulses and a synchronous motor neurone discharge. Even minor dysfunctions of peripheral nerves cause either or both afferent or efferent impulses to become asynchronous and the tendon reflex is consequently lost.

Myasthenic disturbance at the neuromuscular junction usually causes no change in tendon reflexes though they may occasionally be temporarily diminished during periods of profound myasthenic weakness.

Lesions within the spinal canal may interrupt the connections between the sensory and motor limbs of the reflex arc and cause loss of reflexes. Absent tendon reflexes, caused for instance by the compression of a tumour, are valuable indications of the segmental level of a lesion involving the spinal cord. An uncommon reflex change, but one which is of precise localising significance, is the phenomenon of *inversion*. The transmission of a tendon tap stretches muscles other than that directly stimulated. In normal circumstances the slight contractions thus evoked are submerged by the major response mediated through the monosynaptic reflex arc. If, however, the arc is interrupted and the direct response is lost, the contractions in other muscles may become clinically apparent. This is sometimes seen after stretch of the biceps or brachioradialis tendons; no response is seen in the stretched muscle but the fingers flex. This is called inversion of the biceps or supinator jerk (usually both are involved together) and it is due to a lesion involving the neural structures arising from the fifth cervical segment of the cord. It should be emphasised that in these circumstances finger flexion occurs in the absence of response of the muscle stimulated. When finger flexion accompanies a brisk biceps or supinator jerk, it is simply an index of hyperreflexia. Less often seen is inversion of the triceps jerk. When this occurs, due to a lesion of the C.7 spinal segmental structures, tapping the tendon of triceps produces no contraction therein but causes a contraction of the biceps.

Other Abnormalities of Tendon Reflexes. In uncomplicated and isolated cerebellar lesions the tendon reflexes are described as pendular; the limb oscillates several times after the initial jerk, before settling again to its original position. This phenomenon is most easily detected in the knee jerk when the patient is seated on the edge of a bed with the feet swinging freely off the ground (Fig. 8.26). It occurs rarely and is not a sign of great clinical value.

Occasionally one will observe a fairly brisk contraction of a muscle in response to a tendon tap followed by very slow relaxation. This delayed relaxation, most often seen at the ankle, is a consistent and reliable sign of hypothyroidism.

SUPERFICIAL REFLEXES

These consist of muscular contractions evoked by cutaneous stimulation. The plantar response is the best known and most important. Others are the abdominal and cremasteric reflexes.

The Plantar Response. In normal people stimulation of the lateral border of the sole of the foot causes plantar flexion of the great toe and usually of the other toes. The stimulus should not cause injury but it should be of noxious character since this is a nociceptive reflex. However it should be remembered that the sole can be very sensitive. A blunted point such as the end of a car key produces an appropriate stimulus. A pin may be used but needs skilful handling to avoid lacerating the skin. The patient should lie supine with the legs extended. The stimulating point should be drawn along the lateral border of the foot from the heel towards the little toe (Fig. 8.27). This type of plantar stimulation in pathological circumstances gives rise to extension (dorsiflexion) of the great toe at the metatarsophalangeal joint. This is the sign described by Babinski who used a goose quill for its elicitation; it is often referred to by his name. The plantar response should, however, be described as 'flexor' when down going, or as 'extensor' when there is dorsiflexion since the use of Babinski's name often gives rise to the solecism of a 'flexor' Babinski response and to the ambiguity of an 'absent' Babinski response. Dorsiflexion of the great toe in response to plantar stimulation is often accompanied by other abnormal phenomena. There may be a sluggish spreading or 'fanning' of the other four toes. Sometimes an extensor plantar response is attended by simultaneous reflex contraction of the flexor muscles of the hip, knee and ankle. This is called the withdrawal response of which dorsiflexion of the great toe is a fragmentary manifestation.

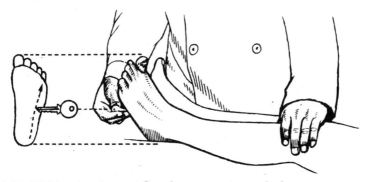

Fig. 8.27 Eliciting the plantar reflex. An extensor response is shown.

INTERPRETATION. There has for many years been extensive investigation into this reflex which is generally accepted as the most significant clinical neurological sign. Doubt has been cast on the precise physiological significance of an extensor plantar response and particularly on the pathways which subserve it. These physiological debates are of interest but they do not detract from the clinical value of the sign. For practical purposes an extensor plantar response indicates a lesion of the complex upper motor neurone system which runs from the motor cortex down to the spinal cord and which is called the pyramidal pathway. It has been averred that in some instances damage to this fibre system does not result in an extensor plantar response, and that occasionally an extensor plantar response is observed in the absence of damage to this system. However, such instances are rare, and ill understood, and there is no reason to abandon the clinical interpretation which regards the extensor plantar response as pathognomonic of a pyramidal lesion. Deductions made on this basis have proved themselves empirically over many decades.

The plantar reflex is normally evoked by stimulation of the sole in the area supplied by the first sacral sensory root. In cases wherein there are widespread and severe lesions of the corticospinal pathways the reflexogenic zone may be greatly enlarged. An extensor plantar response may then be produced by a number of techniques. Rubbing over the crest of the tibia, squeezing the Achilles tendon or a tap over the lateral malleolus may each induce dorsiflexion of the great toe. These signs have eponyms attached to them but are of little clinical importance since when they are obtainable the routine method of scraping the foot invariably elicits a significant response. One accessory sign of damage to the pyramidal pathways may sometimes be useful since it depends not on dorsiflexion of the great toe but on plantar flexion thereof. This is *Rossolimo's sign* where the distal phalanges of the toes are flicked into extension by the examiner's fingers and then allowed to fall back into their normal position. A positive response is a brisk plantar flexion of the great toe. This is a sign of pathological hyperreflexia and does not depend on the same mechanism as the extensor plantar response. It is the counterpart in the lower limbs of Hoffman's sign and can be helpful when an extensor plantar response cannot be obtained because of a concurrent lesion causing paralysis of extensor hallucis longus.

Occasionally no response is obtained to a nociceptive stimulus applied over the lateral border of the foot. Most commonly this is due to coldness of the feet and the test should be repeated after warming the patient. If no reflex movement is elicited despite warming there may be an impairment of cutaneous sensibility over the S.1 distribution or there may be paralysis of the long flexors or extensors of the great toe. The plantar response may be absent immediately after a complete transection of the spinal cord during the phase of spinal shock.

The Abdominal Reflexes. Normally a contraction of the muscles of the anterior abdominal wall is provoked when the skin of the abdomen is stroked or scratched. These responses are polysynaptic nociceptive reflexes. The patient should lie warm and relaxed in a supine position with a low pillow supporting the head. It is common to test four abdominal quadrants whose cutaneous nerves derive from the eighth to twelfth thoracic spinal segments. Upper and lower quadrants on each side are stimulated by drawing a pin towards the midline, parallel respectively with the costal margins and with the inguinal ligaments (Fig. 8.28). A pin is the

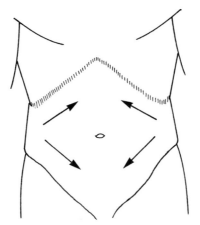

Fig. 8.28   Abdominal reflexes. Sites of stimuli for their elicitation.

implement which most effectively elicits abdominal reflexes but it should be used with care. It should be drawn lightly over the abdominal wall at an acute angle to the skin. If the pin be held vertically it frequently cuts the skin; there is never a need to penetrate the skin when testing the abdominal reflexes. If heavier pressure needs to be applied it is best to use instead a key or the end of the shaft of the tendon hammer.

INTERPRETATION. In most people the muscles underlying the area stimulated will contract briskly. However when the abdominal wall is lax in women who have borne many children and in obese patients the reflexes may be absent without there being any associated neural lesion. The abdominal reflexes may occasionally be lost because of impaired pain sensation in the skin or because of lower motor neurone lesions affecting the abdominal musculature. In most instances absence of responses in a young relaxed patient with good abdominal muscles strongly suggests an upper motor neurone lesion. The reflexes may be lost on one or both sides, reflecting unilateral or bilateral upper motor neurone involvement. While loss of abdominal reflexes is by no means invariable in upper motor neurone lesions, when multiple sclerosis damages upper motor neurones, the abdominal reflexes are consistently absent. Their loss is often a very early manifestation of upper motor neurone disruption in this disease. In upper motor neurone lesions due to motor neurone disease the abdominal reflexes are usually preserved. These empirical observations are sometimes useful in differential diagnosis, but they are not immutable laws and undue weight should not be attached to them. The pathophysiology underlying the differing vulnerability of the abdominal reflexes in different diseases is ill understood. Loss of abdominal cutaneous reflexes probably results only if other pathways, as well as the upper motor neurones, are interrupted and such widespread lesions are liable to occur in multiple sclerosis.

The Cremasteric Reflexes. These are sometimes tested in male patients. Stroking or scratching the inner aspect of the upper part of the thigh normally provokes an elevation of the testis on the same side. This reflex response may be lost as a result of an upper motor neurone lesion.

MISCELLANEOUS TESTS

Under this heading are included those tests which, although not carried out routinely, are often indicated and may yield most important information in special circumstances.

Signs of Meningeal Irritation

Inflammation of the meninges due to infection or blood in the subarachnoid space evokes a reflex spasm in the paravertebral muscles. In the cervical region this manifests itself by *neck rigidity* which impedes passive flexion of the neck. In any patient in whom meningitis or subarachnoid haemorrhage is a possibility neck flexion should be tested (Fig. 8.29). The neck initially should be slowly flexed but in the early stages of a meningeal reaction spasm may be more easily demonstrated if the neck is flexed abruptly. Normally the chin can be made to touch the chest without causing discomfort.

Meningeal irritation causing spasm in the lumbar region can be demonstrated by passive movements of the lower limbs (*Kernig's sign*). The patient lies supine with one leg extended; the leg to be tested is flexed at the hip and knee. Whilst the hip

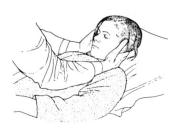

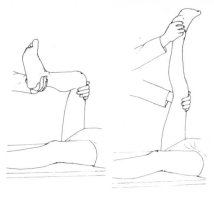

Fig. 8.29 Testing for meningeal irritation (neck rigidity).

Fig. 8.30 Testing for meningeal irritation (Kernig's test).

joint remains flexed the knee is extended as shown in Figure 8.30. When there is meningeal irritation involving the posterior roots in the lumbar area it will be impossible fully to extend the knee because of spasm in the hamstring muscles. Brudzinski's test is used in children (p. 398).

Signs of Nerve Root Irritation

When lumbar and sacral nerve roots are pressed upon by a prolapsed intervertebral disc, stretching of the sciatic nerve or the femoral nerve may give rise to pain. These nerve stretching tests are described on page 343.

Signs of Tetany

In tetany a low serum calcium (or ionised calcium) causes an increased excitability of nerves. Sensations of pins and needles in the hands, feet and round the mouth often precede painful muscle cramps. *Carpopedal spasm* is the characteristic finding. The hands spontaneously take up the position known as the *main d'accoucheur*, in which there is opposition of the thumb, extension of the interphalangeal and flexion

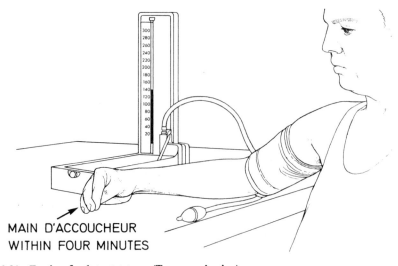

MAIN D'ACCOUCHEUR
WITHIN FOUR MINUTES

Fig. 8.31 Testing for latent tetany (Trousseau's sign).

of the metacarpophalangeal joints. In latent tetany the same position can be induced within four minutes by inflation of the sphygmomanometer cuff to a level above the systolic blood pressure — *Trousseau's sign* (Fig. 8.31). A tap over the facial nerve in front of the ear provokes a brisk momentary contraction of the facial muscles, pulling the mouth to that side in latent tetany, but also in some normal subjects — *Chvostek's sign.*

Signs Elicited by Palpation, Percussion and Auscultation

Palpation of the skull and of the spinous processes occasionally reveals local destructive lesions due to tumours or irregularities due to trauma. Percussion may elicit localised tenderness in the spinous processes overlying an epidural abscess.

Pulsation in the carotid arteries in the neck should be palpated and any asymmetry noted. The juxtaposition of the internal and external carotid arteries means that major lesion in the former may be disguised by normal pulsation in the latter. Auscultation of the neck may reveal a bruit due to stenosis in a carotid, vertebral or subclavian artery. To be significant such a murmur should be localised and not one conducted from the heart. Bruits may arise in internal or external carotids either on the side of a stenotic lesion or on the side opposite the narrowing because of increased flow in the other carotid system. Palpable or audible changes in the neck vessels may suggest a vascular cause for an intracranial lesion but precise anatomical interpretation of such abnormalities is often impossible.

A bruit which is audible over the skull or over the spine may on rare occasions be a most valuable sign. Aneurysms, particularly arteriovenous malformations, may produce murmurs which can be heard over the skull vault, or orbit, or, very rarely, over the spine. When clinical features suggest the presence of an arteriovenous anomaly a careful search for the characteristic continuous murmur should be made in quiet surroundings.

SUMMARY OF EXAMINATION OF THE NERVOUS SYSTEM

Intellect, Speech, Gait.

Cranial Nerves. 1. Sense of smell. 2. Ophthalmoscopy; visual acuity and fields. 3, 4, 6. Inspection, esp. lids and pupils; pupillary reflexes; ocular movements; nystagmus. 5. Facial sensation; corneal reflex; muscles of mastication; jaw jerk. 7. Facial movements; taste anterior $\frac{2}{3}$ tongue. 8. Hearing. 9. Sensation posterior $\frac{1}{3}$ tongue; gag reflex. 10. Phonation; movement of palate and pharynx. 11. Sternomastoid and trapezius muscles. 12. Inspection of tongue and its movements.

Motor System. Inspection of muscles; involuntary movements; tone; clonus; power; co-ordination; fine movements; dyspraxia.

Sensory System. Touch; pain; temperature; position and vibration senses; cortical sensory function.

Reflexes. Tendon and superficial.

Supplementary Tests. e.g. Tests for meningeal or nerve root irritation or tetany.

FURTHER INVESTIGATION

The clinical examination of the nervous system is an integral part of the general medical examination. Similarly, neurological investigations cannot be considered in isolation. In some instances a blood count which reveals a macrocytic anaemia may implicate vitamin B_{12} deficiency as the cause of spinal cord lesions. A leukaemic blood picture or glycosuria may suggest the aetiology of varied neurological pictures. These examples could be multiplied. They emphasise the frequent need to utilise supplementary tests other than those which directly explore the central nervous system in order to evaluate neurological problems.

The intelligent selection of appropriate investigations is based on the clinical picture and should always take account of the discomforts and dangers attendant upon the investigative techniques. In a few cases extreme clinical urgency will demand that the definitive test, even if painful, be performed immediately. In most instances it is wise to instigate those investigations which are least disturbing and only later to proceed to uncomfortable, hazardous or invasive tests.

Some tests which are occasionally indicated do no more than refine and supplement clinical examination; for example slit lamp examination of the eyes may reveal a brownish band at the limbus characteristic of Wilson's disease (p. 74).

Radiological Examination

Plain radiographs are important preliminary investigations in many neurological problems. A chest radiograph may reveal a bronchial carcinoma and hence explain a wide variety of metastatic and non-metastatic neural complications. Plain radiographs of the skull are indicated when the clinical picture is suggestive of an intracranial lesion. They may show erosions caused by tumours; thickening of the vault of the skull may be provoked by a subjacent meningioma. Lesions such as gliomas, tuberculomas and arteriovenous malformations may be delineated by abnormal calcification. Radiographs of the spine should be performed whenever a lesion of the cord or nerve roots is suspected. The vertebral bodies, the pedicles and the disc spaces may display abnormalities which would localise the site and suggest the cause of compression of the spinal cord.

More complex radiological investigation is discussed on pages 301 to 303.

The Cerebrospinal Fluid

An examination of cerebrospinal fluid (CSF) used to be almost a routine procedure in the investigation of neurological disorders. It still often provides information of value, but with the development of non-invasive methods of investigation the indications for its use are fewer. A lumbar puncture is essential when acute or chronic infection of the brain or meninges is suspected, and whenever subarachnoid haemorrhage is a possibility. It should usually be performed in patients suffering from multiple sclerosis or the Guillain-Barré syndrome. It is seldom of primary importance in the diagnosis of cerebral tumours or in the investigation of epilepsy. Lumbar puncture should not be carried out if there is a suspicion of raised intracranial pressure.

Note should be made of the appearance of the fluid. Normally clear and colourless, the CSF becomes turbid if it contains many cells. If blood-stained, the fluid should be collected in three successive tubes to differentiate between a traumatic puncture in which the later collections will be less contaminated, and a subarachnoid haemorrhage in which successive tubes will be uniformly red. Blood-stained fluid should also be centrifuged to see whether the supernatant fluid has a yellow tinge (xanthochromia). The CSF may also sometimes be yellowish in deeply jaundiced patients or when its protein content is much increased.

Laboratory examination of the CSF should include a cell count, estimation of the protein and glucose content and serological examination for syphilis. In appropriate circumstances microbiological studies, bacterial or viral, should be carried out.

Cell Count. The total number of cells and the different cellular components should be counted. Normal CSF contains less than five lymphocytes per cubic millimetre. In bacterial meningitis the cell count may rise to many hundreds or several thousands per cubic millimetre with a marked predominance of polymorphs. Lymphocytosis of moderate degree is found in tuberculous meningitis and viral meningitis, though in the initial stages of these conditions there also may be an increase in polymorphs. A slight to moderate rise in the lymphocyte count may be found in viral encephalitis, in active neurosyphilis and sometimes in multiple sclerosis.

Protein. The total protein content in normal CSF lies between 0.2 and 0.5 g/l. A moderate elevation of protein may be found in many intracranial diseases including acute infections, neurosyphilis, vascular lesions and many cases of cerebral tumour. Very high protein contents are found in the Guillain-Barré syndrome and when compression of the spinal cord blocks the CSF flow. A few systemic diseases, notably diabetes and hypothyroidism, may also be accompanied by a rise in CSF protein.

The total protein in most cases of multiple sclerosis is within normal limits, but the IgG level (normally 6 to 12% of the total protein) is significantly raised (greater than 20%) in approximately two-thirds of patients with multiple sclerosis whether or not the disease is active. The IgG is also increased (usually accompanied by a rise in total protein) in neurosyphilis, in sarcoidosis and in some disorders of connective tissue.

Glucose. The CSF normally contains between 2.2 and 4.5 mmol of glucose per litre (40 to 80 mg/100 ml). The CSF glucose is related to blood glucose being approximately 1.7 mmol per litre below the blood level. A high glucose content, therefore, may be found in diabetes. A marked reduction in CSF glucose is a feature of bacterial meningitis; in severe cases glucose may be absent. A moderate reduction in glucose is found in tuberculous and carcinomatous meningitis. The glucose content is usually normal in viral meningitis.

Serology. The Wasserman reaction, which is a complement fixation test, and the Venereal Disease Research Laboratories flocculation test are still often performed, but the most reliable routine test is the fluorescent treponema antibody test (FTA).

Microbiological Investigation. Whenever infection is suspected the CSF should be centrifuged and the deposit examined microscopically after Gram staining, and, if tuberculous meningitis is suspected, after Ziehl-Neelsen staining. Cultures should also be prepared from the CSF in cases of suspected infection and antibiotic sensitivities determined. Occasionally fungi and cryptococci are found in the CSF and the latter is best demonstrated by staining with Indian ink. If the initial bacteriological examination is negative, but the clinical suspicion of bacterial meningitis remains high, lumbar puncture should be repeated several times in order to identify the responsible organism.

In certain instances viruses may be cultured from the CSF, but often the diagnosis of viral infection depends on rising antibody titres found in paired sera rather than by isolation of the virus in the CSF.

Miscellaneous Tests. In certain situations, more specialised and refined examinations of the CSF may be carried out. For example in carcinomatous meningitis examination of a fresh CSF specimen after cyto-centrifugation may reveal malignant cells. In cases of severe meningitis antibiotic levels may be measured in the CSF as a guide to treatment. Amine metabolites can be measured in the CSF; homovanillic acid (HVA) content is usually low in patients suffering from parkinsonism.

INVESTIGATION IN RELATION TO SITE OF LESION

The choice of more sophisticated and specific investigations is determined by the site of neurological lesions.

Muscles and Peripheral Nerves

The investigation of primary diseases of muscle may require extensive biochemical testing. Of general applicability is the estimation of serum enzymes such as aldolase, lactic dehydrogenase and, most specifically, creatine phosphokinase whose concentrations reflect the rate and extent of muscle fibre disintegration.

Peripheral nerve disorders may also require a range of biochemical investigations such as vitamin assays, blood urea, urinary porphobilinogen and glucose tolerance tests to determine the primary cause.

Electromyography is useful in the investigation of disorders of muscles and also of peripheral nerves. It records muscle action potentials, using a needle electrode and an oscilloscope display system. This procedure will demonstrate denervation and differentiate neural from myopathic lesions. The estimation of conduction velocity in nerve trunks will gauge the extent of dysfunction in neuropathies and will define the site of localised compressions of peripheral nerves, as in the carpal tunnel.

Spinal Cord

Myelography is often required for the investigation of localised damage to the spinal cord and radiculography is used to outline abnormalities of the nerve roots. A radio-opaque dye is introduced into the subarachnoid space via a lumbar puncture needle. The dye is then manoeuvred along the spinal canal, by tilting the patient. Deformation of the column of dye will reveal compressive lesions and suggest their nature. A water soluble, non-ionic dye, metrizamide, is widely used. It gives high definition, outlines root pockets and is absorbed and excreted. It thus causes far fewer complications than myodil which is not absorbed.

Intracranial Disease

A wide variety of techniques is available for investigation of intracranial lesions; harmless, non-invasive tests should be employed first.

The Electroencephalogram (EEG). This records the electrical potentials of the brain after they are attenuated by passing through the skull and scalp. Potential changes are recorded simultaneously over several areas. Intracranial disease may cause normal electrical rhythms to be suppressed or more commonly, abnormal wave forms may be engendered. Such abnormalities may be generalised or localised. EEG abnormalities are more marked with acute lesions such as cerebral abscess than with slowly progressive or chronic lesions. Lesions within the substance of the brain such as gliomas produce more marked and earlier abnormalities than lesions such as meningiomas or angiomas lying outside the brain tissue. The EEG is more precise in its definition of lesions lying in the cerebral hemispheres than it is in lesions lying within the posterior fossa. The EEG will often reveal epileptic discharges but it alone cannot make a diagnosis of epilepsy.

Radionuclide Cerebral Scanning. This is an innocuous and useful investigation. An injected radioisotope (such as technetium) is often taken up differentially by diseased intracranial tissue compared to normal brain substance. Differing intensities of radio activities are recorded through the skull and abnormal areas mapped. In this way tumours, particularly meningiomas, can be localised and areas of infarction defined.

Computed Tomography. (CT scan). This radiographic technique detects and displays the differing X-ray densities of cranial structures. Computed absorption co-efficients of the cranial structures are translated in analogue form to a cathode ray tube where they are displayed as differing shades of grey. White and grey matter and the fluid filled spaces can be visualised and examined in much the same way as conventional radiographs. The sensitivity of the technique can be increased by the intravenous injection of a water-soluble contrast agent containing iodine which increases the absorption coefficient of some intracranial lesions. The technique is atraumatic, takes about half an hour and the patient is exposed to rather less radiation than that required for a conventional radiograph of the skull. It is an accurate and sensitive tool and, with contrast enhancement, will reveal the vast majority of cerebral tumours, cerebral haemorrhages, and abscesses and also cerebral atrophy (Fig. 8.32). It has reduced the need for arteriography and markedly reduced the demand for pneumoencephalography. However, it is not an infallible method of investigation. Small low-density lesions such as infarcts and some gliomas may be missed. Arteriovenous malformations, small subdural haematomas and intrinsic lesions in the brain stem may also be undetected.

Emission Computed Tomography. Emission computed axial tomography (ECAT), one form of which is position emission tomography (PET), is a technique of imaging in which technetium-labelled radionuclides are injected intravenously and the emitted radiation from the brain is recorded by scintillation detectors. As with radiation transmission computed tomography, (CT scanning), a computer is used in order to construct a two dimensional image of the brain. The technique is

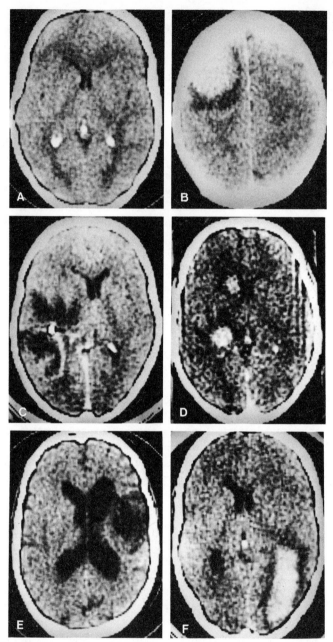

Fig. 8.32 CT scanning as a diagnostic aid. (A) Normal, showing ventricles, choroid plexuses and pineal gland. (B) Meningioma. (C) Tumour with metallic body at biopsy site. (D) Metastases. (E) Infarct with dilated ventricles and sulci due to cerebral atrophy. (F) Cerebral haemorrhage. (*Courtesy of Dr A. A. Donaldson*).

highly sensitive and exposes patients to much less radiation than conventional CT scanning. It can reveal morphological abnormalities and can also define changes in function preceding structural alterations, as in vascular lesions. The equipment is costly and used primarily for research.

Nuclear Magnetic Resonance (NMR) Imaging. This is a procedure which utilises the magnetic properties of hydrogen nuclei within the brain. The brain is exposed to a magnetic field and the hydrogen nuclei within it are excited by radio frequency radiation and the signals thus produced are detected and computed. The brain is scanned to produce images of brain slices similar to those of conventional CT scanning.

Since grey matter contains much more water (and hydrogen nuclei) than white matter this technique vividly differentiates grey and white matter. It produces imaging of the posterior fossa which is superior to that of conventional CT scanning. As well as revealing space occupying lesions it will demonstrate small lesions within white matter such as those in multiple sclerosis (Fig. 8.33). It will be particularly valuable in the diagnosis of demyelinating diseases and in those metabolic and toxic conditions where demyelination is a feature.

Cerebral Angiography. With the advent of the CT scan, angiography is rarely the primary investigation in cases of cerebral tumour. However, it still has a place in defining precise anatomy when a mass has been demonstrated on the CT scan and operation is contemplated. It is also the appropriate investigation when clinical signs point to a lesion of a blood vessel such as an aneurysm or stenosis. Carotid arteriography and less often vertebral arteriography are performed. These investigations are uncomfortable and potentially hazardous and should be performed only if there are appropriate indications.

Pneumoencephalography. This procedure is now rarely performed. Air, introduced into the lumbar subarachnoid space, rises into the basal cisterns and into the ventricles where it can show displacement due to tumour, or dilatation due to hydrocephalus or cerebral atrophy. Pneumoencephalography should not be performed if intracranial pressure is raised. It is frequently followed by severe headache for several days.

Echoencephalography. This procedure utilises the reflection of a beam of ultrasound from the mid-line structures of the brain. It is subject to many inaccuracies and with the advent of more precise imaging techniques is now rarely employed.

THE METHODS IN PRACTICE

Three examples have been chosen. Two of these are general and one is highly specific. The diagnostic process is first discussed and then the examination of the unconscious patient is described. Finally an account is given of the diagnosis of brain death.

1. THE DIAGNOSTIC PROCESS

The completion of the neurological examination is followed by the correlation and interpretation of all the available information in order to reach a diagnosis. This must be based on logical thought processes. There are a number of shorthand

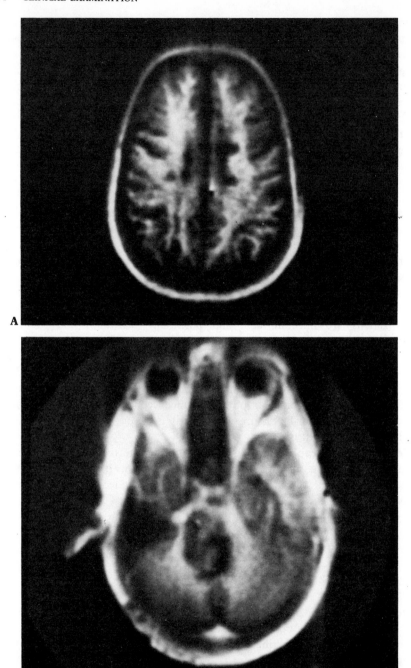

Fig. 8.33   NMR imaging as a diagnostic aid. This technique (T_1 dependent) differentiates much more clearly between grey and white matter than does CT, as is demonstrated in (A), a brain scan, just above the ventricles, which also shows well circumscribed, centrally placed, filling defects in the white matter due to multiple sclerosis. (B) Scan of the posterior fossa showing a large glioma of the pons. (*Courtesy of Professor R. E. Steiner*).

formulae in neurology as for instance the equation of dissociated anaesthesia with a diagnosis of syringomyelia, the attribution of bilateral clawing of hands and feet to peroneal muscular atrophy, the diagnosis of motor neurone disease because of obvious fasciculation and the labelling of any episode of weakness or paraesthesiae in a young adult as multiple sclerosis. There is, of course, an expression of meretricious statistical probability in each of these assertions; diagnoses based on them will often be correct. But they are shibboleths. A quick gamble, even at favourable odds, is not a sound prelude to the best possible management of a patient. The diagnostic formulation should comprise a careful and orderly assessment of the nature of the patient's dysfunction. The neural systems and pathways damaged are then adduced. Next the distribution of lesions is defined Finally the most likely pathological diagnosis is inferred. In other words what is disturbed, where and why?

(i) Disturbance of Function

The patient complains of the end results of disordered physiological functions whose nature is reflected in the abnormal signs revealed during the examination. This process is exemplified in the analysis of motor disturbances on pages 276 and 277. The signs found are correlated by the clinician so that the neural structures disrupted can be identified. The combination of signs attributable to lesions of different parts and paths of the nervous system need to be understood and memorised.

Upper Motor Neurone (pyramidal tract) Lesions. These cause (1) weakness or paralysis of movement; (2) increase of tone of 'clasp-knife' type; (3) increased amplitude of tendon reflexes; (4) diminution of abdominal reflexes; (5) an extensor plantar response.

Lower Motor Neurone Lesions. These give rise to (1) weakness or paralysis of muscles; (2) wasting of muscles; (3) there may be fasciculation in the involved muscles; (4) if many muscles in a limb are wasted, tone will be reduced therein; (5) if affected muscles subserve tendon reflexes, these will be diminished or absent.

Cerebellar Lesions. Damage to the posterior lobe of the cerebellum or of its connections with the brain stem are accompanied by (1) ataxia of gait; (2) intention tremor of limbs; (3) jerking nystagmus; (4) dysarthria of staccato or scanning type; (5) dysmetria and past pointing; (6) impaired alternating movements; (7) hypotonia and pendular tendon reflexes; (8) occasionally, smooth movements may be broken up into their constituent parts producing jerking, marionette-like, decomposition of movements.

Generalised Polyneuropathies. These often cause (1) diminution of superficial sensation affecting the distal aspect of limbs over 'stocking' and 'glove' distributions; (2) wasting and weakness of distal limb musculature; (3) early loss of tendon reflexes.

Spinal or Cranial Nerve Damage. This results in combinations of signs which depend on the area of supply of the individual nerves.

Muscles. Primary affections of muscle fibres lead to wasting and weakness of muscles usually (but not invariably) in the proximal parts of limbs. Fatty infiltration of muscle may cause an apparent increase in size of the affected muscles. Reflexes are preserved until muscle wasting is very marked.

Sensory Tracts. Interruption of *dorsal columns* causes (1) ataxia of gait and limb movements aggravated by eye closure; (2) impaired position sense; (3) diminished appreciation of vibration. Lesions of the *spinothalamic* system cause impairment of pain and temperature sensation.

It is emphasised that these combinations of signs are those of fully developed pictures. Every abnormality is not to be expected in every case and the clinician must be prepared to deduce that a tract has been damaged when incomplete patterns of signs have been demonstrated.

(ii) Distribution of Lesions

The identification of damaged neural structures is followed by the definition of the site or sites of their involvement.

Single Lesions. All the observed signs may be due to a localised lesion affecting adjacent structures.

Impairment of specialised functions of the *cerebral cortex* result in dementia, dysphasia, apraxia, astereognosis and other forms of agnosia. Upper motor neurone lesions at the cortical level cause signs similar to those due to interruption of the pyramidal tract at more caudal sites but since the upper motor neurones are spread over a wide area in the cortex, lesions here typically affect only part of the opposite side of the body. A paresis confined to one limb (monoplegia) or to one side of the face is likelier than a hemiplegia. Bilateral upper motor neurone signs result from solitary cortical lesions only in the rare instance of a parasagittal affection. Lesions here, such as a meningioma, may impinge on both hemispheres on the neurones which lie close together on each side of the sagittal plane and which supply the legs. The demonstration of cortical abnormalities will often enable the extent of a lesion to be mapped out fairly precisely.

Localisation within the *cerebral hemispheres* is helped if a pattern of visual deficit has been elucidated; thus an upper quadrantic homonymous hemianopia points to a lesion in the temporal lobe on the side opposite the field defect (Fig. 8.2).

A profound hemiplegia equally affecting face, arm and leg, associated with loss of sensation of all modalities on the paralysed side suggests a lesion affecting the *internal capsule* where the upper motor neurone and sensory pathways are packed closely together.

Lesions of the *brain stem* are characterised by ipsilateral impairment of one or more cranial nerves with concurrent contralateral affection of one or more long tracts usually the upper motor neurones. Which cranial nerves are implicated will depend on which part of the brain stem is affected. A midbrain lesion is suggested if there is a third nerve palsy on one side and signs of upper motor neurone involvement on the other. Pontine damage is indicated by sixth and seventh nerve signs accompanied by contralateral upper motor neurone signs. Occasionally other tracts such as the spinothalamic pathway are interrupted. Examples of lesions involving the midbrain, pons and medulla are given in Figures 8.34, 8.35 and 8.36.

Spinal cord damage is localised by correlating motor, sensory and reflex changes.

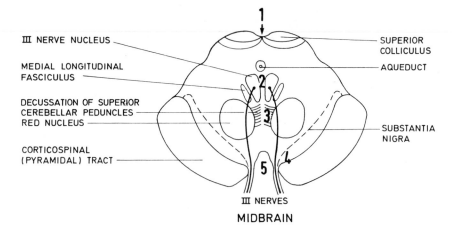

MIDBRAIN

Fig. 8.34 Lesions of midbrain. Lesions at (1), e.g. pressure from a pineal tumour, cause weakness of upward gaze which may first be manifest as nystagmus in a vertical plane. Lesions at (2) produce bilateral, partial lesions of the third nerve and anterior internuclear ophthalmoplegia, p. 250, (damage to medial longitudinal fasciculus). Lesions at (3) cause ipsilateral third nerve palsy and contralateral cerebellar signs (damage to decussating cerebellar peduncles) and/or tremors and athetoid movements (damage to red nucleus). Lesions at (4) cause ipsilateral third nerve signs and contralateral pyramidal involvement. Lesions at (5) cause bilateral third nerve palsy and bilateral pyramidal signs.

Lesions which affect the midbrain immediately below this level may also implicate the fourth nerve.

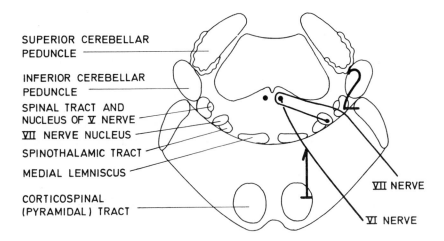

Fig. 8.35 Lesions of the pons. Lesions at (1), e.g. haemorrhage, cause ipsilateral sixth and/or seventh nerve palsies and contralateral pyramidal signs. Lesions at (2), e.g. basilar thrombosis, cause ataxia on the side of the lesion (damage to the cerebellar peduncles). There may also be impaired sensation on the ipsilateral side of the face (spinal tract and nucleus of fifth nerve) and on the contralateral side of the body (spinothalamic tract) and occasionally a seventh nerve lesion. Lesions in the pons often cause posterior internuclear ophthalmoplegia (p. 250) and ataxic nystagmus.

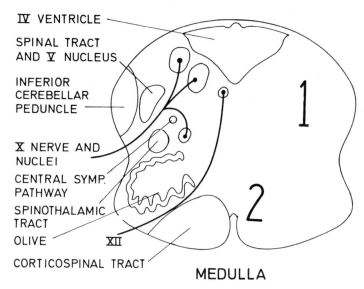

Fig. 8.36   Lesions of the medulla. Lesions affecting lateral medulla (1), e.g. thrombosis of posterior inferior cerebellar artery, cause ataxia and intention tremor on ipsilateral side, jerking nystagmus on turning eyes to the side of the lesion (damage to the spinocerebellar tract in the inferior cerebellar peduncle); analgesia on ipsilateral side of face and contralateral limbs (affection of spinal tract of fifth nerve and the lateral spinothalamic tract); Horner's syndrome (involvement of the central sympathetic pathway); dysphonia, dysphagia and weakness of soft palate and paralysis of vocal cords on the side of the lesion (damage to the tenth nerve).

Lesions affecting the paramedian area (2), e.g. infarction, cause a crossed paralysis — wasting and fasciculation of ipsilateral side of tongue (damage to twelfth nerve) and contralateral pyramidal signs.

Upper motor neurone signs arising from cord lesions are often, but by no means always, bilateral. The location of the site of upper motor neurone lesions can be made only very roughly on the basis of upper motor neurone signs alone; if they are present in the arms then the lesion must be above the fifth cervical segment; if the abdominal reflexes are all lost then a segment above the eighth thoracic must be implicated; signs in the legs indicate a lesion above the conus medullaris.

The site of upper motor neurone damage is localised much more precisely if the offending lesion also involves the anterior horn cells or motor roots. Lower motor neurone signs, with wasting in a segmental distribution define the cord lesion accurately. Sensory signs may help to delineate the position of cord lesions; thus impairment of sensation over a segmental dermatome will indicate the level of a lesion on occasion. Interruption of sensory tracts may give rise to a level of sensory loss which sometimes corresponds to the site of the spinal lesion but often extends only to a more caudal level (p. 287). Spinal cord lesions disrupt reflex arcs and loss of tendon reflexes will reflect the segments which have been damaged.

Often the segmental level and the cross sectional areas of a spinal cord lesion may be gauged (Fig. 8.37). Below a hemisection of the cord on the ipsilateral side there will be found (1) upper motor neurone signs, (2) impaired position and vibration senses, (3) signs of vasomotor disturbance. On the contralateral side there will be reduced sensation to pain and temperature. This composite picture is called the *Brown-Séquard syndrome.*

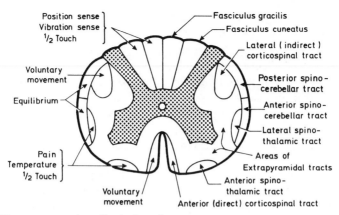

Position sense ⎤
Vibration sense ⎬
½ Touch ⎦

Fasciculus gracilis

Fasciculus cuneatus

Lateral (indirect)
corticospinal tract

Voluntary
movement

Posterior spino-
cerebellar tract

Equilibrium

Anterior spino-
cerebellar tract

Lateral spino-
thalamic tract

Pain ⎤
Temperature ⎬
½ Touch ⎦

Areas of
Extrapyramidal tracts

Anterior spino-
thalamic tract

Voluntary
movement

Anterior (direct) corticospinal tract

Fig. 8.37   Transverse section of spinal cord.

Multiple Lesions. The analysis of a patient's signs may show that they cannot be explained on the basis of a single lesion. Two or more separated, *discrete lesions* may be defined, as for instance when lesions in optic nerves are found concurrently with evidence of spinal cord damage in multiple sclerosis.

Lesions may be systematised, i.e. similar types of fibres or cells may be affected in different parts of the nervous system. A symmetrical polyneuropathy is a systematised affection of peripheral nerves. Damage may be confined to groups of upper and lower motor neurones as in motor neurone disease or to dorsal root ganglion cells as in one form of carcinomatous neuropathy. Spinal tracts may be selectively damaged, singly or in combination as when dorsal and lateral columns are disrupted by vitamin B_{12} deficiency.

Diffuse damage may be demonstrated when disorders affect wide areas of grey and white matter traversing structural and functional boundaries. Thus syphilis may cause a generalised loss of cortical neurones; it may interrupt the central prolongations of dorsal root ganglion cells and hence cause wasting of the dorsal columns; it may damage the pyramidal and extrapyramidal motor systems and may cause transverse cord lesions and cranial nerve palsies. All of these disturbances do not present concurrently but combinations of several such lesions are commonly found in the same patient. Repetitive head injuries also cause randomised, diffuse cerebral affection which results in the dementia, cerebellar ataxia and parkinsonism of the 'punch-drunk' state. The recognition of the patterns of neural lesions, whether single or multiple and, if multiple, whether discrete, systematised or diffuse, provides part of the information needed to make the final aetiological and pathological diagnosis.

(iii) Pathological Diagnosis

The most efficient prediction of the pathological process requires the integration of all the information gained from the patient's history, the general medical examination, and the neurological examination.

In the first instance the course of the development of the illness is reviewed and interpreted in order to estimate the general nature of the neural lesion. More specific clues to aetiology may be contained in the history. The story of an antecedent head injury in an elderly patient with a progressive intracranial lesion may suggest the likelihood of a subdural haematoma. A previous history of gonorrhoea or of a primary chancre may point to a diagnosis of neurosyphilis. A family history of epilepsy, muscle disease or ataxia may clarify the nature of a patient's illness. Circumstantial evidence from the general medical examination may indicate that the neural lesion is due to the same process which involves other systems. Thus evidence of peripheral vascular disease or of a cardiac arrhythmia might imply that a cerebral lesion was of vascular nature. Clinical evidence of anaemia and a smooth tongue would implicate B_{12} deficiency as the likely cause of a myelopathy.

Finally the nature and distribution of neurological signs might inferentially suggest the probabilities of some causal lesions and help to exclude others. If a patient has signs of intracranial damage together with papilloedema then a space occupying lesion, such as a tumour, is likely. The reflex changes of the Argyll Robertson pupil have been found occasionally in patients with midbrain encephalitis or tumours, but their presence, in company with neurological deficit of almost any type, should suggest syphilis as the probable diagnosis. Patients with marked neurological abnormalities, particularly drowsiness and nystagmus, which disappear after a period in hospital may well be suffering from intoxication by either alcohol or drugs.

If the patient with neurological disease is approached in this manner it is often possible to make a firm diagnosis on clinical grounds alone. On those occasions when the information is insufficient for a confident inference to be drawn the probable causes may be deduced and a rational scheme of investigation can be designed. Many neurological investigations cause discomfort and some are hazardous and they should be performed only if they are essential in order to define potentially curable lesions. There is no justification for subjecting patients to angiography or lumbar puncture as a substitute for an adequate clinical examination.

Conclusion. The clinical examination of the nervous system is a medical technique of precision and elegance which can provide a recurrent intellectual stimulus to the clinician and more importantly it is an essential prerequisite to the proper and efficient management of patients.

2. THE EXAMINATION OF THE UNCONSCIOUS PATIENT

The usual orderly and logical approach of history taking, followed by examination and leading to a diagnosis, must be abandoned if the patient's conscious level demands it. Before making any attempt to examine an unconscious patient any inadequacy of the respiratory or circulatory function should be rectified. If circumstances suggest even the remote possibility of hypoglycaemia, glucose should be given intravenously. These measures may be life saving, or may minimise cerebral damage.

After dealing with these overriding preliminaries the diagnostic process can begin. Impaired consciousness is due either to diffuse lesions of the hemispheres or to malfunction of the central structures in the brain stem. Five categories of disease may cause these disturbances:

1. Epilepsy.
2. Impairment of oxygenation or blood supply to cerebral structures.
3. Large supratentorial lesions causing tentorial herniation, and secondary damage to the brain stem.
4. Lesions which impinge directly on the central core of the brain stem.
5. Metabolic diseases which diffusely depress brain function.

In principle the problems of causation can thus be usefully classified. In practice, however, the possible diagnoses are legion, ranging from such common causes as trauma, epilepsy, drug or alcohol intoxication and cerebrovascular disease to rarities like water intoxication and (in Britain) heat stroke. Other conditions like diabetes, hypoglycaemia, cerebral tumours and infections, cardiorespiratory, hepatic and renal failure also need to be considered. This list is far from exhaustive but it indicates that disease of almost any system may impair consciousness. It is therefore essential to narrow down the possibilities rapidly.

History. Even though the patient cannot give a history, an account of the circumstances and development of the unconscious state should, if feasible, be obtained from relatives or other witnesses, or second-hand from the police or ambulance drivers. Enquiry may reveal a history of trauma or of drug ingestion which will make the diagnosis clear. The story of an abrupt loss of consciousness may suggest such possibilities as epilepsy or a cardiovascular lesion, whilst a history of headache, confusion and drowsiness gradually deepening over days or weeks into coma is a pointer to such possibilities as a cerebral tumour of infection, or a chronic subdural haematoma.

Information about the patient's past medical history should be sought from any available source including the patient's family doctor. A history of previous fits, diabetes, cardiovascular disease, hepatic, renal or endocrine lesions may indicate the likely diagnoses.

General Observation. The most important aspect of the examination is a critical observation of the patient. Much may be learnt by looking, listening and smelling.

An unkempt and dirty patient may have become so because of addiction to drugs or alcohol, or because of long standing psychiatric or intracerebral disturbance. Marks of recent injury, particularly to the head, should be observed. External laceration and bleeding will be obvious, but closer inspection may reveal blood or CSF in the nostrils or ears from a fractured skull.

The skin should be inspected carefully. Cyanosis, anaemia, polycythaemia or pigmentation may indicate possible causative factors. Spider telangiectasia may point to long standing alcoholism. Needle punctures may be due to injections of insulin or drugs of addiction. In the latter case the marks will be concentrated around veins, some of which may be thrombosed. Sweating may be profuse in hypoglycaemic coma and diminished in hyperglycaemia.

The pattern of respiration should be watched and heard. Deep regular breathing occurs in postictal states and when rapid may be due to metabolic acidosis. Shallow, rapid respirations are a feature of barbiturate intoxication. Cheyne-Stokes rhythm may result from cardiorespiratory disease, raised intracranial pressure or brain stem lesions. A disorganized irregular pattern is a sign of severe damage to the medulla.

The patient's breath may be revealing. The smell of alcohol may suggest that this has caused unconsciousness. It should be remembered, however, that patients who have been drinking may also have sustained a head injury, a myocardial infarction or any of a variety of other lesions. The smell of acetone may be the result of diabetic ketoacidosis. A characteristic fetid breath may indicate liver failure.

Assessment of Consciousness. For clinical purposes consciousness is defined as the patient's awareness of, and response and reaction to, the environment. Degrees of impairment vary and can be graded into numerical levels of consciousness, e.g. deep coma (grade 4), semicomatose state (grade 3), stuporous patients (grade 2), and drowsy or somnolent patients (grade 1). It is now recognised that the best method of assessment of impaired consciousness is the ranking of behavioural responses by the Glasgow Coma Scale. Motor response, verbal response and eye opening are evaluated independently of each other. The responses may be graded numerically (in parentheses below).

Motor response. Appropriate motor responses to commands are the best response possible (6).

If commands are not obeyed then painful stimuli are applied. Responses in the arm are most useful and firm pressure applied to the nail bed with a pencil pressed on a finger nail is a suitable initial stimulus. Painful stimulation by pinching is then applied to all four limbs, the trunk and the head and neck. The patient may attempt to pull the examiner's hand away (5). Painful stimuli at several sites may cause the limb to move away from the pain. This is called a localising response (4).

A flexor response varies from rapid withdrawal with abduction of the shoulder to an assumption of a hemiplegic posture with adduction of the shoulder (3).

Extensor posturing is the term used for adduction and internal rotation of the shoulder with pronation of the forearm in response to a painful stimulus (2). No response indicates the most severe form of impairment (1).

There may be differences between the responsiveness of the arm on one side and that on the other because of focal cerebral lesions. For the purposes of assessing the degree of altered consciousness, the best response that can be obtained during a given period of examination should be recorded.

Verbal Responses. The patient's speech is assessed. The highest ranked response applies to the patients who converse normally and know who and where they are (5).

Confused speech is used to describe the situation where patients can respond to questions but their responses indicate confusion (4).

Inappropriate speech is used to describe the speech of patients who use intelligible words but in a random, exclamatory manner. Continued verbal interchange between the examiner and patient is impossible (3).

Incomprehensible speech refers to unintelligible noises made by the patient (2). The patient may be silent (1).

Eye Opening. Spontaneous eye opening is scored highest in this aspect of behavioural assessment. It implies normal opening of the eyes with normal arousal (4). Opening of the eyes in response to the examiner's speech is the next lower rank (3). Eye opening in response to pain should be tested by painful stimuli applied to the limbs (2). The patient may not open the eyes at all (1).

PROCEDURE. Each of these parameters should be measured repetitively at intervals of a half to two hours, depending on the severity of the clinical situation.

Sometimes because of trauma, one or other of the responses cannot be assessed but the examination should be as complete as possible on each occasion.

The results of serial examinations can be plotted on a simple chart so that progress can be easily seen. Alternatively the ranks in the various categories can be added together. It has been shown that this form of assessment is reproducible and gives a valuable guide to prognosis. Of those patients with a total score of 4 or less, nearly a half will die. Death is rare in those with a score of 13 or more.

Physical Examination. A clinical examination of all systems should be completed. Neurological assessment will, of necessity, be constrained in comatose patients. Higher functions, speech and gait obviously cannot be tested; examination of the cranial nerves is restricted and sensory testing comprises only the crude responses to stimuli outlined above. Particular attention is given to examination of the optic nerve head and to reflex activity. Despite these limitations it is often possible to localise neurological lesions.

Conclusion. With a methodical approach a firm diagnosis can often be made but, if not, a plan of investigation and management can be formulated in the light of clinical findings.

3. THE DIAGNOSIS OF BRAIN DEATH

It may seem macabre and unnecessary to discuss the diagnosis of death but it has important ethical and legal implications. It has long been accepted that death has occurred when respiration and circulation have ceased. It is now possible to maintain these functions artificially for long periods. It is also generally agreed that permanent cessation of brain function constitutes death and criteria have been established which usually enable this diagnosis to be made with confidence. The need for decision will arise in deeply comatose patients in whom curable causes of coma have been excluded.

Examination. The brain stem reflexes are carefully tested and should be absent. The pupils are unresponsive to bright light, fixed either in wide dilatation or in the mid-position (approximately 5 mm in diameter). The corneal reflex is absent. Twenty ml of ice cold water is slowly injected into each external auditory meatus in turn. If no eye movement occurs the vestibuloocular reflexes are absent. The gag and cough reflexes are absent. The patient should show no spontaneous movement nor any reaction to the environment. Spinal reflex activity, though usually absent, may be preserved, but this does not constitute evidence of persisting cerebral function. Usually the patient is hypotonic.

No spontaneous respiration occurs if the patient is removed from a mechanical ventilator long enough to ensure that arterial carbon dioxide rises above the threshold for stimulating respiration. Blood gases should be measured to ensure that this level (6.6 k Pa; 50 mmHg) has been achieved.

Electroencephalography is not an essential prerequisite for the diagnosis of brain death, but if available it can provide supporting evidence thereof. The EEG shows no sign of any electrical activity of cerebral origin in recordings made at high amplification.

It is customary to repeat the testing after an interval, usually a day later. If any doubt still remains then further examinations should be made in succeeding days.

Conclusion. Brain death should be diagnosed only after consultation between two medical practitioners who are experts in the field. One at least should be a consultant and the other a consultant or senior registrar. Each should establish that the pre-conditions noted above — a deeply comatose patient in whom curable causes of coma have been excluded — have been met before testing is carried out. The length of time before the pre-conditions can be satisfied varies. It is rarely less than twenty-four hours, and may be as long as several days.

The two doctors concerned may carry out the test separately or together. If the tests, on the first occasion, confirm brain death they should none the less be repeated. The duration of the interval between tests varies but it should allow adequate time for explanation to be given to relatives and friends of the patient.

REFERENCE

Macleod J (ed) Davidson's principles and practice of medicine, 13th edn. Churchill Livingstone, Edinburgh

9. The Locomotor System

And so, from hour to hour, we ripe and ripe,
And then, from hour to hour, we rot and rot;
And thereby hangs a tale.

Shakespeare, *As You Like It*

Examination of the locomotor system is often only a part of the assessment of a patient with other complaints. Approached in this way it is not difficult to confirm that all is well. It is necessary only to determine that normal posture and a full painless controlled range of active movements are present. An awareness that posture and the normal range of movement change throughout life is an important point, well taken by Touchstone in *As You Like It*. However, where the general examination reveals an abnormality or when the patient's symptoms indicate involvement of the locomotor system, a more detailed study of the affected area is required. In the first part of this chapter a simple but comprehensive method is set out which can be incorporated with the routine physical examination. This is designed to achieve a rapid assessment of the patient, indicating which region or regions require more detailed review should any abnormality be found.

The second part of the chapter deals with the detailed examination of the various regions. The junior student should initially limit study to Part 1 of this chapter and thereafter refer to the regional examination in Part 2 as specific problems arise.

Part I GENERAL EXAMINATION

THE HISTORY

PAIN PATTERNS IN LOCOMOTOR DISORDERS

Pain, the principal symptom of lesions involving the locomotor system, should be analysed as described on page 30. It often has a characteristic pattern in time or in relation to certain activities. This is frequently so clear that the diagnosis can be made from the history alone, and indeed must be when the clinical signs are few or absent, as may occur, for example, in the carpal tunnel syndrome.

The pattern of complaints can be delineated by taking the patient through a typical day. The following questions cover most activities without suggesting any replies. How do you feel on rising and dressing? How long can you remain comfortably on your feet? How far can you walk? (It is useful to refer to a well-

315

known local thoroughfare to estimate distance. In Edinburgh we are fortunate in having Princes Street as our 'measured mile'.) How long can you sit in comfort? How do you feel at the end of the day? How do you sleep? What makes the pain worse? What makes the pain better?

This routine also gives an estimate of the patient's abilities which can be compared with the findings at a later date. When organic disease is present a consistent story unfolds in contrast to the vague indifference of the hysteric and the aggressive resentment of the malingerer who fears too detailed interrogation.

The following notes provide a guide to the characteristic features of pain encountered in the locomotor system.

Traumatic Lesions

Sprained Ligaments. After the initial acute phase when pain may be severe and constant, pain occurs only with movement which stretches the damaged structure and is relieved when the ligament is relaxed.

Chronic Strain of Ligaments. In weight-bearing ligaments, in the back or the foot for example, the patient is most comfortable when rising in the morning. As the day goes on the supporting muscles tire and an aching pain develops which is relieved by rest.

Fracture. The student must be familiar with all the signs and symptoms of a fracture but only three are present in all fractures—pain, local tenderness, and interference with function to a greater or lesser degree. Crepitus must never be elicited in the conscious patient. Pain occurs on any movement if the fracture is not impacted.

Inflammatory Lesions

Acute Lesions. The pain steadily increases, even at rest, is throbbing in character, and the patient becomes ill and febrile, especially if there is formation of pus and the building up of tension in a structure such as a joint or the bone marrow. Remissions of pain and fever occur if pus escapes. When a joint is involved, all movement is inhibited by protective spasm of the controlling muscles. Any attempted movement, active or passive, causes pain. If the patient sleeps deeply, this spasm may relax and the patient wakens with a characteristic cry as some movement occurs causing pain. When there is infection in bone near a joint, movement of that joint may be inhibited by spasm. Gentle examination, however, will demonstrate that a small range of movement is present. In infants, localising signs are less easy to discover but immobility of the affected part is commonly present, often accompanied by irritability, crying and vomiting.

Chronic Lesions. The features are similar but more prolonged than in acute inflammation and the local and general reactions are less severe. Some movement will still be possible in an early low grade infection of a joint. In rheumatoid arthritis pain and stiffness are characteristically worse in the morning. The patient may take several hours to 'get going'.

Degenerative Lesions

Osteoarthrosis. This term indicates 'wear and tear' whereas '*osteoarthritis*' infers inflammation. Joints so affected are stiff and difficult to move after disuse, but move more freely with use. Thus pain and stiffness after rest, relieved by activity but recurring as the patient tires, are characteristic of osteoarthrosis. This pain is often not immediately relieved by rest and the patient may have difficulty in settling comfortably.

Prolapsed Intervertebral Disc. The pattern of pain may be spread over years. Before the acute episode there is frequently a period of vague aches and pains, often accepted by the patient as a normal reaction to activity. An acute episode occurs when bending or lifting, or on the day following such activities, or with no discernible cause. The pain subsides with rest, but may take several weeks to disappear. Thereafter periods of comfort are interspersed with major or minor episodes of pain. Gradually this characteristically episodic pattern merges into the pattern of osteoarthrosis.

Ischaemia. Intermittent claudication is described on page 135.

Spinal Stenosis. Narrowing of the spinal canal or neural foramina, usually caused by degenerative changes, can result in back pain with radiation to the legs. In the latter site the pattern is similar to that of intermittent claudication in its relation to activity.

The pain of intermittent claudication is however localised to the muscle group involved in the leg, is cramp-like and not accompanied by numbness or tingling. It is relieved by standing still. The pain of spinal stenosis is often diffuse, accompanied by tingling and numbness and by malfunction of the muscles, all of which the patient finds difficult to describe. The symptoms increase with standing and walking and are relieved only by stooping, sitting or lying down.

Instability. Unstable lesions, for example spondylolisthesis, are associated with increasing pain as the day goes on. After rest the muscles and ligaments are relaxed. As the supporting muscles tire the related ligaments stretch and pain increases. The pain is aggravated by standing, returning to the erect posture from stooping and by active, especially bilateral, straight leg raising.

Tumours

With the possible exception of osteoid osteoma, benign tumours do not cause pain unless by pressure on neighbouring structures. Pain is not an invariable feature of malignant tumours but, when present, is not related to any special activity, is not relieved by rest and may even be worse at night driving the patient from bed. A pathological fracture may occur as a result of minor trauma and cause sudden acute pain.

Secondary Gain or 'Compensation' Pain

There is an astonishing constancy in the history and pattern of pain associated with claims for compensation. The patient can recall the accident in minute detail, including the date and time almost to a second, even if it occurred years before. The accident was always some other agent's fault. The pain is constant with dramatic exacerbations, always vividly described. It shows no sign of improving and may even be worsening. The patient remains off work and is often accompanied by the spouse or some other supporter who will testify to the worrying amounts of analgesics which has to be consumed to relieve the pain.

THE PHYSICAL EXAMINATION

There are three main components, namely the examination of (1) posture, (2) gait, and (3) limbs and spine. The ideal arrangement is that the patient is observed walking into the consulting-room, thus allowing an early assessment of posture and gait. Good lighting and adequate space are essential. The examination couch should not lie alongside a wall. It must be accessible from both sides and there must be no obstacle preventing a full range of movements of the patient's limbs.

1. Posture

For adequate assessment the patient should be able to stand and walk. Where this is not possible some idea of the posture can be gained by examination of the patient in the supine and prone positions. Normal posture varies from age to age, passing through a cycle of change as we 'ripe and rot' (Fig. 9.1). *In utero*, and for a short time after birth, there is a generalised dorsal convexity of the spine, or *kyphosis*. When the child holds up its head the cervical spine develops a curve convex ventrally—a *lordosis*. When the child begins to walk, a second lordosis develops in the lumbar region, often an exaggerated amount, and the legs remain flexed and abducted at the hips and flexed at the knees. Only in the juvenile and young adult does the typical human erect posture pertain, but pregnancy or adiposity again exaggerates the lumbar lordosis. Thereafter the lumbar discs degenerate and the lumbar lordosis is lost; the flexion of the hips dating from the previous era is unmasked and with sticks a second quadruped stage is reached. The cervical discs degenerate further and, finally, the general kyphosis of the fetus is reproduced in the wheelchair. In prehistory the cycle was often completed by burial in the womb posture of the fetus.

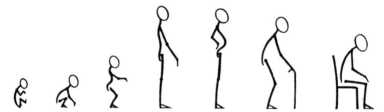

Fig. 9.1 The seven ages of man. Posture changes.

Thus variations in the curves of the spine are to be expected throughout life. When exaggerated, or when angular rather than curved, they become abnormal.

Viewed from in front or behind, the pelvis should be level, the iliac crests being on the same horizontal plane, and the spine in a vertical line. Lateral curvature (*scoliosis*) is always abnormal. In the cervical region it is termed torticollis, or wry-neck. Scoliosis may be due to faulty posture and be correctable, it may be due to protective spasm where a painful lesion is present, or it may be due to structural changes and be permanent. These can be differentiated by asking the patient to bend forwards keeping the legs straight. A postural scoliosis will then be corrected; scoliosis due to a painful condition will be associated with limited flexion to a greater or lesser degree; a curve due to a painless structural lesion will persist even on flexion, and a hump will be revealed on the convex side of the curve. This is because lateral curvature is accompanied by rotation of the vertebrae at the apex of the curve (p. 339).

The posture of the limbs varies in the sexes when seen from in front. In the male the shape is of an inverted triangle. The arms hang straight from the shoulders. The pelvis is narrow so the femora do not have to converge sharply to allow the tibiae to be parallel and together (Fig. 9.2).

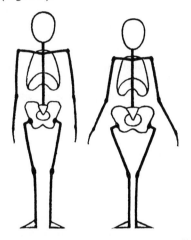

Fig. 9.2   Skeletal differences in male and female.

The female is pear-shaped. To clear the broad pelvis the forearm is abducted at the elbow. This abduction (valgus) at the elbow is known as cubitus valgus, or the carrying angle. The terms *valgus* and *varus* are applied to deviations, of a part distal to a joint, respectively away from (valgus) and towards the midline (varus), the body being in the anatomical position. Because of the width of the female pelvis the femora slope more acutely to the knee giving a greater angulation of the tibia on the femur. Where this is exaggerated and the tibiae no longer lie parallel it is known as genu valgum, or knock-knee deformity. Where the reverse angulation, or varus, is present the tibia is adducted on the femur and the deformity of genu varum, or bow-leg deformity, is produced.

2. Gait

The normal human gait is a complex phenomenon in which movement occurs in several joints simultaneously in three dimensions. Biped gait would be expected to result in abrupt oscillation of the body up and down and from side to side. It is converted into an even undulation of small amplitude, at least in the male, by movements occurring between the spine and pelvis, at the hip, knee and ankle.

Interference with the proper action of one of these components can usually be compensated by extra movement at the others and might be overlooked unless the patient is examined wearing little clothing. Interference with more than one results in an obvious limp.

Although there are great variations in normal gait and in the degree of abnormality of abnormal gaits, the latter can first be divided into two types—those that are painful and those that are not.

Painful Gait. The rhythm more than the contour of the gait is disturbed. The patient takes weight off the painful limb as quickly as possible and the timing is dot-dash, dot-dash, painful-normal, painful-normal. When pain is severe the limb, flexed at hip, knee and ankle, is put delicately to the ground and the patient hops quickly on to the sound leg. The painful region, if it is within reach, is supported by one hand and the other arm is outstretched as a counter-balance. At the other extreme the only sign may be a shortening of the stride on the affected side.

Painless Gaits. The contour rather than the rhythm of the gait is abnormal. The different varieties can be classified as follows:

1. Osteogenic—due to shortening or deformity of bone.
2. Arthogenic—due to joint stiffness, laxity or deformity.
3. Myogenic—due to weakness of muscle.
4. Neurogenic—due to organic disorder of the nervous system.
5. Psychogenic—due to psychiatric causes.
6. Prosthetic—due to wearing an artificial limb.

1. OSTEOGENIC GAIT. When the patient is clothed and wearing special footwear there may be little or no evident disturbance of gait, but when stripped for examination no difficulty should be encountered in detecting the cause of the abnormal gait.

2. ARTHROGENIC GAIT. Complete loss of movement, ankylosis, of the hip or ankle, when not accompanied by deformity, results in very little disturbance of gait and may pass unnoticed in the clothed patient. In the common deformity of fixed flexion of the hip the gluteal region becomes prominent as the leg extends, and the gait is awkward. If the hip has an abduction deformity, an unsightly gait results as the leg has to swing out and round at each pace. When the hip is fixed in a few degrees of flexion and neutral abduction-adduction, the contour of the gait is little disturbed and the patient can climb and descend stairs in a normal manner.

The effect of a stiff knee is immediately obvious and the patient has to mount the stairs one step at a time with the sound leg leading, and descend with the stiff leg leading.

A stiff ankle or foot, if not accompanied by deformity, causes little interference with the normal gait. If the foot is plantar flexed, in equinus (p. 358), the gait will resemble that of a 'drop foot' (p. 236) but this may not be obvious if high heels are worn.

3. MYOGENIC GAIT. The effect of muscle weakness will depend on its site and degree, e.g. in muscular dystrophy or as a result of myopathy in severe osteomalacia in the elderly, there is the characteristic waddling gait, described below, due to involvement of the gluteal muscles.

4. NEUROGENIC GAIT. *Spastic paralysis.* The scissor gait is typical of the 'spastic'

patient whose brain has been severely damaged from birth. The arms are adducted at the shoulder and flexed at the elbow and wrist. The posture is stooping with the legs flexed and adducted at the hips and flexed at the knee and ankle. The patient hitches each knee round and past its neighbour with a jerk, scraping the plantar flexed foot along the ground. In the mildly affected patient the only noticeable abnormality will be the curious impression that the patient is wearing heavy boots which are found difficult to raise off the ground at the beginning of each step.

The gaits of patients suffering from hemiparesis or paraparesis are described on page 236.

Flaccid paralysis. In contrast to the gaits of an ankylosed hip or foot the corresponding gaits in muscle paralysis are very obvious. Paralysis of the muscles controlling the knee, however, can be compensated by the hip and calf muscle and there may be no limp.

(i) Hip. If the abductors of the hip are paralysed, the pelvis cannot be held level when the weight is on the affected limb. The pelvis tilts towards the opposite side and to counteract this the patient has to lean the trunk towards the affected side (Fig. 9.34). This gives the impression of the patient lurching or dipping towards the paralysed side. A similar gait is seen in congenital dislocation of the hip. When both limbs are involved a waddling gait results.

(ii) Knee. If the extensors of the hip and the calf muscles are functioning, paralysis of the muscles controlling the knee will not result in a limp as the joint can be locked in full extension by the action of either when taking the body weight. If the hip extensors are also weak, the patient may push back on the thigh at each step and with the hand to lock the knee in extension. If in addition the calf muscles are weak the patient will be unable to walk without a supporting caliper.

(iii) Ankle and Foot. Paralysis of the dorsiflexors of the foot results in the drop-foot gait (p. 236). When the foot and ankle flexor muscles are paralysed the gait lacks 'spring' and a peg-leg gait results.

Cerebellar and extrapyramidal lesions. The characteristic gaits from these causes are described on page 236.

5. PSYCHOGENIC GAIT. Hysteria may be suspected if the gait is bizarre or if the patient appears to be strangely unmoved by the disability. The malingerer, on the other hand, is more likely to mimic a painful gait but usually fails to achieve the typical rhythm, tending to linger on the painful limb and creating an impression of great agony while doing so.

6. PROSTHETIC GAIT. Clothed, a patient with a 'below-knee' prosthesis is difficult to detect. With an 'above-knee' prosthesis the patient hitches the whole leg forwards, snapping the knee into extension and bringing the foot heavily to the ground. The most characteristic feature may be the sound of the artificial leg striking the ground or the creaking of the supporting straps and hinges.

3. Initial Examination of the Limbs and Spine

This assessment can be carried out as an entity or in stages while other systems are being examined. It will indicate either that all is well or that there is a local abnormality which will require more detailed review as described in Part 2 of this chapter. The methods used are inspection and palpation.

Inspection. The examination begins with inspection of joints and of active movements. Note is taken of any deformity, swelling, discolouration or muscle wasting. Active movements are performed and compared with those of the normal limb, or with the examiner's if both sides are affected. Junior students often make the mistake of beginning by seizing a patient's limb and forcing it through a wide range of movements, until halted by the patient's protests.

HANDS. These should be inspected as described on page 64. Hand movements are normal if the patient can fully extend and 'spread' the fingers then fully flex them to form a closed fist (Fig. 9.3).

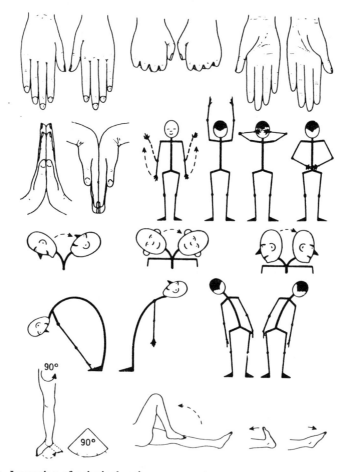

Fig. 9.3 Inspection of principal active movements.

WRISTS. After inspection the patient is asked to put the hands in the position of prayer and then lower the hands, keeping the palms together. This demonstrates the extreme of dorsiflexion. The backs of the hands are then placed together and the arms raised to demonstrate the extreme of flexion, the two sides being compared. If these movements are normal, others need not be checked.

ELBOWS. The patient is instructed to bend and straighten both elbows simultaneously, limitation in this range being revealed by comparison of one with the other side. The patient then pronates and supinates the forearms as demonstrated by the examiner. At the same time the elbow must be kept at the patient's side to prevent movement at the shoulder. Deformity or limitation of movement indicates the need for careful palpation of the joint.

SHOULDERS. The patient is asked to raise the arms forwards to the fullest extent and should be able to do so to the vertical. Abduction, external rotation and internal rotation of the shoulder are tested by the patient touching the back of the neck and then bring the arms down to touch the small of the back keeping the arms in the coronal plane as they descend (Fig. 9.3). Any limitation of movement or painful arc of movement is noted.

SPINE. Any deformity or abnormality of posture will be noted on inspection. The patient is asked to touch each shoulder with the chin and then with each ear. Up to the third decade at least, both should be possible. The patient is then asked to touch the toes without bending the knees. The level which can be reached is noted and whether this movement is achieved by a smooth general flexion of the spine. Protective spasm or structural change will be unmasked. If forward flexion is impaired, later flexion, rotation and extension should also be tested.

HIPS. If rotation of the hip is unimpaired, it is unlikely that other significant limitation is present. Rotation is measured by attempting to put the extended lower limb through the normal arc of 90° using the foot as an indicator. If rotation is impaired, then the range of flexion, extension, abduction and adduction should be measured and recorded.

KNEES, ANKLES and FEET. Inspection of the knees is followed by requesting the patient to move the joint from full extension to full flexion. The ankle joints are similarly flexed and extended by the patient and the feet inverted and everted. Inspection of the feet will show any abnormality such as flattening of the arches, callosities or deformities.

If no abnormality is detected on inspection it is not usually necessary to proceed further.

Palpation. This supplements the findings on inspection. Any points of tenderness should be localised by firm palpation and if possible the involved tissue identified by putting stress on the structure thought to be affected (p. 325). The temperature of a swollen joint should be compared by touch with that of the other limb. Active movements can be repeated while the joints are palpated to detect crepitus or clicks. Passive movements may then be assessed and compared with the active range. During these manoeuvres the patient's face should be watched for any indication of pain which is the commonest cause of limited movement.

Measuring the Movement of Joints

Limb Joints. Movements of the joints of the limbs can be measured directly and objectively recorded by the use of a goniometer (Fig. 9.4). Such records are useful, while descriptions of movements as good, fair or bad are useless. There are various methods of recording the range of movement, but the Neutral Zero Method is recommended as it is simple and generally accepted.

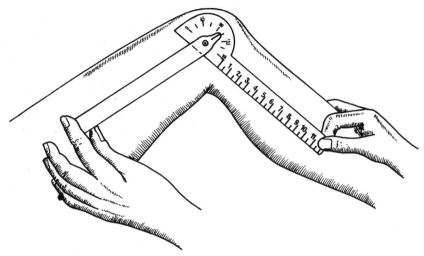

Fig. 9.4   Goniometer.

In this method all the joints are considered to be in neutral position when the body is in the classical anatomical position, with two exceptions. Firstly, the hands are flat against the thighs in the sagittal and not the coronal plane. Secondly, the feet are at right angles to the leg in the sagittal plane, not plantar flexed (Fig. 9.5).

In certain joints, such as the elbow and knee, movement can normally occur only in one direction from neutral, e.g. flexion 0° to 150° or extension 150° to 0°. Extension past 0° normally does not occur and is therefore referred to as hyperextension 0° to ?°. In other joints, such as the wrist and ankle, movement normally occurs in both directions from zero and is defined as palmar or plantar flexion 0° to ?°, and the dorsiflexion or extension 0° to ?° (Fig. 9.5). Finally, certain joints such as the shoulders and hips allow movement in all directions from neutral. Such movements are defined as flexion, extension, abduction, adduction, internal and external rotation, all from neutral. Combined they result in circumduction.

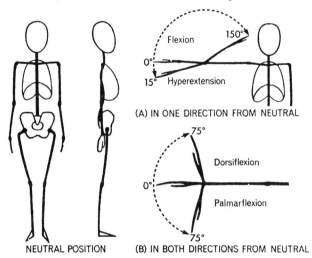

Fig. 9.5   Measuring movements of joints.

Both the active and passive movements are measured and separately recorded if they differ. Where limitation of movement is present it is best described by the arc of movement present. For example, if a patient lacks 30° of extension of the elbow and can flex to 90° from there, the range of movement is described as flexion 30° to 90°.

Spinal Movement. Direct measurements of the movement of the spine is difficult. Indirect methods, however, can be useful and are described with the examination of the components of the spine.

If an accurate measurement of spinal flexion alone is required, uninfluenced by flexion of the hip joints, a mark is made on the skin at the lumbosacral joint, level with the dimples of Venus. Other marks are made 20 cm above and 5 cm below the original mark. On flexion the increase in the distance between the marks is measured and should be significant above the mark and nil below (Fig. 9.6).

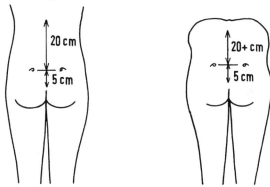

Fig. 9.6 **Measuring forward flexion of spine.**

The Interpretation of Abnormal Joint Movement

The movements of a joint can be restricted or increased by changes in the bone, cartilage, synovial membrane, capsule, ligaments, muscles, and related nerves. By the systematic examination of each structure in turn, the cause of the abnormal movement can be found.

Bone, Articular Cartilage and Synovial Membrane. Inflammatory change, whether traumatic, rheumatic, degenerative, or infective in nature, causes diminished movement in all directions (Fig. 9.7). The degree of limitation corresponds to the acuteness of the process. Tenderness, if present, is general over all the joint.

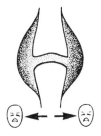

Fig. 9.7 **Inflammation of a joint.**

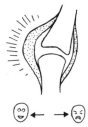

Fig. 9.8 **Sprain of capsule or ligament.**

Complete lack of movement accompanied by pain is due to acute inflammation or recent trauma. These are differentiated by the history.

Complete lack of movement without pain means ankylosis or fusion of the joint (arthrodesis).

Capsule and Ligaments. A strained or sprained capsule or ligament is painful when stretched by active or passive movement towards the opposite side of the joint, and movements in this direction are restricted by protective spasm of muscles. Movement towards the strained ligament relieves the painful tension and is not limited (Fig. 9.8). Tenderness is localised to the sprained area. An effusion may be present as the capsule is intact.

A ruptured ligament is initially painful on movement towards the opposite side of the joint. This movement is excessive in degree. Movement towards the same side 'closes' the joint and relieves pain. Any fluid in the joint escapes and causes swelling over the ruptured ligament (Fig. 9.9).

Intra-articular Structures. A structure, such as a torn semilunar cartilage, displaced in a joint is compressed by movement towards it. Pain is localised over the structure and that movement is restricted. Movement away from the object is not painful or reduced (Fig. 9.10). An effusion is usually present in the joint.

Muscle. *Painful Lesion in Muscle.* Active contraction, even when no movement takes place, causes pain. Active movement involving the muscle causes pain and is restricted. Passive movement in the same direction relaxes the muscle, relieves pain, and is not restricted to the same extent.

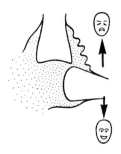
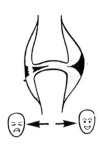
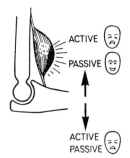

Fig. 9.9 Rupture of capsule or ligament. **Fig. 9.10 Rupture of semilunar cartilage.** **Fig. 9.11 Painful lesion in a muscle.**

Both active and passive movements in the opposite direction cause pain and are therefore restricted (Fig. 9.11).

Pain arising in a strained ligament can be differentiated from pain arising in a muscle close to the joint by making the suspected muscle contract without movement of the joint (isometric contraction). This will cause pain if the muscle, not the ligament, is the cause. For example, in tennis elbow passive extension of the elbow is painful but this stretches both the capsule of the elbow and the extensor muscle origin. The patient now clenches the fist without moving the elbow, thus contracting the extensor muscles, and pain results, localised to the extensor origin, proving that this is the source of the pain.

When examining a muscle which acts over two joints, the same principles apply.

When movement at one joint influences the range of movement at a neighbouring joint, derangement of such a muscle is suspected. For example, if there is fixed equinus or flexion of the ankle joint when the knee is extended, this could be due to changes in the ankle joint itself or to contracture of the gastrocnemius muscle or soleus muscle. Flexion of the knee relaxes the gastrocnemius muscle and has no effect on the soleus muscle or the ankle joint. If dorsiflexion is now possible, the gastrocnemius muscle must have prevented it when the knee was extended (Fig. 9.12).

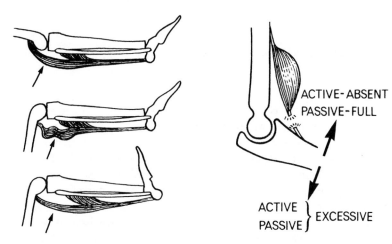

Fig. 9.12   Lesion of gastrocnemius muscle.   Fig. 9.13   Rupture of a muscle.

Rupture or Paralysis of a Muscle. When a muscle is paralysed or its tendon divided, active movement towards the muscle is abolished but passive movement, initially, is unaffected (Fig. 9.13). Active and passive movement in the opposite direction is excessive and, if no treatment is initiated, the uncontrolled antagonist muscles will pull the related joint into an abnormal posture.

The Nerves. The effect of paralysis on joint movement is discussed on page 320. Abnormal tension on a nerve will result in limitation of both active and passive movement which would increase that tension. The nerve stretching tests described on page 343 illustrate how such limitation of movement in the case of a prolapsed lumbar intervertebral disc can be differentiated from that caused by joint or muscle lesions.

PART II REGIONAL EXAMINATION

Another man, Adwyne by name, in the town of Dunwych, that dwelled on the sea-shore, was so contracted that he could not use the free office of hand or foot. His legs were cleaving to the hinder part of his thighs so that he could not walk, and his hands were turned backward. Nothing could be done by them. The extremities of his fingers were so rigorously contracted in the sinews that he could not put meat to his mouth. In this grievous sickness he passed his young age.

> Anon (Quoted from Griffith, E. F. 1951. *Doctors by Themselves*. Cassell: London.)

The above quotation, the earliest recorded account of the admission of a patient to St Bartholomew's Hospital, was written in the twelfth century and is a graphic but extreme example of the complexities which occur in the locomotor system in neglected patients. A very detailed examination may be required for the elucidation of each local disability. Expert help is often required as is indicated by the large numbers of patients attending orthopaedic and rheumatic clinics. While the treatment of traumatic damage from the increasing number of road accidents is frequently a specialised procedure, the initial assessment may have to be carried out by any doctor. However, undergraduates need not be overawed by what confronts them if their methods are based on an understanding of the anatomical features and the pathological conditions commonly encountered in the various regions. A competent history will also do much to clarify the problem.

THE UPPER LIMB

THE HAND, WRIST AND FOREARM

Some of the many abnormalities to be found in the hand have been outlined on pages 65 to 70, notably its involvement in arthritis and the changes of diagnostic value to be seen in the fingers (Fig. 4.1 p. 65) and in the nails (Fig. 4.2 p. 68). In this section the function of the hand is the primary consideration.

The hand's function depends on mobility and the smooth gliding of part on part, tendon in sheath. This makes it liable to a special group of friction syndromes involving its tendons — tenosynovitis. The hands are unusually liable to injury, for obvious reasons. So intimate is the relationship of the skin, bones, joints, tendons, nerves and vessels that it is seldom that injury involves a single structure. Because the hand is constantly contaminated by the environment, open injuries often become infected. Once established, infection may spread in the natural tissue spaces in the hand or along its tendon sheaths.

Anatomical Features

The Skin and Deep Fascia. In the palm both structures are thickened and bound together at the skin creases. On the dorsum the skin and the deep fascia are thin and elastic. Because of these differences any generalised swelling of the hand will be more evident on the dorsum. The skin has a very abundant nerve and blood supply on both aspects of the hand.

Muscles. The muscles in the forearm are the powerhouse of the hand and wrist. Without the help of the intrinsic muscles of the hand, however, neither a proper grip nor fine movements are possible. If the intrinsic muscles are paralysed the long muscles acting alone cause clawing of the fingers. Such a hand is useful only as a paperweight or a hook.

Joints. The interphalangeal joints allow only flexion and extension; the metacarpo-phalangeal joints in addition to flexion and extension allow abduction and adduction, but only when extended. The wrist joint allows flexion and extension, radial and ulnar deviation, and circumduction.

Rotation of the Forearm. This movement depends on the integrity of the superior and inferior radio-ulnar joints and on the concavity of the volar aspects of the shafts of the radius and ulna. In pronation these two concavities fit into one another. Rotation will be limited if this curve is distorted, as may occur after a fracture.

Nerve Supply. The radial, ulnar and median nerves are all implicated in normal functioning of the hand.

The *radial nerve* supplies the wrist and finger extensors and an insignificant area of sensation on the dorsum of the index metacarpal. Damage to the nerve is liable to occur in the spiral groove on the shaft of the humerus, resulting in a 'drop wrist'. The grip is considerably weakened because the flexors now have no antagonist to steady the wrist.

The *ulnar nerve* supplies sensation on the ulnar border of the hand. Its motor contribution is most important in the hand, where it supplies all the small muscles except the short flexor, abductor, and opponens of the thumb, and the lumbrical to the index and sometimes the middle finger. The nerve may be damaged at the elbow or the wrist, resulting in the clawhand deformity (Fig. 4.3 p. 69). The ring and little fingers are clawed, and wasting of the muscles between the metacarpals is most evident in the cleft between the index and thumb. The clawing — extension at the metacarpo-phalangeal joint and flexion at the interphalangeal joints — is the result of the unopposed action of the long flexors and extensors.

The *median nerve* supplies the main bulk of the flexor muscles in the forearm and the small muscles of the thumb, as well as the lumbricals to the index and middle fingers. The common site of damage is at the wrist, causing paralysis of the muscles supplied in the hand. The muscles of the thenar eminence waste and the thumb falls into the flat, ape-like or simian deformity. Although this interferes significantly with hand function, the most disabling component of the injury is loss of sensation on the volar aspect of the thumb, index and middle fingers (Fig. 9.14). It is from this area that so much information is received about the environment. Activities such as dressing and sorting coins in the pocket can no longer be performed unless under direct vision.

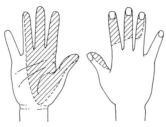

Fig. 9.14   The use of diagrams in case recording. Area of anaesthesia in a patient with a lesion of the right median nerve.

Variations in the distribution of the nerve supply, particularly between median and ulnar, are very common in the hand.

Examination of the Hand, Wrist and Forearm

This consists of inspection (p. 66) and palpation. Particular attention is paid to the assessment of the function of the hand. The hand distal to any wound must be carefully examined. An apparently trivial laceration may involve tendons, nerves or joints. Some authorities consider the thumb, others the index finger, as the first digit. In order to avoid confusion, therefore, the digits must never be numbered but must be specified by name — thumb, index, middle, ring, and little finger. This may be tedious, but it will reduce the risk of the wrong finger being treated, or even amputated. Diagrams showing scars, amputated portions, or other deformities make an accurate and easily understood record (Fig. 9.15).

Assessment of hand function. This involves examination of the active and passive movements of the wrist and digits. Where movement is limited, it is assessed as described on page 325 and the cause is identified. A long time may be required to complete the examination of the whole hand and record the findings.

The integrity of individual tendons is tested by observing if their normal action is present.

Flexor digitorum profundus flexes the proximal and the distal interphalangeal joints. It is the only muscle which flexes the distal interphalangeal joints and its action is therefore tested by flexion of this joint while the finger is held in extension at the proximal joint and in flexion at the metacarpo-phalangeal joint.

Flexor digitorum sublimis flexes the proximal interphalangeal joints. When testing this tendon the action of profundus can be eliminated by extending all the fingers not being examined. The flexor profundus has a muscle belly common to all the fingers; if three of the fingers are extended, the muscle controlling the fourth finger will be unable to contract significantly. If the finger then flexes at the proximal interphalangeal joint this is due to the flexor sublimis.

The lumbricals cause flexion at the metacarpo-phalangeal joint and extension at the interphalangeal joints; they are tested by asking the patient to do this following the example of the examiner.

The *interossei* assist the lumbricals in the movements noted above, and abduct (dorsal interossei) and adduct (palmar interossei) the fingers from the midline of the middle finger. Abduction is tested by asking the patient to spread the extended fingers against resistance. Adduction is tested by the ability to hold a card between

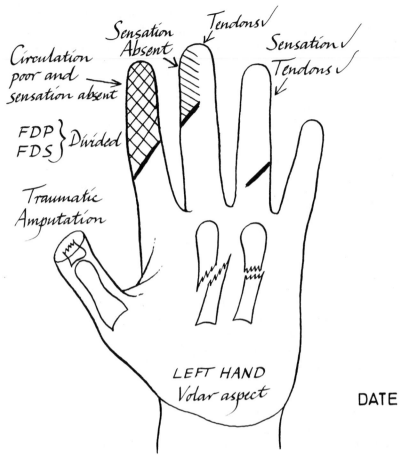

Fig. 9.15   The use of diagrams in case recording. This diagram summarises at a glance the following mass of information: (1) Traumatic amputation obliquely through the distal phalanx of the thumb. (2) Deep laceration of the index finger over the middle phalanx running obliquely from the radial side to the ulnar side of the finger. The digital nerves, arteries and both flexor tendons have been divided. (3) Deep laceration of the middle finger obliquely over the radial aspect of the middle phalanx. The digital nerve on the radial aspect has been divided. The tendons are intact.
(4) Superficial laceration of ring finger over the ulnar aspect of the proximal phalanx without damage to tendons or nerves. (5) Closed fracture of the metacarpal of the middle finger obliquely through the mid-shaft with displacement. (6) Closed fracture of the metacarpal of the ring finger transversely through the mid-shaft without displacement.

the fingers in competition with the examiner. The fingers must be in extension, and in order to ensure this, the test is best carried out with the hand on a flat surface.

The intrinsic muscles (interossei and lumbricals) frequently waste and become fibrosed and contracted in rheumatoid arthritis, and produce an exaggerated version of their normal action. The metacarpo-phalangeal joints are flexed, the proximal interphalangeal joints extended, and the distal joints flexed — the 'swan neck' deformity. In the later stages of this disease several of the joints may become dislocated.

Thenar muscles supplied by the median nerve. The abductor brevis and opponens combine to produce opposition. Difficulty may be encountered in differentiating between true opposition and adduction which is produced by the ulnar supplied adductor pollicis. Observe the nail of the thumb from the palmar aspect. On adduction (ulnar nerve) it is seen in side view. In opposition it has rotated and is now in full view (Fig. 9.16).

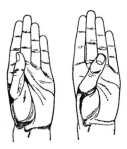

Fig. 9.16   Adduction and opposition of the thumb.

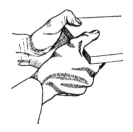

Fig. 9.17   Normal and paralysed adductor pollicis.

Thenar muscles supplied by the ulnar nerve. Paralysis of adductor pollicis is accompanied by muscle wasting in the palm between the thumb and the index finger. The patient is asked to hold a thin book between the radial side of the clenched fingers and the extended thumb. When the adductor is not functioning the thumb cannot be held extended and flexion at the metacarpo-phalangeal and interphalangeal joints occurs. This is because the adductor cannot hold the head of the metacarpal against the index finger (Fig. 9.17).

Extensor tendons. Assessment of paralysis is not difficult, but these tendons are liable to rupture at any of three sites. (1) Separation may occur from the distal phalanx with or without a fragment of bone. This results in mallet finger deformity. (2) The central slip of the extensor which inserts to the bone of the middle phalanx may rupture, producing the 'boutonniere' deformity as the lateral portions slip to each side of the finger. The proximal interphalangeal is then flexed and the distal joint extended. (3) The extensor pollicis longus occasionally ruptures at the wrist after a Colles' fracture, or in rheumatoid arthritis, causing loss of extension at the metacarpo-phalangeal and interphalangeal joints.

Trigger finger and thumb. Flexion is not limited, but extension of the inter-phalangeal joints is, until straightening of the finger suddenly occurs, accompanied by a click felt over the thickened part of the flexor sheath at the level of the metacarpal head. In babies the condition is often not noticed until extension at the inter-phalangeal joints is permanently limited. The thumb is most frequently involved at this age and the thickened flexor sheath is easily palpable over the matacarpal head.

THE ELBOW

Congenital abnormalities are not commonly found in the humerus but this bone is not infrequently the site of acute osteomyelitis in the young. Fractures occur at all ages, and the intimate relationship of the humerus with three nerves — the circumflex at its neck, the radial in the mid-shaft and the ulnar at the elbow — may result in injury to these nerves. Fracture at the supracondylar level may damage the brachial artery and cause ischaemic changes in the flexor muscles in the forearm (Volkmann's ischaemic contracture).

The elbow is not a common site of congenital deformity or degenerative change, but next to the knee it is the most frequent site of osteochondritis dissecans. The reaction of the elbow to trauma is unpredictable. Minor trauma may be followed by complete stiffness, whereas gross disorganisation of the joint may be compatible with excellent function. One stiff elbow, provided it is not too extended, is not a great handicap, but stiffness of both elbows causes severe disability. Patients with rheumatoid arthritis use the elbows to prop themselves up in bed and the resultant pressure is a factor in the production of the nodules which are frequently found over the upper posterior aspect of the ulna in these circumstances.

Anatomical Features

The joint is composed of two parts, that between the humerus, radius and ulna, and the superior radio-ulnar joint. The former allows flexion through a range of 150°, and the latter allows rotation of the wrist through 180°. In the female, in the anatomical position, the forearm is abducted on the humerus to form the carrying angle, cubitus valgus and some degree of hyperextension is common. Where this angle is increased, by fracture of the capitellum for example, the ulnar nerve becomes stretched and its function may be impaired.

The joint between the humerus, radius and ulna is stable, and is not dislocated easily. The head of the radius, however, particularly in children, may dislocate, but cause surprisingly few symptoms.

Examination of the Elbow

Inspection. With both arms exposed, deformity is detected by inspecting the elbow from behind with the arm flexed and extended. The relationship of the olecranon and the lateral and medial epicondyles in the abnormal joint is compared with that of the normal side. The hollow over the head of the radius is filled in when an effusion is present. A flexion deformity cannot be easily differentiated from a valgus deformity. By the same token, the degree of valgus or varus cannot be accurately measured with the elbow even slightly flexed.

The patient should flex and extend both arms at the same time, when the range of each can be compared. The patient is then asked to flex the elbow to a right angle and keep the elbow touching the side while supinating and pronating both hands. Care must be taken to ensure that the elbow is kept to the side when measuring pronation because the movement can be simulated very easily by abduction at the shoulder.

Palpation. This is conducted for bony contour, local tenderness, or signs of inflammation. In tennis elbow tenderness is well localised in the region of the lateral epicondyle at the extensor origin. Pain is reproduced by gripping, by resisted extension of the wrist, and by passive extension of the elbow while the forearm is pronated and the wrist flexed. The patient can lift objects with the hand supine, but experiences pain when lifting the same object with the hand pronated. An effusion in the joint is most easily felt over the head of the radius on the postero-lateral aspect of the joint. Here the head of the radius lies almost subcutaneously and is easily palpated if the forearm is rotated at the same time. Loose bodies are seldom palpable as they tend to collect in the coronoid and olecranon fossae which are covered by muscle. The collateral ligaments can be tested only when the elbow is fully extended. The ulnar nerve is palpated and compared with the normal side to determine any enlargement, tenderness or excessive mobility.

THE SHOULDER

The alignment of the upper limb has changed little from that of the reptile. Most of man's activities involve the use of the hands within an oval limited above and below by the orifices of the alimentary tract, sideways by little more than the breadth of the shoulders, and forwards by the extent of the reach. The emphasis is on mobility rather than stability, despite which congenital dislocation of the shoulder is virtually unknown. In the young adult, dislocation readily occurs following injury and thereafter the tendency to recurrent dislocation is very great. In the older patient the joint has a marked tendency to become stiff, because of little understood changes in the soft tissues of the shoulder. Whatever the cause, this condition, conveniently and graphically described as 'frozen shoulder', is so common from early middle age onwards that it must be kept in mind when examining a patient suffering from any painful condition from the neck to the finger-tips. The shoulder will stiffen if movement of the joint is not maintained because of pain in the neck or arm, after myocardial infarction or following a hemiplegia. In contrast to the frozen shoulder, osteoarthrosis and inflammatory lesions are relatively uncommon in the shoulder region.

Anatomical Features

Movements. Movements of the shoulder is a complicated synthesis of motion at four joints. The glenohumeral and scapulothoracic joints each account for about half of the total range, and it is necessary to measure the contribution made by each. Movement at the acromio-clavicular joint is not important and at the sternoclavicular joint only little more so.

Rather than define the range of movement and try to explain the complex relationship between rotation, flexion and abduction, the reader is invited to demonstrate these movements personally. The range of movement varies with the rotation of the arm. This can be shown with the elbow flexed to a right angle and the forearm acting as an indicator of rotation. Abduction can proceed only a little beyond 90° with the arm in neutral rotation. If the arm is externally rotated, full abduction is possible. In full internal rotation almost no abduction is possible. When limitation of movement is present, the glenohumeral and scapulothoracic contributions must be separated. This is achieved by holding the inferior angle of the scapula with one hand and abducting the arm with the other (Fig. 9.18).

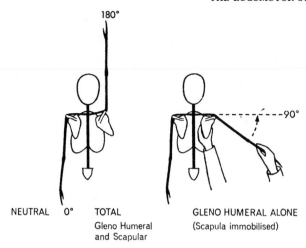

NEUTRAL   0°   TOTAL   GLENO HUMERAL ALONE
                 Gleno Humeral   (Scapula immobilised)
                 and Scapular

Fig. 9.18   Movements at the shoulder joint.

Rotation can be demonstrated again by using the forearm as an indicator. With the arm by the side in neutral rotation and the elbow flexed to 90°, the forearm will be directed medially by some 20° and not in the sagittal plane; 90° of rotation should be possible from this position in both directions. The forearm cannot quite reach the coronal plane in external rotation, but the patient should be able to touch the small of the back in internal rotation. With the arm in full external rotation and the elbow flexed at 90°, abduction of the shoulder will bring the hand up to the back of the neck. A reasonably accurate measurement of full rotation, therefore, is the ability to touch the small of the back and the back of the neck.

Rotator Cuff. This term is applied to the fused tendons of supraspinatus, infraspinatus and teres minor. These, with the tendon of subscapularis, form a hood-like structure covering the head of the humerus, holding it into the socket of the glenoid and initiating glenohumeral abduction. This structure, and especially the supraspinatus tendon, is the most common site of pathological change in the shoulder. When swollen and tender it affects the movement of the shoulder in a characteristic way. As abduction proceeds the swollen portion becomes compressed under the acromion and causes pain. Once it has passed this point painless movement is continued. Patients very quickly learn to avoid this by externally rotating the humerus as abduction proceeds so that the tender area is not compressed under the acromion.

When rupture of the rotator cuff occurs, attempts to abduct the shoulder produce only a shrugging of the shoulder as a whole, the arm barely leaving the side. The deltoid can only pull the humerus in its own axis up against the acromion. If, however, the humerus is passively abducted to 45°, the deltoid can now abduct the rest of the way. Patients learn trick movements to compensate for loss of the initial abduction by passively swinging the arm from the side and 'catching it' with the deltoid to complete abduction. Soon after injury when the shoulder is painful it is impossible to tell whether abduction is inhibited by pain or prevented by rupture of the rotator cuff. Abolition of the pain by injection of local anaesthetic resolves the problem as the patient can then initiate abduction if the cuff is intact.

The long head of the biceps may be involved in lesions of the rotator cuff. This lesion is suspected when resisted flexion of the elbow causes pain in the shoulder.

Nerve Supply. The spinal segments which supply the shoulder girdle contribute to the phrenic nerve. In painful lesions affecting areas subserved by the phrenic nerve, such as the central part of the diaphragm, pain may be referred to the tip of the shoulder in the area of C4, owing to the fact that the greater part of the phrenic nerve is derived from this root.

Points in the History

Lesions in the neck, pericardium and the pleura and peritoneum covering the central parts of the diaphragm may cause pain in the shoulder. Theoretically this should cause little difficulty because no limitation of movement or other abnormality should be found on examination of the shoulder. However, this reasoning may be confounded by the tendency of the shoulder in the elderly to become stiff when immobilised by pain from other sites. Painful lesions in the root of the neck, and the most sinister is an apical bronchial carcinoma, tend to cause pain radiating down the inner side of the arm.

Occasionally ischaemic lesions of the heart cause shoulder pain, but the clinical features of the pain, especially if it is induced by exercise which does not involve the use of the arms, should resolve any doubt about its true origin. Phrenic pain referred to the tip of the shoulder from the diaphragm may be aggravated by deep breathing. True shoulder pain tends to radiate to the insertion of the deltoid muscle and seldom extends beyond the elbow. When a calcified deposit in the rotator cuff ruptures into the sub-acromial bursa the pain is so severe that immediate operation may be required if injections of local anaesthetic and hydrocortisone fail to relieve the pain.

Examination of the Shoulder

Inspection. When only one shoulder is affected much may be learned by simple inspection and comparison with the normal side.

Anterior dislocation of the sterno-clavicular joint is not uncommon and except in the early stages after injury, does not interfere with shoulder movement. The deformity caused by the prominent medial end of the clavicle is easily seen or palpated. Posterior dislocation is less common and is usually accompanied by severe pain and commanding symptoms, including difficulty in swallowing and extreme pain on lifting the head when supine. The deformity, however, especially in the early stages when accompanied by swelling, is not obvious even on radiological examination.

Fracture at the mid-shaft of the clavicle presents little difficulty in diagnosis. Dislocation of the acromio-clavicular joint may be confused with fracture at the lateral end of the clavicle; both cause a distinct 'step' between the acromion and the upwardly displaced clavicle or medial fragment. Neither injury causes much disturbance of shoulder function except in the early stages.

Anterior dislocation of the shoulder poses few diagnostic problems because the humerus displaces downwards as well as forwards. The normal smooth curved contour of the shoulder is replaced by the ugly angular projection of the acromion process of the scapula. Posterior dislocation is frequently not diagnosed immediately after injury, even with the help of radiological examination. A nearly normal contour of the shoulder is preserved because the head of the humerus displaces directly backwards and not downwards. If the patient is muscular, this and the swelling after an injury may be accepted as the reaction to a strain of the joint. Inferior dislocation is rare, the patient being in the sorry plight of not being able to bring the arm to the side. This 'I am a teapot' posture may amuse the onlooker, but not the patient.

SCAPULAR MOVEMENTS. The ability to shrug the shoulder up, backwards and forwards is noted. Weakness of the serratus anterior will be made obvious if the patient raises the arms forward to press against the wall with both hands. Where the muscle is weak, the medial border of the scapula projects backward, producing 'winging' of the scapula.

GLENO-HUMERAL MOVEMENTS. Standing behind the patient, the examiner steadies the scapula by grasping the inferior angle and then putting the shoulder through both active and passive movements.

TOTAL RANGE OF MOVEMENTS. The patient is asked to raise the arm forwards and upwards to the limit, and then to the same end point through abduction. Any painful arc of limitation of movement is noted.

ROTARY MOVEMENTS. By flexing the elbow to a right angle, the forearm acts as an indicator. The shoulder is externally and then internally rotated with the arm at the side. The easiest way to demonstrate a full range of rotation is to ask the patient to touch the back of the neck and the small of the back.

Palpation. Careful palpation may be required to confirm what is suspected on inspection. Local tenderness must be accurately defined, especially in lesions of the rotator cuff. This structure can be more fully explored if the patient clasps the hands behind the back during the examination. Occasionally, in a lean subject, a gap may be palpable where the rotator cuff has ruptured.

THE SPINE

Before considering the cervical, thoracic and lumbar segments separately, it is worth again remarking on the posture of the spine as a whole. At all times the normal spine should present as a straight line viewed from the front or the rear. As seen from the side, posture varies with the patient's age, depending mainly on the state of the intervertebral discs after maturity.

CERVICAL SPINE

The cervical spine is the most mobile section of the vertebral column. While the posture changes steadily throughout life, the neck is seldom in the same position for any length of time, waking or sleeping. Degenerative changes are therefore common but are not necessarily accompanied by symptoms. This mobility is also a factor in the liability of this part of the spine to injury. Congenital deformity is not uncommon, but when present is easy to detect. Infection in the cervical vertebrae is rare in contrast to the soft tissues of the neck where enlarged lymph nodes are commonly found as a result of infection from the mouth or pharynx.

Anatomical Features

In the cervical spine the transverse process projects laterally from the body of the vertebra, protecting the more easily crushed cancellous bone of the body in the event of injury. The facet joints, however, lie more horizontally than at other levels of the spine; thus forced flexion of the neck is unlikely to produce a crush fracture of the body, and more often results in forward dislocation of the upper vertebrae.

The vertebral canal is almost filled by the cervical enlargement of the spinal cord. The emerging cervical roots pass between the articular facets and the intervertebral disc. Prolapse laterally of a cervical disc may produce compression of these roots; a central prolapse may produce pressure on the cord itself. Osteophytic outgrowth from the vertebral body with or without similar change in the facet joint is a common cause of root irritation in the lower cervical region (cervical spondylosis).

Of the movements in the neck, rotation takes place mainly at the atlanto-axial joint, nodding of the head at the atlanto-occipital joint, and flexion-extension in the mid-cervical joints.

Examination of the Cervical Spine

Because of the close relationship of the bones, joints, blood vessels, spinal cord and nerve roots, a lesion of the cervical region may produce symptoms both locally and widely referred. Examination of the neck must therefore include a neurological examination of the upper limbs and elsewhere as indicated.

Inspection. Deformity is easily detected. Where a painful lesion is present, the gait is characteristic. The patient walks with care to avoid jarring the neck, moving the whole body to look to the side. The chin may be supported by the hand. Torticollis (wry-neck) is the most common deformity and is emphasised on movement. If it has been present for several years asymmetry of the face will have developed. The patient is asked to touch each shoulder in turn with the chin and then the ear. Any limitation of active movement is noted and compared later with the passive range of movement. Forward flexion and extension are tested by putting the chin on the chest and by bending the neck backwards. Nodding tests movement at the atlanto-occipital joint.

Palpation. The bone contour is explored; in the root of the neck accessory ribs may be palpable or even visible. Local tenderness, skin temperature and the condition of the cervical lymph nodes are assessed, the latter with the neck slightly flexed. Movements are repeated while palpation continues, to detect crepitus. Passive movements are carried out if there is any impairment of range. An accessory rib may obliterate the radial pulse if traction is applied to the arm with it by the patient's side. Contraction of an abnormal scalenus anterior muscle may obliterate the radial pulse when the patient turns the head to the affected side and then takes and holds a deep breath (Fig. 6.2, p. 163).

The *foraminal compression test* (Fig. 9.19) is performed if a cervical disc lesion is suspected. The examiner's hands are placed on the patient's head, with the patient standing or sitting, and gentle downward pressure applied. If no pain is produced, the manoeuvre is repeated with the neck flexed to either side, in forward flexion and in extension. The test confirms the presence of root compression if it causes the characteristic reference of pain.

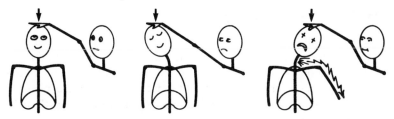

Fig. 9.19   Foraminal compression test.

THORACIC SPINE

This segment of the vertebral column is the least mobile, and throughout life maintains a kyphosis. In contrast with its immobility is its tendency to develop gross deformity whatever the cause — congenital, developmental, or a variety of diseases.

Congenital lesions are not common, for at this level the neural canal and arch are closed at an early stage. Developmental lesions (e.g. epiphysitis), and infection commonly affect this segment. Tuberculosis usually involves several vertebral bodies and, before the introduction of specific chemotherapy, resulted in gross destruction of the bodies and an angular kyphosis. When idiopathic scoliosis or scoliosis secondary to poliomyelitis occurs at this level, the deformity may be very severe. The rotation element of scoliosis is best seen in the thoracic spine. At the apex of the lateral curve the vertebral bodies no longer face ventrally, but are directed towards the convex side of the curve. The ribs, instead of projecting laterally, are now, on the convex side of the curve, directed dorsally, becoming sharply angulated to cause a 'razor-back' deformity. This results in narrowing and distortion of the chest cage and may interfere with the action of the heart and lungs. Such patients experience little pain but have a limited expectation of life.

Anatomical Features

The movements of the thoracic spine consist of flexion and extension and a slight degree of lateral flexion and rotation. The range of movement is small and difficult to measure. The movement of the ribs, however, is easily assessed and can be affected by disease of the spine, such as ankylosing spondylitis, which not only stiffens the spine but may also immobilise the ribs.

Special Points in the History

Pain in the thoracic spine is less common than in either the cervical or lumbar spine. Disc lesions are infrequent, but can occur and be accompanied by girdle pain radiating into the chest and mimicking the pain of cardiac disease. In the younger patient infection of bone, pyogenic or tuberculous, has to be kept in mind although it is much less frequently encountered in Britain than formerly. In middle and old age pathological fracture associated with either osteoporosis or malignant disease is a common cause of pain.

Examination of the Thoracic Spine

Inspection. With the patient standing, the posture is inspected from the front, back and side, and any deformity noted. The ranges of movement on forward and lateral flexion and on extension are recorded. Particular note is taken of the effect movement has on any deformity present. If it is due to faulty posture, it will correct on forward flexion. If due to structural changes, it will be unaffected. The movement of the chest on breathing is also inspected.

Palpation. The bony contour is first examined and areas of tenderness defined. Where local tenderness is not immediately obvious, gentle percussion with the fist may elicit it.

LUMBAR SPINE

This segment of the spine falls heir to many infirmities. The lumbosacral region is a common site for congenital anomalies which seldom cause trouble. Trauma frequently results in damage at the upper end of the lumbar spine where the mobile lumbar segment joins the less mobile dorsal spine. Ankylosing spondylitis, as its name implies, can cause marked limitation of movement (Fig. 4.11 p. 87). Osteoporosis may be marked in the lumbar spine and cause vertebral collapse, a condition often precipitated by corticosteroid therapy. Degenerative changes develop in the lower intervertebral discs in the third decade and osteoarthrosis in the facet joints by middle age. Although these changes and related ligamentous stresses provide the commonest explanations of low backache, this may also be due to gynaecological or psychological causes. Lesions in the lumbar spine may cause symptoms in the lower limbs, with or without accompanying back pain.

Anatomical Features

In the adult the spinal cord ends at the level of the second lumbar vertebra. At the dorso-lumbar level, a common site for injury, the neural canal contains the spinal cord and lumbar nerve roots. Injury at this level may seriously damage the spinal cord, which will not recover, and nerve roots which may recover.

The transverse processes of the lumbar spine are analagous to the ribs and abnormalities are common at the upper end of the lumbar spine; vestigial ribs may be mistaken for a fracture on radiological examination. The sacrum is formed by the fusion of five segments of the spine. The last lumbar segment not uncommonly fuses partially or completely with the first sacral segment — sacralisation of the fifth lumbar vertebra. Conversely the first sacral segment may fail to fuse to the remainder of the sacrum — lumbarisation of the sacral segment. The two can be differentiated only by count of the remaining segments of the spine.

The intervertebral disc consists of a tough outer ring of fibrous tissue, the annulus, and a central jelly-like nucleus with a very high water content. The depth of the disc varies during the day. A fit young adult may be about 2 cm shorter by the end of the day, due mainly to changes in the disc. By the third decade degenerative changes begin in the lower lumbar discs, setting the stage for disc lesions to follow. They take the form of tears of the annulus with or without extrusion of the nucleus and are accompanied by pain. The disc does not, however, slip in and out of place. Less dramatically, this degenerative change may result in permanent narrowing of the disc. The corresponding facet joints between the vertebrae develop osteoarthrosis. Such changes are 'normal' in most individuals by the fifth decade, but are not always accompanied by symptoms; indeed this stiffness may result in stability and resolution of pain. Many individuals achieve a 'do-it-yourself' spinal fusion of the vulnerable joints.

Pus from a chronic infection of the lumbar spine may collect in the sheath of the psoas muscle, forming a palpable tumour in the iliac fossa before tracking farther down the sheath of the muscle to present as a swelling or a sinus in the groin. Acute infection causes spasm of the muscle and flexion of the hip. Active flexion of the hip aggravates the pain and passive flexion relieves it. This contrasts both with infection in the hip where all movements are painful, and with a lesion causing tension of the femoral roots (p. 344) where active and passive flexion of the hip relieves pain.

Special Points in the History

The mode of onset and the pattern of lumbar pain are particularly significant. The acute pain of a disc protrusion comes on suddenly when bending or on the day after such activity. This so overshadows the occasional backaches to which the patient has become accustomed during the preceding period of disc degeneration that these are often not mentioned. Careful enquiry will reveal the pattern of minor backache, the acute episodes which settle with rest, followed by further minor aches, acute episodes, or both. Disc lesions, therefore, cause episodic pain with periods of freedom from symptoms. Recurrences can very often be related to stooping or lifting. Osteoarthrosis in the lumbar region causes the usual pattern of pain and stiffness after rest relieved by activity and recurring when the patient tires. Chronic ligamentous strain and spinal instability, in contrast to osteoarthrosis, cause pain on standing and at the end of the day with freedom from pain at the start of the day.

Spinal stenosis (p. 317) results in backache with or without leg pain. Intermittent claudication is often wrongly diagnosed because the symptoms of both conditions are related to standing and walking and are relieved by rest. Differentiation is discussed on page 317. Ischaemia is a rare cause of gluteal pain and is usually accompanied by other features such as impotence.

Pain not relieved by rest suggests a more serious lesion, such as infection or spondylitis in the younger patient, and in the older groups primary or secondary malignant disease. However, if there is a long history of constant pain unrelieved by rest, an organic cause is unlikely.

Low lumbar or sacral pain may be due to pathological conditions in the pelvis, especially in the female.

Examination of the Lumbar Spine

Inspection. With the patient standing, the posture is observed from behind. The spine should be straight. The most common cause of deviation at this level is a lumbar disc lesion which causes the patient to list to one or other side. If the prolapse is lateral to the adjacent root the patient leans towards the opposite side and pain is aggravated by lateral flexion towards the same side as this pulls the root against the prolapse (Fig. 9.20). If the prolapse is medial to the root, in the 'axilla' between root and dura, the patient lists to the same side as the lesion. Therefore the direction to which the patient deviates depends on the relationship of the disc prolapse to the adjacent root and not on which side the disc prolapse occurs.

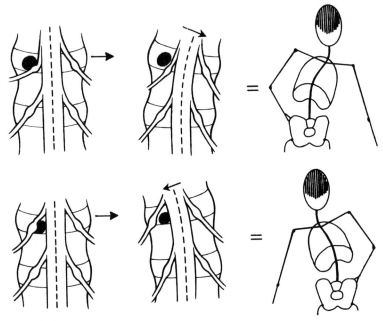

Fig. 9.20 Deviation of spine in prolapsed intervertebral disc.

The patient is then inspected from the side and the presence, accentuation, absence or reversal of the normal lordosis noted. Where a painful lesion is present the lordosis is obliterated or even reversed. The patient is asked to bend forwards and to each side. The level reached and the influence of movement on the lumbar spine are noted. Finally the patient is viewed from in front.

Palpation. This is performed with the patient erect and prone, and again the contour of the spine, the presence of tenderness, and the skin temperature are assessed. Measurement of spinal flexion is described on page 325.

If firm pressure by the thumb is applied between the laminae over a prolapsed disc the pain will be aggravated and radiation of the pain produced (Fig. 9.21). This may not happen immediately, and pressure may have to be maintained for some seconds. When negative, no tenderness or radiation of pain is caused by the test. In France a positive reaction is known as the door bell sign.

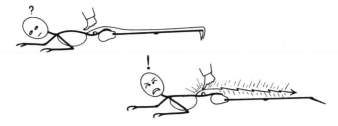

Fig. 9.21 Prolapsed intra-vertebral disc. Local and referred pain.

Nerve Stretching Tests

Sciatic Roots. Usually the fifth lumbar or first sacral root is involved in a lumbo-sacral disc prolapse. Tension is put on these roots by flexing the hip with the knee straight, so-called *straight leg raising.* Normally 90° of flexion at the hip should be possible. Where the root is stretched round or over a prolapsed disc, the same amount of straight leg raising will not be allowed (Fig. 9.22a & b). When the limit of straight leg raising has been achieved, further tension on the root is caused by dorsiflexing the ankle, so pulling the ultimate component of the sciatic nerve, the posterior tibial nerve 'round' the ankle; if positive, the pain is aggravated and is felt in the back of the leg radiating into the lumbar region in some instances (Fig. 9.22c). This test differentiates limitation of straight leg raising due to disc prolapse from that due to short hamstring muscles or a lesion in the hip.

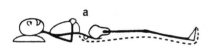

a

Neutral. Nerve roots slack.

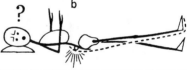

b

Straight leg raising limited by tension of root over prolapsed disc.

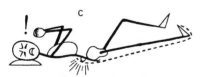

c

Tension increased by dorsiflexion of foot. (Bragaard Test).

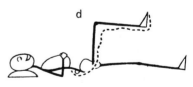

d

Root tension relieved by flexion at knee and ankle.

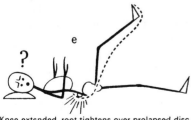

e

Knee extended, root tightens over prolapsed disc causing pain radiating to the back. (Lasegue Test)

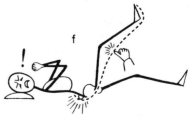

f

Pressure over centre of popliteal fossa bears on posterior tibial nerve which is 'bow stringing' across the fossa causing pain locally and radiation into back.

Fig. 9.22 Stretch tests — sciatic nerve roots.

THE 'BOWSTRING SIGN'. This test is even more accurate and selective and may be useful in diagnosing malingering. Straight leg raising is performed as described above. At the limit the knee is flexed, reducing tension on the sciatic roots and the hamstrings. Unless the hip is stiff, further flexion at the hip will now be possible. Having achieved more flexion at the hip, the knee is again extended until pain is produced (Lasègue's sign, Fig. 9.22d & e). At this stage the posterior tibial nerve is stretched like a bowstring across the popliteal fossa. Firm pressure is applied with the thumb first over the hamstring tendons nearest the examiner, then in the middle of the popliteal fossa and finally on the other hamstring tendon. The patient is asked which caused pain, the first, second or third and if the answer is the second, is asked where the pain was felt. The test is positive only if the pain radiates from the knee into the back or down to the foot.

FLIP TEST. This is a further test of sciatic root tension carried out at the end of the examination if it is suspected that the complaint may not be genuine. The patient sits with the hips and knees flexed to 90° and the knee jerks are tested again. The knee is extended, ostensibly to examine the ankle jerk. Where there is genuine root tension the patient will 'flip' backward to relieve that tension. The 'bogus' patient, distracted by attention to the ankle jerk test, will permit full extension of the knee which is the equivalent of 90° straight leg raising or forward flexion to the toes when standing (Fig. 9.23).

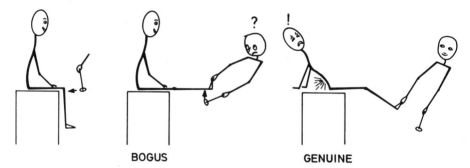

BOGUS   GENUINE

Fig. 9.23 Stretch test — sciatic nerve roots. In the 'flip test' when attention is diverted to the tendon reflexes the genuine patient will still not permit full extension of the leg.

Femoral Roots. Disc prolapse at higher levels may involve the roots of the femoral nerve (L2, 3). The femoral nerve passes into the thigh in front of the pubic ramus, and straight leg raising will relieve any tension on these roots. They are stretched by extending the hip with the knee flexed. This is done with the patient lying prone. Where there is a large disc prolapse or a painful flexion deformity of the hip, the patient may not be able to lie prone, but the test can then be performed with the patient lying on the unaffected side. In either case the knee is flexed. This may be enough to reproduce the pain and cause the patient to flex the hip to relieve the tension on the root. Where limitation of extension is due to changes in the hip, knee flexion should have no effect on the pain. If knee flexion alone causes no pain, the hip is extended with the knee still flexed. If the test is positive, it will cause pain radiating into the back (Fig. 9.24).

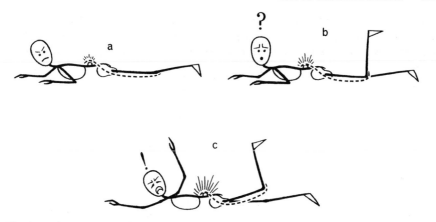

Fig. 9.24 Stretch test — femoral nerve. (a) Patient prone and free from pain because femoral roots are slack. (b) When femoral roots are tightened by flexion of knee pain may be felt in the back. (c) If still no pain, femoral roots are further stretched by extension of the hip.

Neurological Signs. Detailed examination of sensation, motor function and reflexes is a most important part of the examination when nerve root involvement by a disorder of the lumbar spine is under consideration.

An example of the integration of the examination of a patient with backache is given on page 364.

SACRO-ILIAC JOINTS

The sacro-iliac joints are involved at an early stage in ankylosing spondylitis, but other lesions are uncommon. Movement of the sacro-iliac joint cannot be measured on clinical examination, but the joints can easily be tested by firm compression and distraction of the iliac crests. Pain is produced in the region of the sacro-iliac joint if the lesion is there.

THE LOWER LIMB

Before considering individual regions it is worth remembering that the posture of the legs varies throughout life, as does the posture in the spine. These changes do in some measure resemble the changes that have occurred in the evolution from the quadruped to the biped stance. The frequency of congenital abnormalities in the leg compared with the arm may reflect these changes in posture and function. Congenital abnormalities are more frequently found in the foot than in the hand.

THE HIP

This large ball-and-socket joint is very vulnerable. Its components may dislocate at birth; epiphysitis (Perthes disease) or infection may develop before 10 years of age.

The hip joint may slip its epiphysis at puberty, dislocate in the active young adult, develop 'spontaneous' avascular necrosis with maturity, wear out in the middle-aged and fracture in the elderly as a result of osteoporosis or malignancy. This last catastrophe can be further complicated by death of the femoral head.

Anatomical Features

Owing to the depth of the normal acetabulum, the hip is a stable joint, but at the same time is remarkably mobile because the femur has developed a neck which is narrower than the maximum circumference of the head. In the adult the acetabulum faces outwards, downwards, and slightly backwards. The neck of the femur is set on the shaft at an angle of 130° and is directed forwards, anteverted, some 30°. The adult hip is most stable when the femur is extended. In the infant the acetabulum is directed forwards; the neck of the femur is set at a greater angle on the shaft and is directed at least 70° anteriorly. The infant's hip is therefore most stable when flexed and abducted and is in danger of dislocation if extended and adducted at this age. In contrast, the adult hip is most liable to dislocation when flexed and adducted, the posture adopted when sitting. This accounts for the increasing frequency of posterior dislocation in car accidents.

The femoral and obturator nerves supply sensory branches to the hip and the knee joint, explaining the frequent reference of pain to the knee from lesions of the hip joint.

Movements. As the hip is a ball-and-socket joint, flexion, extension, abduction, adduction, rotation and the combined movement of circumduction are possible. The actual range changes throughout life, as does the posture of the joint. As age increases, the first movements to decrease are extension and internal rotation, then abduction.

Special Points in the History

Pain arising from the hip is most commonly situated in the groin, but may radiate down the thigh to the knee or be present in this joint alone. Any patient who cannot accurately localise pain in the knee should be suspected of having a disorder of the hip. Gluteal pain and pain down the back of the thigh suggest the spine as a source of the symptoms.

Examination of the Hip

Gait. This should be observed with the patient lightly clad, otherwise the disability from a stiff hip may pass unnoticed. When adequate inspection is possible it is obvious that the pelvis moves with the leg in this condition. The gait of gluteal dysfunction, whatever the cause, has been described (p. 320).

Posture. If the hip is mobile and one leg is short, the pelvis tilts down towards the shortened side and a scoliosis develops (Fig. 9.25), or the patient simply flexes the hip and knee of the longer leg. A 'raise' under the short leg corrects the posture of the hips and the back (Fig. 9.25). A series of wooden blocks, ranging from $\frac{1}{2}$ cm to 6 cm in depth, is used to determine the comfortable amount of elevation required by a standing patient to compensate for a shortening of a leg.

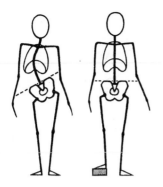 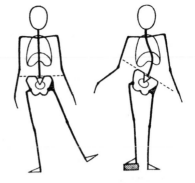

Fig. 9.25   Posture changes in short leg.   **Fig. 9.26   Abduction deformity of the hip.**

A fixed abduction deformity causes apparent lengthening of the leg. The patient can adjust the posture by flexing the knee on the affected side and decreasing the lordosis, or by wearing a raise under the normal but apparently short limb, allowing a scoliosis to develop (Fig. 9.26).

Fixed adduction of the hip causes apparent shortening of the leg. Bending the other knee or using a raise on the affected side does not correct the scoliosis (Fig. 9.27).

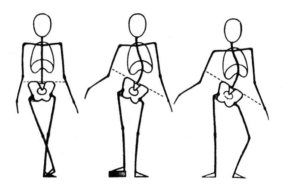

Fig. 9.27   Adduction deformity of the hip.

A fixed flexion deformity will cause apparent shortening, but the patient will be able to compensate by increasing the lordosis and no scoliosis will occur. A raise under the affected leg will allow the spine to return to normal lordosis (Fig. 9.28). A single deformity seldom occurs. The most common combination is adduction and flexion of the hip.

Inspection of the Supine Patient. When the patient lies on the examination couch it is difficult to detect deformity of the hip, because the pelvis can tilt to compensate for a considerable malposition of the hip. The pelvis must first be positioned so that the iliac crests are on the same horizontal plane and at right angles to the spine. Any fixed abduction or adduction will immediately be revealed.

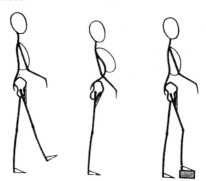

Fig. 9.28   Flexion deformity of the hip.

A flexion deformity will be masked by the patient tilting the pelvis forwards, increasing the lumbar lordosis. The *Thomas test* consists of obliterating the lumbar lordosis by flexing the unaffected hip to its limit and then continuing flexion to straighten the lumbar spine. The affected leg will then be raised off the table, revealing the amount of flexion deformity present.

Inspection is completed by looking for swelling, signs of inflammation, muscle wasting or sinus formation. Although it is impossible to see distension of the hip joint when an effusion is present, the limb takes up the characteristic posture of slight flexion, abduction and external rotation. If an infective process has caused destructive changes in the joint, flexion, adduction and internal rotation will develop.

Measurement of Leg Length. Accurate measurement can be achieved only by special radiological techniques, but clinical examination gives a reasonable assessment of any discrepancy. Where a fixed deformity of the hip joint is present and the legs are brought parallel, the limbs will apparently be unequal in length as shown in Fig. 9.29. The amount of *apparent shortening* is measured between a fixed point, the xiphoid process or the umbilicus, and the tip of the medial malleolus.

True shortening is measured from the anterior superior iliac spine to the medial malleolus (Fig. 9.30). The normal limb must be measured in a comparable position to the abnormal one, in respect of adduction or abduction, if reasonable accuracy is to be achieved.

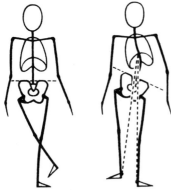

Fig. 9.29   Measurement of apparent shortening of the leg.

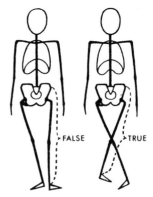

Fig. 9.30   Measurement of true shortening of the leg.

Palpation. In adults it is difficult to detect anything other than gross swelling around the hip joint. Palpation can localise tenderness and so give some indication of the source of the symptoms.

Measurement of Movement. FLEXION. The pelvis must be immobilised in order to be certain that the movement being measured is that of the hip alone and not also of the pelvis on the spine. The iliac crest is stabilised with one hand while the other grasps the leg (Fig. 9.31). The Thomas test is then carried out to see if any fixed flexion is present. This routine is performed first on the normal side and the range compared with the abnormal.

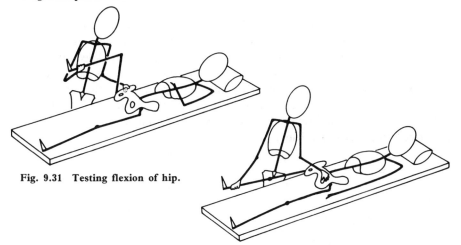

Fig. 9.31 Testing flexion of hip.

Fig. 9.32 Testing abduction and adduction of hip.

ABDUCTION AND ADDUCTION. Movement of the pelvis must again be eliminated. With the patient supine the examiner grasps the opposite iliac crest and lays that forearm across the pelvis over the anterior-superior iliac spine on the nearer side (Fig. 9.32). Abduction and adduction are then carried out. At each extreme the pelvis will be felt to turn with the limb.

ROTATION. This movement should be carried out with the hips first extended and then flexed. With the patient supine, and using the patellae as indicators, the legs are rolled on the couch and the range measured by the excursion of the patellae. A more accurate method is performed with the patient prone. The knees are flexed to a right angle and the tibiae then act as indicators of the arc of rotation. The range of rotation of the flexed hips is measured by flexing both the hip and the knee to a right angle as the patient lies supine. Again the tibiae act as indicators of the degree of rotation.

The accurate measurement of rotation is particularly important if slipping of the upper femoral epiphysis is suspected. An increase of external rotation at the expense of internal rotation is one of the earliest clinical findings. Conversely, a tendency to congenital dislocation is accompanied by more internal than external rotation.

Tests of Stability of Hip. Instability is encountered in congenital dislocation in infants, slipped epiphysis in adolescents, traumatic dislocations in adults, and fractures of the neck of the femur in the elderly and in certain neurological and muscular disorders.

IN INFANCY AND CHILDHOOD. Congenital dislocation of the hip must be diagnosed as soon as possible after birth, certainly many months before the child walks. Thus many of the classical signs are useless. The three most obvious features are:

1. Shortening and external rotation of the limb. The mother may remark that the child does not move the affected leg as much as the other.
2. Asymmetry of the thigh and buttock folds.
3. Limitation of abduction: 90° of abduction in each hip should be possible in an infant.

If any of these signs are present, Ortolani's rest should be performed. This test is now carried out on newborn infants as a routine in many maternity units.

Ortolani's Test (Fig. 9.33). With the infant supine, the hips and knees are flexed to a right angle and the knees brought together. Pressing gently backwards the hips are slowly abducted and extended. If the hips are unstable, the first part of the manoeuvre will push the head of the femur out of the acetabulum. As abduction proceeds the head of the femur will be felt to click back into place. This test can be performed on the newborn baby.

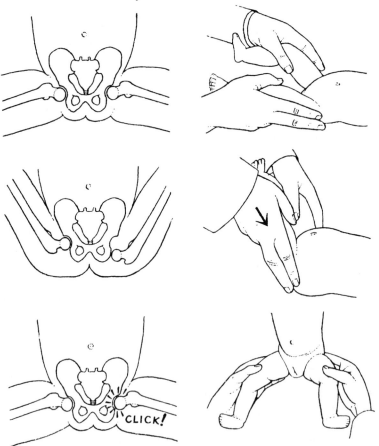

CLICK!

Fig. 9.33 Ortolani's test.

Testing for 'telescoping' of the limb depends on an established dislocation and is therefore a late sign. The term vividly describes the sensation of the limb apparently sinking into the trunk as it is thrust in the axis of the limb itself towards the trunk.

Trendelenburg's Sign. This sign demonstrates that the hip abductors are not functioning, and is useful in the late stages of congenital dislocation of the hip when the patient is walking, and in assessing the disability in poliomyelitis involving the lower limbs. When the normal subject stands on one leg the glutei contract so that the opposite side of the pelvis is tilted up slightly. If the patient stands on the affected leg when the actions of the glutei are deficient, the opposite side of the pelvis will tilt downward and balance can be maintained only by leaning over towards the side of the lesion (Fig. 9.34). The test is performed with the patient's back to the examiner. The patient stands on the normal leg and with the hip extended flexes the knee of the other leg to a right angle. The pelvis remains level or tilts up slightly on the other side. The patient then stands on the abnormal leg and the pelvis tilts down on the opposite side. When walking, the patient compensates for the lack of abduction by leaning over to the affected side so that the centre of gravity is as nearly as possible over the hip. This causes the patient to dip, or lurch, towards the affected side.

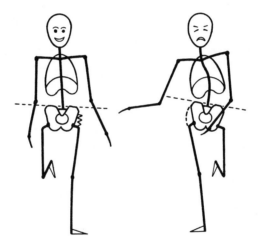

Fig. 9.34 Trendelenburg's sign.

IN PUBERTY AND IN ADULT LIFE. Instability associated with slipped upper femoral epiphysis (adolescent coxa vara), traumatic dislocation of the hip, and fracture in the region of the neck of the femur is apt to occur at a particular age period and is associated with characteristic postures:

1. *Slipped upper femoral epiphysis.* This occurs at puberty. The limb is externally rotated, adducted and shortened.

2. *Traumatic dislocation.* This occurs mainly in mature patients.

(i) Posterior dislocation in which the limb is flexed, adducted and internally rotated is the more common.

(ii) In anterior dislocation the limb is flexed, abducted and externally rotated.

3. *Fracture in the region of the neck of the femur.* This is common in elderly women.

The limb is externally rotated, adducted and shortened. This is the same deformity as in slipped epiphysis because the same mechanism is involved.

THE KNEE

The knee is particularly prone to injury by twisting owing to the fact that its stability through a range of movement of 150° is entirely dependent upon the control of muscles and ligaments. In addition, its exposed position renders it liable to direct injury. Repeated kneeling brings both a tendency to traumatic bursitis and a risk of direct infection of the joint by puncture wounds. Inflammation due to rheumatoid arthritis commonly involves the knee joint. Over the years the stress of weight-bearing often leads to degenerative changes, especially in the obese. Serious congenital abnormalities are rare.

Anatomical Features

There is normally a degree of valgus, or abduction, of the tibia on the femur when the knee is fully extended. In this position, because of the shape of the condyles of the femur, the tibia externally rotates on the femur. This in turn causes the collateral ligaments and the anterior cruciate ligament to become stretched. In this situation the tibia is 'screwed home' on the femur and the joint is 'locked' in full extension and able to sustain the body weight with minimal muscle action. With a few degrees of flexion the external rotation is undone, and the ligaments are relaxed. It is now possible to abduct, adduct and rotate the tibia on the femur, or vice versa. When the ligaments are tight in full extension, they are particularly liable to injury.

The semilunar cartilages, attached by their periphery to the capsule, are relatively mobile structures. When the tibia is abducted, adducted, or rotated on the femur, the cartilage is sucked between the bones on the 'open' side of the joint. A sudden change of position then may trap the cartilage, which tears from its periphery. The torn portion, resembling a 'bucket handle', comes to lie between the condyles of the femur. The knee is then said to be locked because extension is obstructed to a varying degree, although flexion may be largely preserved. Occasionally one end of the bucket handle separates from its attachment and a 'parrot beak' tear results. This is liable to become caught momentarily between the tibia and femur. The patient is aware of a sensation of the knee being about to give way, or it may actually do so. This is in contrast to the 'locking' of a bucket handle tear. Both incidents are usually related to movement involving flexion and rotation while taking the body weight, for example changing direction when running or twisting round when kneeling.

The quadriceps is the most important group of muscles controlling the knee. When these muscles contract they tend to pull in a straight line from the greater trochanter to the tibial tubercle. Because of the normal valgus of the knee, this tends to displace the patella laterally. This tendency, however, is controlled by the action of the obliquely disposed vastus medialis muscles. The more valgus the knee, the greater the tendency to lateral displacement of the patella and the more important the action of the vastus medialis.

Special Points in the History

The anatomical features which have been discussed underline the importance of a detailed history of the mechanism of any injury of the knee. The menisci are liable to be torn by twisting injuries, especially when playing football. Possibly because of the greater valgus at the knee in the female, lateral dislocation of the patella with spontaneous reduction is not uncommon. The history will be identical with a medial cartilage injury. Sudden pain with the sensation of something giving way on the inner side of the joint is felt as the knee is bent with or without rotation. Inspection soon after this episode will settle the diagnosis. With both injuries bleeding occurs. With a cartilage injury it is confined within the joint and no bruising is seen. With dislocation of the patella, the retinaculae on the medial side are torn, blood escapes into the subcutaneous tissues, and bruising is visible.

A violent blow applied to one side of the knee in extension is liable to cause partial or complete rupture of the opposite collateral ligament. The quadriceps muscles react rapidly to injury, infection or lack of use by wasting. The knee itself responds differently according to the degree of injury. Moderate violence, or slight violence often repeated, causes an effusion of varying degree.

Severe violence results in bleeding into the joint which becomes distended — a haemarthrosis. The history is often the only means of differentiating between a large effusion and a haemarthrosis. An effusion takes some hours or even a day to develop; a haemarthrosis develops immediately. Aspiration of the joint settles the issue.

Very severe violence will rupture ligaments. Bleeding will occur, but, because the synovium in addition to the capsule and ligament will be torn, the blood will escape from the joint and present as swelling and bruising about the damaged side of the joint; no fluid will be detected in the joint.

Arthritis is common in the knee joint; in osteoarthrosis the pain and stiffness after sitting may be described as 'locking' by the patient. This underlines the importance of finding out exactly what the patient means and of not accepting such terms uncritically. Rupture of a cyst in the popliteal fossa associated with arthritis, may be mistaken for deep vein thrombosis (p. 139).

Pain may be referred to the knee from elsewhere, notably the hip. Where pain arises in the knee itself, the patient can usually indicate its site accurately. When the patient points vaguely to the front of the lower thigh and knee, one should suspect that the hip is the source of the pain.

Examination of the Knee

Inspection with Patient Erect. The characteristic gait of a stiff knee is immediately evident (p. 320). Provided there is reasonable control of the hip or foot, a patient can walk even when all the controlling muscles of the knee are paralysed, because of the locking mechanism described above.

Abnormalities of posture are most evident when the patient stands. The most difficult problem is to determine when knock-knee (genu valgum, p. 319) becomes abnormal in degree in the two- to four-year-old child. The distance between the medial malleoli when the child stands with the feet parallel and the knees just touching is a useful measurement to record for comparison in the future. It is not possible to give an absolute figure for any particular age, but in the majority the deformity corrects spontaneously by the age of six to eight years. Over this age separation of the malleoli by more than 5 cm is a deformity which is unlikely to correct itself. Before predicting that spontaneous correction will occur, it is wise to inspect the mother's knees unobtrusively. Asymmetrical genu valgum is abnormal at any age.

Inspection with Patient Supine. Deformity can again be reviewed, and in particular the amount of genu valgum measured, as noted above. Wasting of the muscles and any swelling of the joint can now be more easily assessed.

Palpation. The bony contour is checked and signs of inflammation are sought. Muscle girth should be recorded in order to follow progress when wasting is present. The level above the patella at which this measurement is made should also be noted.

Tenderness must be accurately localised. The whole extent of both collateral ligaments and the joint line must be palpated. This latter cannot be localised accurately with the knee extended, but in flexion the joint line becomes visible in the thinner subject and is at least palpable in obese patients.

EFFUSION. A *trace of effusion* can be detected only by the massage test. With the knee straight, any fluid in the antero-medial compartment of the knee is massaged up into the suprapatellar pouch. Then by pressure over the suprapatellar pouch and lateral compartment with the fingers and thumb of the opposite hand the fluid is squeezed back into the antero-medial compartment. The normal depression medial to the patellar tendon is seen to bulge as the fluid accumulates there.

A *moderate effusion* gives rise to a *patellar tap*. With the knee straight the suprapatellar pouch is emptied by pressure with one hand, and the parapatellar compartment by pressure with the other hand, leaving the index finger free to elicit the tap. With this finger the patella is pressed sharply against the femur. If there is sufficient fluid to 'float' the patella off the femur it will be felt to tap against the femur.

A *large effusion* outlines the suprapatellar pouch as an inverted crescentic swelling immediately above the patella and a tap may be easily elicited. By squeezing this swelling while palpating on each side of the patella with the other hand an effusion can be differentiated from synovial thickening by the transmission of a fluid impulse from hand to hand when an effusion is present.

LOOSE BODIES. A careful examination of the knee is required where there is a history of locking. If this symptom results from a particular movement, a meniscus injury should be suspected. When its occurrence is unpredictable, locking is likely to be due to loose bodies. A palpable loose body can move in all directions and usually disappears between the condyles of the femur. Thick patellar retinaculae may be mistaken for loose bodies as they roll under the examining finger. Their position and the fact that they can be moved from side to side and not up and down helps to identify them.

Movements of the Knee. The normal range in the adult is zero to 150° of flexion. In some subjects a few degrees of hyperextension are possible. This is found more frequently in females.

When fully extended no abduction, adduction or rotation of the tibia on the femur is possible. With only a few degrees of flexion, abduction, adduction and rotation through a small range are possible.

When only one knee appears to be affected the active range is examined first in the normal and then the abnormal joint. The passive range is then performed in the same order, and during this examination a hand is placed on the knee to detect the presence and character of crepitus. The site of any pain and its relationship to a particular arc of movement are noted. Care is taken to detect even a few degrees of limitation of extension. When a bucket handle cartilage tear is displaced, passive extension of the knee is blocked. The sensation is of pushing against a firm rubber stop, and the knee recoils as soon as pressure is released. The patient usually complains of pain at the site of the torn cartilage. This 'rubbery' block to extension can be mimicked by an effusion in the knee, but passive extension then does not cause the same localised pain.

The most accurate method of demonstrating a few degrees of loss of extension is to lie the patient prone with the legs projecting over the end of the examination couch, supported only by the thighs. The level of the heels can be compared as an indication of unequal extension of the knees.

Tests of Stability. To test the *collateral ligaments* the knee must be fully extended. The patient's ankle is held between the examiner's elbow and side, leaving both hands free to abduct and adduct the tibia on the femur while keeping the knee straight (Fig. 9.35). Normally no movement should be detected. Where a ligament is strained no movement occurs, but pain is localised over the damaged ligament when it is stretched. When a ligament is lax, the knee 'opens' when pushed from the opposite side and is felt to 'close' with a click when pressure is released.

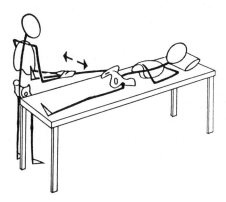

Fig. 9.35 Testing the collateral ligaments of the knee.

The *cruciate ligaments* are tested with the knee flexed to a right angle. This position is maintained by the examiner sitting on the patient's foot (Fig. 9.36). The patient should be warned before doing this because the polite patient withdraws the foot, and the less polite complains. With both hands now free the examiner first checks by palpation that the hamstring muscles are relaxed; otherwise the test is invalid. To test the anterior cruciate the tibia is grasped just below the knee and is drawn forwards. To test the posterior cruciates this movement is reversed. Starting with the normal knee the degree of anteroposterior glide of the tibia is noted as the normal for that patient. Any movement in excess of this in the suspect knee is abnormal. Excessive anterior 'glide' or 'draw' is due to laxity of the anterior

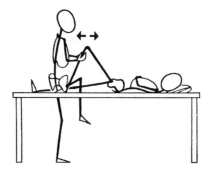

Fig. 9.36 Testing the cruciate ligaments of the knee.

cruciate, and posterior displacement is associated with laxity of the posterior cruciate ligament. Gross instability of a cruciate ligament is usually associated with laxity of one of the collateral ligaments and vice versa.

The McMurray Test. The object of this test of stability of the semilunar cartilages is to induce a torn cartilage to engage between the tibia and the femur by reproducing the mechanism which originally caused the displacement. When this happens, the patient experiences the typical symptoms and a palpable, and occasionally audible, 'click' or 'clunk' results. There is a risk that the examiner will lock the patient's knee and be unable thereafter to free it again.

The patient must be able to relax. To examine the right knee the examiner stands on the right side of the couch, grasps the patient's right heel with the right hand and steadies the knee with the left hand. The knee is flexed to the limit the patient will tolerate. While pressing on the outer side of the knee with the left hand the knee is extended while the tibia is alternately internally, and externally rotated by the right hand (Fig. 9.37). If positive, a 'clunk' accompanied by some discomfort to the patient is felt over the displacing cartilage. If this does not produce the characteristic response, the manoeuvre is repeated while the left hand presses on the inner side of the knee. The former technique is more likely to be positive where a medial cartilage is displaced, and the latter where the lateral cartilage is involved.

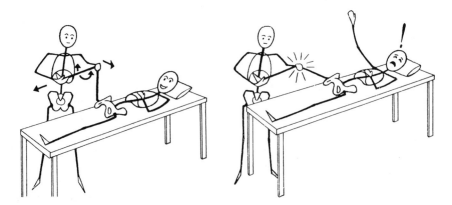

Fig. 9.37 The McMurray test of the semilunar cartilages.

Stability of the Patella. With the knee extended, the patella is grasped and moved from side to side. An impression of excessive mobility may be gained when this is compared with the normal knee. Passive flexion of the knee while the patella is pressed laterally may reproduce the patient's symptoms or may even dislocate the patella.

Tests for Degenerative Change in the Knee. During active and passive movement of the knee palpation may detect crepitus or a grinding sensation, if osteoarthrosis is present. The character of the crepitus varies and the coarser it is the more extreme will be the degree of wear and tear in the articular cartilage.

Where the osteoarthrosis is localised to the patello-femoral compartment of the knee, moving the patella up and down against the femur (patellar grinding) will be painful and will be accompanied by crepitus. Similarly if the patient contracts this quadriceps muscle while the patella is pressed firmly against the femur, characteristic pain will be produced if the patella is the site of osteoarthrosis or of chondromalacia in the younger patient.

THE LEG, ANKLE AND FOOT

The human foot has undergone great evolutionary change. The tarsal bones have become massive and disposed in two layers. The metatarsophalangeal segments now lie roughly parallel and instead of the central segment being the longest, the medial segment, or hallux, has become the longest and strongest component of the forefoot. Many feet fail to achieve this ideal and the first metatarsal remains relatively short and deviated medially (varus). The phalanges then deviate in the opposite direction and hallux valgus results. This is only one example of the many congenital defects found in the feet. In addition to this tendency to congenital abnormality, the feet have to bear the stress of the body weight on hard unyielding surfaces, often cramped and confined by fashionable footwear. For these reasons many problems are encountered in the feet.

Anatomical Features

The two feet placed side by side resemble an inverted soup-plate. Each foot corresponds with half a plate. The inner border of the foot is raised to form the longitudinal arch. The outer border, corresponding with the rim of the plate, lies on the ground. When the feet are placed together an arch, lying across the mid-tarsal region, is formed. When not bearing weight a further lesser transverse arch lies under the metatarsal heads. The arches of the foot act as shock absorbers when the foot takes the body weight and give spring to the gait. The flattened outer border gives stability when standing.

When the patient is standing, the long axis of the talus, navicular, medial cuneiform and first metatarsal should lie in a straight line. This can be seen accurately only on radiological examination with the patient standing, but clinical examination will give some idea where this longitudinal axis is broken in foot deformity. As an aid to the understanding of various deformities, the foot may be considered to have three main components — the talus, the calcaneus and the forefoot. The last includes the navicular, cuboid, cuneiforms, metatarsals and phalanges.

Description of Foot Deformities. *Talipes* is derived from the words talus and pes, inferring that there is a deformity involving the ankle and foot, and must be further qualified to have any meaning. *Talipes equinus* means that the foot and ankle are plantar flexed, like the foot of a horse which walks on the tip of one 'finger'. *'Talipes equino varus'* means that in addition the hind foot is adducted and that the forefoot also is adducted or inverted at the midtarsal joint (Fig. 9.38). This is the typical clubfoot deformity. *Talipes calcaneus* indicates that the heel projects towards the sole of the foot (Fig. 9.39). When combined with valgus of the other parts of the foot, *talipes calcaneo valgus*, it is the other common congenital foot deformity.

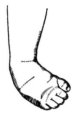

Fig. 9.38   Talipes equino varus.

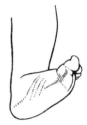

Fig. 9.39   Talipes calcaneus.

Either of these deformities may be associated with deformity of the longitudinal arch. If flattened, the deformity is described as *planus*. If raised or increased, the deformity is described as *cavus*. It is possible, therefore, to have a talipes equino-cavovarus, etc.

Pes means foot and implies deformity involving the foot only and that the position of the ankle joint is normal. *Pes planus* means flat-foot. The axis of the longitudinal arch passing as a straight line through talus, navicular, medial cuneiform and first metatarsal may sag at either the talo-navicular, medial naviculo-cuneiform joint or both. The most severe degrees of flat-foot are usually associated with the former. The normal heel is vertical when viewed from behind. In pes planus the heel is often abducted (valgus, p. 319) and the whole foot pronated.

In *pes cavus* the longitudinal arch is raised and the heel seen from behind is often adducted (varus). In this position the foot is supinated and the toes are usually clawed. This deformity may be associated with abnormalities of the central nervous system, e.g. Friedreich's ataxia.

Claw toes are usually found with a pes cavus. The toes are extended at the metatarso-phalangeal joints and flexed at the interphalangeal joints. All the toes are commonly affected and eventually dorsal dislocation occurs at the metatarso-phalangeal joints.

Hammer toe often involves only the second toe and is not associated with other deformities of the foot. The metatarso-phalangeal joint is extended, the proximal interphalangeal joint is flexed and the distal interphalangeal joint is extended. A painful corn develops over the proximal interphalangeal joint.

Hallux valgus is probably the most common deformity in a shoe-wearing community. In addition to valgus deformity of the phalanges the metatarsal is often shorter than normal and deviated in the opposite direction — metatarsus primus varus et brevis (p. 357).

In *hallux rigidus* the big toe is often longer than the other toes and, perhaps because of this, develops degenerative change or osteoarthrosis in the metatarsophalangeal joint. At first extension is diminished, but in the extreme instances the toe may become permanently flexed — *hallux flexus*.

Special Features in the History

In children pain in the feet directly related to the musculo-skeletal structures is not common. When not associated with obvious deformity or inflammatory changes the cause is usually epiphysitis involving the calcaneus, navicular or the metatarsal heads.

In the adult, pain localised to the foot usually has its origin there, but pain arising in the foot may be referred up the leg. The character and pattern of the pain will give some indication of the cause. Osteoarthrosis has the familiar pattern of pain and stiffness after rest and relieved temporarily by activity. Aching pain which gradually gets worse the longer the patient is standing suggests chronic ligamentous strain. Pain of a burning, tingling character radiating into the third and fourth toes and into the foot suggests a digital neuroma in the cleft between these toes. The patient notices that removing the shoe relieves this pain; on examination there is tenderness in the affected toe cleft, and sensation is depressed in the same toe cleft. Ischaemia of the feet can cause distressing pain at night (p. 136). Special enquiry should be directed at the condition of the feet in elderly patients as severe but remediable disability can be caused by minor abnormalities such as callosities or overgrowth of a nail (onychogryphosis).

Metatarsalgia (pain in the forefoot) is commonly associated with claw or hammer toe deformity where the fibrofatty pad normally under the metatarsal head comes to lie under the toes, leaving the metatarsal heads unprotected. The patient very appropriately describes pain as walking on the bones themselves, or likens it to walking on stones. This situation also develops in rheumatoid arthritis. Other causes of metatarsalgia are stress (march) fractures of the metatarsal shafts, and epiphysitis of the second metatarsal head in adolescence.

Examination of the Leg, Ankle and Foot

Gait. Stiffness without pain causes little alteration in the gait. Equinus deformity, like the drop-foot, causes a high stepping gait in order to clear the ground, but differs from it in that the foot is fixed in the former but loose and flapping in the latter. The gait of talipes calcaneus lacks spring — a peg-leg gait.

Posture. Apart from the effects of the congenital deformities already described, abnormal posture of the foot may result from a poor general posture. Surprising correction of flat-foot deformity is achieved by correcting the typical slouching, knee flexed, pronated feet stance of the disinterested adolescent.

Inspection and Palpation. This is best performed with the patient sitting on the examination couch with the legs dangling over the edge. The calf is relaxed and foot movement is freer when the knee is flexed. The examiner sits on a low stool in front of the patient. The colour, texture and temperature of the skin give useful information concerning the circulation and nutrition of the foot. The condition of the nails is noted. The toes are separated and the area between them is inspected for evidence of fungal infection, in which condition the skin becomes thickened, whitish, sodden and fissured. Particular note is made of the site of any callosity as an indication of abnormal pressure. Tenderness or other signs of inflammation are accurately localised. The pulses are palpated in the dorsalis pedis and posterior tibial arteries.

Movements. While the patient is erect, the ability to stand on the toes, on the heels and on the inner and outer borders of the feet is tested. The active range of non-weight-bearing movement is then noted and finally the range of passive movement is reviewed.

FLEXION AND DORSIFLEXION OF THE ANKLE. The foot is in the neutral position when it is at right angles to the long axis of the tibia. The true position of the foot in relation to the leg is more easily appreciated when viewed from the outer side. In dorsiflexion the broader anterior surface of the talus is engaged in the ankle mortice and no other movement can take place in the ankle joint. In plantar flexion the narrower portion of the talus is engaged and some abduction and adduction can take place. In practice this cannot be differentiated from movement in the subtalar joint.

INVERSION AND EVERSION OF THE HIND FOOT. The examiner holds the heel with the foot at right angles to the leg (Fig. 9.40). The heel is then adducted and abducted. These movements take place mainly in the subtalar joint.

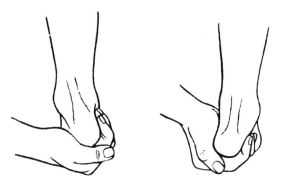

Fig. 9.40 Inversion and eversion of the hind foot.

INVERSION AND EVERSION OF THE FOREFOOT. The heel is held in one hand and the forefoot in the other and the forefoot is adducted and abducted in relation to the hind foot (Fig. 9.41). These movements take place in the mid-tarsal joint, between the talus and calcaneus posteriorly and the forefoot anteriorly.

TARSO-METATARSAL MOVEMENT. The range is so small that it cannot be assessed on clinical examination.

Tests of Stability. TENDO ACHILLIS. The diagnosis of ruptured tendo achillis is often missed, perhaps because it is not realised that the foot can still be plantar flexed by the toe flexors. The classic signs are a palpable gap in the tendon,

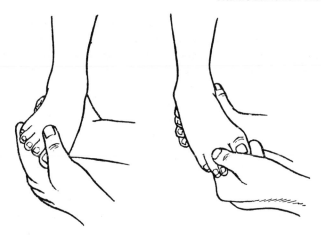

Fig. 9.41   Inversion and eversion of the forefoot.

excessive active and passive dorsi-flexion of the foot, and inability to stand on tiptoe on the affected foot. However, these signs may be difficult to assess because of pain and swelling at the time of injury. The *squeeze test* does not suffer from this handicap. With the patient prone or kneeling, the calf is firmly but gently squeezed just distal to its maximal circumference. Where the tendon is intact the foot plantar flexes. Where the tendon is ruptured, no plantar flexion occurs. This test will also differentiate ruptured tendo achillis from the other common injury to the calf — avulsion of the medial head of the gastrocnemius muscle, as it causes pain at the site of the latter and none when the tendo achillis is ruptured.

LATERAL LIGAMENT OF ANKLE. It is impossible on clinical examination to know if this ligament is ruptured because abnormal movement at the ankle joint cannot be differentiated from subtalar movement. Radiological investigation is required (p. 362).

Foot Prints. Observation of the patient's footprints is occasionally useful in diagnosis. A good imprint can be obtained from a damp foot by standing on brown paper. This is immediately outlined in pencil or ink and affords a permanent objective record of the state of the patient's foot.

Footwear. An abnormality of gait may be suspected or confirmed by irregularities in the pattern of wear on the soles or heels of shoes or boots. Unfortunately this information may not be available as patients often come to the doctor wearing their best and newest footwear.

FURTHER INVESTIGATION

Examination of the Blood. Estimations of haemoglobin, leucocytes, ESR, plasma urate, and rheumatoid and antinuclear factors are used in the differential diagnosis of arthritis. Plasma calcium, phosphate and alkaline phosphatase provide information about the metabolism of bone, and acid phosphatase about bone metastases from carcinoma of the prostate gland.

Radiological Examination and other Imaging. *Radiological examination* plays a very prominent part in the further investigation of abnormalities involving the locomotor system. It is essential, for clinical and medico-legal reasons, if a fracture is suspected. At least two views must be taken, in planes at right angles to each other, to demonstrate the position of the bone fragments. If only one view is taken, the fragments may appear to be in good position when, in fact, they are overlapping and the bone ends are not in contact with each other. Two views may fail to show a crack fracture. When a fracture of the carpal scaphoid is suspected, at least four views are taken. If none is visible but the clinical findings suggest that a fracture is present (p. 70), a plaster is applied and the radiological examination is repeated three weeks later. The alternative is to carry out a radionuclide bone scan before committing the patient to treatment.

In children the epiphyseal cartilage may be confused with a fracture, especially in the elbow. Comparable views of the normal joint will clarify the situation.

When examining the radiographs of the skeleton the opportunity should be taken to look at the whole film for other abnormalities, as, for example, at the apices of the lungs in antero-posterior views of the cervical spine. Similarly, the examination of films of the lumbar spine should include a scrutiny of the soft tissue shadows of the psoas muscles, the abdominal viscera and the diaphragm.

The extent of injury to the soft tissues can be demonstrated by special radiological techniques. Rupture of ligaments allows the related joint to dislocate to a lesser or greater degree and this abnormal position can be shown on a radiograph. For example, a sprained lateral ligament of the ankle cannot be differentiated from a rupture of that ligament on clinical examination. An antero-posterior view of the ankle is required with the foot held in forced inversion. If the lateral ligament is ruptured the talus will be seen to be tilted in the ankle mortice as compared with the normal side. In recent injuries this may have to be performed under an anaesthetic.

If loose bodies are present in a joint, more than the routine antero-posterior and lateral views will often be required. For example, in the knee additional intercondylar views are necessary. Special oblique views may be required for the adequate demonstration of certain joints particularly in the spine, for example the sacro-iliac joints which are involved in the early stages of ankylosing spondylitis and the facet joints when spondylolisthesis is suspected.

Arthrograms can demonstrate abnormalities in the intra-articular structures; air, a radio-opaque fluid or both is injected into the joint. This technique may be used in injuries to the semilunar cartilages in the knee and in defining the position of the labrum of the acetabulum in congenital dislocation of the hip.

Discograms are occasionally helpful. A fine needle is inserted into the disc nucleus and a dye injected. This outlines the disc and may also reproduce the patient's symptoms, helping to confirm the diagnosis in some instances.

Myelograms and *radiculograms* may be used to outline spinal cord and nerve roots respectively (p. 300).

Radionuclide bone scanning (Fig. 9.42) can demonstrate fractures, inflammatory and neoplastic lesions in bones and joints at a stage when they are not visible on radiographic examination.

Computed tomography may be used to define lesions of the vertebrae and related soft tissues (Fig. 7.3, p. 199) difficult to demonstrate by radiographs.

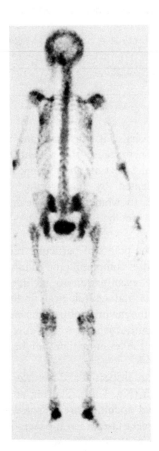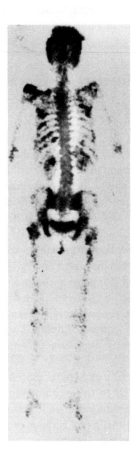

Fig. 9.42   Radioisotope scans (radionuclide imaging) as a diagnostic aid. Uptake of the radioactive tracer is a function of the rate of turnover of bone. In the normal (A) this is greatest in the weight-transmitting parts of the pelvis and spine and around joints (exaggerated in this patient's ankles by arthritis). The other patient (B) has multiple metastases in the ribs and elsewhere, Paget's disease of the skull and a calcific tendinitis of the left shoulder. A bone scan (scintograph) shows the presence of the abnormalities. Radiographs are necessary to make the differential diagnosis. (*Courtesy of Dr M. V. Merrick*).

Ultrasonography provides a rapid non-invasive means of excluding the presence of spinal stenosis.

Other Investigations. *Synovial Fluid.* The properties of fluid aspirated from a joint are helpful in the diagnosis of traumatic, metabolic and inflammatory lesions. In the first haemorrhage can be differentiated from an acute effusion. In the second specific crystals can be seen in gout or pseudogout. In the third leucocytes are found and the infecting organism and its sensitivity can be determined.

Arthroscopy. This is carried out under general anaesthesia and aseptic conditions and has greatly extended the accuracy of diagnosis in certain joints, especially the knee. *Synovial biopsy* is used in the investigation of tuberculosis and tumours.

Choice of Investigation. This will depend on the individual problem, the facilities available and the invasiveness or otherwise of the procedure. As has been stressed in other chapters, discussion of the investigative problem with an expert, for example in imaging techniques, is often essential.

THE METHODS IN PRACTICE

BACKACHE

This example has been chosen mainly because it illustrates one way in which various tests may be integrated in order to cause the patient the minimum inconvenience and to economise on the clinician's time and motion. It also serves to exemplify some of the problems presented by malingering which is not uncommonly encountered with backache. In women, backache may be due to gynaecological difficulties which it would not be appropriate to discuss in this chapter.

History and Examination. Some of the points of particular relevance in the history have been discussed on page 317. After completing the taking of the history it is necessary to plan a comprehensive examination to include checking in particular posture, gait, spinal movements and neurological findings. Methods must be efficiently but rapidly executed as the majority of patients will have few or no signs. The sequence employed by the author is shown in Figure 9.43 to 9.53. When positive findings are encountered the examination can be expanded as appropriate.

First the posture and spinal movements are inspected and next the gait when the patient proceeds to the examination couch (Fig. 9.43). Starting at the head and working downwards, the neck, breasts and abdomen are palpated to check the possibility of a malignant tumour causing metastases; then the sacro-iliac joints are stressed and rotation of the hips tested (Fig. 9.44). Next sciatic and tibial nerve stretching, knee and plantar reflexes, sensation and peripheral pulses are examined (Figs. 9.45 and 9.46). The patient is then carefully observed on turning over on to the prone position (Fig. 9.47). The femoral nerve is stretched, the spine palpated and active extension of the spine observed (Fig. 9.48 & Fig. 9.49). A rectal examination, if indicated, can conveniently be carried out at this stage (Fig. 9.50). If there is doubt about the patient's authenticity the 'flip test' (Fig. 9.23) is performed as the patient is about to descend from the couch (Fig. 9.51). Other tests in this category, for example the foraminal compression test (Fig. 9.19) can be carried out when the patient is again standing (Fig. 9.52). Finally when there are suspicions about ankle weakness, the patient is asked whether walking on the heels or on tiptoe makes the pain worse — not if he or she can walk on the heels or on tiptoe. The malingerer can do both but in apparent agony.

Interpretation of the Findings. The history combined with the clinical signs will establish the diagnosis or indicate what further investigations are required. In the majority there will be few or no positive findings, for example in osteoarthrosis, spondylolisthesis, spinal stenosis and early malignancy, but the history will indicate the probable diagnosis.

In the minority there may be a plethora of clinical signs, for example in the presence of a prolapsed intervertebral disc, an abscess or an advanced malignancy.

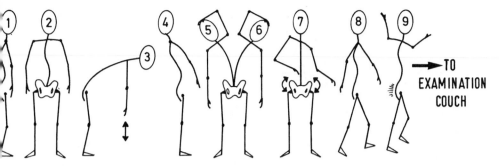

Fig. 9.43 Observe: posture — (1) lateral and (2) postero-anterior; (3) flexion; (4) extension; (5 & 6) lateral flexion; (7) rotation; (8 & 9) gait.

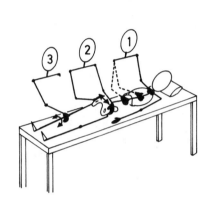

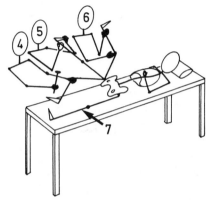

Fig. 9.44 (1) Palpate neck, breasts and abdomen. (2) Stress sacroiliac joints. (3) Rotate legs to check hip rotation.

Fig. 9.45 (4) Knee jerks (5) Straight leg raising and ankle dorsiflexion test. (6) Posterior tibial nerve stretch test. (7) Check active straight leg raising.

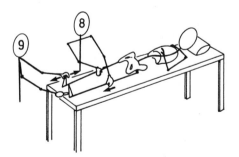

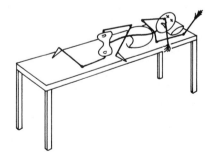

Fig. 9.46 (8) Test sensation from thigh to foot. (9) Plantar reflex; dorsi and plantar flexion of foot; peripheral pulses; girth of calf and thigh if wasting.

Fig. 9.47 Patient turns over; observe performance and posture — patient with femoral root tension cannot lie prone (first stage femoral stretch test).

Fig. 9.43 to 9.47   Backache: integration of examination. First stage.

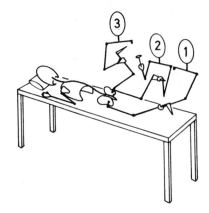

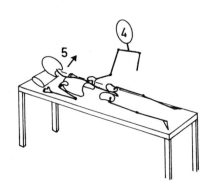

Fig. 9.48 (1) Flex knee (2nd stage femoral stretch test). (2) Ankle jerks. (3) Extend hip with knee flexed. (3rd stage femoral stretch test).

Fig. 9.49 4(a) Palpate spine in midline for contour and local tenderness. (b) Palpate asymptomatic then painful side for tenderness and 'door bell' sign. (5) Check active extension of spine.

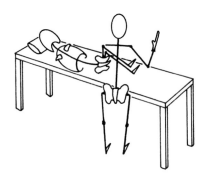

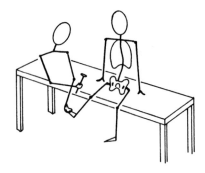

Fig. 9.50 Patient on left side for rectal examination if required.

Fig. 9.51 Flip test to confirm authenticity of sciatic stretch tests.

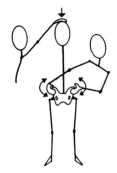

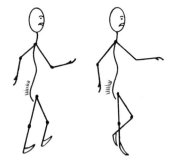

Fig. 9.52 Simulated rotation and axial compression in suspect patients.

Fig. 9.53 Ask patient with suspect ankle weakness if walking on heels or tiptoe makes pain worse.

Fig. 9.48 to 9.53 Backache: integration of examination. Second stage.

They will present a consistent and anatomical pattern and again the history will indicate the underlying pathological lesion.

Hysteria and malingering may also produce a wealth of clinical signs, often easily recognised by their bizarre nature and inconstant and non-anatomical pattern. These inconsistencies include strange postures, a painful gait without the appropriate rhythm, restricted movement when standing and lying which returns to normal when sitting, widespread and variable weakness unaccompanied by measurable wasting, sensory changes of a stocking distribution and widespread and acute tenderness of a regional rather than an anatomical distribution. The affect of the hysteric is one of indifference while the malingerer is on the defensive and often aggressive. In the latter the typical history is one of prolonged continuous pain, even at rest, unaccompanied by any deterioration in general health (p. 317).

It is always important to maintain an impersonal and friendly manner throughout the examination especially when dealing with the last group of patients. Nothing is gained by attempting to browbeat such individuals. Nevertheless all doctors must be aware of the existence of factitious illness. It is of course by no means confined to the locomotor system. Attention has been drawn to Munchausen's disease (p. 3), and to the subterfuges practised by drug addicts (p. 96). Other examples are puzzling fevers produced by thermometer manipulation and symptoms, such as persistent diarrhoea, due to drugs, self-administered with the intent of deceiving the doctor. The reason for such abnormal behaviour should be determined by an evaluation of the patient's personality as described on page 24.

10. The Infant and Child

Children are not men nor women; they are almost as different creatures, in
many respects, as if they never were to be the one or the other; they are as
unlike as buds are unlike flowers, and almost as blossoms are unlike fruits.

W. S. Landor, *Eighteenth Century English Poet*

GENERAL CONSIDERATIONS

In previous chapters the main emphasis has been on the adult, on the elucidation of
symptoms and signs of disease as they present when physical and mental maturity
are well advanced or have been achieved. In this chapter we are dealing with the
infant and child, with the epoch in life preceding the attainment of adulthood but
progressively leading towards it. Further, we are dealing here with all systems.
Paediatrics is a speciality bound by age and not by system. It concerns itself with a
whole individual undergoing rapid growth and change.

In turning at this stage to the clinical examination of the child we are following
the practice which has long pertained in undergraduate clinical teaching —
consideration of the adult first and of the infant and child subsequently. Although
chronologically illogical this practice can be justified. The adult patient is in the
main a more co-operative subject on whom the student's clinical art may be
practised and does not exhibit the wide variations in physique, mentality and
psychological status shown by the child. In adult life physiological normals are
much more constant and are confined within a much narrower range than is the case
in infancy and childhood. Weight is an obvious example of this. The variations
within infancy and childhood may necessitate considerable adaptation of standard
methods of approach, or new methods, and considerable modification or extension
of the techniques of clinical examination. The student who does not appreciate this
may come to have a seriously distorted approach to the clinical examination of
children. It may be felt that the child is merely an adult reduced in size, and,
thinking in this purely quantitative way, the great qualitative differences which
exist are not appreciated. The student may not understand the need to orient
thinking towards growth and development, which are such essential parts of
paediatrics, and away from the established physical and mental status and
degenerative processes which are inherent in adult medical practice. There may be
failure to interpret symptoms and signs and physical measurements in infancy and
childhood against the wide range of physiological normals appropriate to the age of
the patient. The student may try to apply to the child clinical methods which are

impracticable or will yield little information, and may fail to employ more fruitful methods. Signs which, bearing pathological significance in the adult, are without significance in the child may be interpreted as indicative of disease and important signs peculiar to infancy and childhood may be ignored.

While the clinical examination of adults and children have much in common there are important differences. Most of what has already been stated in preceding chapters is relevant to children. This chapter would be inadequate, however, if it indicated merely those points where the clinical examination of the child differs from that of the adult. A disjointed collection of notes and comparisons would result and would give little guidance to the important considerations of emphasis and sequence. It would be difficult on this basis to present the methods of clinical examination of children in proper perspective. Accordingly, an attempt has been made to write a comprehensive chapter with the emphasis on signs and symptoms peculiar to, or of special significance in, infancy and childhood.

A few examples may illustrate some of these points. A static weight in a child is abnormal and may be a sign of disease; in the adult it is normal; vomiting in a baby may have little significance or it may be of great import, whereas in the adult it is likely to have a much more constant pathological significance; a liver edge which is palpable one to two centimetres below the costal margin could indicate hepatomegaly in an adult while it would be normal in a young child; the anterior fontanelle is available for examination in infancy only; on the other hand, mapping of the visual fields in infants and toddlers may be impossible; head retraction is more likely to be associated with meningitis in the older child or adult than in the infant, in whom it tends to be a late sign of meningeal irritation but a common one in association with respiratory infection (meningism); slowly rising intracranial pressure in the infant is likely to reveal itself by increasing head size without papilloedema, and in the older child and adult by headache and vomiting with papilloedema; an extensor plantar response below one year of age has a different significance from such a response beyond this age; haemoptysis in a child is most commonly related to nasopharyngeal bleeding or to the traumatic effect of coughing, and hardly ever to pulmonary infarction which would be a likely possibility in the adult; the trachea is much more mobile in children than in adults and tracheal deviation does not have the same significance in younger patients; measurements of the distance of the apex beat from the midline which are suitable for adults, are inapplicable to children; rigors are rare in childhood and febrile convulsions common, whereas the reverse is true in older patients.

Age Periods

It is convenient to divide the period of infancy and childhood into certain age periods:

Infancy	First year of life
Neonatal period	First month of life
Childhood	1–15 years
Pre-school child	1–4 years
School child	5–15 years.

THE HISTORY

The history of disease in childhood is seldom obtained directly from the patient but usually through an intermediary, commonly the mother. This does not mean that the child should be ignored as a source of information. While infants and young children clearly can give little or no history, the older child may give a very accurate account of symptoms and will usually answer questions accurately and without bias. Where appropriate, a supplementary history should be obtained from the child. The examiner will also have to decide whether the history from the parents should be taken in the presence or absence of the child. The wishes of the parent, the age of the child and the nature of the complaint will determine this.

That so much of the history of childhood illness has to be obtained through a second party creates certain problems. The parents may seek to place their own interpretation on symptoms and signs rather than to describe these precisely as they occur. Further, parents may fail to realise the misinterpretation which children may put on words. For example, a young child may generalise from past experience and use a phrase such as 'sore tummy' to describe pain or discomfort anywhere, but the parents may not appreciate this. Only careful questioning on the part of the examiner, a shrewd appreciation of the degree of insight which the parents have into their child's symptoms, and experience, will enable these difficult differentiations to be made. Further problems may be created by previous medical advice. The doctor who feels that a specific diagnosis must be offered even when this is not possible may be storing up trouble for the future. If in the presence of an unexplained fever — a common situation in childhood — the convenient but erroneous label 'tonsillitis' is frequently attached, the parents may be inclined to attribute all other pyrexias to the tonsils and may recount a long list of attacks of 'tonsillitis' which on closer questioning and examination are unsupported by any real evidence of pain in the throat, tonsillar inflammation or enlargement of the tonsillar lymph nodes. Such parents, presenting with the confident assertion that, 'It is the tonsils, Doctor', may themselves be deceived and may mislead the examiner who is not aware of such pitfalls.

History of Present Illness

There are two main aspects of history-taking. In the first place the parent or parents should be encouraged to give a spontaneous account of the child's illness subject only to such curbs on irrelevancy or verbosity as the examiner deems expedient. Secondly, there are specific questions from the examiner designed to amplify and clarify the parents' description. These may include the following:

AGE AND SEX. Date of birth and sex should be ascertained.

THE SYMPTOMS OR ABNORMALITIES COMPLAINED OF, AND THEIR DURATION. These may require clarification and more precise definition.

THE PRECISE ORDER OF SYMPTOMS. This should include current symptoms and also the order of events in repeated episodes, as in asthma or epilepsy.

CHANGES NOTED SINCE THE ONSET OF THE ILLNESS. This question is designed to bring out the main presenting aspects of the child's illness by contrasting the present condition with that prior to the onset of symptoms.

ACTIVITY OR APATHY. These may be gauged by the child's performance in normal household activities and in play, willingness to walk to school or to the shops and interest in people and things. Is the child active in the house or tend to sit or lie about? Does the child tire easily or return early from play?

FEEDING AND APPETITE. Determine whether the appetite is temporarily or persistently impaired, and if necessary calculate the caloric intake. With bottle-fed babies, an accurate account of the total daily intake of milk (number of scoops of dried milk powder and volume of water or volume of cow's milk or evaporated milk) can usually be obtained. With older children where there is a complaint of poor appetite enquiry should be made about the type and amount of food and liquid actually taken daily. A child who, according to the mother, eats nothing, may be drinking two pints of milk each day and almost completely satisfying caloric needs from this source alone.

Food fads and dislikes on the part of the child or any unusual ideas regarding diet on the part of the parents should be explored, as should the intake of vitamin supplements such as cod liver oil, orange juice, and proprietary preparations.

DIFFICULTY IN SWALLOWING. This is unlikely to be of organic origin in children. The most common cause is over-persuasion of an unwilling child to eat, resulting in choking and gagging.

THIRST. Where there is any suggestion of thirst an attempt should be made to obtain a quantitative estimation of the total daily intake of fluid.

VOMITING. If vomiting has occurred, the amount, frequency and duration should be ascertained. Is it effortless, forceful or projectile? Is there associated pain or screaming as in appendicitis or intussusception? Is the vomiting accompanied by diarrhoea as in gastro-enteritis, or by constipation as in intestinal obstruction or pyloric stenosis? What is the nature of the vomitus, and is it stained with bile or blood? If the patient is a baby, are there unusual movements of the mouth prior to vomiting (as with rumination)? Is there abdominal distension? Has the child been fevered?

ABDOMINAL PAIN. What is the evidence that abdominal pain is or has been present? Enquire about the nature and timing of the pain. Does it interfere with ordinary activity? What is its duration? Is it constant or intermittent? Is it precisely located or is it of a general character? Does it radiate? Is the pain aggravated by breathing or by movement? Is there any relationship to bowel movement or to micturition? Is there associated diarrhoea, melaena, constipation or vomiting? Is appetite affected? Sore throat may be associated with mesenteric adenitis, cough with pneumonia, and petechial haemorrhages with the abdominal lesion of anaphylactoid purpura.

ABDOMINAL DISTENSION. Gross degrees will be evident to parents. Intermittent distension may be reported (e.g. due to obstruction by congenital bands). The degree of distension and any associated symptoms should be ascertained.

STATE OF BOWELS AND CHARACTER OF STOOLS. The infant's stool is semi-solid and mustard-coloured and several are passed each day. The frequency of bowel movement should be ascertained routinely in terms of number of stools daily and enquiry made into any involuntary faecal soiling (encopresis) or any unusual reactions to defecation such as reluctance to allow the bowels to move or crying during the act (as in anal fissure). Questions should be asked about the character of the stools — are they hard or soft, watery, accompanied by mucus, blood-streaked or mixed with blood, bulky, normal in colour or dark or pale, floating on water or not, or malodorous?

LOSS OR GAIN IN WEIGHT. Few mothers are aware of the exact weight changes of their children. They will be able to say whether a child has appeared fatter or thinner, whether the clothing has become too tight or too slack recently, whether the limbs have wasted or have become swollen, whether the eyes have become sunken or the face puffy, and whether these processes have been of sudden or gradual onset. Thus will genuine weight loss or obesity or oedema become evident.

DISCHARGE FROM EYES, EARS, NOSE OR OTHER SITES. Enquire about the duration and note the character of the discharge, e.g. purulent, watery or blood-stained, profuse or scanty, continuous or intermittent.

SORE THROAT. This is likely to be a symptom only in older children. Younger children may have obviously painful lesions in the throat and yet make little in the way of localising complaint.

COUGH. This is one of the most common symptoms in childhood. For how long has the cough lasted? Is the cough 'dry' as in the early stage of pneumonia or bronchitis, or 'moist' as in the later stage of these diseases? Is it continuous or does it occur in paroxysms? Is it more severe by day or by night and does it disturb sleep? Is there any associated wheezing? Is there a whoop or accompanying vomiting? If there is sputum does the child swallow this or expectorate it and what is the character of the sputum — watery, mucoid, mucopurulent or blood-stained? Is there any pain on coughing as in pleurisy, or associated dyspnoea as in asthma or severe respiratory infection? Is there any associated nasal discharge or obstruction as in chronic sinus infection or gross adenoidal hypertrophy?

BREATHLESSNESS. If present, does this occur only on exertion or also at rest? Is it persistent as in some types of congenital heart disease or intermittent as in asthma? If intermittent, do attacks come on gradually or suddenly? Is breathlessness worse at night? Is breathing noisy or not? Is there any breath-holding? Is there any associated cyanosis, wheeze or cough? Ascertain the degree of breathlessness and the amount of exertion of which the child is capable.

MOUTH BREATHING AND STRIDOR. Does the child sleep with the mouth open or shut? Is a crowing noise made when breathing, indicating stridor? What is the duration of the stridor? Is it associated with other symptoms such as dyspnoea or cough?

WHEEZE. Does this occur or not? Is the onset sudden or gradual, at night or by day? Does any particular factor or group of circumstances precipitate attacks of wheezing? Is there accompanying cough or dyspnoea? Does the child tend to put things in the mouth (and therefore run a greater risk of aspirating a foreign body into a bronchus)?

ABNORMALITIES OF THE BREATH. Has the breath been abnormal, e.g. due to acetone, or to fetor in certain mouth infections?

LOCALISED SWELLINGS. Site, size (including variations in size), shape and consistency as noted by the parents, should be recorded, as should the presence of local pain or tenderness on palpation.

RASHES OR OTHER SKIN LESIONS. When and where did the rash occur and how has it progressed? What was its appearance, e.g. colour, size, shape and number of lesions, their nature and duration? Was the rash itchy? In the case of ulcers, site, size and duration should be known.

JAUNDICE. Note time of onset and whether intermittent, static, diminishing or increasing. Has any paleness of the stools or darkness of the urine been noted? Have there been any accompanying symptoms such as vomiting or hepatic tenderness?

CYANOSIS. Bluish shadows under the eyes are frequently described by mothers where no significant disease is present. Enquiry should be directed to determine the distribution of the blueness, e.g. extremities only or generalised, and the circumstances in which it occurs, e.g. in response to cold, exercise or respiratory infection. Blueness of the lips and tongue (central cyanosis) indicates severe arterial oxygen desaturation, as in cyanotic congenital heart disease.

PALLOR. Many healthy children are pale, but pallor tends to cause anxiety in mothers. Is the pallor intermittent or permanent? Intermittent pallor, such as may occur in a sleeping infant or in a child exposed to cold, will be much less significant than persistent pallor.

STATE OF THE MUSCULATURE. In infancy this is most likely to be appreciated by the mother's experience on handling the child. Hypotonicity is likely to be revealed by the fact that the infant is 'floppy' and tends to slip through the mother's hands when being lifted or bathed, hypertonicity by the fact that she feels that the limbs are rather stiff. With older children the development of muscle weakness will show itself by inability to perform activities which were previously possible, such as walking upstairs.

CHANGES IN POSTURE OR IN WALK. Does the child hold the head or trunk in any unusual way (e.g. torticollis or scoliosis)? Has there been any change in the manner of walking or in the way of rising from the sitting position (e.g. the broad based unsteady gait of cerebellar ataxia or the 'climbing up the legs' method of rising in muscular dystrophy)?

CO-ORDINATION OF MOVEMENT. Have things been dropped or fluids spilled from cups? Can fine movements such as writing and buttoning clothing be performed? Has there been any change in speech? These questions may be important, for instance in differentiating chorea from a tic.

INVOLUNTARY MOVEMENTS. Obtain a full description of the nature of the movements. Are the same movements repeated (tic) or is there a series of movements, for example jerky varied movements (choreiform) or writhing movements (athetoid) or a combination of these (choreo-athetoid)? Has the child suffered any injury as a result of the movements? Does emotional stress aggravate them?

CONVULSIONS. Obtain a full description, including the state of the child prior to the convulsion, and apparent precipitating factor (such as pyrexia), any premonitory symptoms, the types of movement observed and the duration of various stages. Was there any localised twitching? Was the child unconscious? Did the child fall down or the eyes roll up? Was there incontinence? Was the tongue bitten or other damage caused? Was the child pale or blue during the convulsive attack? Was there any associated pyrexia? Did the child fall asleep? Was there disorientation afterwards or were previous activities continued?

DEFECTS IN VISION. In a baby we are concerned with a gross assessment, (e.g. are moving objects followed with the eyes?) and in older children with selective visual changes. Can print be read? Is thee any difficulty in reading the blackboard at school?

HEADACHE. Young children seldom complain of headache. With older children the site of the headache, manner of onset, duration, severity (e.g. does the child have to leave the school class or stop play) and accompanying symptoms such as vomiting, are relevant.

HEARING. Does a baby turn to various noises such as the mother's voice when she is out of sight; with an older child is there any apparent inability to understand the spoken word, or to hear common noises such as the door bell?

DYSURIA. Enquiries should be directed to ascertain whether any pain which might be dysuria is in fact related to micturition.

FREQUENCY OF MICTURITION. Enquire about frequency both by day and night.

BED WETTING AND DIURNAL INCONTINENCE. Have these symptoms always been present or developed recently? How frequently does the bed wetting or diurnal incontinence occur? Are the symptoms both diurnal and nocturnal? Is more urine passed than normal? Are there any circumstances which aggravate the symptoms or alleviate them? Is there an associated dysuria, increased frequency of micturition or thirst? What are the parents' reactions to the child's symptoms?

VOLUME OF URINE. In the presence of frequency of micturition or incontinence the mother may have gained an exaggerated impression of the amount of urine passed per day. Statements of an excessive or a diminished output of urine should be carefully assessed.

CHARACTER OF URINE. What is the colour — amber, red, smoky, 'like tea', etc.? Bacterial decomposition of urine in napkins gives an ammoniacal odour.

BEHAVIOUR AND MOOD. It may be more appropriate to question a mother alone about her child's behaviour in the home, in school, or in play with other children. She may describe disobedience, negativeness, aggressiveness, reluctance to go to school, withdrawal from company and from social activities, inability to go to sleep, fear of the dark, nightmares and night terrors, sleep walking, abnormal jealousies, increased tendency to show emotional disturbance in the face of difficulty, nail biting and thumb sucking. The child's natural disposition should be ascertained, whether carefree or anxious, fastidious or careless, 'highly strung' or placid, volatile or stolid. An account of the child's relationship with parents, siblings and other children may be revealing as may reactions to school and relationships with teachers.

TREATMENT ALREADY GIVEN. Any treatment already given to the child for the present illness should be noted even though the mother may not know its precise nature.

SELECTIVITY OF QUESTIONING. Obviously not all of the questions indicated above will be asked in every instance. Some are secondary and dependent on a positive answer to a primary question, while others will be irrelevant to the current symptoms. It is always better to ask too many rather than too few questions as a wide interrogation may uncover aspects of an illness which the parent or child may not have mentioned because they were considered irrelevant or had been forgotten.

Previous History

HISTORY OF THE BIRTH. The manner of birth may have a profound effect on an infant's subsequent health and development. A history of the birth should thus be obtained for all infants and most children presenting for examination, and in certain types of disease such as cerebral palsy, mental retardation or epilepsy this will be of particular importance.

Enquiry should be directed to any illness or accident from which the mother suffered during pregnancy. She should be asked about drugs taken or exposure to radiation. Memory for events early in pregnancy is likely to be less accurate than that for later pregnancy, yet the profound effect which certain disorders such as rubella may have in early pregnancy makes enquiry into events at this time important.

Although the mother's knowledge of the duration of her labour, of the presentation of the fetus, of the type of delivery (e.g. forceps) and of any difficulties during delivery may be incomplete, an adequate account of these facts may be relevant and important. It may be necessary to obtain precise information from those who were responsible for the delivery.

Most mothers are aware of their children's birth weights — fathers can very seldom supply this information. The birth weight, the length of the period of gestation and the place of delivery should always be recorded.

Information should also be sought about the neonatal period. How long after birth was respiration established? Did the child suffer from convulsions, breathing difficulties, blueness, jaundice, vomiting or any other abnormality? Was any special treatment required e.g. oxygen therapy or mechanical ventilation?

FEEDING. A history of past feeding can be combined most conveniently with the present history as discussed above. In infancy we are concerned with questions such as difficulty in the establishment of feeding in the neonatal period, the duration of breast feeding, the type of artificial feeding, and the composition, volume and frequency of the feeds. With older children information on diet, on the past state of the appetite and on the amount of vitamin supplements should be recorded. Attention should be paid to any peculiar dietary habits.

PREVIOUS ILLNESSES. The date, the duration and severity of previous illnesses and operations should be recorded. The mother may require some time to recollect the necessary information.

CONTACT WITH INFECTIOUS ILLNESS. Questions should be asked about infectious illness in other members of the family and in playmates. In such enquiries the symptoms of the more common infectious illnesses may have to be specified e.g. rash, diarrhoea, spasmodic cough or jaundice. Threadworms often have a familial distribution. A knowledge of contact with animals may be relevant, e.g. in the presence of lymphadenopathy due to toxoplasmosis.

RESIDENCE ABROAD. A history of periods of residence abroad may indicate the need to consider the possibility of imported diseases.

IMMUNISATION. Any prophylactic inoculations or vaccinations which the child has received should be recorded, including their approximate dates.

Developmental History

A knowledge of a normal child's develppment (p. 466) is crucial to the diagnosis and evaluation of many childhood disorders. When did the child first smile, appear to see, first sit up without support, crawl, stand with and then without support, walk, say single words and then phrases, undress, feed using the hands, go up and down stairs, dress, count up to ten, etc.?

Age of control of bladder and bowels. At what age did the child become dry by day and at night? When was control of the bowels gained? Does the mother have any strong views about 'pot training'?

Family History

The ages, present stage of health, past health and possible consanguinity of the parents should be ascertained. The ages and sexes of other children in the family (and thus the position of the patient in the family), the occurrence of any stillbirths or miscarriages and past and present illnesses of siblings should also be noted. If any child in the family has died, the age at death and cause of death should be ascertained. Is there anything to suggest child abuse? Illnesses in the parents or in other relatives living with the family should be recorded. With certain disorders (e.g. allergic disorders, bleeding diseases or mental disorder) specific enquiries may require to be made about a much wider circle of relatives than the patient's immediate family. In the case of an adopted child, any available medical history about the natural parents should be noted.

Social and Environmental History

The occupations of the parents, their attitude to each other and to their children, their parental responsibilities, divorce or separation, and the financial status of the family are all relevant.

Many disorders in childhood have a psychological basis. In understanding such disorders history is of paramount importance. For example, in tics, changes in behaviour and mood, enuresis, encopresis, cyclical vomiting, migraine and emotional disturbances the most rewarding investigation may well be the unravelling of the psychological interrelationships of the patient with other members of the family, friends and personal contacts in school and at play. An appreciation of the stresses which the environment, both at home and school, imposes, and of intelligence, particularly as it affects the ability to meet the demands of education, will also be relevant. A great variety of social and environmental factors may cause psychological disturbance in childhood but there are certain provoking situations which recur — a new baby in the home, the death of an immediate relative, absence of one or other parent from the home, first attendance at school, a change of school class or a new teacher, change of residence to another district with loss of playmates, bullying at school, scholastic difficulties, too rigid enforcement by parents or others of a desired pattern of behaviour.

Enquiries should also be made about the size and conditions of the home, including the number of occupants and about any special environmental circumstances of possible physical or psychological significance.

PHYSICAL EXAMINATION

The examination of infants and children is an art demanding qualities of understanding, sympathy and patience, and at times finesse and subtlety. The paediatric patient who enters the consulting-room or who is ill in bed may be a bawling infant whom nothing will pacify, a toddler clinging to his mother and burying a tearful face in her lap at the slightest movement of the examiner towards him, a more robust young man of early school age who stoutly and persistently resists all attempts to remove his clothing particularly his trousers, a mentally retarded hyperactive child who moves rapidly round the room deploying a destructive interest against the furniture, the torch or the doctor's spectacles, or an apprehensive schoolgirl who just retains her self-control during questioning but recoils in terror at the production of a sphygmomanometer or an ophthalmoscope. In contrast there are many children who exhibit exemplary co-operation and self-control. Experience, practice and understanding of children enable much to be done to overcome difficulties. The clinician must not be too conscious of personal dignity; impatience or irascibility is only likely to close the door to much of the information which might otherwise be available. Children are quick to sense the doctors attitude, and respond best to a friendly, tolerant and gentle approach. The opportunity to observe, appreciate and conduct a relevant clinical examination is increased immeasurably.

It would be impossible to describe an all-embracing technique to meet the manifold problems of approach which occur in the clinical examination of children; a few suggestions will suffice. During the history-taking the doctor should be able to gauge the type of child and to judge the approach accordingly. A decision may have to be made whether the child should be examined on the mother's knee or on a couch. Although it is desirable to remove the child's clothing for an adequate physical examination, this may require to be done in stages in certain instances. The examiner must remain patient and confident. The concern which mothers commonly experience that a fractious child's behaviour is annoying or in some way outside the doctor's normal experience should be allayed. Loud noises tend to alarm children. A soft persuasive voice is much more likely to be effective than stentorian exhortations. With active noisy babies and toddlers, gentle stroking of the skin with one finger may result in a brief cessation of movement and of noise. The doctor's attitude and conversation should be attuned to the level of the patient's understanding. A great deal of examination and manipulation can be carried out without the child being very aware of it if attention is held, and to achieve this the clinician may well have to appear to identify with an appropriate current interest of the child — a rattle, a torch, a teddy bear, the recent exploits of a popular space-man, or the current fashions in the dressing of dolls. With older children, simple explanations about the various aspects of an examination should be given. The examiner must be prepared to depart from an established routine as circumstances demand. Procedures which tend to frighten children, such as inspection of the throat or recording the blood pressure, can usually with advantage be carried out at the end of the session.

GENERAL INSPECTION

The assessment of a child from both physical and mental aspects begins from the moment of first meeting. Much may be learned from the child's appearance, demeanour, reaction to the environment and to the examiner, relationships to parents, any sounds uttered or even any accompanying smells.

The general inspection will give information on size relative to age, state of nutrition including obesity or wasting, state of activity whether increased or decreased, posture and bodily habitus whether upright or recumbent or associated with torticollis, short neck, head retraction or scoliosis, and obvious deformities. Major external injuries and haemorrhage will be evident.

The facial expression may reveal pain or anxiety, the blankness of mental retardation or the spasmodic localised movement of the tic. It may show evidence of weight loss, dehydration or oedema or the characteristics of mongolism or cretinism. Pallor, cyanosis, jaundice or other features outlined on page 57 may be observed.

Any rash should be observed and its character inspected. Light touch will determine whether the rash is raised or not. An erythematous rash, blanching on pressure, can be differentiated from a purpuric rash, recognised by its colour and by its failure to blanch. Petechiae can be differentiated from larger macules, macules from papules, papules from vesicles. The content of any vesicles, whether serum, pus or blood, should be observed. The distribution of a rash will be noted, for example flexural in eczema, centripetal in chicken-pox, on the legs and buttocks particularly in anaphylactoid purpura and interdigital in scabies. Scratch marks will indicate whether the skin is itchy or not. A characteristic rash such as that of measles may provide an immediate diagnosis. A rash such as that of erythema nodosum may suggest several diagnoses. There may be other abnormalities of the skin; ulceration; evidence of septic infection such as pustules, boils or impetigo; abnormal formation, as in the dry scaling of ichthyosis or the papery appearance of the neonatal placental insufficiency syndrome; angiomas, pigmentation. Sweating may be prominent. In dehydration the skin is dry and remains in loose folds when plucked up instead of flattening immediately as in the normal elastic state. The shiny tenseness and pitting on pressure of oedema may be noted. There may be visible external swellings.

A first glance will reveal much of the patient's level of consciousness, whether fully conscious, semi-conscious or unconscious. A few moments observation may tell much about a child's psychological make-up and intelligence — whether nervous, excitable, distractible, withdrawn, intelligent or dull — and about difficult emotional relationships with the parents.

Abnormal respiratory rate, pattern and effort may be visible. Abnormal sounds such as a high-pitched cry, cough, wheeze, stridor or whoop may be heard. Body odours may reveal lack of cleanliness; the breath may smell of acetone; to those with an acute sense of smell a mousy odour may suggest phenylketonuria. In older children bodily form, character of the voice and manner will help differentiate between states of pre-pubescence, pubescence and adolescence.

The importance of an adequate general inspection cannot be overemphasised. It is unwise to rush this or curtall it in the premature pursuit of more direct methods of examination, such as palpation, auscultation and the use of instruments. It is probably true that with children (in developed countries) a much higher proportion show no abnormality on application of these procedures than with adults. The frequent paucity of specific localised physical signs in the child as compared with the adult results in a relatively greater contribution to diagnosis being made in the former by the history and general inspection.

PHYSICAL MEASUREMENTS

Weight. The most useful single measurements of physical development in infancy and childhood are weight and height. A comparison between actual and expected weight should be routine in any examination. Expected weight according to age can be calculated in a number of rough and ready ways or may be determined more accurately from tables: In the early weeks of life the average infant should gain approximately 30 g (1 oz) per day after the tenth day, at which time the birth weight should have been regained. Thus at six weeks the expected gain in weight would be almost 1 kg (2 lb). By five months of age the birth weight should have doubled and by a year should have trebled. For the next few years the expected weight can be calculated approximately from the formulae — age in years plus four, multiplied by two, for kilogrammes, or age in years plus three, multiplied by five, for pounds. Average weights for infants and children from birth to 15 years are given in the Appendix. In using this table, it should be remembered that the average is not necessarily the normal for any individual. The normal weight for a child of small parents may be well below the average and an average weight for another child, with parents of large stature, may be below normal. Thus weight in the individual child must be interpreted against a number of background factors. Changes in weight of the individual child have a more specific significance.

Length. Length is the other valuable parameter of growth. It can be measured as standing height in toddlers and older children and as crown-heel length in infants who are recumbent. Average heights from birth to 15 years are given on page 477. In regard to length the same considerations concerning 'normal' and 'average' apply as with weight.

Under certain circumstances a crown-rump length or sitting height (stem length) may be of value for comparison with crown-heel length or standing height, for example in achondroplasia where there is shortening of the limbs. In the recumbent position (e.g. in the infant) the crown-rump length is measured from the top of the head to a board placed against the extremity of the buttocks with the thighs at right angles to the trunk and the knees flexed. A table of crown-rump lengths will be found on page 448. After the age of 3 years sitting height rather than crown-rump length is usually measured.

A correlation normally exists between height and weight. A knowledge of the expected weight for any particular height and an appreciation of any dissociation between these measurements may be of value. In hypothyroidism, for instance, height may be reduced and weight normal, in Marfan's syndrome height increased and weight normal. In a wasting disorder height may be normal and weight reduced, in obesity height normal and weight increased. A correlation of these parameters can be made from tables or from charts such as those shown in the Appendix (p. 449), where the normal ranges for expected height and weight at different ages are charted. Such charts have as their primary function the recording of serial estimations of weight and height.

Head Size. Head size both above and below normal may have considerable significance in respect of childhood disease. Average occipito-frontal head circumferences for different ages with the measuring tape placed round the maximal occipito-frontal circumference are given on page 448.

Temperature. In the presence of any constitutional upset one of the most common instrumental observations made either in the home or in the hospital is that of temperature. For most purposes skin temperature is adequate, but the site selected should not have been unnaturally cooled by exposure or heated by any artificial means. In infants the groin is probably the best site with the thigh held flexed on to the abdomen; in older children the axilla is more suitable. Some prefer the rectal temperature in infants. Where the temperature does not record on a standard clinical thermometer, as for instance in so-called neonatal cold injury, special low-reading thermometers covering the range from 30° to 43°C should be used routinely. The accepted dividing-line between normal and abnormal temperatures, namely 37°C, is appropriate for infants and children; where a skin temperature is taken the normal rectal temperature would be higher by about 0.25°C. Somewhat lower temperatures are normal in premature infants.

EXAMINATION OF INDIVIDUAL REGIONS AND SYSTEMS

It is easiest to consider the examination of individual regions and systems in sequence but it is not always possible to examine them in this way. Certain children, particularly younger ones, tire easily during an examination and in such cases it may be expedient for the clinician to begin with the system which is likely to yield the most valuable information. Thus it may be advisable to auscultate the heart before a child becomes fractious and cries. On the other hand it may be necessary to delay cardiac auscultation until a child has stopped crying. As a general rule those systems which can be examined most by observation should be dealt with first, proceeding thereafter to systems where handling and instrumental examination are more necessary but may result in emotional upset and loss of cooperation. The examiner must remain flexible in approach and exploit any advantageous opportunities as they arise.

HEAD AND NECK

Cranium. Observe the size and the shape, e.g. brachycephaly, scaphocephaly, plagiocephaly, oxycephaly, microcephaly or hydrocephalus (Fig. 10.1). Head shape and size may have special associations with certain developmental disorders and disease processes, e.g. brachycephaly with Down's syndrome; plagiocephaly with prematurity; microcephaly with mental retardation; scaphocephaly and oxycephaly with craniostenosis; hydrocephalus with spina bifida. Measure the occipito-frontal head circumference. Note the amount, colour and consistency of the hair. A lowered hair line posteriorly may be a feature of such diseases as the Klippel-Feil syndrome and Turner's syndrome. Fair hair, blue eyes and a 'mousy' odour may accompany phenylketonuria (p. 405).

The *fontanelles* are peculiar to infancy and the anterior fontanelle in particular may provide information of the greatest value. The posterior fontanelle normally is not more than 0.5 cm wide at birth. This fontanelle closes shortly after birth. Its persistence beyond this time or an increase in its size beyond normal may indicate increased intracranial tension or an abnormality of the cranial bones. The anterior fontanelle normally measures approximately 2.5 cm by 2.5 cm at birth and does not close until 15 to 18 months. Delay in closure beyond 18 months may be another pointer to diseases such as rickets, increased intracranial tension or abnormal development of cranial bones. Early closure may occur in premature synostosis. Fontanelle tension should be assessed at the same time as fontanelle size. Increased tension in the fontanelle can be detected chiefly by palpation, but also in some

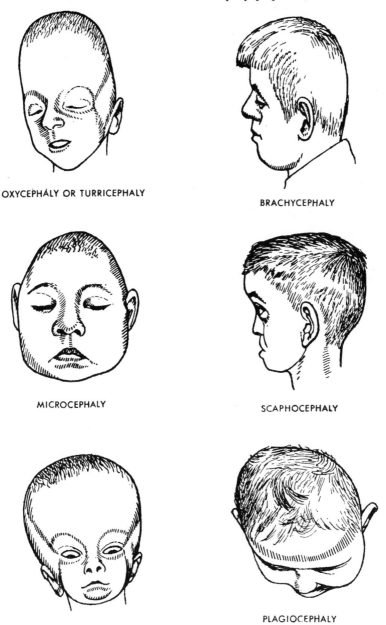

OXYCEPHÁLY OR TURRICEPHALY

BRACHYCEPHALY

MICROCEPHALY

SCAPHOCEPHALY

HYDROCEPHALUS

PLAGIOCEPHALY

Fig. 10.1 The cranium as a diagnostic aid. The disorders associated with these changes are discussed on page 380.

instances by the observation of bulging. Decreased tension with a sunken fontanelle — as in dehydration — is likely to be visible and palpable. An abnormally large fontanelle under increased tension and a large head may be associated with long-standing increased intracranial pressure as in hydrocephalus. Increased fontanelle tension without significant increase in head size is likely to indicate an acute process such as meningitis or intracranial haemorrhage.

In conjunction with increased fontanelle tension the cranial *sutures* may be abnormally wide. At birth the main sutures such as the sagittal and coronal are easily palpable but the bone edges are not widely separated. Premature fusion of the sutures, often palpable as prominent ridges, occurs in cranial synostosis.

Alteration in the consistence of the *cranial bones* is seen most commonly in infancy in, for instance, prematurity or rickets. The phenomenon of *craniotabes* is detected by placing the infant's head, face towards the examiner, between the examiner's hands and exerting pressure over the parieto-occipital region with the tips of the fingers. 'Give' in the bone, such as would be experienced on pressure on a table-tennis ball, indicates craniotabes. Palpation of the skull will also reveal other *structural defects* in cranial bones, lacunae, swellings or local tenderness, e.g. over the mastoid process.

Cranial bruits may be audible on auscultation over the vertex of the skull, the occiput or the temporal region in, for instance, arterio-venous malformations or severe idiopathic hypercalcaemia.

Ears. The external ear may be congenitally deformed as an isolated lesion or in conjunction with congenital abnormalities in other sites, such as the renal tract. Low-set ears, abnormal formation and size of the external ear or deformity of the external meatus may be found (Fig. 10.2).

Infection in the ears is common in childhood and auriscopic examination is an important procedure (Fig. 4.6, p. 75). The speculum used should be appropriate to the size of the auditory canal. Wax or purulent discharge should be noted and also any other obstruction such as a boil. Further inspection may not be possible until wax has been removed by a loop, or discharge by dry mopping with cotton-wool on an orange stick. The drum should be examined for colour, bulging, retraction and perforation. It will appear dusky and injected in the presence of acute infection and there may be some distortion of the cone of light normally extending forward from the tip of the handle of the malleus. A bulging drum appears to be displaced towards the examiner and the light reflex is usually lost. With retraction the malleus is unduly prominent. Perforations may occur in any part of the drum but are most likely to be present in the upper part. They may be of pin-hole size or large, involving almost all of the drum.

Face. Many aspects of disease may be reflected in the face. The expression may indicate the emotional state of the child and reveal something of the psychological make-up. Facial tics may be evident. A specific diagnosis such as cretinism, Down's syndrome (mongolism) or gargoylism may be obvious at once (Fig. 10.2). Many other features may be of diagnostic value — the shape of the forehead, whether prominent as in certain types of cranial dysostosis, narrowed and receding as in microcephaly, or bossed as in rickets; the position of the eyes, especially an increased distance between them (hypertelorism) as in some cases of pulmonary stenosis or mental retardation; the shape and angle of the palpebral fissure and the

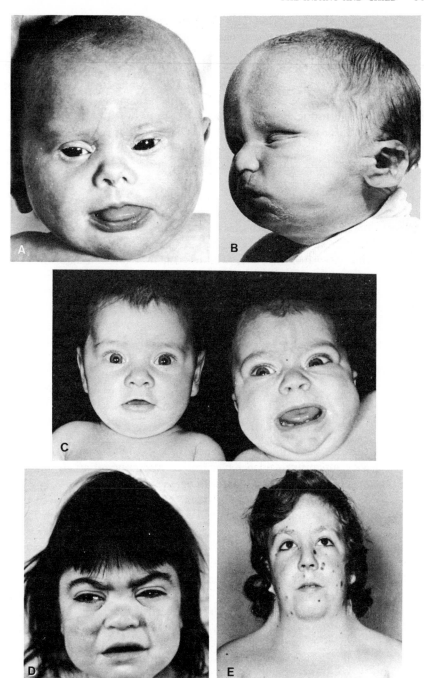

Fig. 10.2   The face as a diagnostic aid. (A) Down's syndrome — palpebral fissures sloping laterally upwards and elongated prominent protruding tongue associated with small mouth. (B) Renal agenesis — small jaw, flattened nose, low set ears. (C) Cretin with normal twin — large tongue, coarse features, bloated cheeks and double chin due to myxoedematous change. (D) Gargoyle — wide nose with depressed bridge, prominent supraorbital ridges and eyebrows. (E) Webbing of neck in Turner's syndrome. Pigmented naevi also present.

presence of prominent epicanthic folds as in mongolism or the Treacher Collins syndrome. Any periorbital oedema or haemorrhage will be noted. The colouring of the conjunctival mucous membrane will give an approximate measure of the haemoglobin level. Examination of the eyeballs will reveal any undue prominence or depression; obvious squint; conjunctivitis; conjunctival jaundice or haemorrhage; congenital defects of the iris (colobomata); abnormal pigmentation or the presence of Brushfield's spots (small whitish inclusions arranged radially between the middle and outer thirds of the iris having the appearance of grains of salt — seen in mongolism); opacities in the cornea, lens, or intra-ocular chambers.

Other examples of the value of the face as a diagnostic aid are given in Figure 10.3.

The *use of the ophthalmoscope* is dealt with in Chapter 11. The difficulties of this examination in children are often considerable. To maintain the young child's gaze in a fixed direction it is usually necessary for a second person to arrange some diversion which for the child has an element of expectancy about it. The examiner, after positioning the patient may say, 'Tell me when the torch flashes', the torch being held in an appropriate position by a helper who may be mother or nurse, or 'Tell me how many fingers nurse has up — how many now?,' the nurse changing the numbers of fingers and thus maintaining the child's attention. With younger children sedation may be necessary and in certain circumstances even a general anaesthetic may be required. Dilatation of the pupil (p. 407) may be necessary. Ophthalmoscopic examination will reveal opacities of the media and gross refractive errors. In the fundus abnormal venous engorgement, haemorrhage, exudate, abnormal pigmentation, cherry-red spots (as in amaurotic family idiocy) and choroidal tubercles may be seen. The optic discs may show blurring of the margins, papilloedema or abnormal coloration.

The shape of the *nose* may indicate racial origins or reveal the sunken bridge of gargoylism or the flattened tip of renal agenesis (Fig. 10.2). Movement of the alae nasi may provide supportive evidence of increased respiratory effort. In the child with a chronic cough, asthma or mouth breathing, the patency of each nasal passage should be tested in turn by blocking the other. Foreign bodies may block nasal passages. Any nasal discharge should be noted along with its amount and character. The state of the nasal mucosa should be observed using an auriscope and wide bored speculum applied carefully to each nostril; is it pale or congested, watery or dry?

Observe the formation of the *lips*, the presence of swelling, as in oedema, pallor or cyanosis, and cracking or ulceration. Check on their function as in whistling or blowing.

Mouth. A child may open the mouth voluntarily. Refusal is likely to be encouraged where there is too much display of shiny instruments and too obvious an indication of intent to use them. Most children will react more willingly to the request to, 'Let me see your teeth', than to, 'Open your mouth', or, 'Show me your throat'. The demonstration of the teeth is more likely to be a matter of some childhood pride. Physical force should be avoided as it breaks the confidence which may have been built up between examiner and patient and will make subsequent examinations very difficult.

With a willing child, inspection of the mouth may reveal possible abnormalities in the *state of the mucosa* — dryness, abnormal colour, ulceration, purpura; the white

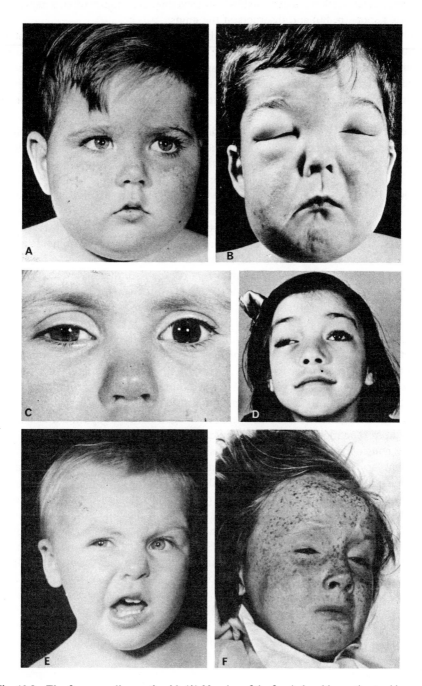

Fig. 10.3   The face as a diagnostic aid. (A) Mooning of the face induced by corticosteroid therapy. (B) Facial oedema in the nephrotic syndrome with peri-orbital involvement almost preventing opening of the eyes. (C) Right-sided Horner's syndrome — smallness of pupil (miosis) enophthalmos and a narrow palpebral fissure. (D) Ptosis (more marked on right side) in myasthenia gravis. (E) Left-sided facial palsy. (F) Risus sardonicus in tetanus; marked freckling of skin.

adherent curd like lesions of thrush which leave bleeding points when scraped off; Koplik's spots (p. 80) and disorders of the gums.

The *teeth* should be observed for number, whether of the primary or secondary dentition, size and shape, discoloration (e.g. yellow colour of the primary dentition of prematurely born children who have suffered from severe neonatal jaundice, or children whose mothers have been given tetracycline during pregnancy), caries and enamel defects. The time of eruption of the teeth may be of some value as an index of normal development (p. 448).

Defects in the *palate* will also be evident. *Tongue* size (large in cretins), shape (elongated and thin in mongols) and surface will be noted. The ease with which the tongue can be examined does not justify the over-importance which in the past was attached to its appearance as an indicator of health.

The *tonsils* should be observed for size (varying with age and maximal at the age of 7–8 years), colour, exudate or pitting, and the peritonsillar region for swelling and inflammation. The posterior pharyngeal wall should be observed for inflammation, swelling, postnasal discharge and the presence of lymphoid tissue.

Oropharynx. At this point, if not earlier, the examiner will probably require to introduce a spatula into the child's mouth in order to see the throat clearly. Some children in saying, 'Aah', will depress the tongue sufficiently to avoid the need for assisted depression. In others a spatula will have to be used. As the child says, 'Aah', the spatula should be placed on the back of the tongue. If the child continues to co-operate, depression of the tongue will reveal the oropharynx. If tense or actively resistant the child will arch the tongue and defy depression of it. It is at this point that the examiner puts the gag reflex to use. By advancing the spatula to touch the posterior wall of the pharynx gagging will be induced, the posterior part of the tongue will be actively depressed and the throat exposed. The exposure is short lived and the examiner must take every advantage of it. One gag should usually be enough, as repetition will upset the child.

The non-cooperative infant or toddler should either be seated on the knee of the assistant or laid on a couch. Movement of the arms should be prevented by wrapping the child in a blanket. If the child is held on the knee, the assistant should place one arm round the child's body to prevent movement of the arms and trunk and the other round the head, holding the forehead. If the child is lying on a couch, the assistant should hold the child's head between two hands and the examiner should restrain movement of the child's arms. The examiner should introduce a wooden spatula between the teeth at the side of the mouth and advance it slowly by gentle levering towards the posterior pharynx. It is possible to do this even although the child is clenching the teeth. When the tip of the spatula reaches the posterior pharyngeal wall the child will open the mouth and gag. In this brief moment, unless the performance is to be repeated, the examiner will have to observe all the features of the mouth which have been mentioned above.

Neck. Inspection from the front and from the back will detect any shortening (as in certain cervical vetebral anomalies), webbing (as in Turner's syndrome, Fig. 10.2), or positional deformity such as torticollis or head retraction. Limitation of movement may involve extension, flexion, rotation or lateral movement. Limitation of flexion (neck stiffness or rigidity) may be an important sign of meningeal irritation due to infection or haemorrhage. It can be tested passively with the patient lying supine on a couch, the examiner placing a hand behind the occiput and gently raising the head. The infant or child may then resist flexion and cry, or the whole trunk may be raised. Alternatively, the child while in the sitting position with the knees drawn up, may be asked to put the nose on the knee. Abnormal swellings such as enlarged cervical lymph nodes should be sought in the anterior and posterior cervical triangles and· over the occipital region. Cystic hygromata are soft and transilluminable, while abnormal thyroid swellings are confirmed by palpation and by observing movement on swallowing. A sternomastoid tumour is a firm nodule or swelling in the sternomastoid muscle seen in infancy. Branchial cleft remnants may also be found.

Lymph Nodes. Enlargement of certain groups of lymph nodes, particularly in the neck and groin is common in childhood. Submental lymph nodes and those in the anterior and posterior cervical triangles should also be examined. Involvement of the axillary lymph nodes is more significant of generalised lymphadenopathy. In palpating these the child's arm should first be held at right angles to the trunk to allow adequate access of the fingers to the axilla, and with the fingers in position the arm returned to a position beside the trunk. Palpable epitrochlear lymph nodes at the elbow is another indication of lymphadenopathy. Examination of lymph nodes will be closely associated with examination of the liver and spleen.

RESPIRATORY SYSTEM

Inspection. In the baby a cross-section of the thorax is roughly circular whereas in the older child and adult it is elliptical. The circular shape confers structural strength to withstand the stresses and strains of delivery, but as a circle cannot be expanded like an ellipse this shape imposes certain functional limitations. Essentially the infant is a diaphragmatic breather.

Acute over-inflation of an infant's chest, as may occur in bronchiolitis, results in expansion of the upper half of the chest anteriorly giving it a distended or 'blown' look. In the older child the antero-posterior diameter should be less than the lateral diameter. Increase in the former relative to the latter is likely to be due to a long-standing respiratory disorder such as asthma. This will also cause an increase in chest circumference.

In children, chest expansion is best determined with a measuring tape at the nipple line. The child is instructed to breathe out fully and then to take a deep breath. Less than 4 cm ($1\frac{1}{2}$ in) expansion probably indicates impairment. Asymmetry of movement on expansion is best detected by observing chest movement during a full inspiration. The method depicted in Figure 6.7 (p. 172) is of little value in young children due to the pliability of the chest wall. Other deformities of the chest, either as a result of previous disease or developmental anomalies, may be evident in childhood such as pigeon chest, pectus excavatum or Harrison's sulcus (p. 166). Precordial bulging may be visible as a result of cardiac enlargement; spindle-shaped thickening at the costo-chondral junctions (the rickety rosary) may be present with rickets; deformity of the costochondral junctions, like the back of a dinner fork, may occur with scurvy.

Observation of the *respiration rate* is of great value in respiratory infection because of the paucity of other signs which may exist in acute respiratory infections in infants and children. Crying or struggling will disturb the true rate and observation must therefore be made with the infant or child at peace, not crying, struggling or feeding. The upper limit of normal of the respiratory rate at various ages is approximately as follows:

0-2 years	2-6 years	6-10 years	Over 10 years
40/min	30/min	25/min	20/min

In addition to the respiratory rate, the *respiratory rhythm* may be disturbed. In the premature newborn infant respiration may be irregular both in time and in amplitude. A similar pattern may occur with asphyxia in the newborn period. With older children the normal relationship between the phases of respiration may be disturbed with the occurrence of respiratory inversion. Normally the order of events in respiration is, inspiration — expiration — pause, whereas in respiration inversion it is, expiration — inspiration — pause. The mother may describe this as a 'catch' in the child's breathing. It is seen particularly with pneumonia. Normally the inspiratory phase of respiration is longer than the expiratory phase but in certain diseases, particularly asthma, expiration is longer than inspiration. Periodic breathing (Cheynes-Stokes respirations, p. 168) may also occur. This is seen most commonly in the neonatal period particularly in preterm babies. Reversion to this pattern of breathing is not uncommon during the course of respiratory tract infections occurring in the early months of life.

The greater mobility and pliability of the infant's thoracic cage make certain signs related to chest movements much more common and significant at this age period. Increased respiratory effort due to obstruction to the free flow of air in and out of the lungs or to diminished lung compliance, is likely to reveal itself by intercostal indrawing and costal margin recession. These signs are frequently found in bronchiolitis, pneumonia, asthma and pulmonary oedema.

There may be abnormal sounds associated with disordered respiratory function. Stridor may be present with laryngeal or tracheal obstruction. In lesser degrees this will be inspiratory only, but in more severe degrees both inspiratory and expiratory. With respiratory infection, breathing may be grunting and with acidosis, hissing. Wheeze indicates the presence of obstruction of the intrathoracic airways, such as occurs in asthma. It gives audible evidence of prolongation of expiration.

Palpation. The flat of the hand laid on the chest may reveal palpable rhonchi or local tenderness or the crepitant sensation of subcutaneous emphysema. It will also reveal the position of the apex beat which is normally felt in the fourth or fifth intercostal space just within the mid-clavicular line. Due to its normal mobility and ready displacement with changes of body posture, deviation of the trachea is not of great value in the infant and young child as an indication of mediastinal displacement.

Percussion. The thinner chest wall of the infant and child usually makes the percussion note in younger patients somewhat more resonant than in adults. Percussion should be lighter, particularly in infants. Alterations of percussion note may be absolute as in pleural effusion or extensive consolidation. Much more commonly, only a relative difference is detected by comparison with other areas of the lung. Fairly large areas of underlying consolidation or collapse can be present, without any change of percussion note, so that impairment of percussion usually indicates an extensive lesion. In respiratory disease the significance of the area of cardiac dullness is usually in respect of reduction or loss as occurs in overinflation of the lungs or pneumothorax.

Auscultation. This may precede percussion in young children as the act of percussion may cause upset or crying. However the fractious crying child as well as the co-operative one can be examined by auscultation. A child cannot cry during the inspiratory phase of respiration and the very act of crying causes a full inspiration. Auscultation is possible during this phase.

The *breath sounds* in infants and children are harsher (broncho-vesicular) than in adults. The auscultatory time relationships are: inspiration, expiration (about one-third of the duration of inspiration), then a silent period of the approximate duration of inspiration. In auscultatory examination the breath sounds themselves should first be assessed. Are they audible and if so are they of normal, diminished (as with a pleural effusion, pneumothorax or obstructive emphysema), or increased intensity (as with some types of consolidation and collapse)? Do they have the harsher quality which is commonly associated with bronchitis and bronchiolitis? Is the relationship of the various phases of the respiratory cycle normal, i.e. is there any prolongation of the expiratory phase of respiration (as with asthma) or is there abolition of the normal silent period, with inspiration and expiration of equal length and of an intense character (bronchial breathing)?

The significance of *added sounds*, i.e. rhonchi, crepitations and friction rubs, does not differ from that in the adult as described in Chapter 6.

Abnormal signs in the cardiovascular system are considered in the succeeding paragraphs. These can indicate respiratory as well as cardiac disease. Displacement of the apex beat, for instance, is as likely to be due to a pulmonary as a cardiac cause. As a corollary dyspnoea in infancy may well have a cardiac aetiology.

CARDIOVASCULAR SYSTEM

Inspection. Inspection of the child may show signs due to a cardiovascular cause such as poor physical development, squatting, dyspnoea, tachypnoea, central cyanosis, oedema, clubbing of the fingers and toes and distension of superficial veins. Precordial bulging associated with cardiac enlargement may be evident and there may be abnormal precordial pulsations. In right ventricular hypertrophy there may be excessive pulsation of the central and superior parts of the precordium leading towards the left sterno-clavicular joint, and in left ventricular hypertrophy an accentuated apical impulse and visible lifting of the precordium. The position of the apex beat, if visible, should also be noted. Assessment of the jugular venous pressure in the neck and of the venous pulse wave may be important (p. 113). In younger children inspection of the neck veins may not be easy because of the relative shortness of the neck and the mobility of the child.

Palpation. Palpation of the precordium may reveal a right ventricular type of parasternal impulse or the heaving apex of left ventricular hypertrophy. It may also reveal the presence of a thrill appreciated better with the palm than with the fingers. The site of maximal intensity of the thrill should be identified. A palpable second heart sound associated with pulmonary hypertension may be felt in the region of the second costal cartilage. The position of the apex beat (point of maximum impulse) should be indentified and in children should normally be within the mid-clavicular line in the fourth or fifth intercostal space.

The radial pulse can be used as an indication of heart rate, but in babies the difficulty of feeling it makes cardiac auscultation a much more reliable method. In older children at least, pulse volume and the presence or absence of a collapsing pulse can be assessed as in adults (p. 109). The pulse can also be used in the detection of arrhythmias. Sinus arrhythmia, i.e. an increase in heart rate on inspiration and decrease on expiration, is a common and normal finding in most children. In any case of suspected congenital heart disease both radial pulses should be palpated to determine any difference between them, and the femoral pulses should also be felt. Absence or weakness of the femoral pulses or delay when they are palpated concurrently with the radial pulses is likely to indicate coarctation of the aorta. In the same condition pulsation of collateral vessels may be detected by palpation in the scapular region.

Percussion. This is not comparable with radiological examination in accuracy of assessment of cardiac size. However, the thinner chest wall of the child makes percussion more suitable than in the adult. The information which is obtainable by percussion of the upper (second intercostal space) and right (mid-clavicular line to right sternal edge) borders of the heart, used in conjunction with the position of the apex beat, is certainly of some value. An overall extension of the area of cardiac dullness indicates cardiac enlargement or pericardial effusion. Displacement of the area may indicate mediastinal shift. Reduction of the area of cardiac dullness is likely to be due to hyperinflation of the lungs.

Auscultation. The auscultatory signs of cardiac disease in infancy and childhood are basically the same as in adults, but as certain types of disease are more common in childhood there is a difference in incidence of the various signs. Congenital heart disease is much more common in infants and children while acquired heart disease is less frequently encountered.

Auscultation of the heart requires silence and a reasonably still patient. These may be difficult or at times impossible to obtain with infants and young children. There are occasions when cardiac auscultation may require to be abandoned till another day.

The heart sounds are usually more readily audible in infancy and childhood than in adulthood. Splitting of the pulmonary second sound on inspiration and a third heart sound are normal findings after the first year of life. The average heart rate varies with age the ranges (rate per min) being as follows:

Newborn	Infancy	Preschool child	School child
70–120	80–160	75–120	70–110

In auscultatory assessment we are concerned with the heart sounds, cardiac rhythm, the presence of any murmurs — with their site, timing, quality, intensity, propagation and variation with position — and the presence of any added sounds such as friction. The scheme of auscultation set out in Chapter 4 can be applied to the child. Murmurs associated with congenital heart disease will preponderate. Thus a loud systolic murmur at the left sternal edge (e.g. ventricular septal defect), a systolic murmur in the pulmonary area (e.g. pulmonary stenosis or atrial septal defect), a systolic-diastolic murmur (machinery murmur or Gibson murmur) at the left sternoclavicular joint (e.g. persistent ductus arteriosus), an ejection systolic murmur transmitted into the neck (e.g. aortic stenosis), and murmurs easily audible over the back (e.g. coarctation of the aorta) are more likely to be heard than the systolic or diastolic mitral murmurs or the aortic diastolic murmurs of established rheumatic heart disease. Mid-diastolic flow murmurs may be heard in congenital heart disease, e.g. at the apex with ventricular septal defect due to increased blood flow through the mitral valve and at the lower left sternal edge with atrial septal defect due to increased blood flow through the tricuspid valve. Presystolic mitral murmurs are relatively rare in childhood. A venous hum (p. 134) is common in childhood and must not be misinterpreted as signifying congenital heart disease.

Blood Pressure Estimation. The normal *auscultatory method* of blood pressure estimation can usually be carried out easily in children over the age of three years. It may be applied, but with more difficulty, to children younger than this. For smaller children narrower cuffs are available of 5 cm (2 in) and 7.5 cm (3 in) widths. As the width of the cuff relative to the length of the upper arm affects the pressure reading (the narrower the cuff relative to the upper arm the higher the reading), a ratio of 2:3 (cuff width:upper arm length) should be preserved. The determination of blood pressure in the legs (e.g. in suspected coarctation of the aorta) by the auscultatory method may be very difficult. The *palpatory method* of blood pressure determination can be extended down to toddlers and babies, but with babies even this may be difficult. In such circumstances the *flush method* may be employed. Two operators are required. A suitably sized cuff is applied loosely round the upper arm or thigh. The limb below the elbow or knee is blanched either by wrapping an elastic bandage around it or by one of the operators compressing it with two hands. The cuff is then inflated by the second operator following which the compression of the limb is released. The limb remains blanched due to the sphygmomanometer cuff preventing entry of blood into it. The sphygmomanometer pressure is allowed to drop quite rapidly. The point at which the blanched lower limb flushes is indicated verbally by the first operator to the second who is watching the sphygmomanometer scale and who notes the pressure. The flush pressure represents a mean pressure approximately midway between the systolic and diastolic levels. Average blood pressure readings (mmHg) in infancy and childhood are as follows:

Newborn	35–85 (flush method)
Infancy	80/55 (auscultation)
Preschool child	85/60 (auscultation)
School child	90/60 (auscultation)

The range of the auscultatory readings is these means plus or minus approximately 20%.

Examination of the Liver. This is described below, but hepatic enlargement is such an important sign of cardiac failure in infancy that it is mentioned here as part of the examination of the cardiovascular system.

ABDOMEN

Inspection. The more distended the abdomen the more shiny and tense will the skin appear. A child who has lost weight may show a retracted (scaphoid) abdomen with the skin of the abdominal wall lax and even wrinkled.

In view of the diaphragmatic type of breathing in normal infants, movement of the abdominal wall is very obvious with respiration. Loss of this movement in infants and also in older children may therefore be an important sign of intra-abdominal disease, such as peritonitis.

Visible peristalsis may be evident through the abdominal wall in obstruction of the alimentary tract. It is seen most frequently during the first three to four months of life in congenital hypertrophic pyloric stenosis — a common disease of male infants. It should be sought while the infant is feeding and placed in such a position that a cross light is shining over the abdomen from the right side. The examiner, seated on the infant's left side and with the eyes just above the level of the abdominal wall, watches for gastric peristalsis moving from left to right across the epigastrium.

In intestinal obstruction there may be abdominal distension, visible peristalsis and a ladder pattern created by loops of gut.

A distended bladder may show itself by a uniform rounded central swelling in the suprapubic region.

Inspection of the abdominal wall will also reveal any abnormality of the umbilicus such as a hernia or infection, and any distension of veins of the abdominal wall as in portal obstruction.

Palpation. Abdominal palpation should normally be carried out with the patient supine and relaxed. The examiner is probably best seated beside the examination couch and the hands should be warm. Relaxation may be assisted by getting the child to draw the knees up and by diverting the child's attention by conversation or by some visual distraction (e.g. a fly crawling on the ceiling). With infants and children who cry on being laid flat it may be better to conduct the abdominal examination with the child sitting on the mother's knee. The abdomen cannot be adequately palpated when a child is crying. If all attempts at pacification fail a limited palpation can be carried out during the few seconds of relaxation when the child stops crying to inspire.

Loss of weight may be indicated by the ability to pick up loose folds of skin.

Tenderness should be sought by gentle palpation covering the whole area of the abdominal wall, progressing gradually to deep palpation. Throughout, the patient's face should be observed for expressions of pain. The extent of the area of tenderness and its site of maximum intensity should be determined. After deep palpation, rebound pain (p. 203) can be sought particularly where any doubtful area of tenderness is discovered. During light palpation any *guarding* (e.g. in early appendicitis) or *boarding* (e.g. in peritonitis or tetanus) of the abdominal wall will become evident.

Palpation for a *pyloric tumour* is an essential part of the diagnosis of congenital hypertrophic pyloric stenosis (Fig. 10.4). Under the same examination conditions and position as for the observation of visible epigastric peristalsis, the examiner palpates with the flat of his left hand on the abdomen, the fingers being directed

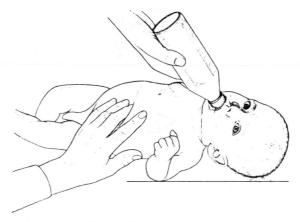

Fig. 10.4   Palpation for a pyloric tumour.

towards the right hypochondrium with their tips lying below the hepatic edge just lateral to the rectus muscle. Gentle depression of the tips of the fingers, using particularly the middle finger, is employed seeking a tumour up to 2 cm in diameter which tends to harden intermittently. It is likely to be impalpable during relaxation and may become firm only once in 10 to 15 minutes. The examination must therefore be conducted for this length of time.

The lower border of the *liver* can normally be felt in infants; to palpate the edge the examiner should place one or both hands flat on the abdomen with their axes directed towards the costal margin and at right angles to it (Fig. 10.5). Palpation is conducted lateral to the rectus abdominis muscle by gentle intermittent depression of the tips of the fingers. The increased resistance to palpation created by the liver can usually be felt just below the costal margin in the normal infant or extending further away from it in the presence of hepatomegaly. As palpation is continued at increasing distance from the costal margin, the edge of the liver will be felt and can be confirmed by approaching the liver from below using moderately deep palpation so that the tips of the fingers are deeper than the liver edge and rolling the tips of the fingers upwards over the edge. In a child who will co-operate, deep breathing assists the examination. On inspiration the liver edge descends and becomes more superficial and the fingers can be rolled more easily over the edge to identify its position. In a crying child the periods of abdominal relaxation between cries will have to be used for these manoeuvres.

The *spleen* may be just palpable in about one in ten healthy children. The technique of palpation does not differ from that in the adult (p. 206). In older children, as in adults, it becomes palpable in the left hypochondrium and enlarges towards the right iliac fossa while in infancy it is more lateral and enlarges towards the left iliac fossa.

The *kidneys* can often be felt in normal children and especially in the newborn infant. Sitting beside the patient, the examiner should place one hand behind on the renal angle and the other in front and conduct bimanual palpation (p. 207). The hands are approximated during expiration and the shape and size of the kidney defined. A rounded pyriform swelling is palpable in the suprapubic region when the *bladder* is abnormally distended.

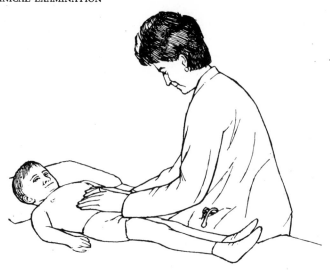

Fig. 10.5 Palpation of the liver in the child.

Other masses of varying size, site and consistency may also be felt. *Faeces* may be palpable along the descending colon. In other cases more extensive scybala may give rise to widespread hard lumps throughout the abdomen. *Mesenteric nodes*, may be palpable as somewhat rubbery masses. *Tumours* such as those due to neuroblastomas and Wilms' tumour are likely to be easily felt. The soft sausage-shaped tumour of an *intussusception* in the upper right quadrant may be much more difficult to feel. It may be associated with a detectable emptiness in the right iliac fossa. *Hernias* may be present — e.g. a soft swelling seen to develop in the inguinal region on crying and reducible by palpation. When strangulated there is likely to be discomfort and a tender, harder, irreducible swelling.

Percussion. The chief value of abdominal percussion lies in the detection of free fluid in the abdomen and in the differentiation of distension due to gas, from solid or liquid containing masses. The technique for percussion in the flanks for shifting dullness is as valid in the child as in the adult (p. 208); so too is the elicitation of a fluid thrill (p. 209). A distended bladder will result in impairment of the percussion note in the suprapubic area.

Auscultation. Bowel sounds, tinkling and crackling in character, are normally intermittently audible on auscultation of the abdomen. These will be accentuated where there is increased peristalsis, as in intestinal obstruction, and will not be heard in the absence of peristalis, e.g. in peritonitis.

Perineum and Genitalia

The *anus* should be examined; anterior positioning may occur or there may be an abnormal opening into the vagina. The formation of the anus should be observed. In ano-rectal atresia it may be noted to be imperforate; in myelomeningocele it may be abnormally open and patulous. The presence of prolapse of the rectum will be obvious. Introduction of the finger may reveal diminished tone, increased tone or stenosis.

Rectal examination is carried out as with adults except that with babies and toddlers the smallest finger should be used to avoid undue stretching of the anus. Gripping of the finger by the narrow rectal segment of Hirschsprung's disease is more likely to be encountered in infants and children than in adults.

The genitalia. In the female, inspection should detect the presence of labial adhesions, enlargement of the clitoris (e.g. in the adreno-genital syndrome), abnormal vaginal discharge or abnormal positioning of the vaginal introitus or urethra.

In the male the size and shape of the penis should be noted, and also any abnormal development, such as hypospadias, or infection, such as balanitis. The position of the testes should be checked (i.e. in the scrotum, palpable in the inguinal canal or not palpable in either of these locations). Any testicular swelling or tenderness or an inguinal hernia or hydrocele will be noted.

NERVOUS SYSTEM

Examination of the nervous system in the older child can be conducted with the same exactitude as in the adult. With the younger child, and particularly with the infant, the central nervous system has not developed the functional precision with which it operates later. Also, mental development has not reached a stage at which full co-operation is possible. Chapter 8 covers the neurological examination as applied to the older child. Here we shall concentrate on the younger child and infant in whom neurological examination is much more objective in its approach and less precise in its application.

Inspection. In the developing child neurological disorder is often linked with disorders of intellect and behaviour. Thus an assessment of these characteristics is important in the neurological examination. After the age of five it usually becomes fairly easy to test *intelligence* separately from motor function. The younger the child the more difficult this is as many of the tests by which intelligence is assessed in infancy and early childhood depend on motor functional ability. This is one of the major difficulties of intelligence testing in children who have suffered neurological damage. The child may appear to be less intelligent than he or she is in the presence of a primary disorder of motor function or, alternatively, the presence of a nervous disorder may be assumed wrongly to explain a poor performance in tests of development when impaired intelligence is the real cause. Bearing these pitfalls in mind, we should as part of the neurological examination attempt to assess the intelligence which a child possesses and likewise observe behaviour and reactions to the environment.

Level of consciousness may be closely related to neurological disease. Hyperexcitability, unresponsiveness, drowsiness, semi-consciousness and unconsciousness may accompany such disorders as meningitis, encephalitis, the post-epileptic state, cerebral injury and others. A somewhat finer appraisal will assess the child's degree of alertness, interest and memory for events in relationship to age.

Disorders of posture and movement may be gross or may be minimal. What position does the child adopt voluntarily — standing, sitting, recumbent, attitude of flexion or attitude of extension? Can the child sit or stand — if at the appropriate age for these activities? Is there an obvious limitation of his ability to carry out certain movements of trunk, head or limbs (e.g. neck stiffness in meningitis, loss of power in poliomyelitis or in nerve inury)? Are there any abnormal movements such as the writhing movements of choreo-athetosis (e.g. following kernicterus), intention tremor on reaching for objects, tics (repetitive involuntary movements) or rolling movements of the eyes (e.g. in blindness)? Are there any convulsive movements associated with impaired consciousness such as generalised convulsions, or localised twitchings, e.g. of the limbs or face? The so-called salaam attacks (myoclonic spasms) are epileptic in nature; the sitting infant suddenly and momentarily falls forward or drops the head abruptly. Does the child in making spontaneous movements exhibit any evidence of inco-ordination or clumsiness (e.g. in certain types of cerebral palsy and cerebral tumour)? Does the gait reveal any abnormality such as the broad-based groping walk of ataxia; or the rather stiff-legged movements of spasticity, associated possibly with inability to put the heels to the ground and excessive wear of the toes of the shoes; or the scissors gait of cerebral diplegia; or the slight outward fling and stiffness of the leg seen in hemiplegia with failure to swing the arm on that side; or the staggering gait of cerebellar disturbance? Has any change been noted in the child's normal hand or foot dominance? Inspection may also reveal some obvious peripheral nerve damage such as facial palsy, wrist drop or Erb's palsy.

Cry and speech may be affected in local and systemic diseases (e.g. the hoarse voice of laryngitis, the gruff one of cretinism and the nasal speech of cleft palate), but neurological disorders probably account for the widest range of abnormality. The infant may have a high pitched cry (e.g. in cerebral birth injury or meningitis), the child's speech may lack intelligibility in varying degree (e.g. in cerebral palsy), speech may disappear (e.g. aphonic chorea), or there may be well marked stammer (e.g. in psychological disturbance) or monotony and lack of expression (e.g. certain post-traumatic states following head injury or with impaired hearing). Delay in the onset of speech may also be noted, as in mental retardation, deafness or infantile autism. The range of vocabulary and language may also give some indication of mental and cerebral functional status.

Cranial Nerves. Specific methods for examining the cranial nerves have been described in Chapter 8. In older children these will be applicable in their entirety; the younger the child the greater will be the limitations imposed by age. Specific appreciation of *smell* does not develop until later childhood. *Vision*, to the extent of appreciation of light and darkness, is probably present at birth. At approximately four weeks infants will watch the mother. By six weeks they will be beginning to watch moving objects, but the arc of visual movement will not be more than 90°; by eight weeks they will be fixing, converging and focusing, and by 12 weeks the arc of visual movement will be approximating to 180°. Thus by six to eight weeks defects in visual perception, and from 12 weeks disordered eye movements, begin to be evident. The accurate testing of visual fields is hardly possible until the child reaches the age of 5 years.

Strabismus. This is common in children. A certain amount of transitory squinting occurs in the early weeks of life. Thereafter a squint becomes significant and we must determine whether the squint is paralytic or non-paralytic (concomitant) in type. In the former the paralysed eye will constantly fail to move in one or more directions, e.g. when a slowly moving light is being followed. Thus the angle between the axes of the eyeballs will vary according to the direction in which the child is looking, e.g. in paralysis of the right sixth nerve the squint will be evident on looking to the right and on this movement the eyeball axes will converge due to movement of the left eye; they will remain parallel when the eyeballs look straight ahead or to the left. With a concomitant squint the two eyes maintain the same relative position in whatever direction the child looks. This type of squint is not necessarily persistent. It may be much more evident at the end of the day when the child is tired or when unwell. The squinting eye can be determined by getting the child to look at an object and covering alternately one and then the other eye. When the dominant eye is covered the squinting eye will look at the object but its gaze will move away from the object when the dominent eye is uncovered. The dominant eye will look at the object both when the squinting eye is covered and uncovered.

The testing of *hearing* is discussed on page 398.

Although testing of *other cranial nerves* is normally carried out with the voluntary co-operation of the patient, some testing can be carried out in younger children incapable of co-operating by observing spontaneous movement. Thus a facial palsy, even of the upper motor neurone type, can be readily diagnosed in the new-born when the infant cries. The normal depression of the corner of the mouth and screwing up of the face with crying does not take place on the affected side. Likewise palatal and tongue movements can be observed.

Motor System. *Muscle Tone.* Handling of the child and passive movements of the limbs will give a general idea of muscle tone. Hypotonia will be indicated by softness of the muscles, floppiness on handling and excessive laxity of the joints due to poor muscle support; hypertonia by excessive firmness of the muscles and stiffness on movement of the limbs. Hypotonicity is usually generalised as in mental retardation, but it may have a local distribution (e.g. in certain types of cerebral palsy). Hypertonicity in children is usually due to an upper motor neurone lesion causing spasticity of 'clasp knife' type (p. 271). Hypertonicity may be generalised but is much more likely to show a specific regional distribution (e.g. unilateral with predominant lower limb involvement in hemiplegia). Certain groups of muscles especially the adductors of the thigh and plantar flexors of the foot are more prone than others to be affected by spasticity.

Motor Power. In the infant, loss of power may be deduced from lack of activity or limited movement without obvious cause. In an older child, active tests of power can be used. An assessment can be made of the grip, flexion or extension at the elbow against resistance, pronation and supination of the forearm, abduction and adduction at the shoulder, raising the knee against pressure while in the recumbent posture, dorsiflexion and plantar flexion of the foot against resistance and abduction and adduction of the hip joint.

Co-ordination. This can be actively tested by asking the child to carry out specific movements requiring co-ordination, e.g. picking up pins, or in younger children by giving them the opportunity to perform similar movements for their own interest. A certain amount of ingenuity will enlarge the range of testing.

Sensory System. In the infant the crying response or the withdrawal response can be used to test pin-prick sensation and muscle tenderness. It may not be possible to test light touch and position sense until the child reaches an age at which co-operation is possible.

Reflexes. A number of reflexes peculiar to infancy are recognised and the absence or impairment of these or their persistence beyond the normal time of disappearance may have diagnostic and predictive value. The *sucking* and *swallowing reflexes* are present in all normal newborn infants and persist until voluntary control of these activities is achieved. The *Moro relfex* may be elicited by a sudden noise or vibration but is probably best stimulated by holding the baby in the supine position with the shoulders, back and buttocks supported on one hand and arm of the examiner, and the head (occiput) in the other hand. If the head is allowed to fall back about an inch while the body remains supported, the arms rapidly abduct then come together again with an embracing movement. This reflex normally disappears at two or three months. The *grasp reflex* is also present in normal newborn babies. It is elicited by placing the examiner's forefingers in the palms of the infant's hands. The baby's hand closes on the examiner's finger. This reflex also disappears at two to three months. The *rooting reflex* is present in normal infants and helps them to find the mother's nipple. When light contact is made with the infant's cheek, the infant turns towards the point of contact. The *tonic neck reflex* is elicited with the baby in the supine position. Rotation of the head to one side produces increased tone in the arm on the same side with partial extension of it and there may be flexion of the knee on the contralateral side. This reflex normally disappears at two to three months. The Moro reflex, grasp reflex, rooting reflex and tonic neck reflex may be absent in a baby suffering from cerebral birth injury or certain types of cerebral dysgenesis. In cerebral palsy or mental retardation they may persist beyond the time at which they normall disappear. The *light reflex* is present almost from birth. The *knee and ankle jerks* are of limited value in the neonate but develop in intensity after a few weeks. The *abdominal reflexes* are present from birth but great patience may be required to elicit them in the newborn. They show the adult pattern of response. The normal adult type *plantar reflex* (p. 292) is seen in children over one year of age. Under one year, an equivocal response with 'fanning' of the toes is normally obtained. In certain disorders (e.g. meningocele) loss of the *anal reflex* (constriction on stroking the perianal skin) may be of some value.

Tests of Meningeal and Nerve Irritation. Kernig's is a late sign in meningitis and should be carried out as in the adult. It may be associated with Brudzinski's sign which is positive (e.g. in meningitis) when on flexing the head the thighs and knees also flex, or with inability of the child, in the sitting position with the knees drawn up, to touch the knees with the nose. The straight leg raising sign — limitation of the angle to which the leg can be lifted due to the development of sciatic pain — may be of use where the lower spinal nerve roots are subject to pressure as, for example, by a spinal tumour.

Hearing. Defective hearing in a child may go unsuspected for years and have a serious effect on the development of speech and education. Ability to hear certain sounds may give the impression of normal hearing whereas partial deafness may be present.

The possibility of deafness may well not have occurred to parents when they describe delayed or abnormal speech, inattentiveness, apparent backwardness or tantrums in their child. The examiner should bear this possibility in mind in the presence of such symptoms. The testing of hearing in infancy and childhood is difficult. If a doctor has reason to suspect impairment of hearing a few simple tests involving a range of common sounds may be carried out but if there is any doubt, the child should be referred for more expert examination.

With an infant or child suspected of deafness, a fairly prolonged period of observation in a peaceful environment in the presence of the mother is likely to be required. Impairment of hearing and of comprehension of speech may reveal themselves by general indifference to sound, lack of response to the spoken word and response to noises rather than voice; vocalisation and sound production may be defective. From about four months onwards babies laugh aloud and vocalise freely with such sounds as 'ba', 'ka', 'goo', etc. At 7 months a tuneful repetitive babble of the 'dad-dad', 'bab-bab', 'mam-mam' variety is to be expected, followed at 10 to 12 months by a few words understandable to the mother only and at 14 months by a few recognisable words. Any delay in reaching these stages of vocalisation should arouse the suspicion of deafness. Sound production may also be abnormal in character, monotonous in quality and indistinct. Laughter may be lessened and pleasure, annoyance and need may be expressed by yelling and screeching.

Loss of hearing may increase visual attention and alertness to gesture and movement. Gestures may be markedly imitative and vehement.

Social rapport and adaptation may be affected. This may be evident in vocal nursery games. The facial expression may be unexpectedly enquiring, surprised or thwarted.

Disturbances of emotion may be evident such as attention-seeking tantrums. Obstinacy, irritability and outbursts of self-vexation may occur because of failure to be understood.

Objective tests of hearing in young children have been developed but require practice and experience and must be carried out exactly as specified to give accurate results. There is a series of more simple tests for infants and children from six months to seven years. These utilise sounds made by familiar objects. For infants of 6 to 14 months a soft-pitched rattle, the crinkling of tissue paper, a small handbell, the stroking of a spoon round the rim of a cup and the spoken voice are used. The sounds are made at half a metre from the infant at a level with the ear and with the examiner outside the range of vision. The child should react by turning the head in the direction of the sound. For children from 15–24 months similar sounds and a series of verbal tests are used. In the latter a number of common objects such as a cup, ball, toy motor-car and doll are displayed and verbally identified. The child is then asked to pick out individual articles when they are named. For two-year-olds further objects are added such as spoon, fork, knife and cubes, and thus the conversation related to the larger group of objects is extended to include a wider range of sounds. The child's own speech and phonetic usage will at this stage further indicate the ability to appreciate sound.

At 3 to 4 years and at 5 to 7 years the general principle is followed of widening the range of sounds addressed to the child via the examiner's voice. By the latter age the child should be capable of co-operating in more formal testing to the extent of covering one ear and repeating a list of words spoken at 3 metres into the uncovered ear, identifying a watch tick, etc. By this age, too, the spoken language of the normal child is usually fluent and correct.

LOCOMOTOR SYSTEM

Examination of the nervous system will inevitably involve some examination of the locomotor system. The more specific examination of this system may reveal other defects.

Fractures. These may be suspected because of bony deformity, crepitus (should not be actively elicited), local pain and tenderness on attempted movement. Bony tenderness and swelling may also be present in other conditions, such as osteomyelitis.

Deformities of the Trunk and Neck. These may take the form of scoliosis, kyphosis or lordosis. They should be sought with the child unclothed and standing erect or lying free. Scoliosis may be suspected if the skin creases in the flanks are asymmetrical and if they fail to disappear when the spine is passively flexed to the opposite side. Absence of ribs may be detected in association with scoliosis, kyphosis and lordosis. Anterior positioning of the shoulders may be found to be associated with absence of the clavicles. Torticollis is excluded by a full range of passive rotation of the head. If a tuft of hair is visible over the lumbo-sacral region, spina bifida occulta may be present and may be palpable.

Deformities of the Limbs. In the upper limbs a number of deformities may be evident. There may be an increased carrying angle at the elbow in Turner's syndrome. In the absence of the radius, severe flexion and lateral twisting of the hand occur at the wrist. There may be other flexion deformities or absence of part of the arms or fingers, extra digits, or incurving of the little finger (as in Down's syndrome), or a variety of other abnormalities. Functional deformities such as the dinner fork deformity of the wrist with the hands outstretched (as in chorea) may be evident.

In the lower limbs examples of deformity would be genu valgum, talipes equino varus (club foot), absence of part of the limbs, and shortening or unequal development, e.g. hemi-atrophy or hemi-hypertrophy. Pes planus is best observed with the child standing, when eversion of the foot and flattening of the normal plantar arch will be evident.

Muscles. The muscles should be examined for evidence of general or local wasting or absence of individual muscles. Hypertrophy may also be noted, as in the calves in the Duchenne type of muscular dystrophy. Assessment of muscle tone has been described on page 397.

Joints. Examination of a joint will assess its range of movement, the presence or absence of deformity, swelling, tenderness, pain on active and passive movement and any local rise of temperature. Swelling of a large joint may be seen in conditions such as rheumatic fever and haemophilia, and of small joints in rheumatoid arthritis. Congenital dislocation of the hip must be diagnosed as soon as possible after birth, on the basis of routine screening using the Ortolani test (p. 350).

DEVELOPMENTAL DIAGNOSIS

The progressive acquisition of the various body movements and motor skills which characterises normal development is closely related to the maturation of all systems but especially to that of the nervous system. The dates of passing so-called milestones of development may be of great diagnostic and predictive value in the assessment of intellect and physical disorders. Some of the stages ('milestones') in normal development from 4 weeks to 5 years of age are given on page 446.

FURTHER INVESTIGATION

Collection of Specimens

Urine. This should be examined routinely in any clinical examination of an infant or child. At the uncooperative ages specimens may not be easily obtained when required. Infants tend to pass uring after feeding so that the chances of success in obtaining specimens are higher at this time. Polythene bags for urine collection are available with an opening surrounded by adhesive material which sticks to the skin round the pubis, groin and perineal areas. These can also be used for the collection of 24-hour specimens. The average daily output of urine at different ages is as follows:

First and second days	30–60 ml
Third to tenth day	100–300 ml
Tenth day to two months	25–450 ml
Two months to one year	400–500 ml
1–5 years	500–700 ml

For bacteriological purposes a mid-stream specimen may be obtainable. The younger the child, the more are patience, luck and a steady hand on the receptacle required. In childhood, however, suprapubic aspiration will often be necessary when it is important to make a bacteriological diagnosis. As the bladder in the infant extends well above the pelvic brim, suprapubic aspiration at this age is not usually a difficult procedure.

Faeces. Specimens of faeces should be collected in sterile containers using a spoon or spatula to transfer the specimen from the pot or the napkin. Where a specimen of faeces for bacteriological examination is unobtainable a rectal swab may be taken but is less satisfactory. An ordinary throat swab is introduced into the anus for an inch or so for this purpose.

Sputum. In younger children sputum, if present, is difficult to obtain. A cough swab may be taken in an attempt to obtain a sample for bacteriological examination. A throat swab is introduced as far back as possible and the child is encouraged to cough. Gastric aspiration may occasionally enable swallowed sputum to be obtained.

Throat Swab. The procedure already described for visualising the oropharynx is employed (p. 386) and the tonsils and pharynx are swabbed.

Gastric and Duodenal Juice. In babies the passage of a fine polythene tube into the stomach through the mouth or nose is easy, as active swallowing is not necessary. In older children, in using a Ryle's tube, persuasion, encouragement and even demonstration may be required. Intubation of the duodenum is not usually easy in young children, but by leaving the tube down for some hours and by placing the child on the right side the passage of the tube through the pylorus will be encouraged.

Blood. Venepuncture is much more difficult in infants due to the smaller size and greater mobility of the veins, and the plumpness of the limbs which is usually present. The external jugular vein, the veins in the antecubital fossa, the femoral veins and scalp veins may be used. The femoral vein lies medial to the femoral artery which can be identified by palpation.

For many purposes an adequate quantity of blood can be obtained by heel puncture (p. 430).

Sweat. In the diagnosis of cystic fibrosis it may be necessary to collect sweat. The skin is first cleaned with distilled water then dried with a gauze swab. A piece of sodium and chloride free filter paper is applied to the skin (usually of the back) and is covered with a piece of polythene which has been washed in distilled water and dried. The polythene is sealed down with adhesive. After some hours the filter paper is removed with forceps and placed in a chemically clean container which is then sealed and despatched to the biochemistry laboratory. Iontophoresis using pilocarpine is a more reliable method of promoting sweating. Ideally the weight of sweat obtained should exceed 200 mg. Diagnostic concentrations of sodium and chloride respectively are 80 and 60 mmol/l of sweat.

Cerebrospinal Fluid. The technique of lumbar puncture is essentially the same in the infant and child as in the adult. Some prefer the child to be in the upright position, others in the lateral position. Smaller lumbar puncture needles are available for infants and toddlers.

THE METHODS IN PRACTICE

The example chosen supplements as well as exemplifies what has been discussed in this chapter.

EXAMINATION OF THE NEWBORN INFANT

The majority of infants born in Britain are now medically examined at birth. If any abnormality is present this may be obvious on casual inspection, as with a gross congenital disorder such as spina bifida, or may be uncovered only after a careful and thorough clinical examination. While the principles and practices described throughout this chapter apply in the main to the newborn infant, there has to be some selectivity in the methods of approach on the grounds of practicability, and the limitations of clinical examination at this age have to be recognised. Underlying disease may be present, but the signs by which it can be recognised may not yet have developed. A gross congenital cardiac defect such as transposition of the great vessels may be present without murmurs, without clinical evidence of cardiac enlargement or cardiac failure and without cyanosis (which will develop later); severe infection may occur with little rise in temperature; gross mental defect may be present yet its recognition may be impossible; vision has not yet developed; the range of facial expression is limited; hypothyroidism may be present without any of the signs of cretinism. While the difficulties have to be recognised, they should not

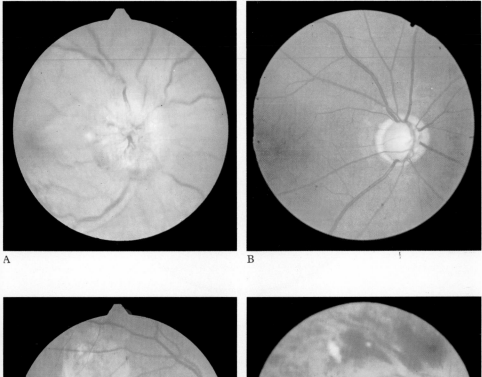

A   B

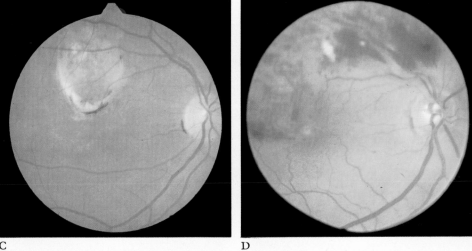

C   D

Plate III   **The fundus as a diagnostic aid.** Retinal photographs showing: (A) Papilloedema. Edge of optic disc blurred and partly surrounded by small haemorrhages; retinal vessels obscured on and beyond edge of disc by swelling of papilla; small dilated vessels on surface of centre of disc in sharper focus than peripheral vessels as these are at different levels. (B) Glaucoma. Vessels emerge from and enter periphery of an atrophic disc over lip of an enormously enlarged and deepened optic cup, in contrast to their level course in primary optic atrophy. (C) Disciform degeneration due to ischaemia. Slightly pigmented scar just above macula. (D) Branch vein occlusion. Superior temporal vein has been occluded and has led to haemorrhages and two white patches of oedema. Several small lakes of blood lie in front of retinal vessels in the vitreous and there are some dilated collateral vessels above the macula. It is more usual in this condition for the blood to lie in the nerve fibre layer and to have a flame-shaped arcuate pattern. Disc and lower retina are normal (*courtesy of Professor I. C. Michaelson*).

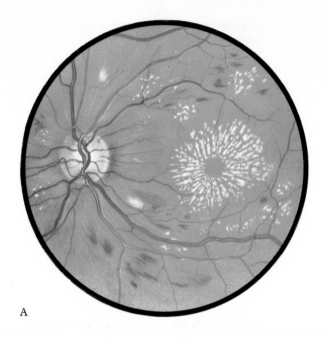

A

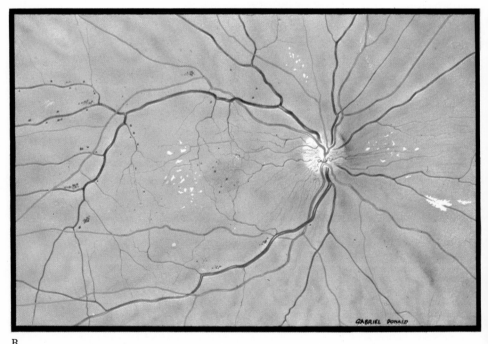

GABRIEL DONALD

B

Plate IV. The fundus as a diagnostic aid. Retinal painting showing: (A) Hypertensive retinopathy. Note haemorrhages, two soft exudates, numerous hard exudates including a macular star and irregularity of the calibre of the arterioles. (B) Diabetic retinopathy. Note microaneurysms and a few hard exudates (*courtesy of Professor I. C. Michaelson*).

discourage the routine clinical examination of the newborn infant. This may reveal much and the information obtained and recorded at this time may be of great value in the future should the infant later develop any abnormality. As the methods have largely been described already this section will indicate chiefly the breadth and scope of the neonatal examination rather than the technique.

The *medical history of the parents and other relatives* is relevant, for example in disorders which have a strong hereditary tendency such as haemophilia, haemorrhagic telangiectasis or the Treacher-Collins syndrome, and those with a weaker but definite hereditary tendency such as cleft lip and spina bifida. The history of the mother's pregnancies may indicate factors such as recurrent prematurity or postmaturity. Her age may be important (e.g. Down's syndrome is common in the elderly mother). Disease such as rubella, syphilis or toxoplasmosis may have affected the mother during pregnancy and may have had a profound influence on the fetus. Enquiry about siblings may reveal familial disease such as cystic fibrosis, the adrenogenital syndrome, mental retardation or albinism. Drugs administered early in pregnancy (e.g. warfarin or phenytoin) may be related to the occurrence of congenital abnormalities.

In the newborn infant the history of previous illness consists largely of the *birth history* (p. 374). This will include information on fetal distress, e.g. slowing of the fetal heart rate or meconium staining of the liquor; early rupture of the membranes; induction of labour; prolonged or rapid labour; difficulties of delivery — forceps delivery or caesarean section; maturity; birth rank; birth weight; asphyxia, such as that associated with delayed onset of respiration or irregular or periodic breathing; respiratory distress with increased respiratory effort and costal margin recession; twitchings and convulsions or disturbances of consciousness; jaundice, pallor or cyanosis.

Weight, length (crown-heel or crown-rump) and head circumference are *standard measurements*. If available, the weight, charted from the time of birth, is valuable.

The following are a few examples of *deformities* which, when present, will be obvious in most cases:

1. Spina bifida or webbing of the neck.
2. Deformities of the limbs such as achondroplasia or hemimelia (arm ends abruptly above or below elbow).
3. Abnormalities in cranial shape and size such as hydrocephalus, excessive moulding or cephalhaematoma.
4. Abnormalities such as the characteristic facies of Down's syndrome or the flattened nose and low set ears of renal agenesis (Fig. 10.2).
5. Absence of digits, ribs, etc.
6. Tumour masses such as sacro-coccygeal teratoma.

Areas of local swelling such as an umbilical hernia or a cystic hygroma should also be obvious.

The *state of consciousness* of the child, for example the unresponsiveness of severe apnoea or the open eyes and hyperactivity of cerebral irritation, will be evident and the response to stimuli, such as pinching of the skin, noted. The amount of spontaneous movement may be significant. Convulsive movements, if present, may be localised or generalised.

The skin is elastic and pink in the healthy infant, but may be cracked and parchment-like in placental insufficiency, abnormally pallid as a result of fetal exsanguination, cyanosed as a result of asphyxia or severe congenital heart disease, jaundiced in hepatic, biliary and haemolytic disorders, loose and inelastic in prematurity, dry and inelastic in dehydration, blemished with superficial angiomata or milia (pinpoint-sized white spots due to retention of sebaceous material) or infected with pustules. Oedema may be present especially in premature infants. The character of the umbilical cord or the presence of umbilical bleeding or infection should be noted. Skin temperature may be roughly assessed by palpation with the dorsum of the middle phalanges; a suspected abnormality should be checked with a rectal thermometer. The temperature should also be recorded in the presence of symptoms such as unexplained loss of weight, anorexia or vomiting.

The *mouth* will be examined for deformities such as cleft palate, drying of the mucous membranes, ulceration, or infection. The size, shape and tension of the *anterior fontanelle* and the degree of closure of the *posterior fontanelle* may be important.

The shape of the *chest*, the pattern of respiration (e.g. regular in time and force, or periodic and of varying depth), the respiration rate, the presence of respiratory distress, respiratory depression as in the failure of establishment of adequate respiration, moisture in the chest (the 'mucousy' baby), abnormalities in the breath sounds such as diminished air entry or added sounds, may all be important observations.

The *heart* will be examined for position, for the presence of any abnormal precordial pulsation and for murmurs. The radial and femoral pulses should be palpated and if indicated the blood pressure estimated in the arms and legs (probably by the flush method).

In the *abdomen* any impairment of the normal movement with respiration will be observed and also the shape of the abdomen — scaphoid in certain types of oesophageal atresia or distended or exhibiting peristaltic waves in intestinal obstruction. The abdomen should be palpated for masses.

The infant may with advantage be watched while *feeding*, for vigour and co-ordination of sucking, character of swallowing, vomiting and evidence of visible abdominal peristalsis.

The *genitalia* will be examined for conditions such as hydrocele or undescended testes in the male or for clitoral enlargement (as in adrenogenital syndrome) in the female. Any imperforation of the anus or malposition of the urethral orifice as occurs in hypospadias will be noted.

In the *nervous system* local pareses, for instance of one side of the face in facial palsy or of the legs in the presence of spina bifida, should be sought. The hemisyndrome is characterised by diminished movement on one side of the body. The Moro reflex and the grasp reflex may be absent in the presence of cerebral injury. The character of the cry may be revealing such as the high-pitched cry of cerebral irritation or the 'cri-du-chat' syndrome. Muscle tone should be assessed. Hypotonia and hypertonia frequently indicate cerebral disturbance. Posture may also have a similar implication, e.g. extension of all four limbs in brain stem injury (decerebrate rigidity) or 'fisting' (hand clenched with thumb against palm) in cerebral irritation.

The performance of certain basic activities in the newborn infant such as sucking, swallowing and crying and a normal sleep pattern (about 20 hours asleep and 4 awake) are dependent on the integrity of the nervous system. Any deficiencies in these abilities or disturbances of pattern raise the question of brain damage. Examination should include observation of the infant's ability to suck and swallow and an appreciation of the pattern of sleep and wakefulness.

In the *locomotor system* any limitation of joint movement such as occurs in arthrogryposis, the click of congenital dislocation of the hip on Ortolani's manoeuvre (p. 350), any reduction in muscle tone as may occur with cerebral damage or specific muscle disease or increase in tone which again may occur with cerebral damage, will be appreciated by handling the infant.

Faeces and Urine. Enquiries can be made about the passage of meconium and the frequency and character of the stools. The latter may be examined. Likewise there may be indications for examining the urine visually, chemically, bacteriologically and for measuring daily volume.

Further Investigations. Biochemical (e.g. plasma electrolytes), bacteriological (e.g. blood culture) or radiological studies (e.g. radiographs of chest or abdomen) may be indicated. The Guthrie test applied after feeding is established as a screening test for phenylketonuria.

Conclusion

The examination of the newborn infant exemplifies fundamental clinical principles even though these are being applied at a time of life when many manifestations of disease are different from those found later. As presenting symptoms in early life are less specific than in adulthood, a full clinical examination is necessary in all infants who appear unwell. Furthermore, if disease in infancy and childhood is to be diagnosed early and reversed early before it causes irretrievable damage, diagnosis must be based on minimal, not gross, signs. For example, a positive Kernig's sign in infancy is likely to indicate not just that the child has meningitis but that the meningitis has advanced to a stage when, if there is recovery, permanent sequelae will result. Clinical examination revealing at an earlier stage that the infant was pyrexial, was off feeding, had unexplained vomiting and was irritable or 'far away' and resulting in a lumbar puncture, would have enabled treatment to be instituted early with a very much higher chance of rapid and complete recovery.

11. The Use of the Ophthalmoscope

The first model was constructed of pasteboard, eye lenses, and cover glasses used in microscopic work. It was at first so difficult to use that I doubt if I should have persevered unless I had felt that it must succeed; but in eight days I had the great joy of being the first who saw before him the human living retina.

Herman von Helmholtz, 1821–1894

The tradition that the ophthalmoscope is difficult to use dies hard. Modern ophthalmoscopes are so constructed that Helmholtz's initial difficulties have long since been overcome and attention to a few simple details of technique will suffice to enable the student to see the fundus without difficulty. In different subjects, the colour and form of the visible structures vary like complexions and faces; familiarity with the range of normal appearances is therefore essential. The ophthalmoscope, like the stethoscope, should be accepted as a necessity at the start of the student's career and inspection of the fundus should be included as part of the routine clinical examination.

Serious or life-threatening conditions, which may be potentially curable such as malignant hypertension, raised intracranial pressure, miliary tuberculosis, or malignant melanoma may be revealed by ophthalmoscopy. Fundal examination may lead to the diagnosis of such lesions as glaucoma and retinal detachment which can cause loss of vision. Inspection of the optic fundus may also help in the diagnosis of a number of systemic disorders, for example, diabetes mellitus and systemic lupus erythematosus.

The Ophthalmoscope

The principles of operation of the ophthalmoscope are simple. A beam of light from a battery-operated lamp is deflected through a right angle by an angled mirror at the top of the instrument. The observer looks through a small hole in the mirror along the pathway of the light, through the pupil, so that the structures of the eye, including the fundus, are illuminated, and can be inspected (Fig. 11.1). Lenses of graded focal length may be placed behind the hole in the mirror and are moved by a milled wheel, conveniently placed so that it can be controlled by the index finger of the hand holding the ophthalmoscope. There is a series of lenses marked with a '+' which are convex and an array of '−' lenses which are concave. Each lens also bears a number which corresponds to its focal length expressed in dioptres. One dioptre is the refractive power of a lens whose focal length is one metre, while two dioptres corresponds to a focal length of half a metre and twenty dioptres to one twentieth of a metre. These lenses are used to compensate for refractive errors (hypermetropia or myopia) in the examiner's or patient's eyes.

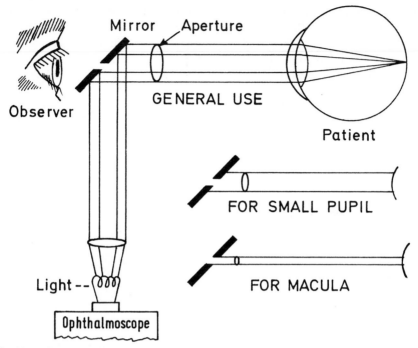

Observer

Mirror   Aperture

GENERAL USE

Patient

FOR SMALL PUPIL

Light

FOR MACULA

Ophthalmoscope

Fig. 11.1 **Ophthalmoscopy: Basic principles.** Some models have a changeable aperture to narrow the beam of light, e.g. for inspection of the macula. Others also have an auriscopic attachment (p. 75).

Technique in the Use of the Ophthalmoscope

During a routine examination, the fundus may be inspected through the untreated pupil. However, if the clinical picture suggests that there may be a fundal abnormality, and always for a thorough examination of the fundus, the pupil must be dilated with a short acting mydriatic. Tropicamide or cyclopentolate drops (0.5–1%) are most widely used. Homatropine should not be instilled since its effects are too prolonged. Mydriatics should not be used if the patient is known to suffer from acute glaucoma. Rarely, dilatation of the pupil by mydriatics may precipitate an attack of acute (closed angled) glaucoma in those patients who have a shallow anterior chamber. An effective estimate of the depth of the anterior chamber may be made fairly simply by shining a light from the margin of the cornea across the iris; if the anterior chamber is of normal depth, the iris will glow around its whole circumference. If the patient has a shallow anterior chamber, only that half of the iris near to the light will be illuminated. If there is any doubt about the depth of the anterior chamber, expert ophthalmological assessment should be made before mydriatics are employed. If this precaution is observed, it is not essential to constrict the pupil after the examination; a drop of 2% eserine sulphate will constrict the pupil if this is thought desirable.

The procedure for the use of the ophthalmoscope itself is as follows:

1. The patient should be examined in a darkened environment if possible. Brightly illuminated conditions should be avoided.

2. If the examiner has a refractive error, the ophthalmoscope may be used while spectacles are worn. Preferably they should be removed and an appropriate correcting lens selected and placed behind the sight hole in the mirror.

3. The ophthalmoscope should be held in the right hand and the right eye should be used to examine the patient's right eye. The examiner's left hand and left eye are used to examine the patient's left eye.

4. The patient should be asked to look straight ahead, to keep an eye fixed on a selected, distant object and to keep both eyes open. Blinking does not interfere with the view.

5. Vision in the eye not being examined should not be obstructed by the examiner's head; otherwise the patient's gaze tends to wander (Fig. 11.2).

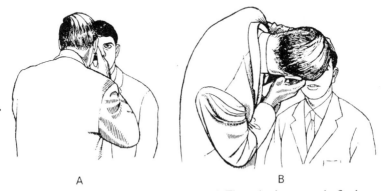

A   B

Fig. 11.2   Ophthalmoscopy. (A) The correct method. The patient's gaze can be fixed on a distant point. (B) The wrong method. The patient's view is obstructed and the gaze cannot be fixed on a distant point.

6. The examiner's eye should be placed as close as possible to the ophthalmoscope. This enables a greater area to be visualised through the sight hole as when one looks through a key hole. The ophthalmoscope should be held steadily by pressing it against the side of the nose and against the superior orbital margin.

7. It is helpful to rest the ulnar border of the examiner's free hand above the patient's superior orbital margin. If the eyes are closed, voluntarily or involuntarily, the thumb may be used to raise the patient's upper lid gently clear of the pupil.

8. The examination should begin with the ophthalmoscope held 20 to 30 centimetres away from the patient's eye with the light directed into the pupil. The pupil will then appear to glow uniformly red in normal circumstances. This is the red reflex.

9. The ophthalmoscope and the examiner's head are moved closer to the patient's eye and during this procedure opacities, appearing as black or glistening silhouetted gaps in the red reflex, may be seen. The ophthalmoscope should come as close as possible to the patient's eye, without touching the eye lashes or cornea.

10. The fundus should be brought into clear focus, using correcting lenses if necessary.

11. The light should always be directed at the patient's pupil even when it is necessary to make lateral movements of the ophthalmoscope. A clear view of the fundus may be hampered by light reflected back from the patient's cornea. This can

be obviated by a slight tilting of the ophthalmoscope. Inexperienced observers often over-accommodate their eyes which impairs clarity of vision. This happens involuntarily because of the closeness of the examiner's eye to the patient. Practice at 'looking into the distance' will enable the observer consciously to prevent this accommodation; it can be compensated for by the use of a low power negative lens in the ophthalmoscope.

Difficulties from Opacities and Errors of Refraction

Opacities causing interruptions of the red reflex may lie in the cornea, the lens or the vitreous. When such an opacity is recognised its site should be determined. Corneal opacities due to scarring are revealed if a light is shone obliquely on the cornea. Opacities behind the cornea may be better defined by inserting convex lenses behind the sight hole of the ophthalmoscope. There may be opacities in the lens due to cataracts.

Opacities in the vitreous are commonly due to irregular, spider-like, drifting black masses. These are known as vitreous 'floaters'. These are extremely common, particularly in myopic patients and the elderly; they are due to precipitation of the vitreous proteins and do not indicate any serious lesion. Vitreous opacities may also be due to haemorrhages and occasionally to persistent fetal hyaloid vessels or their vestiges which lie between the optic disc and the posterior pole of the lens.

Opacities of the refractive media may be localised by slight lateral movements of the ophthalmoscope. Opacities in the cornea will then appear to move in the direction opposite to that of the light of the ophthalmoscope. Opacities of the lens will not move at all. Opacities in the vitreous seem to move in the same direction as the light.

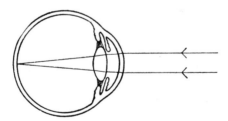

Fig. 11.3   The emmetropic (normal) eye. The retina is in focus without a lens in the ophthalmoscope.

Errors of Refraction. If there are no opacities, close in to the normal position and adjust the lenses if necessary until the retinal vessels are in sharp focus. If the observer's and the patient's eyes are both normal then no lens ('0') is required; the fundus, although only about 3 cm from the examiner's eye, is in perfect focus owing to refraction by the cornea, lens and vitreous body amounting in all to about 60 dioptres (Fig. 11.3). The need to employ a plus lens to focus on the fundus indicates hypermetropia, while a minus lens is required for a myopic eye (Figs. 11.4, 11.5).

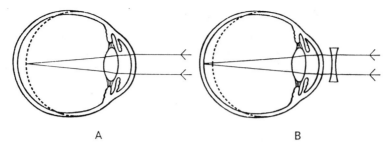

Fig. 11.4   The myopic (short-sighted) eye. (A) The eye is too long and the retina is not in focus when no lens is used. (B) The use of a concave (minus) lens brings the retina into focus.

Myopia is common, and in very short-sighted persons it may be necessary to use a − 20 lens or more before a clear view is obtained. Many ophthalmoscopes have no more than a − 20 lens so that exact focus may not be possible.

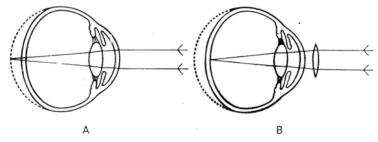

Fig. 11.5   The hypermetropic (long-sighted) eye. (A) The eye is too short and the retina is not in focus when no lens is used. (B) The· use of a convex (plus) lens brings the retina into focus.

The cornea, vitreous and the lens combine to magnify the features of the fundus. In an emmetropic eye the optic disc appears about four times its true diameter. If the lens of the eye has been removed for cataract it will be noted that the retina of a previously emmetropic eye is now in focus with a + 10 lens, a large area of the fundus is in view, the disc and vessels look very small and the inevitable little movements of the patient's eye do not have the usual adverse effect on one's ability to see the fundus. On the other hand, in a myopic eye, a strong minus lens is required, only a small area of the fundus may be in view, the disc and the vessels appear very large, and any little movement is magnified. A very myopic patient can be asked to wear spectacles while the *optic disc* and the central parts of the retina are examined; the features are more readily seen. Unfortunately, the reflection off the glass makes it impossible to examine the peripheral parts of the retina in the usual way. A good area may, however, be examined by asking the patient to look up, down, to the right and to the left, though patches are liable to be missed.

Gross astigmatism may also cause some difficulty. If the curvatures of the cornea and of the anterior and posterior surfaces of the lens of the eye are segments of perfect spheres, the fundus is magnified without distortion. However, there is commonly some degree of astigmatism, a term applied when the curvature of any of these surfaces varies in different planes. The effect of severe astigmatism is to distort the image just as one sees distortion on looking through a window pane that is slightly defective. Particular difficulty then arises in trying to recognise segmental narrowings of the retinal arterial blood columns.

Inspection of the Optic Fundus

It is important to adhere to a fixed routine when examining the fundus of the eye.

1. The *optic disc* should first be inspected (Fig. 11.6). It lies slightly to the nasal side of the optical axis of the eye and looks paler than the surrounding retina. It can be located by following the course of an artery or vein. The acute angle between a main vessel and its branches or tributaries points towards the disc.

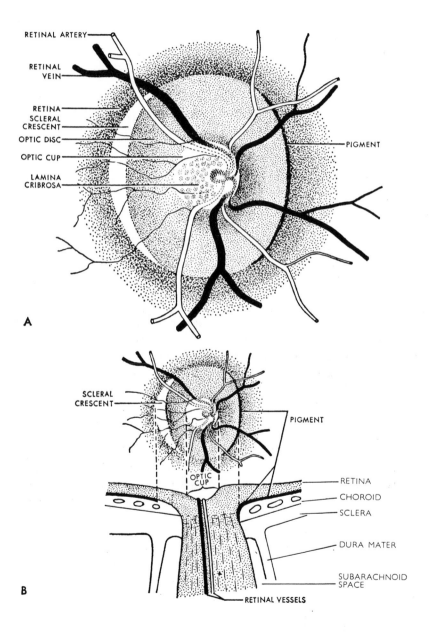

Fig. 11.6   The normal right optic disc.

2. The *arteries and veins* should be inspected next. Note whether they are straight or tortuous and examine their width and colour, the light reflex along the centre of the arterioles and the appearance at arteriovenous crossings. The artery usually lies on the vein and blood columns should not be distorted by the crossing. The light reflex is normally the only evidence of the vessel wall. If the ophthalmoscope is quite steady, it is possible in most subjects to see pulsation of the retinal veins as they lie on the optic disc. Absence of this venous pulsation is not necessarily abnormal but is sometimes a feature of papilloedema.

3. The appearance of the *fundus background* should be studied systematically by radiating from the disc to the periphery right round the fundus in a clockwise or anticlockwise manner. The position of any abnormality such as alteration of pigment, or haemorrhages, exudates, tubercles or underlying choroidal changes should be noted as if the fundus was a clock with the optic disc as its centre.

4. Finally the *macula and its surroundings* should be examined. Unless the pupil is dilated, it is probable that a narrow beam will be required for inspection of the macular area (Fig. 11.1). It can be seen at once if the patient looks directly into the light. The macula is situated about two discs' width to the temporal side of the lower pole of the optic disc. It appears as a small dull red patch, darker than the remainder of the fundus. In the centre there is often a little glistening white dot which is due to reflection of light from the fovea. Lesions in this area tend to cause serious loss of vision.

Interpretation of Ophthalmoscopic Appearances

The Optic Disc and its Immediate Surroundings. Attention should be paid particularly to the colour of the optic disc, the physiological cup and the disc margin.

A normal optic disc (Fig. 11.6) is a variable shade of pink because of the interlacing capillaries which lie among the translucent nerve fibres. The surrounding retina is a duskier shade of red than the disc owing to the underlying pigment layer. There are fewer capillaries over the temporal half of the disc which, in normal people, tends to look paler than the nasal half. Capillaries covering the base of the optic cup are sparse and the cup, therefore, appears whiter than the rest of the optic disc.

The physiological cup, recognised by its pallor, varies in depth and diameter in different individuals. It usually occupies about a quarter of the area of the optic disc. Although in some normal people it may extend almost to three quarters of the disc's area, enlargement of the physiological cup is a cardinal sign of chronic glaucoma (Plate III). In the depths of the cup lies the lamina cribrosa which often can be seen as a very faintly chequered appearance (Fig. 11.6).

The margin of the optic disc is usually well demarcated from the rest of the retina. Sometimes, in normal people, the periphery of the nasal side of the disc lies slightly above the level of the surrounding retina and this leads to obscuring of the disc margin in this area. There is commonly a line of pigment around part of the disc's edge which is of no pathological significance (Fig. 11.6).

In *myopia* the optic disc appears large and the stretching of the inner coats of the eye frequently causes degenerative changes in the adjacent choroid. The disc may become surrounded by a white crescent. Large irregular white patches may occur due to the shift or disappearance of pigment and to atrophy of the choroidal vessels so that the sclera is visible; pigment may be seen in or around these white areas.

In *hypermetropia* the disc appears small and may also look a deeper shade of pink than is normal.

In *papilloedema* (Plate III) the disc usually looks pinker than normal and the margins of the disc become blurred (p. 239); later the overlying blood vessels are obscured. The discs of patients with hypermetropia often look as though they may be swollen and the blurring of the margin on the nasal side of a normal disc also sometimes leads to a mistaken diagnosis of papilloedema.

An occasional congenital abnormality, of no pathological significance, is the *persistence of myelination* around some nerve fibres. These fibres are opaque and white, display irregular edges and usually lie contiguous to the disc margin. Rarely they may be seen in more peripheral parts of the retina.

Pathological pallor of part or all of the disc means that there is *optic atrophy*, i.e. there is loss of some of the capillary network and glial proliferation. Optic atrophy is discussed on page 238. The normal pallor of the temporal half of the disc is sometimes mistaken for partial optic atrophy as are myopic crescents, large optic cups, and myelinated nerve fibres abutting on to the disc.

Blood Vessels. In the retinal arteries and veins only the blood is visible. Light is reflected off the vessel wall and is seen as a thin bright white line running along the centre of the arteries in particular.

Thickening of vessel walls is mainly recognised by narrowing of the blood column. The arterioles may show pallor and diffuse or segmental narrowing, widening of the light reflex and sometimes sheathing due to hypertensive sclerosis. Sometimes a vessel may be white. This is due to extreme thickening so that the blood column can no longer be seen, or to total occlusion. Atheroma is rare; it shows as a dense yellowish-white opacity obscuring part or the whole of the blood column and sometimes projecting beyond it.

Emboli are sometimes seen in retinal arteries. Glistening spots which seem to lie on the arterial wall are due to cholesterol emboli. A platelet embolus appears as a white spot in an artery, obstructing blood flow; it often breaks up and disappears within a few hours.

Dilatation of the veins appears especially in chronic respiratory failure, papilloedema and diabetes. A ratio of 2:3 between the normal artery and vein is approximately valid but only when branching of the vessels is comparable as in the superior temporal quadrant of Figure 11.6. Changes in the ratio may be due to narrowing of the arteries or dilatation of the veins.

Ateriovenous crossings. The artery and vein share their media and adventitia at these crossings. Hypertensive sclerosis therefore commonly distorts or obscures the venous blood column. Senile arteriosclerosis with thickening of the adventitia may cause similar appearances so that the arteriolar changes already described provide the more direct evidence of hypertension. However, distension of the vein distal to the crossing usually indicates arteriosclerosis; it is apt to be complicated by venous thrombosis.

The Background. The red background of the fundus is due largely to blood in the massive meshwork of choroidal vessels whose detail is fogged by the retinochorodial pigment layer on which the rods and cones lie. If the pigment layer is missing, as in the albino, or is thin, as in some fair haired people, then the choroidal vessels will be clearly seen lying on a white background of sclera. In contrast, dense pigment, commonly present in dark skinned or black haired people, is often arranged in streaks between the main choroidal vessels and gives a tigroid appearance to the fundus. The pigment also tends to become finely granular with advancing years, and the retina loses the shiny appearance seen in the child and young adult.

Nerve fibres, interspersed by their cell nuclei, run vertically from the light receptors in the deepest layers of the retina until they reach the internal limiting membrane where they turn horizontally and converge upon the optic disc. The retinal vessels lie in the anterior horizontal layer of nerve fibres and nourish the inner third of the retina while the choroidal vessels supply the outer-two-thirds. Consideration of these facts explains the shapes of haemorrhages according to their depth.

Background abnormalities may be red, white or black.

RED LESIONS. These are due to haemorrhages, microaneurysms or new vessel formation.

Haemorrhages. Superficial haemorrhages are linear, or fan- or flame-shaped because they track along the horizontally arranged nerve fibre layer. This type of haemorrhage prediminates in arterial hypertension (Fig. 11.7 and Plate IV).

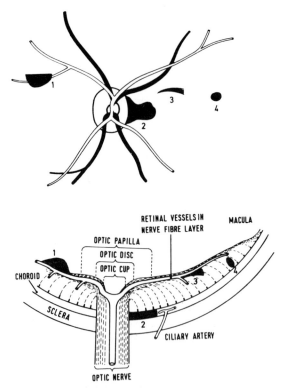

Fig. 11.7   Sites of retinal haemorrhages. (1) Subhyaloid haemorrhage. (2) Choroid haemorrhage. (3) Haemorrhage in nerve fibre layer. (4) Deep haemorrhage in diabetes mellitus.

Haemorrhages which lie in the deeper layers of the retina, where the tissues are arranged vertically, do not spread laterally and so appear as small dots or blobs, a particularly common feature of diabetic retinopathy (Fig. 11.7 and Plate IV).

A choroidal haemorrhage is less common; it is often large with a wavy, map-like margin, and dark owing to the fact that it lies beneath pigment of variable density (Fig. 11.7). It may be mistaken for a melanotic tumour but, like all other haemorrhages in the fundus, it tends to disappear without trace in a few weeks.

A subhyaloid (preretinal) haemorrhage bulges forward and lies between the retina and the vitreous. A light reflex may be seen somewhere near its centre. Roundish at first, it usually sediments to give a flat topped lesion (Fig. 11.7). The blood may burst into and mix with the vitreous, and obscure the fundus by total darkness. Alternatively it may cause streaky pools in the vitreous which are seen to lie in front of the retinal vessels. Vitreous haemorrhages may become organised by fibrous tissue. A subhyaloid haemorrhage is most often seen in company with subarachnoid haemorrhage, especially one arising from the anterior communicating artery, but may also be observed in almost any other condition in which retinal haemorrhages occur.

Occlusion of a retinal vein is accompanied by masses of linear haemorrhages and sometimes also by patches of oedema in the affected segment (Plate III).

Microaneurysms. These are dark red, small, dense, well circumscribed 'dots' which may rupture to form 'blot' haemorrhages (Plate IV). They are persistent in contrast to haemorrhages of comparable size which disappear within two weeks. Microaneurysms occur characteristically as an early feature of diabetic retinopathy but they may also be found with arterial hypertension and macroglobulinaemia or following occlusion of a retinal vein.

Neovascularisation. New vessel formation is seen in diabetes mellitus, first as fine tufts of delicate vessels forming arcades on the surface of the retina. These vessels are fragile and readily leak, causing retinal, preretinal or vitreous haemorrhages. Later a connective tissue reaction (*retinitis proliferans*) is seen first as a white cloudy haze among the network of new vessels. This extends to obliterate the vessels and cover the surrounding retina in a dense white sheet. At this stage bleeding is less common but retinal detachment occurs. In Britain diabetic retinopathy is now the single most common cause of blindness in the middle aged.

WHITE OR WHITISH LESIONS. These are due to exposed sclera, exudates, colloid bodies, miliary tuberculosis, fibrous tissue and other causes.

Sclera is exposed in albinos, in congenital and myopic crescents around the disc, and in choroidal lesions such as congenital gaps (colobomata) or post-inflammatory or degenerative changes (Plate III).

Exudates are white lesions. They are usually described as hard or soft. Both types are soft and friable. The terms refer to visual appearances which suggest degrees of hardness.

Soft exudates (Plate IV) are fluffy and ill-defined and look rather like small pieces of cotton wool. They are due to infarcts caused by arteriolar occlusions. They often displace or obscure retinal vessels indicating that they lie superficially. They occur in arterial hypertension, diabetes mellitus and other microvascular diseases such as systemic lupus erythematosus; they are also seen in severe anaemia. Soft exudates often disappear within a few weeks.

Hard exudates which are small, intensely white, spots lie deeply and consist of lipid deposits. They are a common feature of diabetic retinopathy.

The arrangement of nerve fibres has a bearing on the distribution of exudative lesions. In the peripheral retina a single nerve fibre is distributed to about 80 light receptors. In the macular region each cone has its own nerve fibre; the number is so great that the fibres have to radiate outwards from the macula before turning towards the optic disc. The deeper inter-connecting fibres which run perpendicularly elsewhere, here lie nearly horizontally. This accounts for the star-like pattern of exudative lesions in this area (Plate IV and Fig. 11.7).

Colloid bodies are hyaline deposits in the deepest layer of the retina; they appear with advancing years and are nearly always present in elderly subjects.

Miliary tubercles, which usually lie in the choroid, are rare in Britain but are important because they may be visible sometimes when a radiograph of the chest shows no evidence of miliary tuberculosis.

Fibrous (glial) tissue occurs, especially in diabetic retinopathy in association with neovascularisation, and the prognosis for vision is poor. In contrast a patch of *myelinated nerve fibres* is a harmless congenital anomaly (p. 413). *Thick or occluded blood vessels* show as white streaks (p. 413).

BLACK LESIONS. The tigroid fundus and the deposits of pigment at the disc edge have been described (p. 414). Occasional black spots of congenital origin occur which are comparable with benign melanomas of the skin. Other pigment disturbances indicate choroidal or deep retinal lesions. Choroidal degeneration in myopia or in healed choroiditis causes irregular clumps of pigment on or around a white background of sclera (Plate III). In the hereditary disorder, retinitis pigmentosa, characteristic pigment patches giving the appearance of bird's footmarks occur in the midzone, while visual acuity relentlessly deteriorates. Lastly, but not least, is the rare but very malignant melanoma which is also sometimes determined by a dominant inheritance.

Fluorescin Angiography. Some abnormalities may not be clearly diagnosable by unaided ophthalmoscopy; this may be then augmented by the technique of fluorescin angiography. The dye, fluorescin, is injected intravenously and the retina is photographed whilst the fluorescin is passing through the fundus. As the permeability of damaged retinal vessels is increased, the fluorescin leaks and gives rise to diffuse and persisting fluorescence.

Conclusion

It would be a fruitless task to attempt to portray adequately in words the manifold appearances of the fundus oculi in health and disease. Although there is no real substitute for direct experience, modern colour photography has much to offer and the student is advised to study an atlas of ophthalmoscopy as an introduction to the clinical appreciation of this field. A few examples have been reproduced in Plates III and IV to illustrate the wide range of information which may be made available by the use of the ophthalmoscope.

REFERENCE

Michaelson I C 1980 Textbook of the fundus of the eye, 3rd edn. Churchill Livingstone, Edinburgh — A very well illustrated book.

12. The Examination of Urine and Blood

First we must consider the nature of man in general and of each individual and the characteristics of each disease. Then we must consider the patient — his mode of life, his mannerisms, his silences, his thoughts, his habits of sleep or wakefulness and his dreams. Next we must note whether he plucks his hair, scratches or weeps. We must observe his paroxysms, his stools, urine, sputum and vomit. We must determine the significance of all these signs.

Hippocrates, 5th Century B.C.

This comprehensive view of the scope of a clinical examination reminds us that it is not complete until observations have been made on the patient's urine and, in appropriate circumstances, on the blood, vomit (p. 191), faeces (p. 217), and sputum (p. 154). In regard to the examination of the urine, simple and convenient tests using commercially prepared strips containing the necessary reagents have become established as reliable alternatives to many of the classical methods. In contrast, in the examination of the blood, the emphasis has passed to the laboratory. Every doctor must know how to make the best use of all these facilities.

EXAMINATION OF THE URINE

The urine should be tested in every case and this is usually conveniently carried out immediately before or after the physical examination. Some diagnoses may become apparent only after this is done; for example glycosuria may be the sole manifestation of diabetes mellitus. Many renal disorders are unattended by any obvious physical abnormality and the patient's complaints may be non-specific. Significant renal disease is almost invariably accompanied by urinary abnormalities and their detection may be the only indication of the origin of the disorder. The development of simple and reliable methods of analyses has also resulted in urine testing becoming an important way in which early diagnosis of some diseases may be achieved by screening groups of the population.

In special circumstances the urine can be submitted to a large number of biochemical and biological investigations of varying degrees of complexity but a few simple observations and tests suffice for routine purposes. These concern the volume, colour, opacity and smell, the measurement of specific gravity and pH, and tests for blood, protein, glucose and micro-organisms. If protein is present or if there are clinical indications of renal disease or disorder of the urinary tract, the centrifuged deposit of a specimen should be examined microscopically. If glucose is present, a test for ketone bodies should be made. When the clinical features point to disease of the liver or biliary tract, tests for bilirubin and urobilinogen are indicated.

All tests should be carried out on fresh specimens and the manufacturer's instructions should be followed exactly when tablets or reagent strips are being used. The latter are available separately for testing for protein, glucose, ketones, bilirubin, urobilinogen, blood and pH in the urine and are also combined in a single strip, *Multistix,* which can be read in 45 seconds.

Volume of Urine

The volume of urine excrèted in 24 hours is determined by the fluid intake, the amount of solute to be excreted, and the capacity of the kidneys to form a concentrated or a dilute urine. In healthy adults and in temperate climates this volume varies within the range of 800 to 2500 ml. Measuring the volume of urine is important in many clinical circumstances both as a guide to the state of hydration and as a means by which oliguria or polyuria may be recognised. When the urine is being collected over 24 hours the bladder should be emptied at a convenient hour immediately before the start of the period, e.g. 8 a.m. All the urine passed in the next 24 hours up to and including the same hour next day is collected in a clean polythene or glass bottle.

Without special attention to detail it is often more difficult in hospital than in the home to collect the total output of urine over a period of 24 hours. A succession of nurses may empty the bedpan, domestics may remove the urinal, and through failure of communication or human memory, specimens are lost. Whenever possible the close cooperation of the patient should be enlisted; even when this can be obtained, a proportion of the urine may be lost unwittingly, especially during defaecation. For some collections a reagent may be required in the container, e.g. HCl for the estimation of catecholamines or their metabolites in the diagnosis of phaeochromocytoma or for the excretion of calcium. For others, such as screening for porphyrins, it is necessary to use a dark bottle.

In some circumstances, as for example after injury or prostatic operations, it is necessary to monitor the urinary flow hourly. This is conveniently done by using a calibrated urinometer draining the bladder.

Appearance of Urine

Normal fresh urine is clear, but its colour varies greatly from one individual to another and from day to day. Dyes in some sweets may make the urine green or it may become pink after beetroot is eaten. Little significance should be attached to colour changes unless they are marked, and no estimate of urinary concentration should be based upon them. Certain definite colour changes should be confirmed by appropriate qualitative tests. These include:

Bile	Brownish 'like beer' with yellow froth.
Blood, haemoglobin or *methaemoglobin*	Red, brown or 'smoky'.
Porphobilinogen	Red on standing if the urine is acid.
Melanogen	Urine darkens on standing.
Homogentisic acid (Alcaptonuria)	Urine darkens on standing.

The colour of urine may occasionally be altered by the presence of certain drugs or their derivatives as follows:

Tetracyclines and riboflavin	Yellow.
Phenindione	Orange.
Phenolphthalein purgatives	Reddish orange, colour disappears on acidification.
Methyldopa	Dark grey.
Iron (intramuscular)	Grey or black.
Rifampicin	Pink.

The urine may be cloudy and a sediment may be present because of the presence of mucus, pus or blood, or because of precipitation of some of its constituents on standing, e.g. phosphates or urates. The nature of such deposits can best be determined by microscopic examination (p. 426). A milky urine may indicate the presence of fat globules as in chyluria.

Smell of Urine

Most people are aware of the peculiar odour of concentrated urine. An ammoniacal smell is the result of bacterial decomposition and is commonly present on babies' napkins or in urine which has been standing for many hours. Food and drugs may cause distinctive smells. For instance, asparagus causes a characteristic odour, while turpentine was consumed by Cleopatra to give her urine the scent of violets. A smell of fish is caused by infection with *Esch. coli*. It may be possible to smell acetone in the urine of patients with ketosis.

Specific Gravity of the Urine

For most clinical purposes and in the absence of glycosuria, determination of specific gravity affords an approximation to the osmolal concentration of urine. Its determination in a random sample of urine is of limited value. It is most useful as a measure of the extent to which renal tubules are capable of establishing on osmotic gradient between the blood and the urine in the collecting ducts under conditions of hydropenia or hydration.

The specific gravity of the urine is usually measured by a clinical hydrometer which is a relatively inaccurate instrument. Errors are less if the urine is allowed to cool to room temperature as hydrometers are calibrated to read at 15°C. The hydrometer should be pushed deeply into the urine and gently rotated, care being taken to see that it floats freely without contact with the wall of the container.

A guide to the specific gravity and osmolality of the urine can also be included in multiple test strips.

Maximal Concentration of Urine. The maximal capacity of the kidneys to concentrate urine may be determined after depriving the patient of fluid for a standard time. In health, fluid deprivation results in a rise in plasma osmolality which acts as a stimulus for release of the antidiuretic hormone, vasopressin, from the posterior pituitary. The urine becomes progressively more concentrated as fluid deprivation is continued, and in experimental subjects increasing values for urine osmolality are found up to three days. This is far too long a period for clinical application and it is customary to determine the degree of urinary concentration after 18 to 24 hours. With this procedure urinary specific gravities of from 1.022 to 1.040 are obtained in healthy individuals corresponding to between 800 and 1200 mosmol/l. Restriction of fluid to this extent is nearly always unpleasant and may be dangerous in severe cases of diabetes insipidus. In these circumstances the test should be discontinued if more than 5 per cent of body weight is lost during the period of restriction. If a random specimen of urine is found to have a specific gravity of 1.020 or more there is clearly no need to carry out formal testing.

When the results obtained are equivocal or more accurate information is being sought, urinary osmolality may be determined in the laboratory following intranasal administration of desamino-arginine vasopressin (DDAVP).

Minimal Concentration of Urine. The minimal concentration of urine that can be attained is determined after the ingestion of one litre of water or the intravenous infusion of one litre of 5% dextrose in water to the fasting subject. No longer than 20 minutes should be taken to drink the fluid and the urine should be collected hourly thereafter for four hours. During this time the normal subject excretes at least 80% of the water load and the specific gravity of at least one specimen should be below 1.004.

Abnormalities in the Concentration of Urine. Diminution in the power to concentrate the urine may be due to (1) an inability to produce vasopressin in response to fluid deprivation such as occurs in diabetes insipidus; (2) failure of the renal concentrating mechanism to respond to vasopressin; this category includes patients with a wide variety of acute and chronic primary renal diseases (e.g. pyelonephritis or glomerulonephritis) and extrarenal conditions such as hyperparathyroidism and lithium intoxication; or (3) the existence of an osmotic diuresis.

Although defects in urinary concentration are usually accompanied by restriction in renal diluting power, this is not invariable and the latter may persist long after concentrating power is lost. This is especially liable to happen in the presence of uraemia.

Reaction of the Urine

In health and on a normal diet, 40 to 80 mmol of acid is excreted daily in the urine. The greater part of this acid is excreted buffered partly in the form of dihydrogen phosphate, which constitutes the bulk of the titratable acidity of the urine, and partly as ammonium ions. A very small amount of free hydrogen ion is also excreted and it is this which is measured when the pH is determined. Little information is gained from the routine determination of urinary pH in random samples. The urine is normally more acid than pH 6.0. Occasionally the finding of a urine with a pH of 7.0 or above is due to the consumption of alkali or a vegetarian diet, or to infection in the urinary tract by organisms other than *Esch. coli.*

The ability of the renal tubules to excrete hydrogen ions is depressed in certain circumstances such as distal renal tubular acidosis occurring either as an inherited or acquired defect. These patients can be recognised by their inability to acidify the urine below pH 5 following the oral administration of ammonium chloride.

Proteinuria

The detection of protein in the urine by either of the two methods described below is always of clinical significance, postural proteinuria being a notable exception. During a febrile illness and in cardiac failure, protein may be found transiently in the urine. Otherwise proteinuria almost invariably indicates the presence of significant glomerular or tubular disease of the kidneys but its magnitude bears no relation to the degree of renal failure. Proteinuria does not usually occur with disease of the lower urinary tract, though a trace of protein may be found in the presence of severe inflammatory or haemorrhagic processes there.

Salicylsulphonic Acid Test. Half a ml of 25% salicylsulphonic acid is added to between 5 and 10 ml urine in a test-tube. In the presence of protein, mucoprotein and Bence Jones proteins (light chains of immunoglobulins), a cloudy precipitate forms. The test is sensitive and detects as little as 100 mg/dl. Positive results are also found in patients taking tolbutamide, sulphonamides, penicillin or para-aminosalicylic acid or who have been given radiographic contrast media such as biligrafin.

Albustix. This is the most convenient method available for the detection of protein in the urine. Albustix is even more sensitive than salicylsulphonic acid; a 'trace' represents 5 mg/dl which is only just above the normal daytime concentration of 1–2 mg albumin/dl urine. The test strips are impregnated at one end with buffered tetrabromphenol blue and are dipped momentarily into the urine. The yellow test end of the strip should not be touched nor should the strip be left in the urine or passed through a urine stream. Protein, if present, is absorbed on to the strip and produces a greenish-blue colour, which should be compared immediately with the appropriate colour chart. The amount of colour change varies roughly with the concentration of protein in the urine, the + colour block corresponding to about 30 mg albumin/dl urine. It is best to read the strip in daylight.

Positive results are occasionally seen in patients receiving large doses of phenothiazine drugs. Urine which has been acidified for purposes of preservation may give a negative reaction although protein is present, and protein-free urine which has become very alkaline through bacterial activity may give a positive reaction. Contamination of the urine with detergents or antiseptics, particularly those containing quaternary ammonium compounds, may give false positive reactions.

Bence Jones Proteins. These are rarely found in urine but they are important because the presence of Bence Jones proteins is practically diagnostic of multiple myeloma, though they are detected in less than 25% of such cases. When Bence Jones proteins are present in concentrations above 150 mg/dl the Albustix test is positive. The technique, however, may fail to detect these proteins in lower concentrations. A sensitive test is to mix five parts of urine with one part of 50% acetic acid and three parts of saturated sodium chloride solution. Bence Jones proteins are precipitated at once at room temperature, dissolve on boiling and reappear on cooling. Other urinary proteins are precipitated by these reagents but do not disappear on boiling.

Glycosuria

Qualitative Test for Glycosuria *(Clinistix)*. The presence of glucose in the urine is best detected using a reagent strip impregnated with glucose oxidase, a peroxidase and a KI chromogen. When dipped into urine containing glucose and withdrawn, the glucose is oxidised by atmospheric oxygen in the presence of glucose oxidase to form gluconic acid and hydrogen peroxide. The latter reacts with the chromogen in the presence of the peroxidase to produce colours which range from green to brown. The colour change is observed in exactly 10 seconds. For all practical purposes the reaction in the test strip is specific for glucose, and is sensitive to quantities greater than 100 mg/dl. Lactose, which may be present in the urine during the latter part of pregnancy and during lactation, and other reducing substances, such as metabolites of salicylates, do not give a positive reaction.

Although specific to glucose, the reaction is affected by such factors as temperature, pH and the amount of ascorbic acid present and, for this reason, the test is not quantitative. Ascorbic acid in the urine of patients receiving this vitamin for therapeutic purposes may be present in sufficiently high concentrations to reduce the sensitivity of the test. False positive reactions can occur if the urine container has been contaminated with hydrogen peroxide, hypochlorite (e.g. household bleach) or detergents containing sodium perchlorate.

Used as a routine screening procedure in infancy and childhood, this enzyme test might lead to failure to recognise the rare condition of congenital galactosaemia, for the adequate treatment of which early diagnosis is essential. For this reason the less specific quantitative test for glucose described below is recommended for infants as screening procedure. In older children and in adults the simple specific enzyme test is adequate since failure to detect rare abnormalities such as pentosuria or fructosuria is not likely to have serious consequences.

Quantitative Test for Glycosuria *(Clinitest)*. Benedict's test has been used for many years to detect the presence of glucose in the urine and as a semi-quantitative method. The test, which depends on a reduction of a cupric to a cuprous ion, has been modified and is available as a self heating tablet. The test is carried out as follows: with the special dropper provided, 5 drops of urine are placed in a clean dry test-tube. The dropper is rinsed and 10 drops of water are added. One Clinitest tablet is then dropped into the test-tube and the reaction mixture effervesces. The tube should not be shaken during this period and the effervescence should be allowed to settle. Fifteen seconds after the effervescence has subsided the tube should be shaken gently and the colour produced compared with the colour scale provided, which ranges from blue (no glucose) to orange (2 g/dl glucose).

If, while the reaction is taking place, an orange colour appears, even for a moment, and then changes to greenish brown, more than 2 g/dl of sugar should be recorded. Failure to watch the reaction and to note the 'orange flash' may mean the final colour is compared with other colours on the scale, with misleading results. When used in this way Clinitest tablets possess the same sensitivity and fallacies as the original Benedict's reaction. The different sensitivities of Clinistix and Clinitest occasionally result in a urine being found to be positive for Clinistix and negative for Clinitest. This result means that glucose is present in the urine in concentrations of between 100 mg/dl and 250 mg/dl.

Apart from glucose, other reducing substances include fructose, lactose, galactose, glucuronides and phenolic drugs such as salicylates. In very concentrated specimens reduction may occur with creatinine or uric acid. Ascorbic acid in high concentrations may also give the reaction and the urine of patients with alcaptonuria has reducing properties. The tablets are very hygroscopic and must be kept in a tightly sealed container; any tablets which have become discoloured should be discarded.

The Determination of Blood Glucose

Test strips such as *Dextrostix* which, like clinistix, contain glucose oxidase, are specific for the presence of glucose in the blood. Read visually they provide an approximate assessment of the concentration of blood glucose and may be used to distinguish between hypoglycaemia, normal or near normal concentrations of blood glucose and high blood glucose. The method is particularly helpful in an emergency or at night in detecting values outside the lower and upper ranges of normal, or in suggesting that the blood glucose may be sufficiently abnormal to account for the occurrence of coma. Confirmation of an abnormal result observed with Dextrostix should be obtained as soon as possible by more accurate biochemical methods. An instrument is available which measures the reflected light from the surface of the reacted Dextrostix and converts the measurement to a direct reading of the blood glucose within two minutes.

Capillary or venous blood may be used, but blood samples to which sodium fluoride has been added should be avoided as the enzyme in the test strip may be inactivated. A large drop of blood is spread over the printed side of the test area of the reagent strip; smears of blood must not be used. After exactly one minute the strip is held vertically and the blood is washed off with a fine jet of cold water conveniently kept in a plastic wash bottle and applied for no longer than two seconds. The colour of the strip is compared immediately with the chart provided. If too short a time is allowed for the reaction, the result will tend to be low; if the timing is greater than one minute the result will be too high. Over and under washing lead to similar errors. A Dextro-Check synthetic control set, consisting of three known levels of glucose, is available. It is helpful for those not familiar with the use of Dextrostix or who use them infrequently.

Dextrostix reagent strips should be kept in their original container and protected from exposure to heat, light and moisture. They should be stored in a cool place (not in a refrigerator). The bottle should be recapped immediately and tightly after use. Any strips with a brown discoloration should not be used.

Ketonuria

The detection and semi-quantitative assessment of ketonuria is of importance in patients with diabetes mellitus and in those suffering from starvation or persistent vomiting. In those conditions acetoacetic acid, acetone and β-hydroxybutyric acid appear in the urine as a result of their increased production. There is no satisfactory method for the urinary detection of β-hydroxybutyric acid and in ketosis acetoacetic acid is present in concentrations about ten times more than that of acetone. For practical purposes only acetoacetic acid is detected by the tests described. Acetoacetic acid is liable to decomposition to acetone which is volatile. Heat or the presence of bacteria rapidly cause the removal of acetoacetic acid from the urine. Refrigeration is the best way of preserving the specimens if analysis is delayed.

Rothera's Nitroprusside Test. This has been modified and incorporated into a reagent strip test (*Ketostix*) and a standardised tablet test (*Acetest*). Ketostix is easier to use but Acetest easier to interpret. Both are reliable for qualitative purposes but both are unsatisfactory when used semi-quantitatively because some observers find difficulty in differentiating the colours induced by ketosis of varying severity. Atypical colours are also produced if the patient is taking levodopa.

Ferric Chloride Test. A 10% solution of ferric chloride in 2 N HCl is added drop by drop to about 5 ml of fresh urine. A precipitate due to phosphate frequently forms but redissolves on further addition of ferric chloride.

If acetoacetic acid is present a reddish brown colour develops rapidly. If this occurs another sample of urine should be boiled for 10 minutes in an open beaker. If the boiled urine when cooled fails to give a positive result the presence of acetoacetic acid is confirmed. Persistence of the colour development after boiling indicates the presence of interfering non-volatile compounds of which salicylates and phenothiazine drugs and their metabolites are the most commonly encountered.

The ferric chloride test is less sensitive than Acetest or Ketostix and covers a wider range of ketone levels. Used semi-quantitatively the depth of colour can be conveniently and easily assessed as varying from a trace to 4 +. The ferric chloride test is therefore the most reliable test in assessing the severity and the response to treatment in diabetic ketosis.

Bilirubin in the Urine

Conjugated bilirubin is water soluble, and appears in the urine whenever there is interference with the excretion of bilirubin glucuronide in the bile, i.e. in extrahepatic biliary obstruction and some cases of hepatocellular disease. In these circumstances bilirubin can be detected in the urine before jaundice can be recognised clinically. Large quantities of bile pigment in the urine make it brownish in colour and a stable yellow froth is easily produced on shaking.

A test for bilirubin is incorporated in Multistix (p. 418). *Ictotest* tablets provide a more specific and a more sensitive test which can detect very small amounts of bilirubin in the urine and which can be used if there is any difficulty in interpreting the reagent strip test.

Urobilinogen and Porphobilinogen in the Urine

These two compounds appear in the urine in entirely different disorders; they are described together because they both give a colour reaction with Ehrlich's aldehyde reagent.

Urobilinogen is present in excess in haemolytic disease and in the early and recovery stages of hepatocellular disease. It is detectable in abnormal amounts in heart failure and often in infectious mononucleosis. Urinary urobilinogen is absent in complete obstruction of the biliary ducts when, of course, bilirubin is detectable in the urine. Determination of urobilinogen and bilirubin is therefore of great value in the differential diagnosis of jaundice.

Porphobilinogen can be detected in acute intermittent porphyria, in variegate porphyria, and in certain drug induced porphyrinurias.

Ehrlich's Aldehyde Test. Two ml of the reagent (2% dimethylaminobenzaldehyde in HCl 7 mol/l) is added to 5 ml of fresh urine. Urobilinogen and porphobilinogen both give a pink colour within five minutes. To distinguish between these substances add 1 ml saturated sodium acetate solution and 2 ml chloroform. Stopper the tube and shake for one minute. Allow the chloroform and aqueous layers to settle. If the pink colour is due to urobilinogen it will be extracted into the chloroform (lower) layer, but if it is due to porphobilinogen it remains in the aqueous (upper) layer. In health the amount of urobilinogen in the urine is usually insufficient to be detected by this method unless the urine is highly concentrated, when a faint pink colour may develop. Several substances interfere with the detection of urobilinogen and prophobilinogen. Positives occur with patients receiving sulphonamides and in the presence of acetone or during treatment with para-aminosalicylic acid.

Urobilistix also detect urobilinogen but, not reliably, porphobilinogen. The strip is dipped into fresh urine for 5 seconds and read in exactly 45 seconds. Results are expressed in Ehrlich units, one unit being equivalent to 1 mg urobilinogen/dl. Commonly a trace (1 mg/dl) is present and the scale rises to 12 units.

Blood and Haemoglobin in the Urine

Red blood cells may be detected in urine by microscopic examination as described on page 427. Chemical methods of detection, however, are equally sensitive and are capable in addition of demonstrating the presence of haemoglobin which may have been released from cells when the urine is hypotonic or has been standing for some time or in haemoglobinuria. Chemical determination depends upon the peroxidase-like action of haemoglobin. In the presence of a peroxide, haemoglobin and its derivatives bring about the oxidation of a variety of substances including o-tolidine. The method is conveniently carried out using *Haemostix* reagent strips, the test end of which is dipped into urine and removed immediately. The colour of the strip is then compared with the appropriate chart after 30 seconds. A positive test goes blue within this period of time.

In health, urine will give a negative result with this method which is capable of detecting as little as 50–100 red blood cells per mm^3 or 15 μg haemoglobin/dl urine. Significant degrees of haematuria below this level are extremely rare. Falsely positive results may be obtained if the urine contains iodide in high concentrations as may occur if, for example, the patient is being given potassium iodide.

Phenylketonuria

Phenylketonuria is a rare genetically determined defect in the metabolism of phenylalanine which, if untreated, may lead to mental deficiency. Hence its early detection in infants is extremely important if the severity of the mental defect is to be minimised. In classical phenylketonuria, phenylpyruvic acid is elevated in the blood; its derivatives are excreted in urine and can be detected by using *Phenistix*. Unfortunately in many cases screening of infants using Phenistix is unreliable and microbiological assay on blood obtained by heel prick is usually now employed, i.e. the *Guthrie test* (p.405).

Drugs, Enzymes and Stones

Phenistix gives a reddish brown colour if salicylates are present in the urine. This reaction may be used as an aid to diagnosis in cases of coma or to ascertain whether patients advised to take paraminosalicylic acid are really doing so. A similar colour change can also be caused by phenothiazine drugs. Many other drugs are excreted in the urine, the detection of which may be helpful, e.g. in cases of self-poisoning.

The estimation of enzymes is also of diagnostic value, e.g. amylase in acute pancreatitis.

Stones should be inspected and analysed chemically when the diagnosis is in doubt. About 70% of calculi are composed of calcium oxalate and/or phosphate. Calcium oxalate stones are small and hard with rough spicules. The calcium phosphate variety may be soft or hard and are yellow-brown. They form most staghorn calculi. Magnesium ammonium phosphate is found in 25% of stones and its presence suggests infection of the urinary tract. Calculi composed of uric acid alone are small, hard, reddish brown and not radio-opaque. Cystine stones are smooth, waxy and yellow in colour.

Miscroscopic Examination of the Urine

Microscopic examination of the centrifuged deposit of a fresh specimen is the only reliable method of detecting the presence of red blood cells, pus and casts. These structures rapidly disintegrate if the urine is allowed to stand and the microscopic appearances become further confused by the appearance of various crystals which deposit as the pH alters and as the urine cools. Patients with significant bacteriuria almost always show bacilli or other organisms.

Microscopy is indicated when certain conditions are under consideration, such as renal colic, urinary tract infections, infective endocarditis, glomerulonephritis or proteinuria. Examination of the deposit microscopically is also occasionally of value in recognising when opacity is due to bacteria. In appropriate geographical areas, microscopic examination of the last few drops of urine passed is the standard method for the discovery of the ova of *Schistosoma haematobium* in bilharziasis (Fig. 12.1). Yeast cells are sometimes found in urine in diabetic patients; the flagellate protozoan, *Trichomonas vaginalis*, may also be recognised in both males and females.

About 15 ml of urine should be centrifuged in a clean tube for two minutes at 3000 r.p.m. The supernatant urine is then discarded by decanting, leaving about 0.5 ml in the centrifuge tube. Any sediment is then mixed by gentle shaking and a drop of this is placed on a clean microscope slide and a cover slip added. The specimen is examined at first with reduced illumination under low-power magnification. It is common in health to detect in each low power field one or two red cells and hyaline casts, an occasional epithelial cell and a few white blood cells. In many pathological states these cellular constituents are present in larger numbers and their nature should be confirmed by examination under higher magnification.

Cells. Cells seen in the urinary deposit are illustrated in Figure 12.1. *Red blood cells* are recognised as round, refractile, non-nucleated discs. Shrunken crenated cells occur in concentrated urine. Enlarged cell 'ghosts' may be seen in hypotonic urine. *Epithelial cells* are two to four times larger than red cells, nucleated and cuboid in shape. *Pus cells* are easily distinguished by their roundness, the refractile granularity of their cytoplasm and by the presence of lobed nuclei. These features may be rendered more prominent if a 10% solution of acetic acid is run under the cover slip. Pus cells very often appear in clumps or groups and are slightly larger than red cells.

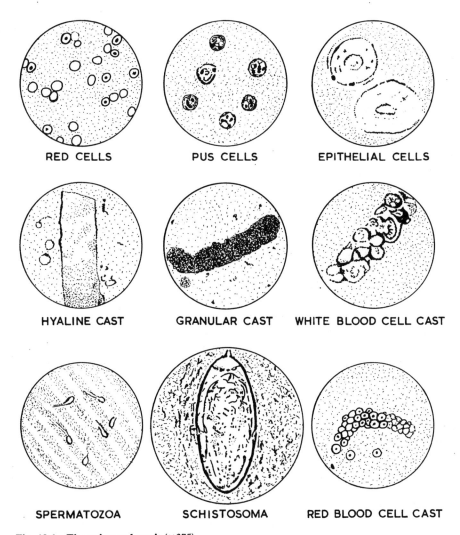

RED CELLS	PUS CELLS	EPITHELIAL CELLS
HYALINE CAST	GRANULAR CAST	WHITE BLOOD CELL CAST
SPERMATOZOA	SCHISTOSOMA	RED BLOOD CELL CAST

Fig. 12.1 The urinary deposit ($\times 375$).

Urinary Casts. These are best seen in subdued light with the microscope condenser at its lowest adjustment and are illustrated in Figure 12.1. Casts are cylindrical bodies of coagulated protein, so called because their shape represents a cast of the renal tubular lumen. Their presence in the urine therefore indicates that the proteinuria has its origin in the kidney. Hyaline casts are transparent, homogeneous structures. Although an occasional hyaline cast may be found in healthy persons, their numbers rise significantly as proteinuria increases. Tubular cells in varying stages of degeneration subsequently adhere to their surface to form epithelial and granular casts. These indicate the presence of tubular damage and desquamation such as occurs in pyelonephritis. Red blood cell casts are composed of masses of conglutinated red cells which give them an orange or brown colour. Leucocyte casts are formed in a similar way. Red blood cell casts always reflect glomerular disease, of which the most common example is acute proliferative glomerulonephritis.

Crystals. A variety of crystals may be visible on microscopic examination of the urine but individual identification is seldom of value. An exception to this is the rare condition of cystinuria, in which hexagonal crystals of cystine are found. While the diagnosis may be suspected on the basis of the microscopic appearance of the crystals, it should always be confirmed by chemical analysis.

Bacteriological Examination of the Urine

For the detection of tubercle bacilli, three or more early-morning or 24-hour specimens should be sent to the laboratory. For all other bacterial infections a fresh, clean-voided, midstream specimen of urine is required, and detailed attention must be paid to the technique of collection. The patient is provided with a sterile container. The specimen is collected by switching the container into the stream of urine. For the ambulant patient the hands should be washed and collection is conveniently made at a urinal or while sitting front to back on a lavatory seat. Women should sit astride the lavatory seat or squat over a bedpan or basin. The vulva should be washed and dried. While the labia are separated by the index and middle fingers of one hand, urine is passed and a wide-mouthed container is then switched into the stream with the other hand. For ill patients of either sex, some assistance and common-sense modifications of these techniques may be required. The collection of urine from infants and children is described on page 401.

The specimens of urine should be conveyed to the laboratory at once. Some bacterial contamination is almost unavoidable, and as each organism may divide into two every 15 to 20 minutes, a false result may be obtained if the urine is not fresh. Furthermore, a large population of contaminant may sometimes suppress the growth of pathogens. If immediate delivery is not possible, the specimen should be quickly cooled, preserved in an insulated container at 0 to 4°C and sent to the laboratory within 15 hours.

Dip Inoculation Culture (e.g. Oxoid dip slide). A slide with nutrient agar on one side and MacConkey's agar on the other is dipped momentarily into a fresh specimen voided into a sterile container. Organisms are caught on the agar surfaces in numbers proportional to their concentration in the urine and the slide is returned to a securely closed sterile vial. Although claims have been made that, after 16–24 hours incubation at 37°C, direct reading of the bacterial growth can be made by comparing the appearance of the slide with colony density models, considerable experience is required if accurate results are to be obtained. Another disadvantage is that no information of antibiotic sensitivity is forthcoming. In spite of these shortcomings the technique offers the considerable advantage that if delay in sending specimens to a laboratory is unavoidable, reliable results are obtained by subculture of the slides after several days. Thus the technique is of particular value in screening tests for urinary tract infection.

Nitrite and miniaturised culture test. The nitrite test is based on the ability of Gram-negative organisms to reduce the nitrate, normally present in urine, to nitrite. About 90% of urinary pathogens produce nitrate reductase which activates this reaction. Best results are obtained by testing urine which has been incubating in the bladder for some hours and for this reason a fresh early morning sample is preferred. The nitrite in the urine reacts with arsalanic acid in the strip to form a diazonium compound which in turn forms a pink colour with naphthyl ethylene diamine. The pink colour is not quantitatively related to the number of organisms and any degree of colouration indicates the presence of at least 10^5 organisms per ml. The nitrite test is available in combination with Multistix as *N-Multistix.*

Microstix is a plastic strip with three separate reagent areas, (1) a chemical test for nitrite, (2) a culture area to support Gram-positive growth and (3) a culture area to support Gram-negative growth. The strip is immersed in fresh urine for 5 sec and the nitrite reaction is read in 30 sec. Thereafter it is inserted into the sterile pouch provided, which is squeezed to exclude air and sealed by pressure at the ends. The strip can be applied to a conventional culture plate at a convenient later time, and the organisms and their antibacterial sensitivity determined. Alternatively, it can be incubated at 35–37°C for 18–24 hours; the great majority of urinary organisms reduce the triphenyltetrozolium, with which the media is mixed, and matching of the culture areas with colours provide a semiquantitative estimate of the number of organisms present.

EXAMINATION OF THE BLOOD

Blood is the most easily biopsied tissue in the body. Its components, both cellular and fluid, can be accurately measured and provide invaluable information in a wide range of clinical circumstances. There follows a description both of the means of obtaining blood samples and of interpreting the results of the laboratory investigations of the cellular components and those of the plasma related to the blood coagulation.

Blood Samples

Venepuncture. This is the best method of obtaining blood for blood counts. Modern counting equipment generally requires volumes of blood that can be collected only in this way. Under certain circumstances, smaller volumes can be used and may be collected by skin puncture techniques.

A tourniquet will be required and should be applied for as short a time as possible to keep haemoconcentration distal to the site of the tourniquet to a minimum. If an accurate platelet count is required the needle must be in the vein before suction is applied. Otherwise tissue fluid will contaminate the sample and cause platelet aggregation which interferes with counting. Blood withdrawn in this way should be transferred immediately to a tube containing potassium EDTA anticoagulant and gently but thoroughly mixed by repeated inversion.

Skin Puncture. Where, for a variety of reasons, blood cannot be obtained by venepuncture, puncture of the skin may be used. Suitable sites are the pulp of the finger, puncturing to one side of centre in order to avoid leaving a tender pressure point, the ear lobe or, in infants the heel, again using the medial or lateral aspect. A disposable sterile stilette, individually wrapped and sealed, should be used for only one patient. The best sample will be obtained if the part is warm, and pre-warming may be required. The skin should be cleansed with an antiseptic fluid, usually spirit-based and allowed to dry. The first drop or two of blood should be discarded and gentle rubbing rather than squeezing used to produce a free flow of blood. The blood may be taken directly into a pipette or allowed to run into a tube containing anticoagulant. Mouth suction should be avoided if at all possible. If essential, the pipette should be fitted with a long extension tube and trap, great care being taken to prevent blood entering the mouth because of the danger of acquiring hepatitis B viral infection which has caused fatalities in laboratory workers.

Storage. Changes in leucocyte morphology occur quickly in vitro but these are slowed if the blood is kept in a refrigerator until it can be examined. It is best to make films within one hour after withdrawal of the blood. After eight hours, considerable distortion appears, and after 24 hours some of the leucocytes may be unrecognisable due to disruption during the spreading of the blood film. Haemoglobin estimation, reticulocyte counting and platelet counting can be done satisfactorily for up to 24 hours after anticoagulation. The sedimentation rate should be measured within 8 hours.

Cleaning and Decontamination of Glassware. Much time can be wasted and many results will be worthless if dirty apparatus is used. All glassware that has been in contact with blood and is not disposable should be immersed first overnight in a detergent solution of a biodegradable type which has no deleterious action on skin or clothing, is non-toxic, non-corrosive and non-inflammable. Thereafter glassware should be washed in running water and dried in a hot air oven at 140 deg. C. Glassware has now been largely replaced by plasticware which is meant to be expendable and used only once.

Quality Control. All blood counting methods require careful quality control. Without this serious errors can creep in. Sophisticated equipment does not ensure accuracy unless it is controlled in this way. Most laboratories conduct internal quality control and also participate in regional and national schemes. Results should be regarded as suspect from any laboratory that is unwilling to divulge its quality control methods and results.

Haemoglobin Determination

Many methods have been devised for the determination of haemoglobin. The majority are based on measurement of the extinction of light at wavelength 540 or

525 nm by a lysate of red cells. The most accurate techniques utilised by automated electronic equipment are suitable only for sophisticated laboratory use. A simplified version of the Gray Wedge photometer may be useful in circumstances where there is no access to a laboratory.

The Sahli method, now used only in circumstances where the above mentioned forms of equipment are not available, can however still provide a useful approximation and is simple to perform. This method estimates oxy- and reduced haemoglobin by their conversion into acid haematin, the brown colour of which can be compared with that of a standard acid haematin solution or a non-fading coloured glass. The test is carried out in a tube calibrated to give a percentage reading, 100% representing 14.6 dl. Blood (0.2 ml) is drawn up in a special 'haemoglobin' pipette and mixed with N/10 HCl which has previously been added to the tube to the level of the '20' mark. One of the disadvantages is that although the colour develops rapidly in the first few minutes it is not fully developed for 40 minutes in the adult and longer in the infant. Each Sahli comparator must therefore be read at the time stated on the instrument, usually five minutes, as the coloured glass is standarised to give the most correct result at this time. Distilled water is then added gradually until the colour matches that of the standard. The accuracy of the standard must be checked in a haematological laboratory every six months. There may be as much as 10% variation between the observations of different individuals. Bilirubinaemia, meth-, sulph- and carboxhaemoglobin influence the final colour.

Erythrocyte Sedimentation Rate (ESR)

The ESR is a very simple test in which anticoagulated blood is allowed to stand in a 200 mm graduated glass or disposable plastic Westergren tube of 2 mm internal diameter, held or suspended vertically. The extent to which the red cells fall in the first hour is read from the graduations on the tube, the blood having been drawn up to the top mark at the start of the test. Usually, the red cells form a clear cut upper level, but in some cases the upper end is diffuse and difficult to read. The test should then be recorded as showing a diffuse end point. Blood anticoagulated with K_2EDTA is used, but it is customary to dilute it with 3.8% sodium citrate (0.5 ml to 2 ml of blood). Alternatively, freshly drawn blood may be anticoagulated using 3.8% sodium citrate without prior anticoagulation with K_2EDTA.

Westergren tubes should not be filled by mouth suction. It is now possible to avoid exposure to blood at all stages by the use of suitably designed polythene containers into which a disposable Westergren pipette may be inserted. If such a system is not available, the pipette should be filled by suction from a device such as a specially constructed syringe which will fit the top of the Westergren tube.

In health the ESR is usually below 15 mm and is, on average, lower in males. Above the age of 60 years, the normal value rises until, over 80 years, levels of up to 50 mm may not necessarily indicate an abnormality.

Inflammatory disease is by far the commonest cause of a raised ESR. This correlates well with fibrinogen and haptoglobin levels in such cases. Reduction in haemoglobin level causes a rise but this tends to be minimal in iron deficiency anaemia. Correction for anaemia is unrewarding because various types of anaemia affect the result in differing degrees.

A very high ESR may be obtained in multiple myeloma, but less than 10% of cases over 40 years of age with an ESR above 100 mm have this disorder. Furthermore, a normal ESR is found in a few patients with multiple myeloma. A normal ESR is generally regarded as reassuring although it should not encourage complacency. Patients in cardiac failure and those with polycythaemia tend to have relatively low readings.

Blood Films

The preparation and staining of blood smears on glass slides is essential for the scrutiny of the morphology of red cells, white cells, platelets and for the determination of the relative numbers of the various types of white cell. Blood smears are also useful for the recognition of certain human parasites such as in malaria and trypanosomiasis.

Preparation of the Blood Film. A chemically clean slide, free from dust, is polished with a grease-free cloth. A small drop of the patient's blood is placed towards one end of the slide. The unbroken, smooth end of another slide or a specially manufactured slide spreader is used to spread the film and is placed at an angle of 45 deg. to the slide bearing the patient's blood (Fig. 12.2). The edge is drawn back until contact with the blood is made. As soon as the blood flows evenly along the edge, the spreader is advanced in an even movement over the surface of the slide until all the blood has been spread. Film thickness can be varied by the speed of spreading. A well-made film will be about 3 cm long and occupy about two-thirds of the width of the slide.

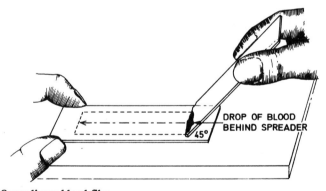

DROP OF BLOOD BEHIND SPREADER

45°

Fig. 12.2   Spreading a blood film.

Staining the Film. Blood films should be dried as rapidly as possible by placing them in front of a fan. Alternatively, they may be waved rapidly in the air. They should be fixed as soon as possible; thereafter staining can be done as required, but it is usual to do so immediately after fixation.

Romanowsky stains are the most universally employed. Staining with May-Grünwald followed by Giemsa provides the most reliable and consistent results. In this combination, Jenner's stain may replace May-Grünwald. Single stains, such as Leishman and Wright's, are more unpredictable in their quality but have the advantage of only one stain being required.

Fixing and staining of blood films is now most commonly done in machines which submerge the slides sequentially in a series of baths. In this way, large numbers of slides can be stained to a high standard. When only a few slides are to be stained, they should be placed on a level staining rack, formed by placing parallel glass rods over a sink or container. Each film is covered with 20 drops of neat May-Grünwald stain, using a pipette. The methyl alcohol in the stain fixes the film. After 2 minutes, an equal volume of buffered distilled water is added producing a 50% dilution of the stain. The water and the stain should be well mixed by sucking fluid in and out of the pipette. After 12 to 15 minutes the slide is washed with buffered distilled water and excess water shaken off. Then, 20 to 30 drops of Giemsa stain, freshly diluted to 5% with buffered distilled water, are added and allowed to stain for a further 12 to 15 minutes before being washed off. The slide is 'differentiated' by flooding it with buffered distilled water for approximately 1 minute and dried at room temperature or in a place where there is gentle warmth.

If Leishman stain is used, the same technique as for May-Grünwald should be employed, but the volume of buffered distilled water added to the stain should be double the volume of the stain on the slide. While the times recommended for these stains may prove to be suitable, further adjustment based on trial and error may be required to establish optimal times for each new batch of stain.

Appearance of the Blood Film. In a well-made blood film there is an area in the centre where the red cells begin to overlap. It is here that red cell morphology should be inspected. Towards the tail the red cells become more widely separated, flattened and show artefactual alteration. At the head of the film, the red cells tend to form rouleux. The white cells are irregularly distributed, the lymphocytes tending to remain in the centre while neutrophils and monocytes are carried to the edges and the tail. Platelets are usually fairly evenly distributed, but where clumping has occurred, these may be seen mainly in the tail. In badly made films there is often an excessive number of white cells in the tail where they may be distorted beyond recognition.

The Red Blood Cells. In health the red cell is a circular biconcave disc showing pallor of staining at the centre. It is described as being *normochromic* and *normocytic*. The former term means that the degree of colouring of the cell is within the normal range and by inference, therefore, the haemoglobinisation of the cell is normal; the latter term indicates that the shape of the cell is also within normal limits. Some degree of variation in size is acceptable, as is the finding of a small proportion of oval cells and occasional slightly misshapen cells. In the first few weeks of life, the number of irregularly shaped cells is greater. Cells which have a bluish tinge (*basophilia*) and which are slightly larger than average are usually young red cells (*reticulocytes*). The presence of many basophilic cells in a blood film produces a multi-coloured effect known as *polychromasia*.

Recognition of morphological abnormalities in red cells has considerable diagnostic value. Iron deficiency leads first to reduction in the size of the cells (*microcytosis*) and when more severe, to thinner red cells, which have a reduced concentration of haemoglobin and appear to have an unusual degree of pallor in the centre (*hypochromia*). There may be variation in size (*anisocytosis*) and varying numbers of elliptical cells are almost always seen. Deficiency of vitamin B_{12} and/or folate leads to increase in the average red cell size (*macrocytosis*) and to both anisocytosis and considerable variation in shape (*poikilocytosis*). The oval macrocyte is a most useful and important cell in drawing attention to the possibility of megaloblastic change. It may be the only significant abnormality as it appears before other forms of poikilocytosis. Unless there is co-existent deficiency of iron, leading to a '*dimorphic*' picture, the cells contain a normal concentration of haemoglobin. Because they are larger cells they may give the impression of being more deeply stained but this should not be taken to represent an increase in haemoglobin concentration. Macrocytosis may be evident in disorders other than megaloblastic blood formation in the marrow. It may occur if there is brisk marrow activity, hypothyroidism, liver disease, invasive disease in the marrow, in association with cytotoxic chemotherapy, excessive or even regular alcohol intake, and occasionally for reasons not understood.

In hereditary spherocytosis, the typical cell appears to be small, round and densely staining (*microspherocyte*); this cell may also be found in acquired haemolytic anaemias, particularly those due to auto- or iso-immune processes, in malaria, in association with extensive burns and indeed in any process which damages the red cell and results in membrane loss.

Fragmentation of red cells (*schistocytes*) together with spherocytes is seen when for one reason or another the red cells are traumatised in the circulation as in the presence of prosthetic heart valves, disseminated intravascular coagulation and the administration of drugs such as sulphasalazine and dapsone. *Target cells* (cells with a central dot of staining) suggest liver disease or the presence of an abnormal haemoglobin, and when associated with a microcytic hypochromic picture, suggest thalassaemia, if iron deficiency has been excluded. The combined presence of target cells and red cells containing nuclear fragments known as *Howell Jolly bodies* and iron containing inclusions (*Pappenheimer bodies*) suggest previous splenectomy or reduced splenic function. Large numbers of elliptical or oval red cells usually indicate hereditary *elliptocytosis*. In 90% of patients the disorder is benign but in the other 10% some reduction of red cell survival may occur.

The White Blood Cells. White cells are seen in the blood as they migrate from the bone marrow to the tissues. Their numbers and their relative proportions vary considerably but are generally within fairly clearly defined limits. The *polymorphonuclear leucocytes* are distinguished from other cells by multilobed nuclei and from each other by the character of the staining reactions of their cytoplasmic granules. The granules of the neutrophil are small, numerous, brownish in colour and have neutral staining characteristics, hence the term neutrophil. The eosinophil stains with the acid stain eosin to give fairly large, even sized, orange granules which fill the cytoplasm. The cell characteristically has a bilobed nucleus, looking like a pair of spectacles. The granules of the basophil, which vary considerably in size and often overlie the nucleus, stain with basic or alkaline stains giving a blue-black colour.

The mononuclear cells (lymphocytes and monocytes) do not have segmented nuclei and the cytoplasm is blue. *Lymphocytes* vary considerably in size depending mainly on the amount of cytoplasm. The nucleus is only slightly larger than a normal red cell, a point that is very useful in gauging red cell size. A few cytoplasmic azurophil granules may be seen in the larger lymphocytes against a clear blue cytoplasm. Some lymphocytes have a deeper blue cytoplasm, indicating an increase in ribosomal content.

The *monocyte* is the largest cell in the blood, and while the nucleus is generally not segmented like the polymorphs, it varies very greatly between being round, kidney-shaped and sometimes lobulated. The cytoplasm has a grey frosted appearance, generally contains many fine azurophilic granules and may be vaculoated.

Differential White Cell Count. This involves counting at least 100 and preferably 200 white cells. Because the cells are irregularly distributed on the slide, the count should be made by scanning longitudinal strips from the tail of the film through the centre. If this is not done, gross distortions of the differential count may be reported.

The Normal Differential Count (Adults)

Neutrophil granulocytes	40–75% (2.0 –7.5 × 10^9/l)
Eosinophil granulocytes	1–6% (0.04–0.4 × 10^9/l)
Basophil granulocytes	Less than 1% (0.01–0.1 × 10^9/l)
Lymphocytes	20–45% (1.5 –4.0 × 10^9/l)
Monocytes	2–10% (0.2 –0.8 × 10^9/l)

The numbers in brackets are the absolute figures for white cell counts within the normal range of 4.0–11.0 × 10^9/l.

In neonates and infants, the number of lymphocytes is considerably greater than in the adult, and these cells may form the majority in the total white cell count. Furthermore, a lymphocytosis may result from infections which would produce a neutrophil leucocytosis in the adult. The appearance of some of the lymphocytes in a young child's blood is different to that in adults (*paediatric lymphocytes*) and to the inexperienced they may be mistaken for primitive cells. The absolute number of neutrophils in the young child is similar to that in the adult.

At all ages, the number of neutrophils may rise in response to pyogenic infections but tends to be unaffected or depressed in viral infections, although in the early stages of some viral infections a neutrophil leucocytosis occurs. Eosinophils are increased in many hypersensitivity reactions and in response to a number of helminth infections. An eosinophilia may be found in polyarteritis and in some cases of Hodgkin's lymphoma. An absolute eosinophil count should always be done before the presence of eosinophilia is accepted.

The Platelets. These cells appear as blue or purple non-nucleated discs, with a granular centre; they vary considerably in size but are generally about a quarter of the diameter of a normal red cell. Up to 15% of platelets may be large without necessarily indicating an abnormality. If platelets are easily found, it can be assumed that the patient does not suffer from significant thrombocytopenia. If scanty, the tail of the film should be searched for platelet aggregates, since the commonest cause of an apparently low platelet count is bad venepuncture technique. Inspection of the film in this way can be of considerable value in the initial assessment of bleeding problems, especially when more sophisticated investigations are not available.

Abnormal Nucleated Cells

Normoblasts, the nucleated marrow precursors of normal red cells, may be found in the blood when there is brisk marrow activity (e.g. after haemorrhage or in the presence of haemolytic disease), and when the marrow is infiltrated by leukaemia, by fibrosis as in myelofibrosis or by secondary carcinoma. Frequently, the appearance of primitive red cells is associated with primitive white cells in the blood and the film is then said to show a 'leucoerythroblastic picture'.

Megaloblasts, unlike normoblasts which have a small round dense nucleus, are larger cells in which the cytoplasm is at a more advanced stage of maturity than the nucleus, which remains primitive with poorly and irregularly condensed chromatin displaying a rather open network. Howell Jolly bodies may be present in the cytoplasm. These cells may appear in the blood and can be fairly easily found if 'buffy coat' preparations are made. In this way, the diagnosis of megaloblastic blood formation may sometimes be established, without recourse to bone marrow examination.

Primitive white cells of all types and stages of maturation are seen in leukaemias. In chronic leukaemia the total white count tends to be higher than in acute leukaemia and frequently exceeds $100 \times 10^9/l$ in untreated cases. Generally the count is higher in chronic granulocytic leukaemia than in chronic lymphocytic leukaemia. Both these leukaemias are recognised by the presence of fairly large numbers of 'mature' cells of the appropriate series, although there may also be varying numbers of more primitive cells, particularly in the granulocytic variety.

About 20% of acute leukaemias do not have raised white cell counts (subleukaemia) and in some there are no abnormal circulating cells (aleukaemic). Acute leukaemias are divided into acute lymphoblastic and acute non-lymphoblastic (myeloblastic or myelomonocytic). They are characterised by the predominance of primitive cells known as blast cells, which are morphologically very similar to the most primitive recognisable marrow elements, and also the fact that there is little evidence of a maturation sequence deriving from these primitive cells. Some mature elements may be present, but there is a maturation gulf between the two. In some acute leukaemias, a moderate degree of maturation does occur, and clinically these patients may present a subacute course. Characterisation of the acute leukaemias has now become a highly sophisticated exercise, requiring methodology available only in the main centres. Since therapeutic decisions are very dependent on the establishment of the type of leukaemia, patients should not be denied the benefit of such investigations.

The platelet count is often helpful in differentiating between acute and chronic leukaemias, being usually profoundly depressed in the former and either raised, normal, or only slightly depressed in the latter.

Buffy coat preparations are useful for monitoring patients with acute leukaemia who have been treated and in whom the number of circulating primitive cells may be very small. They can also be used to detect other abnormalities, such as cancer cells, difficult to detect in ordinary blood films.

Plasma cells are seldom found in the blood in adults, but are not uncommon in children, particularly during febrile illnesses such as measles. They are usually found in association with 'Turk' cells or proplasmacytes and reflect an immunological reaction. Myeloma cells may be found circulating and constitute plasma cell leukaemia.

Large mononuclear cells are frequently found in infectious mononucleosis and some other viral infections. Characteristically they are bigger than the large lymphocyte and may show patchy blue staining of the cytoplasm. The cells are usually irregular in outline, and may appear to form pseudopodia. Some of these large mononuclear cells may appear very primitive, with obvious nucleoli, and mislead the inexperienced into diagnosing leukaemia. They are thought to be transforming T lymphocytes.

Miscellaneous Findings. In a well-made film of blood from a healthy individual, *rouleaux formation* occurs only when the film is thick. Widespread rouleaux formation in all areas of the film is abnormal. It occurs in conditions in which the ESR is considerably raised, generally in association with high levels of globulin and fibrinogen in the plasma or the presence of red cell antibodies. Thus, it is frequently seen in inflammatory diseases, myeloma, septicaemia and autoimmune haemolytic disease, particularly those associated with 'cold' autoantibodies. Rouleaux formation may also occur for a time after the intravenous infusion of dextran; this observation explains why the giving of dextran may temporarily interfere with blood grouping and cross matching.

TROPICAL DISEASES. The spirochaete of relapsing fever, and the parasites of malaria, filariasis, trypanosomiasis, kala azar and other forms of leishmaniasis may be seen in the blood stained by Romanowsky dyes. A textbook of tropical diseases should be consulted for the recognition of these organisms in the blood (p. 444).

Blood Cell Counts

It is now recognised that cell counts using conventional counting chambers are subject to considerable error. In unskilled hands this may be as much as + or − 10% and in the case of red blood cell counts such errors may render the results valueless. It is for this reason that red cell counts should normally be carried out only by laboratories equipped with electronic counting apparatus.

The White Blood Cell Count. The white cell count is subject to the same errors as the red cell count. However, an error of + or − 10% (i.e. the difference between 5×10 and 6×10 cells/l) has much less clinical significance than with the red cell count. A 1 in 20 dilution of blood in 2% (20 ml/l) acetic acid coloured pale violet with gentian violet is obtained by using either a white cell bulb pipette or the much less expensive haemoglobin pipette. The cell suspension is then thoroughly mixed and added to the counting chamber (improved Neubauer) under the special glass cover slip. When applying the coverslip to the counting chamber the observer should look for the appearance of Newton's rings on the glass supports; these indicate that the cover-slip is properly and firmly in position. Ordinary thin glass cover-slips must not be used; they bend and thereby alter the volume of fluid in the chamber. Fluid must not be spilled into the moat around the edges of the counting area. The count should be undertaken after allowing 3 minutes for the cells to settle.

The counting area is best located with a ×10 objective lens. The ruled area of the improved Neubauer counting chamber is illustrated in Figure 12.3. It will be seen that there are nine large squares each 1×1 mm and that the central area is subdivided into 25 squares each of which is further divided into 16 small squares. If the ruled area of the counting chamber is faint, better definition of the lines may be achieved by reducing the light intensity by lowering the condenser of the microscope or rubbing gently before use with a very soft lead pencil and then polishing to remove excess graphite.

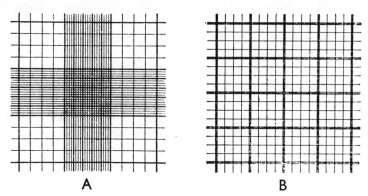

A   B

Fig. 12.3   Counting chambers. (A) Improved Neubauer for white blood cell and platelet counts. (B) Fuchs-Rosenthal for CSF and absolute eosinophil counts.

The cells are counted in the 1×1 mm large squares preferably in all nine large squares in the ruled area. One cubic millimetre of blood contains the total number of cells counted multiplied by 200 and divided by the number of large squares counted.

The normal total white count in adults is from $4.0-11.0 \times 10^9/l$. It tends to be higher in infants where values of up to $18 \times 10^9/l$ are found and up to $25 \times 10^9/l$ in the first 24 hours of life.

The Reticulocyte Count. Young red cells freshly liberated from the marrow have a faint blue tinge when Romanowsky stains are used. This reflects residual ribosomal material in the cells. They can be recognised with certainty, however, only by using a supravital stain such as a brilliant cresyl blue. When this is done, the ribosomal material is aggregated and can be clearly seen as blue reticular material.

A reticulocyte preparation is made by mixing a drop of blood with several drops of a 1% solution of brilliant cresyl blue in physiological saline in a small test tube which is then allowed to stand for at least 15 minutes at room temperature. A small button of cells sediments to the foot of the tube and can be pipetted off and a smear prepared. It is customary to count a thousand red cells, noting the number of reticulocytes among them, and expressing this number as a percentage of the total. The normal figure is usually less than 2%. Since results expressed as percentages lend themselves to misinterpretation it is now customary to report the reticulocyte count as an absolute figure $\times 10^9/l$. Reported in this way the normal range is up to $100 \times 10^9/l$. Red cells which show basophilic stippling in Romanowsky stained preparations are also reticulocytes which have been altered by harmful substances, for instance, lead. However, an occasional stippled cell may be found in health. They are also commonly found in thalassemia and in myelodysplastic syndromes.

An increase in circulating reticulocytes is an excellent measure of increased erythropoietic activity and is encountered in all those conditions in which there is increased red cell production. The very high reticulocyte count found during the initial response to haematinic therapy (e.g. vitamin B_{12}) is due to the fact that in such a deficiency state the marrow contains an accumulation of cells in maturation arrest. When the appropriate haematinic is administered, all the arrested cells develop simultaneously and appear in the circulation in vast numbers. These do not reflect genuine marrow activity which can be assessed only after the initial flush of cells has passed. Very low reticulocyte counts usually indicate a degree of erythropoietic failure. From these facts it should be obvious that the reticulocyte count is an extremely useful measure in the investigation of any anaemia.

The Platelet Count. The platelet count may be carried out by making a 1 in 100 dilution in formol citrate red cell diluent or a 1 in 20 dilution in ammonium oxalate diluent. The latter has the advantage of lysing the red cells and making it easier to see the platelets. The disadvantage is that there is the possibility of red cell debris being mistaken for platelets. In the former technique, platelets have to be counted among the red cells. Phase contrast microscopy improves the ease and accuracy of counting. The diluted blood is placed in a Neubauer counting chamber in the same manner as for the white cells and the calculation differs only with respect to the degree of dilution. The normal range is 150 to 400 × 10^9/l.

Electronic means of counting platelets are widely used and are generally satisfactory. However, they may be unreliable for very low counts and should then be checked by visual means.

Measurements of the Red Blood Cells

Haematocrit (Packed Cell Volume, PCV). The haematocrit expresses the percentage volume of red cells in whole blood. Being an accurate determination, it is useful as a screening test for anaemia. The haematocrit is also essential for the calculation of absolute values such as the mean corpuscular haemoglobin concentration. When estimated by manual techniques, the haematocrit is usually obtained by centrifuging the blood either in a microhaematocrit capillary tube or a Wintrobe haematocrit tube. However, when electronic means of cell counting are used, such as the Coulter counter, the haematocrit may be a derived value calculated from the red cell count and the mean cell volume, both of which are measured directly. This results in a slightly different and probably more accurate estimation of the true haematocrit because no allowance has to be made for trapped plasma.

When manual techniques are employed, the packing must be adequate and can be monitored by testing if the red cell layer is translucent to transmitted light. If not, packing is incomplete, and the reading will be erroneous. It should be remembered that the buffy coat, which is made up of the white cells and platelets, is above the red cell layer and is not included in the haematocrit. It may be of considerable depth in patients with leukaemia. The normal range of the haematocrit, expressed as a percentage, is 47 + or −7 in men and 42 + or −5 in women.

Mean Cell Volume (MCV). This is inaccurate when calculated from results obtained by manual techniques. However, electronic counters measure the mean cell volume directly and accurately and provide an outstandingly valuable parameter. In healthy adults the range of normal is between 82 and 98 fl. although some authorities accept a figure down to 76 as normal. Generally, values below 80 indicate microcytosis, and in the vast majority of cases this reflects iron deficiency. Values above 100 suggest a macrocytic state, and above 110 the cause is most often megaloblastic erythropoiesis. Values between 100 and 110 occur in developing megaloblastic disorders but are also commonly found in patients in whom the consumption of alcohol is excessive, and in patients receiving cytotoxic chemotherapy. The MCV may be in the normal range when causes of both macrocytosis and microcytosis occur together. Iron should not be prescribed when the MCV is within the normal range without further investigation such as estimation of the serum iron and iron binding capacity.

Mean Corpuscular Haemoglobin Concentration (MCHC). This value is derived from the haemoglobin and the haematocrit and is effectively a statement of the grams of haemoglobin found per decilitre (100 ml) of red cells. It must be appreciated therefore that the MCHC is not the grams of haemoglobin in one decilitre (1 dl) of blood but in 1 dl of pure red cells without plasma. The grams of haemoglobin in 1 dl of blood is the patient's haemoglobin level. If a patient has a haemoglobin of 15 g/dl and a haematocrit of 0.45 (45%) it follows that there are 15 g haemoglobin in 45 ml of red cells. Divide 15 by 45 to obtain the haemoglobin in 1 ml of blood and then multiply by 100 to obtain the value in 1 dl. The result is 33.3. This is the MCHC.

The normal range for the MCHC is 32.5 + or − 2.5 g/dl. When the MCHC is less than 30 it means that the red cells contain less than the normal concentration of haemglobin. Iron deficiency is by far the commonest cause, but any other disorder of haemoglobin synthesis may reduce the level. The concentration of haemoglobin in the red cell cannot be increased beyond 38 g/dl and values above this invariably indicate extracorpuscular haemoglobin (haemoglobinaemia). This parameter, when produced by electronic counters is less sensitive to the changes associated with iron deficiency and more truly reflects the fact that haemoglobin saturation of the red cell does not drop off until iron deficiency is moderately advanced. It follows that when measured by electronic means a lowered MCHC is even more convincing evidence of reduced haemoglobin formation.

Mean Cell Haemoglobin (MCH). This value is derived from the haemoglobin and red cell count. The result was not reliable until electronic counting equipment made it possible to obtain accurate red cell counts. In health it is remarkably constant having a value of 29.5 + or − 2.5 pg. Any disorder which reduces red cell size reduces the amount of haemoglobin in the cell and lowers the MCH. Likewise disorders increasing cell size raise the value. The MCH is also affected by the MCHC since a reduction in concentration will lower the value. This is most often seen in association with a reduction in red cell size. In practice the estimation is probably of less value than the MCV as it is influenced by two variables.

Tests for Sickle Cell Haemoglobins

Haemoglobin S, the cause of sickling of red cells, is the most common abnormal haemoglobin. The vast majority of cases are found in negroes, and the incidence of the abnormality is high in vast areas of West, Central and East Africa, and the distribution corresponds to the areas in which falciparum malaria is rife. It is common elsewhere among people of negro extraction but is also seen among peoples from the Middle East and India. Haemoglobin S is found in the carrier state (heterozygote) where it provides approximately 30% of the total adult haemoglobin in each red cell. The patient, who inherits the abnormality from both parents (homozygote), suffers from sickle cell anaemia, and all the red cells contain approximately 98% haemoglobin S. In other patients, the inheritance of haemoglobin S is associated with that of haemoglobin C to give rise to haemoglobin SC disease, a less severe form of sickle cell disease. The problems associated with haemoglobin S have now become important in those areas of Britain where there is a large immigrant community of Negro extraction.

Sickling Tests. Sickling of red cells containing haemoglobin S may be demonstrated by depriving them of oxygen. This may be done simply by sealing a wet film of the patient's blood under a coverslip with petroleum jelly or wax, and incubating at 37 deg. C. Negative and positive controls are also required. A positive control, that is a blood specimen which will sickle under the conditions of the test, is essential if a negative result on the test sample is to be meaningful. The positive control provides evidence that the test works. Distortion of the red cells into elongated spiked shapes is seen after two hours, especially in sickle cell anaemia. In haemoglobin SC disease, the appearance of the red cells resembles holly leaves.

Sickling may be induced more rapidly by suspending the patient's red cells in a freshly-made 2% solution of sodium metabisulphite. This test also requires positive and negative controls, and otherwise is performed in the same way as the sickling test described above, except that sealing of the coverslip is not necessary if the slide is incubated in a moist chamber. The test can be read in half an hour.

In the absence of suitable control bloods, it is safer to establish the presence of haemoglobin S by performing a haemoglobin S solubility test. This test is based on the greater solubility of haemoglobin A than haemoglobin S in phosphate buffer, to which sodium dithionite is added just prior to performing the test. Haemoglobin S, if present, forms a precipitate. The likelihood of false positive results is remote. Commercial test kits are available.

A positive sickling test indicates only that haemoglobin S is present and will be positive in sickle cell anaemia, sickle cell trait, haemoglobin SC disease and sickle cell/thalassaemia. Sickle cell anaemia can, in the majority of cases, be recognised from a stained blood film where the sickle cell forms, resembling the blade of a sickle, are seen and are virtually diagnostic. The additional presence of target cells, polychromasia, and nucleated red cells indicates a fairly severe and sustained haemolytic process. Haemoglobin SC disease may be suspected by the holly-leaf pattern of sickling, but requires electrophoresis for confirmation. Sickle cell trait is a benign disorder usually associated with normal health, a normal haemoglobin level and no distinctive blood film abnormality.

Tests In Haemorrhagic Disease

The great majority of bleeding disorders require specialised laboratory investigation. When a bleeding problem arises a clotting screen should be undertaken. Normally this would include a platelet count, a thrombin time, a prothrombin time, a partial thromboplastin time with kaolin and a measurement of the fibrinogen level and fibrin degradation products. The prothrombin time monitors the final common pathway and the extrinsic coagulation mechanism. The partial thromboplastin time will detect abnormalities in the intrinsic system in which factor VIII and factor IX play a key role. The thrombin time will reflect low levels of fibrinogen and heparin-like activity in the plasma and the level of fibrin degradation products will give a clue to the degree of fibrinolytic activity in the blood. Abnormalities detected by the screen can then be investigated in greater detail if necessary.

Where the patient's problem is thrombotic rather than haemorrhagic, antithrombin III estimations should be undertaken and the patient's ability to mount a normal fibrinolytic response should be evaluated with venous occlusion techniques.

If none of the above estimations are available a few relatively simple tests outlined below may be used but it is emphasised that these are of limited value as they frequently miss the less severe abnormalities.

The Whole Blood Clotting Time. Ideally this test should be performed using blood which has been withdrawn into a plastic syringe or siliconised glass syringe and in tubes which are kept at 37 deg. C. A clean venepuncture is essential. Four ml of blood are required. One ml is delivered into each of four unsiliconised glass tubes of 10 mm external bore and a stop watch started. At half minute intervals the tubes are tilted. The end point is when a tube can be tilted through more than 90 degs. without spilling blood. The average of the times taken by the blood in the four tubes to clot is the whole blood clotting time. The normal range is 4–9 minutes. If the test is performed at room temperature (20 deg. C.) the times of the normal range almost double.

If a whole blood clotting time is abnormal, it is a clear indication of a fairly major coagulation disturbance, due either to a deficiency of factors or the presence of inhibitors, and among these, the administration of heparin is probably the most common.

The Bleeding Time. This is undoubtably a useful test, if carefully done. It is prolonged in thrombocytopenia and usually abnormal in capillary defects, although a normal bleeding time does not necessarily exclude the latter. Coagulation factor deficiencies produce either no prolongation or only modest prolongation of the bleeding time which is often normal in, for instance, haemophilia.

The Ivy method is recommended. A sphygmomanometer cuff is placed round the patient's upper arm and inflated to a pressure of 40 mmHg. Three punctures are made with a disposable lancet in the flexor aspect of the forearm to the depth of the lancet hilt, avoiding veins and scars. A stopwatch is started as the stabs are made, and the exuded blood absorbed with the edge of filter paper without touching the skin, until all bleeding ceases. It is convenient to blot the exuding blood every 15 seconds on the filter paper. This provides an additional time check and is very useful if a stop watch is not available. The longest time taken for the bleeding to stop from the three puncture wounds is the 'bleeding time'. The normal value is between 2 and 8 minutes.

The 'template' method of doing the bleeding time has now been introduced and is widely regarded as the most satisfactory and reproducable way of doing the test. It employs a simple device in which a tiny blade is made to cut the skin. The depth and the width of the cut is carefully controlled and provides a more accurate result.

The only disadvantage is that the cut can produce tiny scars but these are usually nearly invisible.

Fibrinogen. Special problems of massive haemorrhage may sometimes arise when the fibrinogen level has been severely reduced by intravascular coagulation and fibrinolysis. In the vast majority of cases, intravascular coagulation initiates overactivation of the fibrinolytic system with the production of the fibrinolytic enzyme, plasmin, to remove the deposited fibrin. Plasmin does not distinguish between fibrin and fibrinogen and the latter is also digested, producing severe deficiency. This problem may be seen in relation to childbirth, particularly with antepartum haemorrhage and intrauterine death of the fetus but also after incompatible blood transfusion, in carcinomatosis, acute hypergranular promyelocytic leukaemia, and in septicaemia. Management of such a condition, which is often associated with other deficiencies such as thrombocytopenia, requires intensive, skilled laboratory support, but in the absence of this, a useful estimate of fibrinogen levels may be made by using the fibrindex qualitative test.

FIBRINDEX QUALITATIVE TEST. Fibrindex is supplied in 1 ml ampoules and is reconstituted by dissolving the contents in 1 ml of normal saline. Place 0.5 ml plasma from citrated or oxalated normal blood in a small test tube, to serve as a control. In a second test tube, place 0.5 ml plasma from the blood to be tested, add 0.2 ml reconstituted Fibrindex (human thrombin diagnostic reagent) solution to each test tube. Start a stopwatch immediately. Mix by shaking gently for 2 seconds or less, and then tilt tube slowly backwards and forwards. Visible fibrin formation will be seen by the fluid in the test tube ceasing to flow evenly. This should be apparent between 5 and 12 seconds if the fibrinogen concentration is normal. After 60 seconds there should be a firm stable clot, extruding no serum and sticking to the test tube well. If the fibrinogen concentration is subnormal, the initial fibrin formation will be delayed beyond the control plasma time. If no fibrin forms in the test plasma within 30 seconds, a severe defect probably exists. If the normal control plasma forms no fibrin within 12 seconds, the test should be repeated with fresh material.

This rather crude test will be of value only if the blood has been drawn without allowing clot formation to take place. Only citrated or oxalated blood should be used and the correct dilution of blood to anticoagulant should be made. Fibrindex solution may be used for further tests within 6 hours; thereafter it should be discarded.

THE METHODS IN PRACTICE

THE USE OF THE HAEMATOLOGY LABORATORY

The routine examination of the blood and the tests described can be carried out by any doctor with a minimum of simple equipment. However, it is now customary for most of these tests, and many others, to be performed by well-equipped haematology laboratories, staffed by experienced medical and technical personnel. The automated equipment in these laboratories produce the basic results to a high level of accuracy, and this together with experienced interpretation of results provides a wealth of useful information for the clinician. It is therefore extremely important that the clinician using this service should be conversant with the data supplied.

Most laboratories now provide a basic screen, which includes a haemoglobin, haematocrit, red cell count, white cell count, MCV, MCH and MCHC. Of these, the haemoglobin, the white cell count and the MCV are probably the most useful. In addition, reticulocyte counts should be available in all cases of anaemia, and platelet counts are of great value in investigating bleeding disorders and in monitoring the progress of cytotoxic therapy. Much can be learnt from a peripheral blood film and the report on this should be scruitinised, as it may well point the way to further investigation.

Haematology laboratories provide reports on bone marrow specimens, estimations of serum vitamin B_{12}, serum folate and red cell folate levels, vitamin B_{12} absorption studies by the Schilling test, red cell survival and iron turnover studies using radioactive tracers, serological testing for glandular fever, prothrombin times, more complex coagulation investigations and more detailed investigation of haemolytic disorders. Many of these investigations require negotiation with the medical staff of the laboratory, and good communications should be encouraged between the clinicians and the laboratory staff in order to obtain the most effective use of these investigative facilities.

General practitioners now use some of these facilities intensively, adding a valuable extension to their diagnostic and management abilities. It is equally important that they, as well as the hospital based doctor, understand the data produced.

REFERENCE

Jeffrey H C, Leach R M 1975 Atlas of medical helminthology and protozoology, 2nd edn. Churchill Livingstone, Edinburgh

13. Appendix

There is no authority except facts. These are obtained by accurate observation.
Deductions are to be made only from facts.

Hippocrates, 5th century B.C.

Contents

1. Stages in the development of infants and children (p. 446).

   (i) 'Milestones'.
   (ii) Average heights and weights of boys and girls (p. 447).
   (iii) Average crown-rump lengths and sitting heights (p. 448).
   (iv) Average head circumference (p. 448).
   (v) Average times of eruption of teeth (p. 448).
   (vi) Charts for recording growth (p. 449).

2. Desirable weights of adults (p. 450).

3. Uses of questionnaires (p. 451).

4. Notes on International System of Units (p. 453).

5. A system of case recording (p. 454).

6. Problem-oriented medical records (p. 458).

7. Continuing medical education (p. 461).

445

STAGES IN THE DEVELOPMENT OF INFANTS AND CHILDREN

'Milestones'

4 weeks
Prone position — pelvis high, knees under abdomen.
Almost complete head lag on pulling into sitting position.
Grasp reflex present.

6 weeks
Head held momentarily in same plane as rest of body on ventral suspension.
Prone — pelvis high, knees no longer under abdomen.
Considerable, but not complete head lag on pulling into sitting position.
Grasp reflex may be lost.
Smiles at mother.
Follows objects with eyes.

3 months
Head held beyond plane of rest of body on ventral suspension.
Prone — pelvis flat on couch.
Only slight head lag on pulling to sit.
Momentary grasping when object placed in hand.
Squeals of pleasure.
'Hand regard' evident, i.e. visual study of own hands.
Turns head to sound.

6 months
Sits supported by own hands.
Supine — spontaneously lifts head off couch.
Bounces when held standing.
Feeds self with biscuit.
Transfers object from one hand to other.
Responds to name.

9 months
Crawls by pulling forward with hands.
Can achieve sitting position.
Sits steadily without overbalancing.
Can stand holding on to furniture.
Can release grasped objects.
Waves 'bye-bye'.

1 year
Walks supported by one hand.
Beginning to throw objects to floor.
May understand simple phrases.
Uses two or three words with meaning.

18 months
Walks up stairs with support.
Seats self on chair.
Builds 3 to 4 cubes on top of each other.
Takes off socks, gloves.
Scribbles with pencil.
Points to parts of body.

2 years
Goes up and down stairs.
Runs.
Turns door knob.
Kicks ball.
Puts on socks, etc.
Turns pages of book singly.
Asks for things.

3 years
Jumps off a step.
Rides tricycle.
Dresses and undresses.
Copies circle with pencil.
Knows nursery rhymes.
Can count, e.g. up to 10.

5 years
Skips on both feet.
Ties shoelaces.
Gives age when asked.
Can name four colours.

REFERENCE

Illingworth R S 1980 The development of the infant and young child, 7th edn. Churchill Livingstone, Edinburgh

Table 13.1   Average heights and weights of boys and girls

Age	Boys		Girls	
	Height cm (in)	Weight kg (lb)	Height cm (in)	Weight kg (lb)
Birth	50.7 (20.0)	3.4 (7.5)	49.8 (19.6)	3.3 (7.3)
2 weeks	51.7 (20.4)	3.4 (7.5)	51.0 (20.1)	3.3 (7.3)
3 months	60.2 (23.7)	5.8 (12.8)	58.8 (23.2)	5.4 (11.9)
6 months	66.6 (26.2)	7.9 (17.4)	64.9 (25.6)	7.4 (16.3)
9 months	71.2 (28.1)	9.2 (20.3)	69.6 (27.4)	8.7 (19.2)
1 year	75.1 (29.6)	10.3 (22.7)	73.9 (29.1)	9.8 (21.6)
1½ years	80.6 (31.8)	11.4 (25.1)	79.1 (31.2)	10.9 (24.0)
2 years	86.2 (34.0)	12.6 (27.8)	84.3 (33.2)	11.9 (26.2)
2½ years	90.5 (35.7)	13.6 (30.0)	89.1 (35.1)	13.0 (28.7)
3 years	94.7 (37.3)	14.6 (32.2)	93.2 (36.7)	14.1 (31.1)
3½ years	98.7 (38.9)	15.7 (34.6)	97.4 (38.4)	15.1 (33.3)
4 years	102.0 (40.2)	16.7 (36.8)	100.9 (39.8)	16.2 (35.7)
4½ years	105.5 (41.6)	17.7 (39.0)	104.2 (41.1)	17.1 (37.7)
5 years	108.6 (42.8)	18.6 (41.0)	107.6 (42.4)	18.0 (39.7)
5½ years	110.4 (43.5)	19.0 (41.9)	110.4 (43.5)	18.9 (41.7)
6 years	112.4 (44.3)	20.0 (44.1)	·113.0 (44.5)	19.8 (43.7)
7 years	118.8 (46.8)	22.4 (49.4)	118.4 (46.6)	22.0 (48.5)
8 years	123.7 (48.7)	24.5 (54.0)	123.3 (48.6)	24.0 (52.9)
9 years	127.9 (50.4)	26.4 (58.2)	127.8 (50.4)	26.3 (58.0)
10 years	133.3 (52.5)	28.9 (63.7)	132.8 (52.3)	28.7 (63.3)
11 years	138.7 (54.6)	31.8 (70.1)	138.4 (54.5)	31.7 (69.9)
12 years	144.7 (57.0)	35.2 (77.6)	144.9 (57.1)	36.3 (80.0)
13 years	150.3 (59.2)	39.5 (87.1)	151.8 (59.8)	41.8 (92.2)
14 years	156.0 (61.5)	44.0 (97.0)	156.1 (61.5)	46.4 (102.3)
15 years	163.3 (64.3)	50.3 (110.9)	159.6 (62.9)	50.5 (111.4)

NOTES. (i) *Crown-heel length* is measured with the child in the position of attention in bed.

(ii) *Height* can be measured as standing height from the age of 18 months onwards, the child standing barefooted with heels and back against a vertical surface or rule. The head should be held upright with the line of sight parallel to the floor. A right-angled block held against the wall or a sliding bar at right angles to the rule should then be moved down until it touches the child's head. One standard deviation from above means would be approximately ± 4%.

(iii) *Weight* should be measured in the nude or with child wearing thin pants. One standard deviation from above means would be approximately ± 12½%.

(iv) Tables 13.1 to 13.4 are derived from the data of Thomson J 1954 Health Bulletin 12: 25; Acheson R M, Kemp F H, Parfit J 1955 Lancet 1: 691; Provis H S, Ellis R W B 1955 Archives of Disease in Childhood 30: 328.

Table 13.2   Average crown-rump lengths and sitting heights

Age	Boys		Girls	
	Crown-rump lengths			
	cm	inches	cm	inches
Birth	34.3	13.5	33.6	13.2
2 weeks	34.8	13.7	34.2	13.5
3 months	39.5	15.6	39.0	15.4
6 months	44.2	17.4	42.9	16.9
9 months	46.5	18.3	45.2	17.8
1 year	48.4	19.1	47.0	18.5
1½ years	51.8	20.4	50.2	19.8
2 years	54.5	21.5	52.9	20.8
3 years	58.4	23.0	57.2	22.5
	Sitting height			
3 years	57.1	22.4	55.3	21.8
4 years	59.9	23.6	57.7	22.7
5 years	61.9	24.4	60.6	23.9
6 years	63.7	25.1	63.0	24.8
7 years	65.8	25.9	65.7	25.9
8 years	67.6	26.6	67.9	26.7
9 years	69.7	27.4	69.6	27.4
10 years	71.8	28.3	71.5	28.1
11 years	73.8	29.0	74.1	29.2
12 years	76.0	29.9	77.4	30.5
13 years	78.6	31.0	81.3	32.0
14 years	81.6	32.1	84.0	33.1
15 years	85.5	33.6	86.2	33.9

Table 13.3   Average head circumference

Age	cm	inches	Age	cm	inches
Birth	35.0	13.8	6 years	51.2	20.2
3 months	40.4	15.9	7 years	51.7	20.3
6 months	43.4	17.1	8 years	52.0	20.4
9 months	45.2	17.8	9 years	52.2	20.6
1 year	46.4	18.3	10 years	52.5	20.7
1½ years	47.7	18.8	11 years	52.9	20.8
2 years	49.0	19.3	12 years	53.4	21.0
3 years	49.6	19.5	13 years	53.8	21.2
4 years	50.0	19.7	14 years	54.1	21.3
5 years	50.7	20.0	15 years	54.8	21.6

One standard deviation from these means is approximately ± 2½%.

Table 13.4   Average times of eruption of teeth in primary and secondary dentitions

Deciduous teeth	Date of eruption	Permanent dentition	Date of eruption
Central incisors	8th month	First molars	6th– 7th year
Lateral incisors	10th month	Central incisors	6th– 7th year
First molars	12th month	Lateral incisors	7th– 9th year
Canines	18th month	First premolars	10th–11th year
Second molars	24th month	Canines	10th–12th year
		Second premolars	10th–12th year
		Second molars	12th year
		Third molars	17th–25th year

Charts for Recording Growth

Charts of the type shown in Figure 13.1 can be used in a variety of ways, for instance (i) to compare a single observation of height or weight with the normal means and ranges for children of similar weight in the community; in interpreting such observations the height, but to a much lesser extent the weight, of the parents should be taken into account — thus a normal height for a child whose parents' heights are below average would be below the means on the chart; (ii) to plot serial observations with a view to detecting any trend; (iii) to make a comparison between height and weight in respect of their relationship to community values, e.g. dissociation between height and weight on the graphs would indicate that a child was light for height or overweight for height.

Similar charts are available for girls aged 1–16+ years and for both sexes aged from 0–5 years.

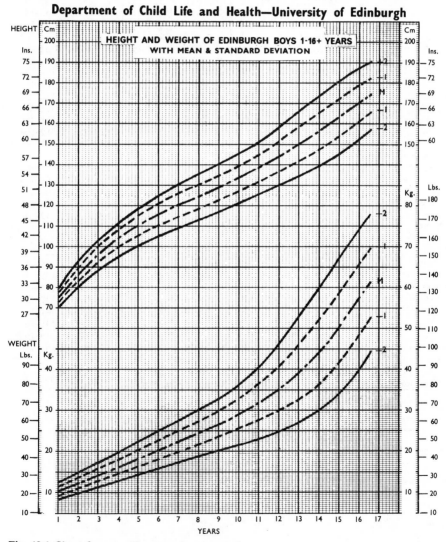

Fig. 13.1 Chart for recording growth: an example.

DESIRABLE WEIGHTS OF ADULTS

Table 13.5   Desirable weights of adults according to height and frame

Height without shoes			Small frame		Medium frame		Large frame	
cm	ft	in	kg	lb	kg	lb	kg	lb
Men								
155	5	1	50.8–54.5	112–120	53.5–58.5	118–129	57.2–64.0	126–141
157.5	5	2	52.2–55.8	115–123	54.9–60.3	121–133	58.5–65.3	129–144
160	5	3	53.5–57.2	118–126	56.2–61.7	124–136	59.9–67.1	132–148
162.5	5	4	54.9–58.5	121–129	57.6–63.0	127–139	61.2–68.9	135–152
165	5	5	56.2–60.3	124–133	59.0–64.9	130–143	62.6–70.8	138–156
167.5	5	6	58.1–62.1	128–137	60.8–66.7	134–147	64.6–73.0	142–161
170	5	7	59.9–64.0	132–141	62.6–68.9	138–152	66.7–75.3	147–166
172.5	5	8	61.7–65.8	136–145	64.4–70.8	142–156	68.5–77.1	151–170
175	5	9	63.5–68.0	140–150	66.2–72.6	146–160	70.3–78.9	155–174
177.5	5	10	65.3–69.9	144–154	68.0–74.8	150–165	72.1–81.2	159–179
180	5	11	67.1–71.7	148–158	69.9–77.1	154–170	74.4–83.5	164–184
182.5	6	0	68.9–73.5	152–162	71.7–79.4	158–175	76.2–85.7	168–189
185	6	1	70.8–75.7	156–167	73.5–81.6	162–180	78.5–88.0	173–194
187.5	6	2	72.6–77.6	160–171	75.7–83.5	167–185	80.7–90.3	178–199
190	6	3	74.4–79.4	164–175	78.1–86.2	172–190	82.7–92.5	182–204
Women								
142.5	4	8	41.7–44.5	92–98	43.5–48.5	96–107	47.2–54.0	104–119
145	4	9	42.6–45.8	94–101	44.5–49.9	98–110	48.1–55.3	106–122
147.5	4	10	43.5–47.2	96–104	45.8–51.3	101–113	49.4–56.7	109–125
150	4	11	44.9–48.5	99–107	47.2–52.6	104–116	50.8–58.1	112–128
152.5	5	0	46.3–49.9	102–110	48.5–54.0	107–119	52.2–59.4	115–131
155	5	1	47.6–51.3	105–113	49.9–55.3	110–122	53.5–60.8	118–134
157.5	5	2	49.0–52.6	108–116	51.3–57.2	113–126	54.9–62.6	121–138
160	5	3	50.3–54.0	111–119	52.6–59.0	116–130	56.7–64.4	125–142
162.5	5	4	51.7–55.8	114–123	54.4–61.2	120–135	58.5–66.2	129–146
165	5	5	53.5–57.6	118–127	56.2–63.0	124–139	60.3–68.0	133–150
167.5	5	6	55.3–59.4	122–131	58.1–64.9	128–143	62.1–69.9	137–154
170	5	7	57.2–61.2	126–135	59.9–66.7	132–147	64.0–71.7	141–158
172.5	5	8	59.0–63.5	130–140	61.7–68.5	136–151	65.8–73.9	145–163
175	5	9	60.8–65.3	134–144	63.5–70.3	140–155	67.6–76.2	149–168
177.5	5	10	62.6–67.1	138–148	65.3–72.1	144–159	69.4–78.5	153–173

Based on weights of insured persons in the United States associated with lowest mortality (Statistical Bulletin, Metropolitan Life Insurance Company, 40, Nov.–Dec. 1959).

THE USE OF QUESTIONNAIRES

With Particular Reference to Sexual Problems in the Male
In a literate society questionnaires constitute an efficient and time-saving method of obtaining information. They can be used for example in health reviews and as a data base in problem orientated case notes (p. 458). Questionnaires can also provide detailed information in special situations. They are particularly useful in assessing sexual problems, for example infertility, because the questions can be posed without the embarrassment of doing so at an interview and the sexual partner can help to answer them.

In sexual problems in the male the questionnaire consists of two parts. In the first the patient fills in details about his past and present health, with appropriate reference to (i) conditions such as sexually transmitted disease, mumps and tuberculosis which may affect the testes, (ii) his marital status including offspring, (iii) current and previous cigarette and alcohol consumption, (iv) medication and drug abuse, and (v) nature of employment and previous occupations.

The second part of the questionnaire contains explicit questions about sexual activities. First a general sexual history is obtained and then more specific information is sought, as, for example, about problems with erection or ejaculation. In all cases psychological factors are also assessed. Examples of such questionnaires are given below.

Sexual Problems Questionnaires *(Part II)*

Sexual History
1. How often on average do you try to have intercourse?
2. Does shift work or absence from home interfere with opportunities to have sex?
3. Do you have any physical difficulties with the sex act that would prevent conception, e.g. pain during intercourse sufficient to prevent penetration?

If the answer to any of the above questions is *yes*, please give details.

Wife/partner
1. Does your wife/partner experience pain during sexual intercourse?
2. If *yes*, is the pain sufficient to make you stop having intercourse on occasions?
3. Has your wife/partner had a sterilisation operation?
4. Has your wife/partner had a hysterectomy?

Problems with Erection
Do you get satisfactory erections of the penis for sexual purposes?
If not please answer the following questions:
1. Which is the situation that most closely resembles your own?
   (i)   No erection of any sort at any time.
   (ii) Incomplete erections occasionally but the penis is not firm enough to allow penetration.
   (iii) Firm erections at first allowing penetration but not lasting long enough for completion of sexual intercourse.
   (iv) Firm erections in the morning or during wet dreams but unable to have erections when trying to have intercourse with partner.
   (v)   Firm erections but the penis is bent when erect making sexual intercourse impossible.
2. When was the last time you had a normal erection firm enough to allow normal sexual intercourse or masturbation?
3. Do you get morning erections?

Problems with Ejaculation

Do you get satisfactory ejaculation of sperm?

If not please answer the following questions:

1. Do you think you ejaculate normally when you have sexual intercourse with your wife/partner?
2. Do you think you ejaculate normally when masturbating?
3. Do you think you ejaculate sometimes during dreams when you are asleep?
4. Do you have a feeling that you ejaculate but the sperm goes the wrong way

    A.   The sperm goes the wrong way.

    B.   I do not ejaculate at all.

    C.   I ejaculate too quickly.

    If you have answered *yes* to option B is this because either:

      You have no sex because you have no erections

      or

      You have normal erections but despite much stimulation no ejaculation takes place?

    If you have answered *yes* to option C please tick the situation that most closely corresponds to your problem.

    I cannot ejaculate near my wife/partner.

    I ejaculate before any penetration of the penis has taken place.

    I ejaculate very soon after penetration of the penis.

Psychological Problems

Do you think that your problem is caused by emotional or psychological difficulties?

If *yes* please try to tell me what these are.

Scrutiny of the answers to the questionnaire quickly identifies the main problem which the clinician can then clarify at an interview with the patient. It must be borne in mind, however, that no questionnaire is complete and that the patient must be given the opportunity to speak about any other related matters.

NOTES ON INTERNATIONAL SYSTEM OF UNITS (SI UNITS)

Volume. The basic SI unit of volume is the cubic metre (1000 litre). Because of its convenience the litre is used as the unit of volume in laboratory work.

Amounts of substance ('molar') concentration (e.g., mol/*l*, μmol/*l*) is used for substances of defined chemical composition. It replaces equivalent concentration (mEq/*l*), which is not part of the SI system. For univalent ions such as sodium, potassium, chloride and bicarbonate the numerical value is unchanged. For divalent ions such as calcium and magnesium the numerical value is halved.

Mass concentration (e.g., g/*l*, μg/*l*) is used for some protein measurements, for substances which do not have a sufficiently well defined composition and for serum vitamin B_{12} and folate measurements. The numerical value in SI units will change by a factor of 10 in those instances previously expressed in terms of 100 ml. Haemoglobin is an exception. It is agreed internationally that meantime haemoglobin should continue to be expressed in terms of g/dl (g/100 ml).

SI units are not employed for enzymes and immunoglobulins.

Metric Equivalents

Volume 28.4 ml (30 ml approx.) = 1 fl oz; 1 pint = 568 ml
Weight 1 kg = 2.2 lb
Length 2.54 cm = 1 in; 30.5 cm = 1 ft; 1 metre = 39 in
Temperature To convert °F to °C, subtract 32 and then multiply by 5 and divide by 9.

A SYSTEM OF CASE RECORDING

Name: Age: Sex: Marital status:
Address: Telephone No:
Occupation: In the case of a married woman give that of her husband and
                   her own if she also works. In the case of a child give the
                   parents' occupation(s).
Family doctor:
Date of admission to hospital:
Date of examination:

HISTORY

Present Illness. Begin by naming the presenting or principal symptoms and the duration of each. Proceed with a chronological account of the mode of onset and course of the patient's illness. *Systemic enquiry:* record any symptoms such as cough, breathlessness, digestive or urinary troubles, pain, insomnia or change in weight. Note any *drugs* taken and any *allergy.*

Previous Health. Illness, operations, accidents, and their dates. Note any travel abroad, prophylactic medication, vaccination and immunisation. Date and result of any previous medical examination (e.g. for life insurance) or radiological examination. History of birth in the case of infants and children.

Family History. Note age, health, or cause of death of parents, siblings, spouse and children (Fig. 1.1, p. 5).

Social and Personal History. Record the relevant information about occupation, housing, and personal habits regarding recreation, physical exercise, alcohol and tobacco, and in the case of children, about school and family relationships.

PHYSICAL EXAMINATION

General Assessment. In an introductory statement comment on the patient's *demeanour* and *general condition,* i.e. physique, nutrition, state of hydration, posture, gait, personality and mental state. Record height and weight. Note any abnormality not recorded under a systemic heading, e.g.:

Hands and arms. Note any information of diagnostic value obtained from inspection of hands and nails. Epitrochlear and axillary lymph nodes.

Head, face and neck. Describe in detail any abnormality such as goitre or enlarged lymph nodes.

Skin. Colour; pallor, cyanosis, pigmentation, jaundice, etc. Specific lesions.

Subcutaneous tissues. Nodules; vascular abnormalities; oedema.

Breasts. Note findings on palpation.

Cardiovascular System

Arterial Pulse and Pressure. Rate, rhythm, wave form and volume of radial pulse. Blood pressure.

Jugular Venous Pulse and Pressure. Note form of the jugular pulse wave and height of the jugular venous pressure.

Heart.

Inspection. Pulsations and deformity of anterior chest wall.

Palpation. Position of apex beat, character of apical impulse and other pulsations; thrills.

Auscultation. First and second heart sounds; added sounds; murmurs.

Peripheral Circulation.

Arterial. Pulsation of limb arteries; skin temperature and colour; local nutrition; bruits.

Venous. Abnormal vessels; signs of inflammation or occlusion.

Respiratory System

Note cough, character and quantity of sputum, wheeze or other respiratory difficulty.

Upper Respiratory Tract. Nose; tonsils; pharynx.

Chest.

Inspection. Shape and lesions of chest wall; respiration rate and depth; chest expansion; mode of breathing.

Palpation. Range of movement; position of trachea.

Percussion. Anterior, lateral and posterior chest wall; hepatic dullness.

Auscultation. Breath sounds, vocal resonance and added sounds.

Alimentary and Genito-Urinary Systems

Mouth. Lips, tongue, teeth, gums and other mucosae. Character and quantity of any vomitus.

Abdomen.

Inspection. Scars; veins; hair. Abdominal wall: shape, general and local changes, e.g. hernias and movement of respiratory, peristalic, vascular or fetal origin.

Palpation. Tenderness; guarding; individual organs and abnormal masses; hernial orifices; inguinal lymph nodes.

Percussion. Fluid, gas, and individual organs.

Auscultation. Frequency and character of bowel sounds; vascular bruits.

Genitalia. *Inspection.*

Palpation. Penis, testes, epididymes and vasa deferens. Vaginal examination in special circumstances only.

Rectum. Inspection of the anus and examination of rectum if indicated; inspection of and testing of faeces for occult blood, if indicated.

Urine. Volume, colour, opacity, odour, reaction, specific gravity; microscopy; chemical tests for protein, glucose and other substances as indicated.

Nervous System

Intellectual Function. See Psychiatric Examination (p. 456).

Speech. Language function, articulation, phonation.

Cranial Nerves.

First. Sense of smell.

Second. Visual acuity; visual fields; ophthalmoscopic examination.

Third, Fourth and Sixth. Eyelids, ptosis, palpebral fissures; pupils, size, shape, symmetry and reflexes; eye movements, diplopia and nystagmus.

Fifth. Facial sensation; muscles of mastication, corneal reflex and jaw jerk.

Seventh. Movements of facial muscles; taste on the anterior two thirds of the tongue.

Eighth. Auriscopic examination; estimation of auditory acuity; tuning fork tests; positional nystagmus.

Ninth. Sensation of pharynx and of the posterior third of the tongue; palatal and pharyngeal reflexes.

Tenth. Phonation; movements of palate and posterior pharyngeal wall; palatal and pharyngeal reflexes.

Eleventh. Sternomastoid and upper trapezius muscles.

Twelfth. Inspection of tongue and its movements.

Motor System. Inspection of musculature; involuntary movements including fasciculation; tone; clonus; power; co-ordination; fine movements; dyspraxia.

Sensory System. Touch, pain and temperature; position and vibration sense; cortical sensory function, e.g. two point discrimination, stereognosis.

Reflexes. Tendon reflexes; abdominal and plantar responses.

Supplementary Tests. Bruits audible in the neck or skull. Meningeal or nerve root irritation. Tetany.

Locomotor System

Spine. Shape and movement of neck and trunk.

Joints of Limbs. Movements, deformity, swelling, tenderness, temperature.

Muscles. Atrophy, contractures, swelling, tenderness.

Bones. Deformity, tenderness.

Psychiatric Examination

The Mental State.
1. *General appearance and behaviour.*
2. *Thought processes. Sample of talk.*
3. *Mood.*
4. *Delusions.*
5. *Hallucinations.*
6. *Obsessions.*
7. *Evidence of intellectual defect.*
   (i)   Orientation.
   (ii)   Memory.
   (iii)   Attention and concentration.
   (iv)   General information.
   (v)   Intelligence.
8. *Insight and judgement.*

Personality Diagnosis.

CLINICAL DIAGNOSIS

Record the differential diagnosis in order of probability.

FURTHER INVESTIGATIONS

It is helpful to outline a plan of any further investigations considered necessary at this stage.

TREATMENT AND PROGRESS NOTES

These should be entered from day to day.

FINAL DIAGNOSIS

SUMMARY

It is advisable to conclude the case recording with a brief summary incorporating the principal symptoms, the main abnormalities on physical examination, the significant findings on further investigation, the diagnosis, the therapeutic measures employed and the decisions regarding further management. Alternatively the summary can take the form of a 'problem list' as described below.

PROBLEM-ORIENTATED MEDICAL RECORDS

The traditional method of case recording has been adapted in some centres to incorporate the problem-orientated medical record developed by Weed and his colleagues (1968). Basic information is collected by the methods described in this book but its recording is orientated around the patient's problems. Weed's system is structured into four main components, the data base, the problem list, the initial plan and the progress notes.

1. Data Base. This consists of:

(a) the principal complaint.

(b) relevant social data and the 'profile'; the latter is a description of how the patient spends an average day. Therapeutic goals can be related to this profile.

(c) the history.

(d) the physical examination.

(e) laboratory and other basic investigations, such as haemoglobin, urea and electrolytes and chest radiography.

2. Problem List. All the patient's problems, past and present, are named and numbered on a *provisional problem list*. Physical problems may comprise a symptom, such as weight loss, a sign such as cervical lymphadenopathy or a pathological condition, such as chronic bronchitis. Other problems may be social, for example cigarette smoking, or psychological such as a grief reaction from a recent bereavement. As the clinical situation is clarified, these problems are transposed to a *master problem list* which is displayed prominently in the front of the case notes. Problems are classified as either active or resolved. The former category includes not only those which have been diagnosed but also any unexplained or ambiguous findings. In the case of hospital patients the master problem list is best prepared about one or two days after admission. It is open ended and is modified as the situation changes. New problems are added as they are recognised. The master problem list serves as a guide to the case notes and provides a summary which helps not only the medical staff but also nurses, physiotherapists, social workers and others to assess the position 'at a glance'. An example of a master problem list is given in Figure 13.2.

3. Initial Plan. For each active problem an initial plan is organised from three aspects:

(a) the collection of further data to clarify the situation.

(b) therapy.

(c) education of the patient in active participation in the management of the disease.

4. Progress Notes. The records are kept up to date by entering all additional relevant information, as it is obtained, under the named and numbered title of the problem to which it pertains. The notes are further structured by sub-headings:

(a) subjective data; prominence is given first to the patient's reactions.

(b) objective data.

(c) interpretation; this includes both decisions and impressions.

(d) therapy; this includes education of the patient.

(e) immediate plans.

Master Problem List   (1.5.83)
Mrs A.B.C.   (Date of birth 1.5.38)

Active	Inactive

1. Acute abdominal pain
   acute cholecystitis (2.5.83)
   cholecystectomy (10.5.83)
2. Obesity
3. Varicose veins
4. Hysterical psychoneurosis
5. Psoriasis
6. Left facial pain
   secondary to 4 (4.5.83)
7. Social deprivation
   (divorced; 4 children;
   2 rooms)
 	
10. Pulmonary embolism
   (16.5.83)
	
	8. Duodenal ulcer (1974)
	9. Penicillin allergy (1972)

Fig. 13.2   Basic features of a master problem list — an example. A glance at this gives an overall view of the current situation in the context of the patient's total medical needs. *Note.* Problems 1 and 6 were redefined when their aetiology became clear on the dates shown. Problem 8 signalled the need for particular care in the use of anticoagulants for problem 10. Problem 9 warned the clinician that ampicillin was contraindicated in the treatment of problem 1. The patient required realistic advice about problem 2 in relation to problem 7 which itself received attention from social workers. Further treatment was planned for problems 3 and 5.

These notes are supplemented by *'flow sheets'* when dealing with fast moving situations such as diabetic ketoacidosis, shock or acute ventilatory failure. Then the inter-relationships of data and therapy are crucial; time, serial measurements, therapy and comment are recorded side by side and repeated as frequently as the situation demands.

Finally a *discharge report* is prepared summarising each numbered problem on the list; particular attention is paid to any problems which may not have been fully elucidated or which may recur.

Conclusion

Weed's original work must be consulted for further information about problem-orientated medical records, including illustrations of these methods in practice and the philosophy on which they are based.

The system presents data in structured ways readily amenable to assessment and audit by others. The methods, however, are time consuming and this has been a barrier to acceptance in their entirety. Many clinicians have found the master problem list useful, particularly in the outpatient follow up of complicated problems, as a flexible, intelligible and up-to-date summary which allows an immediate grasp of the medical and social situation and reduces errors of omission and commission in treatment. Weed's methodology also reminds us that the quality and scope of medical care is reflected in its recording.

REFERENCES

Weed L L 1968 Medical records that guide and teach. New England Journal of Medicine 278: 593 and 652.
Weed L L 1970 Medical records, medical education and patient care — The problem-orientated record as a basic tool. Press of Case Western Reserve University, Cleveland, Ohio

CONTINUING MEDICAL EDUCATION

Medical Audit and Self-assessment

In the introductory quotation to this book, Sir George Pickering states that the true aim of education is an understanding of method rather than a knowledge of fact. Once the student has learned how to learn, the accumulation of knowledge must continue, particularly in a discipline like medicine where scientific advances are continuous and often rapid. In clinical practice the acquisition of reliable methods of examination is the essential prerequisite and these must be kept under constant review. Medical students have their skills scrutinised and constructively criticised by their tutors, a means of learning particularly applicable to the acquisition of techniques of interviewing psychiatric patients (p. 17). When clinical methods have become established they can be tested by medical audit and self-assessment.

Medical audit has become national policy in the United States to evaluate standards of clinical practice; it will no doubt play an increasing part in Britain and other countries. Audit is most effective when criteria are agreed beforehand and where the aim is educational; it is potentially abrasive and counter-productive when it is conducted by an independent body and where it carries a punitive threat.

Self-audit involves a conscious effort of appraising one's own clinical practice; it should be an integral part of medical care. A practical example of audit by others in the clinical field is when two or more clinical teams (firms, cliniques, etc.) take part. Notes are chosen at random from among patients recently discharged from hospital and these are subjected to scrutiny by the other team. They may be studied from the point of view of errors of omission or commission in the clinical record and they may bring to light lack of information, for example about smoking habits, or faulty judgements such a decision to treat 'hypertension' on the basis of a single estimation of blood pressure. Such studies conducted in a friendly atmosphere and in good faith can provide an excellent climate for learning and lead to a general improvement in performance.

The use or abuse of ancillary services can also be assessed by audit. It has been demonstrated, for example, how limited is the value of routine chest radiographs in patients under 40 years of age without pulmonary symptoms. Furthermore medical audit can evaluate the safety and efficiency of new drugs and the optimum use of limited resources in relation to new, and often costly, techniques.

It would however be incorrect to suggest that audit by others is ever totally without threat, that it is yet generally accepted, or that there is agreement as to whether clinical judgement, for example, is capable of being assessed.

Self assessment is another aspect of continuing education. One simple method involves a written diagnostic analysis of each patient at the time of initial interview, followed by a critical reappraisal once the results of investigations are available. There are now many self assessment programmes (SAPs) which attempt to assess both factual knowledge — a relatively easy task — and judgement, and such programmes are becoming available. Skills can also be tested by multiple choice questions (MCQs) and this textbook is supplemented by a separate publication specifically designed to perform such a task.

Conclusion. The critical scrutiny of both practice and records by one's peers and by oneself provided by medical audit and self assessment will be welcomed by those interested in establishing that their professional standards have kept up with progress in medical skills and knowledge. These methods are logical developments in a scientifically orientated discipline; they constitute a responsibility and a challenge in the continuing study of medicine.

REFERENCE

Fleming P R et al 1980 1200 MCQs in medicine. Churchill Livingstone, Edinburgh

Index

Abdomen, acute, examination of, 224
  auscultation of, 209
  contour, 201
  examination of, 200
    in childhood, 392
  hair, 201
  in newborn, 404
  inspection of, 200
  mass and respiration, 204
  movement, 201
  pain in, 190
  palpation of, 202, 204
  percussion of, 208
  radiographic examination, 217
  reflexes of, 294
  regions of, 200
  skin lesions, 201
  tumours in childhood, 394
  veins, 201
Abducent nerve, 241
  lesions of, 250
Accommodation reflex, 245
Acetest, 424
Acetone, in breath, 60
  in urine, 423
Achondroplasia, 61
Acidosis, metabolic, 42, 168
  renal tubular, 420
Acne vulgaris, 88
Acromegaly, hands in, 66
Addiction to drugs, 96
Addison's disease, pigmentation in, 58, 79
  skin in, 58
Adenoma sebaceum, 230
Aegophony, 178
Aerophagy, 195
Aggression, 27
Agnosia, 306
Agranulocytosis, 80
Air hunger, 42, 44, 168
Airways obstruction, 42, 169
Albinism, 58

Albuminuria, 421
Albustix, 421
Alcohol, in breath, 60
Aldosterone and oedema, 51, 53
Allergy, 4, 13
  and respiratory system, 159
  and skin, 94
Alopecia areata, 71
Alphafetoprotein, 221
ALT, 221
Alveolitis, 160
  crepitations in, 182
Amylase, in urine, 426
  serum, 222
Anaemia, external features of, 57
Anal reflex, 398
Anarthria, 234
Anasarca, 52
Aneurysm, of aorta, pain in, 102
  student's, 136
Angina, decubitus, 101
  pectoris, 100
Angiocardiography, 144
Angiography, cerebral, 303
  pulmonary, 185
Angioma, 95
Angio-oedema, 55, 90
Anisocytosis, 433
Ankle, examination of, 323, 359
  jerk, 289
  lateral ligament of, 361
Anorexia, 195
  nervosa, 63
Anosmia, 237
Anthropometry, 60
Anticoagulants, 13
Anuria, 196
Anus, examination of, 212
  in childhood, 395
Anxiety neurosis, 28
Aorta, coarctation of, 111, 137
Aortic valve, 122, 129, 132

463

Aortography, and renal arteries, 223
Apex beat, 120
Appendicitis, 33
Apraxia, testing, 275
Arachnodactyly, 66
Arcus, lipidus (corneal), 74
Argyll Robertson pupil, 248
Arm, examination of, 330
Arrhythmia, sinus, 108, 390
Arteries, examination of, 135
Arteriography, carotid, 303
Arteriovenous anomaly, 297
    murmurs, 134
Arteritis, in connective tissue disorders, 70
    cranial, 71
Artery, fetal hyaloid, 409
    retinal, 412, 413
Arthritis, psoriatic, 68
    rheumatoid, 68
Arthrogram, 362
Arthroscopy, 363
Ascites, 208
Aspergillosis, 158
Assessment, of clinical skills, 461
AST, 221
Asthma, bronchial, 43
    cardiac, 43
    cough in, 153
    physical signs, 183
Astigmatism, 410
Ataxia, cerebellar, 273
    sensory, 273
Athetosis, 270
Atrial septal defect, murmurs of, 130
Atrophy, cerebral, 302
    optic, 238, 413
Attention, 24
Audiometry, 260
Audit, medical, 461
Auditory acuity, 259
Auriscope, 75
Auscultation, in infancy and childhood, 389,
        390
    of abdomen, 209
    of arteries, 138
    of heart, 121
    of lungs, 176
    of swellings, 50
    of thyroid gland, 82
Austin Flint murmur, 134
Autoantibodies, and liver disease, 221
Automatism, 40
Ayre spatula, 215
Axilla, examination of, 83

Babinski, 293
Backache, examination of, 364
Baker's cyst, 139
Barber's chair sign, 284
Barium enema, 218
    meal, 218
Barrel-chest, 166
Basophilia, 433

B.C.G. vaccination, 158
Bed wetting, 374
Behaviour, in childhood, 374
Bell's palsy, 257
Bence Jones proteins, 421
Benedict's test, 422
Beriberi, oedema in, 54
Biceps jerk, 289
Bilharziasis, 426
Biliary tract, radiography of, 221
Bilirubin, 221
    and complexion, 58
    in urine, 424
Bimanual examination, of abdomen, 204
    of pelvis, 215
Biopsy, from alimentary tract, 218
    of kidney, 223
    of liver, 222
    of lung, 186
    of lymph node, 186
    transbronchial, 186
Birth, history of, 374, 403
Blackhead, 88
Blackouts, 37
Bladder, urinary, neurological disturbances of,
        197
Bleeding time, 442
Blepharitis, 73
Blepharospasm, 72
Blood, examination of, 429
    film, 432
    gases, 186
    in faeces, 217
    in urine, 425
    pressure, 112
        in childhood, 391
    samples of, 402, 429
Borborygmi, 196
Boutonniere deformity, 332
Bowel sounds, 209
Bow-leg deformity, 319
Brachio-radialis jerk, 288
Brachycephaly, 380
Bradycardia, 107
Bradylalia, 235
Bragaard test, 343
Brain, death of, 313
    stem, lesions of, 288
    syndrome, acute, 28
    tumour of, 302, 310
Breast, abscess of, 84
    examination of, 84
    tumour of, 84
Breath sounds, 177
    amphoric, 178, 181
    bronchial, 177, 181
    in infants and children, 389
    interpretation of, 181
    vesicular, 177
Breathing, periodic, 168
    sterterous, 168
Breathlessness, 41 *see also* Dyspnoea

Bronchiectasis, cough in, 153
  physical signs, 183
Bronchitis, cough in, 153
  physical signs, 183
Bronchography, 186
Bronchopneumonia, physical signs, 183
Bronchoscopy, 186
Bronchus, carcinoma of, cough in, 153
  obstruction, physical signs, 183
Brown-Séquard syndrome, 308
Brudzinski's sign, 398
Bruit, abdominal, 210
  carotid, 297
  cranial, 297
Brushfield's spots, 384
Buffalo obesity, 62
Buffy coat, 436
Bulla, 90
Burning feet syndrome, 287
Butterfly rash, 94

Café au lait patches, 95
Calculus, salivary, 79
Caloric tests, 261
Campbell de Morgan spots, 92
Cannon waves, 116
Capsule, internal, lesion of, 306
Caput Medusae, 201
Carbon dioxide, partial pressure, 186
Carboxyhaemoglobin, 57
Carcinoid syndrome, 103, 210
Carcinoma see individual organs
Cardiomyopathy, 103, 131
Caries, dental, 77
Carotene, and complexion, 58
Carotid, artery, kinked, 136
  shudder, 130
  sinus, hypersensitivity, 38
    massage, 109
    reflex, 117
Carpal tunnel syndrome, 70, 315
Carpopedal spasm, 296
Cartilage, semilunar, 326, 353
Case recording, 13, 454
Casts, urinary, 428
Cataplexy, 41
Cataract, 409
Catheterisation, cardiac, 144
Causalgia, 287
Cavernous sinus, lesions of, 250
Cells, in urine, 427
Cerebello-pontine lesions, 258, 261
Cerebellum, lesions of, 276, 305
Cerebrospinal fluid, 298
Chagas' disease, 73
Chancre, primary, 80
Cheilosis, 76
Chemosis, 74, 162
Chest, auscultation of, 176, 181
  examination of, 166
    in childhood, 387
  expansion, 168
    in childhood, 387

frozen, 172
in newborn, 404
injured, 187
injuries and operations, 158
inspection of, 166, 170
palpation of, 170
percussion of, 173
physical signs, 170, 183, 184
radiography of, 184
radioscopy of, 185
shape of, 166
tomography of, 185
wall, lesions of, 167
Cheyne-Stokes breathing, 168
  in infancy, 388
Childhood, 369
Children, examination of, 376
Chloasma gravidarum, 58
Cholangiography, 221
Cholecystitis, 206
Chorda tympani, 255, 258
Chorea, 269
Choroid, pigment, 413
  tubercles, 416
Choroiditis, 416
Chvostek's sign, 297
Cigarette smoking, 160
Clasp-knife spasticity, 271
Claudication, intermittent, 135
Clavicle, fracture of, 336
Clawhand, 329
Click, ejection, 127
  mid-systolic, 127
  pneumothorax, 180
Clinistix, 422
Clinitest, 422
Clonus, 271
Clubbing of fingers, 161
Coagulation, disseminated intravascular, 443
Coal miners' marks, 66
Cocaine sniffing, 76
Cochlear nerve, 259
Cogwheel rigidity, 271
Coin test, 182
Colic, 34
Collapse of lung, physical signs, 183
Collateral circulation, 92
Colloid bodies, 416
Colobomata, 384
Colon, palpation of, 203
Colonoscopy, 218
Coma, grading of, 312
Comedone, 88
Communication, non-verbal, 2
Complexion, 57
Compulsion, 24
Concentration, 24
Confrontation, visual, 241
Congenital abnormalities, 403
Conjunctiva, inspection of, 73
Conjunctivitis, 73
  phlyctenular, 162
Connective tissue disorders, and skin, 94

Consciousness, level of, 312
  in childhood, 395
  in newborn, 403
Consolidation, physical signs in, 183
Constipation, 194
Convulsions, in childhood, 373
Coordination, 273
  in childhood, 373, 397
Cornea, 409
  inspection of, 74, 409
  reflex of, 253
Cor pulmonale, 147
Cortex, cerebral, lesions of, 288, 306
  sensory functions of, 284
Corticosteroids, 13
  and obesity, 62
Cough, 102, 152
  bovine, 264
  in childhood, 372
  in heart disease, 102
  syncope, 38
Courvoisier's law, 206
Coxa vara, adolescent, 351
'Crackles and wheezes', 178
Craniotabes, 382
Cranium, examination of, 71
  in childhood, 380
Cremasteric reflex, 295
Crepitations, 179, 182
Crepitus, in fracture, 316
  in subcutaneous emphysema, 167
Cresyl blue, 438
Cretinism, 61, 382
Crown-rump length, 379, 448
Cry, cerebral, 396
Crystals, in urine, 428
CSF, 298
CT scans see Imaging, diagnostic
Cushing's syndrome, 62
Cyanosis, 105, 161
  in childhood, 373
Cyclopentolate, 407
Cyst, meibomian, 73
  popliteal, 353
  sebaceous, 95
  ultrasound in diagnosis, 220
Cystic fibrosis, 402
Cystinuria, 426
Cystocele, 197
Cystoscopy, 223

D and C, 223
Deafness, 261
  in childhood, 398
Death, of brain, 313
Defecation, 194
  in childhood, 371
Deformity, in infancy and childhood, 400
  in newborn, 403

Dehydration, 64
Déjà vu phenomenon, 40
Delirium, 28
Delusion, 23
Demeanor, 56
Dementia, 28
Denial, of disease, 84
Depression, endogenous, 28
  reactive, 29
Dermatitis artefacta, 95
  contact, 73
  of hands, 67
Descent, x and y, 115
Desquamation, 90
Development, psychological, 21
Development, physical, record of, 449
  stages in, 446
Dextrocardia, 120
Dextro-Check, 423
Dextrostix, 423
Diabetes mellitus, 63, 423
  retinal changes in, 415
Diagnosis, 15
  developmental, 400
  psychiatric, 25
Diagrams, in case recording, 13
  in hand injuries, 330
Diarrhoea, 194
Diastole, murmurs in, 131
Differential white cell count, 435
Digestion, disorders of, 196
Dinner-fork deformity, 271
Diphtheria, 80
Diplopia, 246
Disc, intervertebral, 317, 341, 342
  optic, 238, 411
Discharge, nasal, 157
  vaginal, 215
Discography, 362
Discrimination, of two points, 285
Dissociated sensory loss, 287
Dizziness, 229
Doctor-patient relationship, 8
Door-stop breathing, 172
Dorsal columns, lesions of, 306
Down's syndrome, 382, 400, 403
Drugs, addiction to, 96
  and history, 4
  in case recording, 13
  in urine, 419, 421, 423, 426
  withdrawal and fits, 40
Ductus arteriosus, persistent, 134
Dullness, shifting, 208
Duodenum intubation, in infancy and childhood, 401
Dupuytren's contracture, 68
Dwarfism, 61
Dysarthria, 233
Dysdiadochokinesis, 274
Dysgraphia, 233
Dyslexia, 233
Dysmetria, 274

Dyspareunia, 199
Dysphagia, 190
  in childhood, 371
Dysphasia, 231
Dysphonia, 234
Dyspnoea, 41
  exertional, 45
  grading, 45
  in heart disease, 99
  paroxysmal nocturnal, 44, 99
Dyspraxia, testing, 275
Dyssynergia, 274
Dystrophy, muscular, 270
  myotonic, 71
Dysuria, 196

Ear, drum, 75
  external, 75
  in childhood, 382
Ecchymosis, 91
Echocardiography, 142
Echoencephalography, 301
Echolalia, 235
Ectropion, 73
Effusion, in knee joint, 353, 354
  pericardial, percussion in, 121
    pulsus paradoxus in, 110
    ultrasonography in, 142
  pleural, physical signs, 183
Ehrlich's aldehyde reagent, 425
Ejaculation, premature, 198, 452
Ejection click, 127
Elbow, examination of, 322, 324, 333
  lesions of, 333
Electrocardiography, 141
Electroencephalography, 301
Electrolyte disturbance, in heart disease, 103
Electromyography, 300
Elephantiasis, 54
Elfin facies, 106
Elliptocytosis, 434
Embolism, massive pulmonary, 44
Emmetropia, 406
Emphysema, mediastinal, 167
  signs of, 183
  subcutaneous, 167
Empyema, physical signs in, 183
Encopresis, 371
Endocarditis, infective, 148
Endocrine system, examination, 56
Endoscopy, alimentary, 218
Enophthalmos, 72
Enteropathy, gluten-induced, 62
Entropion, 73
Epididymis, 211
  pain in, 198
Epigastrium, pulsation in, 118
Epilepsy, 39
  drugs causing, 40
  focal, 39
Epiphysis, slipped, 351
Epiphysitis, 339, 345, 359

Epistaxis, 157
Epithelioma, 96
ERCP, 221
Erection, problems with, 451
Erythema, 90
  ab igne, 88
  multiforme, 95
  nodosum, 94
  palmar, 70
Erythrocyte sedimentation rate (ESR), 431
Escutcheon, male, 71
Examination see also individual organs
  physical, environment and equipment, 10
  method of, 11
Exanthemata, 93
Exophthalmos, 72
Expression, facial, 57
Exteroception, 277
Extrapyramidal lesions, 277
Extrasystole, 107
Exudate, retinal, 415
Eye, in respiratory disease, 162
  inspection of, 72
  movements of, 242
    testing of, 245
  disorders of, 249
    neurological lesions, 249
Eyebrow, 72
Eyelashes, inspection of, 73
Eyelid, inspection of, 72, 245
  retraction of, 72
  swelling of, 72

Face, expression of, 57
  inspection of, 72
Facial nerve, 254
  lesions of, 257
Facies, adenoid, 76
  in childhood, 378, 382, 385
Faeces, examination of, 217
  impaction of, 194
  in childhood, 371, 401
  in newborn, 405
  inspection of, 194
  palpable, 203
Failure, cardiac, 145
Fainting, 37
  lark, 38
Family history, 5
Fasciculation, 268
Fat, abnormalities of, 62
  subcutaneous, measurement of, 61
Feeding, in infancy, 371, 375
Femoral nerve stretch test, 344
Femur, fracture of neck of, 351
Ferric chloride test, 424
Fetor hepaticus, 60
FEV/FVC ratio, 187
Fibrillation, atrial, 108
Fibrindex qualitative test, 443
Fibrinogen, 443
Fibrosis, pulmonary, physical signs in, 183

Filariasis, blood in 437
Finger, clubbing, 161
  flexion jerk, 290
  nose test, 274
  to finger test, 274
Fits, 39, 373
Fleas, 93
Fluctuation, testing for, 49
Fluid, cerebrospinal, 298
  interstitial, 51
  thrill, 209
Fluorescein angiography, in papilloedema, 416
Fluoroscopy, 140
Fluorosis, teeth in, 77
Flush, pressure, 391
Flutter, atrial, 108
Fontanelle, 380
Foot, arches of, 357
  deformities of, 358
  drop, 236
  examination of, 323, 359
  print, 361
  wear, 361
Foramen compression test, 339
Forced expiratory time, 182
  volume, 186
  vital capacity, 186
Forearm, examination of, 328
Foreign body, in ear, 76
  in eye, 73
  in lung, 159
Forgac's 'crackles and wheezes', 178
Fracture, radiological examination of, 362
  signs of, 316
Fragilitas ossium, 74
Fremitus, vocal, 172
Frequency of micturition, 196
Friction, pericardial, 135
  pleural, 179
  pleuro-pericardial, 182
Fructosuria, 423
Fuchs-Rosenthal counting chamber, 438
Fundus oculi, 412
Fungus, infecting nail, 67
Funnel-chest, 167

Gag reflex, 262, 386
Gait, 235
  abnormalities of, 319
  cerebellar, 236
  drop foot, 321
  festinant, 236
  in childhood, 373, 396
  in hysteria, 321
  in malingering, 321
  peg-leg, 321, 359
  prosthetic, 321
  scissor, 320
  spastic, 320
  waddling, 236, 320
Galactorrhoea, 84
Galactosaemia, congenital, 422

Gall bladder, pain in, 206
  palpation of, 205
  radiography of, 221
  ultrasonography of, 221
Gallop rhythm, 126
Gap, auscultatory, 112
Gargoylism, 382
Gastrocnemius, lesion of, 327
Gaze, coordination of, 244
Genitalia, examination of, 211
  in childhood, 394
  in newborn, 404
  investigation of, 223
Genu valgum, 353
  varum, 319
Geriatric patients, faecal impaction in, 194
  feet of, 359
  frozen shoulder in, 334
  history in, 3, 4, 6, 7
  multiple lesions in, 10
  pathological fracture in, 341
  physical examination of, 10, 11
  postherpetic pain in, 93
  purpura in, 91
  scleromalacia in, 74
  skin in, 201
  teeth in, 77
Giemsa stain, 432
Gigantism, 61
Gingivitis, 77
Glabella reflex, 256
Glasgow coma scale, 312
Glassware, cleaning of, 430
Glaucoma, 412
  intraocular tension in, 75
Globus hystericus, 191
Glossopharyngeal nerve, 262
Glucose, in blood, 423
  in CSF, 299
Glycosuria, 422
Goitre, 81
  lingual, 81
Gout, tophi in, 75
Graham Steell murmur, 133
Grand mal, 39
Granulocyte, 434
Graphaesthesia, 285
Grasp reflex, 398
Grey Wedge photometer, 431
Grip, 66
Groin, examination of, 210
Growth record, 449
Guillain-Barré syndrome, 258, 299
Gum, examination of, 77
Guthrie test, 405
Gynaecological examination, 214
Gynaecomastia, 84

Habit spasm, 269
Haemangioma, 92
Haematemesis, 191

Haematocrit, 439
Haematoma, subdural, 310
Haemoccult test, 217
Haemoglobin, abnormal, 440
  and complexion, 57
  estimation, 430
  in urine, 425
Haemoptysis, 102, 154
Haemorrhage, cerebral, CT in, 302
  retinal, 414
  subconjunctival, 74
  subhyaloid, 415
Haemorrhagic disease, tests in, 441
Haemorrhoid, 214
Haemostix, 425
Hair, 71
  of abdomen, 201
Halitosis, 60
Hallucination, 23, 39
  olfactory, 238
Hallux, flexus, 359
  rigidus, 359
  valgus, 357, 358
Hammer toe, 358
Hand, anatomy of, 329
  assessment of function, 330
  examination of, 65, 322, 330
Harrison's sulcus, 166, 387
Head, circumference, 448
  examination of, 70
    in childhood, 380
  size, 379
Headache, 34, 36
  in childhood, 373
Hearing, 259
  in childhood, 374, 398
Heart, apex of, 120
  auscultation of, 121
  block, 108
  disease, congenital, 390
  failure, 145
    oedema in, 53
  fluoroscopy of, 140
  in childhood, 389
  in newborn, 404
  inspection of, 118
  palpation of, 120
  percussion of, 121
  radiography of, 140
  rate, in infancy and childhood, 390
  sound(s), 124
    due to prosthetic valves, 127
    ejection, 127
    first, 124
    fetal, 50
    fourth, 126
    second, 124
      splitting, 124
    third, 126
  valve areas, 122
Heartburn, 192
Heberden's nodes, 68

Heel-knee test, 274
Height, 60
  in infancy and childhood, 379, 447
  sitting, 379, 448
Hemianopia, 240
Hemiballismus, 270
Hemiplegia, 236, 267
Hemisphere, dominant, 231
Henoch-Schönlein syndrome, 92
Hepatitis B surface antigen, 219
Hepatomegaly, 205
Hernia, epigastric, 202
  examination of, 202
  femoral, 210
  incisional, 202
  inguinal, 210
  reduction of, 210
  umbilical, 202
Herpes simplex, 93
  zoster, 93, 254
Hess's test, 91
Hiatus hernia, pain of, 192
Hip, anatomy of, 346
  dislocation of, 351
    congenital, 350
  examination of, 323, 346
  lesion liability and age, 345
  measurement of movement, 349
  tests of stability of, 349
Hippocratic succussion, 183
Hippus, 245
Hirschsprung's disease, 395
Hirsutism, 71
History, 1
  developmental, 375
  dietetic, 7
  family, 5, 20
    in childhood, 376
    in newborn, 403
    in respiratory disease, 159
  from third party, 4
  in alimentary disease, 189
  in childhood, 370
  in cardiovascular disease, 98
  in locomotor disorders, 315
  in neurological disease, 229
  obstetric, in heart disease, 104
  occupational, 6, 160
  of birth, 374, 403
  of current illness, 2
  of previous health, 4
  psychological, 7
    in childhood, 376
  social, 6
    in childhood, 376
    in respiratory disease, 159
Hoarseness, 157
Hoffman's sign, 290
Holmes-Adie syndrome, 249
Holter monitoring, 39
Homatropine, and pupil, 407
Homogenistic acid, in urine, 418

Horner's syndrome, 248
Howell-Jolly body, 434
Hum, venous, 134, 391
Hutchison's teeth, 77
Hydration, state of, 64
Hydrocele, 211
Hydrocephalus, 380
Hydrometer, clinical, 419
Hygroma, cystic, 387
Hyperacusis, 258
Hyperaemia, reactive, 136
Hypercapnia, 41
Hyperhidrosls, 89
Hypermetropia, 409, 413
Hypertelorism, 382
Hypertension, systemic, 148
  retina in, 414
Hyperthyroidism, eyes in, 72
Hypertonia, 270
  in childhood, 397
Hypertrophy, left ventricular, 118, 120
  right ventricular, 118, 120
Hyperventilation, 38, 42
Hypochromia, 433
Hypoglossal nerve, 265
Hypoglycaemia, 40
Hypogonadism, hair in, 71
Hypoparthyroidism, teeth in, 77
Hypopituitarism, hair in, 71
  hands in, 66
  pallor in, 58
Hypoproteinaemia, oedema in, 53
Hypospadias, 395
Hypotension, postural, 38
Hypothermia, 64, 88
Hypothyroidism, 59, 72
  tendon reflexes in, 292
Hypotonia, 271
  in childhood, 397
Hypoxia, 41, 42
Hysteria, 28, 41
  and backache, 367
  gait in, 321
Hysterical personality, 26

Ichthyosis, 88
Ictotest, 424
Imaging, diagnostic
  computed tomography (CT) of
    abdomen, 219
    brain, 305
    lung, 185
    spine, 362
  emission computed tomography (ECAT), 301
  nuclear magnetic resonance, 303
  radiography see individual organs
  radionuclide (radioisotope) scanning
    brain, 301
    bone and joint, 362
    heart, 142
    liver, 221
    lung, 185

thyroid, 82
ultrasonography of
  abdomen, 219
  gall bladder, 221
  heart, 142
  kidney, 223
  liver, 221
  pancreas, 222
  pregnancy, 223
  spine, 363
  thyroid, 82
Immunisation, 375
Impotence, 198, 225
Incontinence, of urine, 197
  stress, 197
Infancy, 369
Infants, examination of, 376
Infarction, cerebral, CT in, 302
  myocardial, pain in, 101
Infection, contact with, 375
Infertility, investigation of, 223
Inflammation, signs of, 55, 316
Injury, chest, 187
  head, 310
Insight, 24
Inspection, in childhood, 377
  in heart disease, 104, 118
  of abdomen, 201
  of arteries, 136
  of chest, 166, 170
  of joints see Ankle, Knee, etc.
  of veins, 138
Intellect, defect of, 24
  functioning of, 231
  testing, 24
Intelligence, 24
  testing, in children, 395
Intention tremor, 274
International System of Units, 453
Interoception, 277
Interrogation of patient, 3
Intra-ocular tension, 74
Intussuception, palpation of, 394
Involuntary movement, 269
  in childhood, 373
I.Q., 24
Iridocyclitis, 162
Iris, inspection of, 74
Iritis, 74, 162
Ischaemia, cardiac, 100
Isotope scanning see Imaging, diagnostic
Ivy's bleeding time, 442

Jacksonian epilepsy, 40
Jaeger card, 239
Jaundice, 58, 192
Jaw jerk, 253
Jenner's stain, 432
Joint(s) see Ankle, Knee, etc.
  abnormal movement of, 325
  examination in childhood, 400
  inflammation of, 325
  inspection of, 322

Joint(s) *(contd)*
  measurement of movement, 323
  palpation of, 323
Judgement, 24
Jugular venous pressure, 113
  pulse, 115

Kala azar, blood in, 437
Kayser-Fleischer ring, 74
Kernig's sign, 295
Ketonuria, 423
Ketostix, 424
Kidney, biopsy of, 223
  function tests, 222
  in heart disease, 103
  pain in, 198
  palpation of, 207
    in childhood, 393
  scanning of, 223
Knee, anatomy of, 352
  arthritis of, 353, 357
  collateral ligaments of, 355
  cruciate ligaments of, 355
  effusion of, 353
  examination of, 323, 353
  haemarthrosis of, 353
  jerk, 289
  loose bodies in, 354
  oesteoarthrosis of, 354
  tests of stability, 355
Knock-knee, 353
Koilonychia, 67
Koplik's spots, 80
Korotkov sounds, 112
Kussmaul's sign, 115
Kveim test, 185
Kwashiorkor, oedema in, 53
Kyphoscoliosis, thoracic, 167
Kyphosis, 318, 339

Laboratory, haematology, use of, 443
Lactose, in urine, 423
Language function, 231
Laparoscopy, 223
Laryngoscopy, 164
Larynx, examination of, 164
  symptoms, 157
Lasègue test, 343
Lead pipe rigidity, 271
  poisoning, gums in, 77
Leg, examination of, 359
  measurement of, 348
  shortening of, 348
Leishman stain, 432
Leishmaniasis, blood in, 437
Length, in infancy, 379
  measurement of, 448
Lens, optic, 409
Leprosy, 70
Leucocyte, 434
Leuco-erythroblastic anaemia, 436
Leuconychia, 67

Leukaemia, gums in, 77
  white cells in, 436
Leukoplakia, 78
Libido, lack of, 198, 225
Lice, on hair, 71
  on skin, 93
Lid lag, 72
Ligaments, pain in sprain or strain, 316
  rupture of, 326
  sprain of, 326
Light reflex, 245
Limbs, initial examination of, 321
Lip, epithelioma of, 77
  examination of, 76
Lipodystrophy, progressive, 63
Lipoma, 63
Liver, biopsy, 222
  enlargement of, 205
  function tests, 221
  pain in 31
  palpation of, 205
    in childhood, 393
  percussion of, 209
  radiography of, 221
  radionuclide scan, 221
  ultrasonography, 221
Locomotor system, in childhood, 400
  in newborn, 405
  radiography of, 362
Lordosis, 318
L.S.D., and fits, 40
Lumbar puncture, 298
  in infancy and childhood, 402
Lung, biopsy of, 186
  cavitation, physical signs, 183
  collapse, physical signs, 183
  compliance of, 42
  consolidation, physical signs, 183
  fibrosis, physical signs, 183
  function tests, 186
  interstitial disease, physical signs, 183
  radiological examination, 184
  surface marking of, 173
Lupus, erythematosus, 94
  arteritis in, 70
  pernio, 163
Lymph node(s), axillary, 83
  biopsy, 186
  epitochlear, 83
  examination of, 82
    in childhood, 387
  mesenteric, 394
  scalene, 163
  supraclavicular, 163
Lymphocyte, 434
Lymphoedèma, 54

MacBurney's point, 203
MacMurray test, 356
Macrocytosis, 433
Macula, examination of, 412
  star at, 416
Macule, 90

Main d'accoucheur, 296
Malabsorption syndrome, oedema in, 53
  tests for, 219
Malaria, blood in, 437
Malingering, and locomotor system, 367
  gait in, 321
  temperature in, 64
Mallet finger, 332
Mania, 28
Marfan's syndrome, 61
May-Grünwald stain, 432
MCH, 440
MCHC, 440
MCQs, 461
MCV, 439
Mean, cell haemoglobin, 440
  cell volume, 439
  corpuscular haemoglobin concentration, 440
Measles, 158
Measurements, in children, techniques, 448
  physical, in childhood, 379
  standard, in newborn, 403
Meatus, external auditory, 75
Median nerve, and hand, 329
Mediastinoscopy, 186
Medulla, lesions of, 306
Megaloblast, 436
Meiosis, senile, 248
Melaena, 194
Melanin, and complexion, 58
Melanogen, in urine, 418
Melanoma, of eye, 416
  of skin, 95
Memory, 24
Menarche, 198
Ménière's syndrome, 261
Meninges, irritation of, 295
Meningism, 369
Menopause, 198
Menstrual cycle, 198
Mental state, 22
Metatarsalgia, 359
Methaemoglobin, 57, 105
Metric system equivalents, 453
Microaneurysms, retinal, 415
Microcephaly, 380
Microcytosis, 433
Microscopy, of faeces, 217
  of urine, 426
Microstix, 429
Micturition, frequency of, 196
  in childhood, 374
  syncope, 38
Midbrain, lesions of, 306
Milestones of development, 446
Milroy's disease, 55
Mitral valve, 122, 130, 131, 133
Mongolism, 382
Monocyte, 435
Mononucleosis, infectious, 437
Mood, evaluation of, 23
  in childhood, 374

Mooning of face, 62
Moro reflex, 398
Motility, alimentary, 219
Motor function, abnormalities, 276
  neurone disease, 268
  pathways, 268
  system, 267
    examination, summary of, 275
    in childhood, 397
Mouth, breathing, in childhood, 372
  carcinoma of, 79
  diseases of, 79
  examination of, 76
  in childhood, 384
  pigmentation in, 79
Movement, abnormal, 59
  in childhood, 395
  choreiform, 269
  dystonic, 270
  fine, assessment of, 274
  involuntary, 269
  voluntary, 269
Multistix, 418
Munchausen's disease, 3
Murmur(s) and Valsalva manoeuvre, 118
  arteriovenous, 134
  Austin Flint, 134
  diamond-shaped, 129
  diastolic, 131
  exocardiac, 135
  flow, 135
  Gibson, 391
  grades of, 128
  Graham Steell, 133
  in childhood, 390
  machinery, 391
  of aortic regurgitation, 132
  of aortic stenosis, 129
  of atrial septal defect, 130
  of mitral regurgitation, 130
  of mitral stenosis, 133
  of persistent ductus arteriosus, 134
  of pulmonary regurgitation, 133
  of pulmonary stenosis, 130
  of tricuspid regurgitation, 131
  of tricuspid stenosis, 134
  of ventricular septal defect, 131
  pansystolic, 130
  presystolic, 131
  systolic, 128
Murphy's sign, 206
Muscle(s), flexor digitorum, 330
  gastrocnemius, 327
  grading of power, 272
  in childhood, 400
  in infancy, 373
  interossei, 330
  lesions of, 305
  lumbrical, 330
  masseter, 251
  ocular, 241
  painful lesion of, 326

Muscle(s) *(contd)*
 palpation of, 270
 paralysis of, 327
 pterygoid, 251
 quadriceps femoris, 352
 rupture of, 327
 sternomastoid, 264
 tone, 270
 trapezius, 264
 wasting, 267
Myasthenia gravis, 258, 273, 292
 ptosis in, 248, 249
Myelination, retinal, 416
Myelography, 300
Myelomatosis, 421, 432
Myoclonus, 269
Myokymia, 269
Myopathy, 248, 249, 258
Myopia, 410, 412
Myositis, 270
Myxoedema, 51
 voice in, 59

Naevus, 95
Nails, examination of, 67
Narcolepsy, 40
Nasopharynx, examination of, 79
 symptoms, 157
Neck, examination of, 80
 in childhood, 386
 in respiratory disease, 162
 rigidity, 295
 webbing of, 386
Neostigmine, 250
Neovascularisation, of fundus oculi, 415
Nephrotic syndrome, oedema in, 53
Nerve(s) cranial
 first, 237
 second, 238
 third, 241
 fourth, 241
 fifth, 251
 sixth, 241
 seventh, 254
 eighth, 259
 ninth, 262
 tenth, 263
 eleventh, 264
 twelfth, 265
 examination in childhood, 396
 examination, summary of, 266
 median, and hand, 329
 opaque fibres, 416
 parasympathetic to eye, 243
 peripheral, lesions of, 286
 phrenic, and shoulder, 336
 radial, and hand, 329
 recurrent laryngeal, 263
 root irritation, 33, 296
 stretch tests, 343
 sympathetic, to eye, 244
 ulnar, and elbow, 333
  and hand, 329

Nervous system, examination, summary of, 297
 in childhood, 395
 in newborn, 404
Neubauer counting chamber, 437
Neuralgia, glossopharyngeal, 263
 trigeminal, 254
Neurofibroma, 95
Neuroma, digital, 359
Neuromuscular junction, lesions of, 276
Neurone, lower motor, lesions of, 273, 276, 305
 upper motor, lesions of, 273, 276, 305
Neuropathy, autonomic
 postural hypotension in, 38
 testicular pain in, 225
 Valsalva in, 118
Neutral Zero Method, 323
Newborn, examination of, 402
Nicotine, stain, 66
Nitrite test, 429
Nocturia, 197
Nodules, in rheumatoid arthritis, 333
Normoblast, 436
Nose, discharge from, 157
 examination of, 76
 in childhood, 384
 obstruction of, 157
 symptoms, 157
Notes, taking of, 9
Numbness, 229
Nutrition, 61
Nystagmography, 261
Nystagmus, 246, 252, 260

Obesity, 62
 buffalo, 62
Observer error, 12
Obsession, 23, 26
Obstruction, airways, 42, 169
 intestinal, 210
 of bronchus, 183
 of veins, 138
 of vena cava, 161, 201
 pyloric, 201
Occult blood in faeces, 217
Occupation, and disease, 6, 160
Oculomotor nerve, 241
 lesions of, 249
Odour, abnormal, 59
Oedema, 50
 famine, 53
 in cardiac failure, 53
 in hypoproteinaemia, 53
 in lymphatic obstruction, 54
 in malabsorption syndrome, 53
 in nephrotic syndrome, 53
 in normal persons, 52
 in respiratory disease, 161
 in venous obstruction, 54
 nutritional, 53
 of inflammatory origin, 55
 pitting, 51
 pulmonary, 43, 99

Oesophagus, 200
  pain in, 192
Olfactory nerve, 237
Oliguria, 196
Ophthalmoplegia, internuclear, 250, 307
Ophthalmoscopy, 406
  in children, 384
Optic cup, 412
  nerve, 238
Orientation, 24
Oropharynx, examination of, 79
Orthopnoea, 44, 99
Ortolani's test, 350
Osler's nodes, 149
Osmolality of the urine, 420
Osteoarthropathy, hypertrophic pulmonary, 162
Osteoarthrosis, of hands, 68
  of knee, 357
  pain in, 317
Osteochondritis, 333
Osteomalacia, gait in, 320
Osteoporosis, 340
Otitis media, 76
  in childhood, 382
Ovary, cyst of, 208
  pain of, 198
Overventilation, 168
Oxoid dip slide, 428
Oxycephaly, 380
Oxygen, partial pressure, 186

Packed cell volume, 439
Paget's disease, of skull, 71
Pain, abdominal, 190
  in childhood, 371
  analysis, of, 30
  biliary, 33, 34
  cardiac, 100
  deep, 381
  duodenal, 32, 35, 36
  epididymal, 198
  foot, 359
  hepatic, 31
  in gastric ulcer, 32, 35
  in osteoarthrosis, 317
  in vertebral disease, 190
  laryngeal, 157
  lightning, 35
  locomotor, 315
  of hiatus hernia, 192
  ovarian, 198
  pleural, 155
  prostatic, 198
  rebound, 203
  referred, 32
  renal, 198
  retrosternal, 100
  sensation, 280
  shoulder, 336
  small intestinal, 35
  testicular, 198, 225
  tracheal, 158
  urethral, 198
  uterine, 198

Palate, 78
  reflex of, 262
  soft, 263
Palilalia, 235
Pallor, in childhood, 373
Palm, erythema of, 70
  pigmentation of, 58
Palpation, dipping, 209
  of abdomen, 202
    in childhood, 392
  of chest, 170
  of gall-bladder, 205
  of heart, 120
  of kidneys, 207
  of liver, 205
  of prostate gland, 213
  of pyloric tumour, 392
  of spleen, 206
  of veins, 138
Palpitation, 102
Palsy, bulbar, 266
  pseudobulbar (supranuclear), 266
Pancreas, radiography of, 222
  scanning of, 222
  tests of function, 222
Pancreatitis, 222
Papillitis, 239
Papilloedema, 239
Papilloma, of skin, 95
Pappenheimer bodies, 434
Papule, 90
Paracentesis, abdominis, 222
  pleural, 186
Parasites, in blood, 437
Parkinsonism, eyes in, 250
  facies, 257
  gait, 236
  glabella reflex, 257
  posture, 267
  rigidity, 271
  speech, 237
  tongue, 266
  tremor, 269
Parosmia, 238
Parotid duct, 79
  gland, swelling of, 47
Patella, grinding, 357
  lateral dislocation of, 357
  stability of, 357
  tap, 354
Patient, approach to the, 1
PCV, 439
Peak expiratory flow rate, 187
  flow meter, 187
Peau d'orange, 54
Pectoriloquy, whispering, 177, 181
Pectus carinatum, 166
  exacavatum, 167
Pediculosis, 93
Pedigree charts, 5
Penis, examination of, 211
Pentagastrin test, 219
Pentosuria, 422

Perceptual rivalry, 285
Percussion, clavicular, 175
 description of note, 176
 of abdomen, 208
 of chest, 173
  in childhood, 388
 of heart, 121
  in childhood, 390
 of liver, 209
 of spleen, 209
 technique, 174
 tidal, 175
Pericarditis, acute, 135
 pain in, 101
Perihepatitis, 210
Perineum, in childhood, 394
Perisplenitis, 210
Peristalsis, gastric, 201
 small intestine, 202
 visible, in childhood, 392
Personality disorders, 26
 evaluation of, 24
Pes cavus, 358
 planus, 358
Petechiae, 91
Petit mal, 39
Peutz-Jegher syndrome, 79
Phaeochromocytoma, 148
Pharynx, examination of, 79
 in childhood, 386
 reflexes of, 262
Phenistix, 426
Phenylketonuria, 380, 405
Phenytoin, and gums, 77
Phobia, 29
Phonocardiography, 122
Phosphatase, alkaline, 221
Photophobia, 72
Physical examination, environment and
          equipment, 10
 method, 11
Pigeon-chest, 166
Pigmentation, of mouth, 79
 of skin, 58
Piles, 214
Pingueculae, 74
Pit, of oedema, 51
Plagiocephaly, 380
Plantar reflex, 292
 in childhood, 398
Plasma cell, 436
Platelet, 435
 count, 439
Pleurisy, 155, 158
Pneumaturia, 197
Pneumoencephalography, 303
Pneumonia, 158
 dyspnoea in, 43
 physical signs in, 183
Pneumothorax, click, 180
 physical signs, 183
 spontaneous, 44
Poikilocytosis, 434

Point discrimination, 285
Poisoning, bullae in, 95
Polyneuropathy, 287, 305
Polyp, nasal, 76
Polyuria, 196
Pons, lesion of, 306
Porphobilinogen, in urine, 418, 424
Porphyria, 425
Port wine stain, 95
Position, sense of, 281
Posture, 267, 318
 in childhood, 373, 395
Precordium, catch, 102
Pregnancy, pigmentation in, 58
 tests for, 223
Pressure, arterial, 112
 jugular venous, 113
 intraocular, 75
Problem-orientated clinical records, 458
Proctoscopy, 214
Prolapse of mitral valve, 131
Proprioception, 277
Prostate gland, pain in, 198
 palpation of, 213
Protein, in CSF, 299
 plasma, 221
Proteinuria, 421
Prothrombin time, 221
Pruritus, 58
Psittacosis, 160
Psoas abscess, 341
Psoriasis, 95
 and arthritis, 68
 of nails, 67
Psychiatric, examination, 16
 history, 19
Psychoneurosis, 28
Psychosis, 27
Pterygium, 74
Ptosis, 246
Pulmonary valve, 122, 130, 133
Pulse, anacrotic, 111
 aortic, 137
 brachial, 109
 cartoid, 109
 collapsing, 111
 deficit, 108
 delayed, 101
 dicrotic, 111
 dorsalis pedis, 137
 ectopic beats, 108
 femoral, 109
 jugular venous, 115
 normal, sites of, 137
 posterior tibial, 137
 radial, 106
  in childhood, 390
 rate, 108
 rhythm, 108
 subclavian, 137
 ulnar, 137
 volume, 109
 wave, 111

Pulsus alternans, 110
  bisferiens, 111
  paradoxus, 110
'Punch-drunk', 309
Pupil(s), constriction of, 248
  dilatation of, 248
  inspection of, 245
  reflexes, 245
    abnormal, 248
    tonic, 249
Purpura, 91
  senile, 91
Pyelography, 223
Pyorrhoea alveolaris, 77
Pyramidal tract, lesions of, 305

Questionnaires, use of, 198, 451

Radial nerve, and hand, 329
Radiography see individual organs
Radionuclide (radioisotope) scanning see
      Imaging, diagnostic
Râle, 179
Rash, in childhood, 372, 378
Raynaud's disease, 136
Razor-back deformity, 339
Rebound pain, 203
Rectum, examination of, 212
Red blood cell, 433
  measurements, 439
Reflex(es), abdominal, 294
  accommodation, 245
  corneal, 253
  cremasteric, 295
  deep, 288
  examination of, 288
  gag, 262, 386
  in infancy 398
  jaw, 253
  light, 245
  nasopalpebral, 256
  palatal, 262
  pendular, 292
  plantar, 292
  reinforcement, 291
  snout, 257
  superficial, 292
  tendon, 288
    abnormalities of, 290
    inversion of, 292
  tonic neck, 398
  vasomotor, 117
Reflux, hepato-jugular, 114
Refraction, errors of, 409
Regurgitation, aortic, 132
  mitral, 131
  pulmonary, 133
  tricuspid, 131
Rehabilitation, 6
Reinforcement, of tendon reflexes, 291
Relapsing fever, blood in, 437

Respiration, accessory muscles, and, 169
  depth of, 168
  in newborn, 404
  inversion, 388
  mode of, 168
  movement, 168, 171
  paradoxical, 169
  rate, 168
    in childhood, 387
  rhythm, in childhood, 388
Reticulocyte, 433
  count, 438
Retina, 411
Retinitis pigmentosa, 416
Rheumatoid arthritis, 68
  deformity in, 331
  nodules in, 333
  pain in, 316
Rhinophyma, 76
Rhonchus, 179, 182
Rhythm, gallop, 126
  triple, 126
Rib accessory, and radial pulse, 338
Rickets, 61
  rosary, 387
  teeth in, 77
Rigidity, 271
  decerebrate, 267
  decorticate, 267
Rinne's test, 260
Rodent ulcer, 95
Romanowsky stain, 432
Rombergism, 281
Rooting reflex, 398
Rosacea, 76
Rossolimo's sign, 294
Rothera's nitroprusside test, 424
Rouleaux formation, 437
Rub, pericardial, 135
  pleural, 179, 182

Sacro-iliac joints, 345
Saddle-nose, 76
Sahli method, 431
Salaam attacks, 396
Salicylates, in urine, 426
Salicylsulphonic acid test, 421
Salivary gland, 79
SAPs, 461
Sarcoidosis, and skin, 94
Scabies, 93
Scalenus, and radial pulse, 338
Scalp, examination of, 71
Scanning see Imaging, diagnostic
Scaphocephaly, 380
Scaphoid, fracture of, 70, 362
Scapula, winging of, 337
Scars, 90
Schistocyte, 434
Schizoid personality, 26
Schizophrenia, 28
Sciatic nerve stretch test, 343

Sclera, inspection of, 74
Sclerosis, multiple, 228, 299, 309
  tuberous, 230
Scleroderma, hands in, 67
Scleromalacia perforans, 74
Scoliosis, 319, 339
Scotoma, 239
Scrotum, 211
Scurvy, 92
  gums in, 77
Segmental innervation, 282
Self assessment, 461
Sensory extinction, 285
  pathways, 278
  system, 277
    abnormalities of, 286
    examination, summary of, 285
    in childhood, 397
Serial sevens test, 24
Sexual development, 21
  disturbances of, 198
  intercourse, 198
Shoulder, anatomy of, 334
  dislocation of, 336
  examination of, 323, 336
  frozen, 334
  movements of, 334
  rotator cuff, 335
Shingles, 93
SI units, 453
Sickling tests, 441
Sigmoidoscopy, 218
Sinusitis, 76
Skin, carcinoma of, 96
  examination of, 86
  hypersensitivity of, 94
  in newborn, 404
  in respiratory disease, 163
  infection of, 93
  infestation of, 93
  lesions, 90
    in childhood, 378
    of abdomen, 201
  metastases of, 96
  of hands, 67
  pigmentation of, 58
  sensitivity tests, 185
  structure and functions, 86
  vascular lesions, 91
  vitamin deficiency in, 94
Skinfold, thickness of, 61
Skull, palpation of, in childhood, 380
  radiography of, 298
Smear, cervical, 215
Smell, sense of, 237
Snap, mitral opening, 127
Sneezing, 157
Snellen types, 239
Snout reflex, 257
Sociopathy, 27
Sounds, abnormal, 59
Spasm, carpopedal, 296

Spasticity, 270
Specimens, collection of, in infancy and
    childhood, 401
Speech, 231
  abnormal, 59
    in childhood, 396
  assessment, summary of, 235
Spermatocele, 211
Spherocyte, 434
Sphygmomanometer, 112
Spider telangiectasia, 92
Spina bifida, 400
Spinal accessory nerve, 264
Spinal cord, lesions of, 287, 306
Spine, cervical, 337
  examination of, 323
  lumbar, 342
  thoracic, 340
Spinothalamic tract, 278
  lesions of, 287
Spleen, palpation of, 206
  in childhood, 393
  percussion of, 209
Splenomegaly, causes of, 206
Splinter haemorrhages, 67, 149
Spondylitis, ankylosing, 340, 345
Spondylosis, cervical, 338
Sputum, 154
  examination of, 185
  in infancy and childhood, 401
Squeeze test, 361
Squint, 246, 396
  in childhood, 396
Stadiometer, 61
Stammering, 235
Steatorrhoea, 194
Stenosis, aortic, 129
  congenital pyloric, 392
  mitral, 133
  pulmonary, 130
  spinal, 341
  tricuspid, 134
Stereognosis, 285
Sterno-clavicular joint, dislocation of, 336
Sternomastoid tumour, 387
Stethoscope, 121
  method in use of, 122
Stomach, aspiration of, in infancy, 401
  carcinoma of, 191
Stomatitis, angular, 77,
  aphthous, 80
  ulcerative, 80
Strabismus, 246
  in childhood, 396
Straight lèg raising test, 343
Strangury, 196
Striae, cutaneous, 90
Stridor, in childhood, 372, 388
  laryngeal, 157
  tracheal, 158
Stuttering, 235
Stye, 73

Succussion, gastric, 202
Sucking reflex, 398
Suicide, thoughts of, 19
Sulphaemoglobin, 57, 105
Supinator jerk, 288
Supraspinatus, lesions of, 335
Surgery, and chest disease, 158
Sutures, cranial, 382
Swallowing reflex, 398
Swan-Ganz catheter, 145
Swan-neck deformity, 331
Sweat, 88
  collection of, in infancy, 402
Swellings, examination of, 46
Symptoms, analysis of, 30
Syncope, 38
  cough, 38
  in heart disease, 102
  micturition, 38
  postural, 38
Synostosis, cranial, 381
Synovial fluid, examination of, 363
Synovial membrane, biopsy of, 363
Syphilis, of mouth, 80
  of nervous system. 310
  of nose, 76
  serological tests, 299
  teeth in, 77
Systole, murmurs in, 128

Tachycardia, 107
  paroxysmal, 108
Talipes, calcaneo valgus, 358
  calcaneus, 358
  equino varus, 358
  equinus, 358
Tamponade, cardiac, 110
Target cell, 434
Taste pathways, 255
Tattoo marks, 67
Teeth, 77
  in childhood, 386
  time of eruption, 448
Telangiectasia, 92
  hereditary haemorrhagic, 92
Temperature, 64
  conversion of °F to °C, 453
  in infancy and childhood, 380
  of skin, 89
  sensation, 280
Tendon, rupture of, 70, 360
Tenesmus, 194
Tennis elbow, 326, 333
Tenosynovitis, 328
Testicle, ectopic, 211
  examination of, 211
  pain in, 198
Tetany, signs of, 296
Texture, identification of, 285
Thalamus, lesions of, 288
Thermometers, clinical, 64
Thomas test, 348

Thoracoplasty, and chest deformity, 167
Thoracoscopy, 186
Thought processes, 22
Thrill, cardiac, 120
  in ascites, 208
Throat swab, in infancy and childhood, 402
Thrombocytopenia, 435
Thrombosis, deep venous, 138
Thrush, 80, 386
Thyroid gland, carcinoma of, 82
  examination of, 81
Thyroiditis, 82
Thyrotoxicosis, tremor in, 59
Tibial nerve stretch test, 343
Tic, 269
Tinnitus, 261
Tiredness, in heart disease, 102
Toes, clawing of, 358
Tomography, computed see Imaging, diagnostic
Tone, muscular, 270
Tongue, abnormalities of, 78
  examination of, 77, 265
  fasciculation, 265
  geographical, 78
  in childhood, 386
  neurological lesions of, 266
Tonsils, examination of, 78
  in childhood, 386
  infection of, 78
  tumours of, 79
Tophus, 75
Torsion spasms, 270
Torticollis, 338
  spasmodic, 269
Touch, sensation of, 280
Trachea, examination of, 164
  symptoms, 158
Transferase, serum, 211
Transference, erotic, 8
Transillumination, 50
Travel and illness, 5
Tremor, 59, 269
  flapping, 59
  intention, 274
Trendelenburg sign, 351
  test, 140
Trichinosis, 73
Trichomonas vaginalis, 215
Tricuspid valve, 122, 131, 134
Trigeminal nerve, 251
Trigger finger, 332
Triple rhythm, 126
Trochlear nerve, 241
  lesions of, 250
Tropicamide, 407
Trousseau's sign, 297
Trunk, as diagnostic aid, 87
Trypanosomiasis, blood in, 437
Tuberculin test, 185
Tuberculosis, 158
  of choroid, 416
  of spine, 339

Tuning fork, 260
Turner's syndrome, 66, 386
Two point discrimination, 285
Tympanum, 75

Ulcer, peptic, pain of, 32, 36
  rodent, 95
Ulnar nerve, and elbow, 333
  and hand, 329
Ultrasonography see Imaging, diagnostic
Unconscious patient, examination of, 310
Underventilation, 168
Urethra, pain in, 198
Urethroscopy, 223
Uraemia, tremor in, 59
Urgency of micturition, 196
Urination, disturbances of, 196
Urine, appearance of, 418
  bacteriological examination of, 428
  concentration of, 418
  in infancy and childhood, 374, 401, 405
  microscopic examination, 426
  midstream specimen, 428
  reaction of, 420
  smell of, 419
  specific gravity of, 419
  stream of, 197
  volume of, 418
Urobilinogen, in urine, 424
Urobilistix, 425
Urography, 223
Urticaria, 90
Uterus, pain in, 198
Uvula, 78

Vagina, discharge from, 199
  examination of, 214
Vagus nerve, 263
Valgus, 319
Valsalva manoeuvre, 117
Valves, of heart, 122
  see also individual lesions
Varicella (herpes) zoster, 93
Varicocele, 211
Varus, 319
Vasomotor reflexes, 117
Vasovagal attack, 37
Veins, collateral, 138
  examination of, 138
  of abdomen, 201
  retinal, 412, 413
  thrombosis of, 138
  varicose, 139
Vena cava, inferior, obstruction of, 201
  superior, obstruction of, 161
Venepuncture, 429
  in infancy and childhood, 402
Ventricular septal defect, murmurs of, 131
Venus, dimples of, 325

Vertebra, pain from, 33
Vertebro-basilar insufficiency, 38
Vertigo, 229, 261
Vesicle, 90
Vestibular function, 260
  nerve, 259
Vibration sense, 284
Vincent's infection, 80
Virilisation, 71
Vision, acuity of, 239
  defects in heart disease, 103
  fields of, 241
  in childhood, 373, 396
  pathways of, 240
Vital capacity, 186
Vitamin B, deficiency of, 309
  in skin, 94
Vitiligo, 58
Vitreous, 409
Vocal cord, paralysis of, 164, 263
Voice, abnormal, 59
  sounds, 177
Volkmann's ischaemic contracture, 333
Volume, measurement of, 453
Vomit, examination of, 191
Vomiting, 191
  in childhood, 371
Vulva, examination of, 214

Waves, venous cannon, 116
Wax, in ear, 75
Weber's test, 260
Weight, 60
  average of boys and girls, 447
  change of, 63
  in childhood, 372, 379
  desirable for adults, 450
  measurement of, 448, 451
Wenckebach's phenomenon, 108
Wernicke's encephalopathy, 250
Westergren tube, 431
Wheeze, 156
  in childhood, 372, 388
'Wheezes', 178
White blood cell, 437
  count, 434
Whooping-cough, 152, 158
Wilson's disease, 74
Wintrobe's haematocrit tube, 439
Wright stain, 432
Wrist, examination of, 322
Wry-neck, 338

Xanthelasma, 73
Xanthochromia, 299
Xanthomatosis, 95
Xerostomia, 59